Atlas of Head and Neck Cancer Surgery

Nirav Trivedi

Atlas of Head and Neck Cancer Surgery

The Compartment Surgery for Resection in 3-D

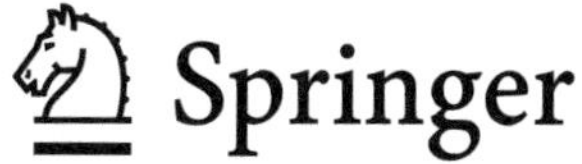

Springer

Nirav Trivedi
Narayana Hridayalaya Multispeciality
Bangalore
India

ISBN 978-81-322-2996-4 ISBN 978-81-322-2050-3 (eBook)
DOI 10.1007/978-81-322-2050-3
Springer New Delhi Heidelberg Dordrecht London New York

Printed on acid-free paper

Springer is part of Springer Science+Business Media (www.springer.com)

Patients Who Suffer From Cancer
Teachers & Colleagues
Parents and Family Whom I Owe Everything
&
To My Loving Wife Nirali and Daughters Anvi and Stuti

Foreword

I have had the privilege and honor of reviewing the book "Atlas for Head and Neck Cancer Surgery – The Compartment Surgery for Resection in 3-D" written and edited by Dr. Nirav P Trivedi. Head and neck cancer is increasing worldwide, representing an important cause of morbidity, mortality, pain, suffering, and use of resources. Few cancers can match such a disturbing and unfortunate interruption to life.

This is a surgical atlas that essentially covers an entire spectrum of open head and neck cancer surgeries. Each section deals with different subsites and focuses on each aspect of ablative and reconstructive surgery. This is a pictorial book where text is kept to a minimum and all the procedures are demonstrated with series of photographs. This gives an impression of actually watching an edited video of procedures, and I am sure that readers will find this experience satisfying. The atlas contains few chapters (surgery for very advanced cancer, surgery in resource-constrained setup) that are completely new and relevant to our clinical practice. The chapter of infratemporal fossa provides clear insight to a difficult area, and the new classification and detailed surgical procedure have a great potential for treating such patients. The photographs are of high quality, very clean, detailed, and systemically arranged.

The basic concept in surgical management of malignant soft tissue tumor is complete en bloc removal of primary tumor with microscopically negative margins. This means removal of primary tumor without visualizing the tumor during the surgical excision by keeping some normal soft tissue all around the tumor. This book's author has conceptualized and practiced the same principle in head and neck cancers. He has coined the word "3-D resection" for the same and proposed a concept of surgical removal of tumor by excising the entire anatomical compartment. This surgical principle to operate exclusively within the normal tissues is to my mind quite unique, innovative, radical, logical, appealing, and most effective in eradicating the disease locally. This concept is also effective for surgically difficult areas like infratemporal fossa and skull base, and I am very impressed with such an approach to remove soft tissues in depth.

Overall, I believe the readers, i.e., both veterans as well as those getting introduced to this specialty as beginners, will find this monogram an easy read. This is an excellent immediate resource of comprehensive, authoritative, well-organized and cleverly written information backed by excellent photographs. The "compartment surgery for resection in 3-D" certainly meets these criteria and is a meaningful work.

Mehsana, India — Pravin H. Trivedi

Foreword

Although there are specific roles for chemoradiotherapy in the overall management of head and neck cancer, the treatment modality that has an overarching bearing in the comprehensive management of head and neck cancer is surgery. It plays a critical role in diagnosis, definitive and salvage treatment, as well as reconstruction and rehabilitation. The discipline of surgery, which is the oldest cancer treatment modality, also has undergone tremendous changes in the recent past: moving from a Halstedian philosophy of "supraradical" to conservative surgery to the present concept of "selective-radical" approach. It is important to recognize that basic surgical principles laid out by William Halsted over a century ago remain the hallmark of surgery even today. That includes (1) gentle handling of tissue, (2) meticulous hemostasis, (3) preservation of blood supply, (4) strict aseptic technique, (5) minimum tension on tissues, (6) accurate tissue apposition, and (7) obliteration of dead space. In oncology surgery, one needs to add the additional fundamental principle of obtaining resection with uninvolved margin. An oncological resection with positive margin cannot be considered more than a "grand biopsy." The principle of obtaining R0 resection cannot be violated. The use of induction chemotherapy prior to surgery to downstage the cancer and the overdependency of chemo-radiotherapy to manage positive surgical margin has not improved the oncological outcome over traditional surgery with uninvolved margin and appropriate adjuvant treatment. Moreover, there are emerging reports to suggest that the surgical ablation following compartmental resection can have improved outcomes.

Dr. Trivedi has to be congratulated for brining out a practical manual that outlines step-by-step principles of head and neck surgical procedures. This should serve as an important reference for head and neck surgeons from trainees to practicing surgeons. He has standardized the common surgical procedures to well-defined steps so that the surgeons do not have to invent a "new technique" but rather follow a proven series of steps that will give predictable results. The surgical procedures once performed in the "operation theater" as an artistic endeavor when the procedure needs to be discovered and improvised is no longer valid. Each surgical procedure can now be considered as a process where one undertakes procedures following well-defined steps, similar to flying an airplane by a well-trained pilot. In this respect, Dr. Trivedi's "surgical manual" may serve similar to the "flight manual" for head and neck surgeons. Once again, I would like to congratulate Dr. Trivedi for simplifying and demystifying head and neck surgery. I am very confident that this book will bring in the much-needed standardization of surgical procedures with long-term goals of embracing a mastery of head and neck surgery by many and improving the outcome of head and neck cancer.

Bangalore, India

Moni Abraham Kuriakose, MD, FRCS, FDSRCS, FFDRCS, Dip AB

Preface

REMOVE THE TUMOR IN A WAY THAT IT DOESN'T COME BACK!

Head and neck cancer is a mutilating disease that causes great pain, agony, and loss of life to patient and family. The incidence is increasing in recent years and is directly associated with use of tobacco. The incidence is more common in developing countries where consumption of tobacco is part of social custom. This results in great burden to person, family, and society. The disease affects organs that serve essential functions for good-quality life. The disease and its treatment can result in great morbidity and even mortality, and the whole process can influence the life of the entire family. It is imperative as clinicians to make considerate decisions for each patient.

This book focuses on surgical aspects of treatment of head and neck cancer. This is an atlas with a demonstration of each surgical procedure with operative photographs in stepwise manner. The book deals with all the subsites of the head–neck region in separate chapters focusing on all points that are relevant for ablative surgery. Each chapter focuses on relevant surgical anatomy of particular sites, potential patterns of tumor spread, and concepts for surgical resection. All possible surgical approaches for tumor in that site are described in detail with operative photographs. An algorithm for the reconstruction of surgical defects further simplifies the procedures and outlines various options. The text content of the atlas is kept to an optimum level mainly to highlight important points. This is a user-friendly operative guide for ready reference before performing any head and neck cancer surgery. I have tried my level best to cover the entire spectrum of head and neck cancer surgeries in this book.

The primary aim of any ablative cancer surgery is to achieve negative margins. It is more difficult to achieve negative margins for soft tissues in depth (compared to mucosa) for advanced and posteriorly located head–neck tumors. The incidence of positive margins for advanced disease varies from 20 to 35 %, and approximately one-third of patients ultimately develop local recurrence. Though there are various factors that can possibly contribute to local failure, a positive margin is the culprit in a majority of cases. In a multidimensional anatomy of the head and neck, none of the traditional surgical approaches have demonstrated consistent results in this regard. This book introduces a concept of dissection in the *3rd dimension* or "The Compartment Surgery." This is not a new surgical technique but a novel approach where we can achieve negative margins all around a tumor with consistency. The concept started to develop when I was working as a fellow. I would feel very uncomfortable and insecure about damaging major blood vessels while clearing deep soft tissues. This would invariably result in close or positive margins, and I would feel guilty all the time. I started to dissect all branches of carotid artery before mobilizing large tumors just to be aware of their location. This would result in mobilization of depth beforehand, and resection started to become easier and resulted in consistent margin clearance. I started using this approach for all moderately advanced and very advanced tumors for various subsites and realized its potential in the head and neck. I can reasonably predict that tumor will not come back locally unless it is a microscopic disease in an intracranial compartment. This approach is developed with work of approximately 5 years, and now I feel confident about its feasibility, utility, and oncological safety. It is also feasible to perform this selectively radical approach for all subsites in the head and neck, and this is described in detail in different chapters.

The entire surgical procedure is actually a summation of multiple small steps, and difficult procedures can be safely performed by following basic surgical principles and keeping things simple. It is the passion, dedication, and intent of a surgeon that is more important than the infrastructure and support structure. I have performed a majority of surgical procedures described in this book in a rural clinic with basic infrastructure and firmly believe that resources are not a hindrance to providing good care. This book has been a journey for me that started from my fellowship days, and I have learned a great deal compiling it. I sincerely hope that my experience will be of help to my colleagues and wish them all the good luck in their professional career.

Bangalore, India Nirav P. Trivedi

Acknowledgment

The work described in this book is carried out in the following departments, and all the consultants and fellows are integral parts of this work. I wish to show my sincere gratitude to all of them for their support.

- *Department of Head and Neck Oncology and Reconstructive Surgery:*
- Mazumdar Shaw Cancer Center and Narayana Health,
- Bangalore, Karnataka, India.
  1. Dr. Moni Abraham Kuriakose (MD, BDS, FDSRCS, FFDRCS, FRCS Ed, FRCS)
     Professor
     Director and Head of Department
  2. Dr. Vikram Kekatpure (MS, MCh)
     Senior Consultant
  3. Dr. Mathan Mohan (MDS)
     Fellow
  4. Dr. Manjula B.V. (MS)
     Fellow
  5. Dr. Dipak Kittur (MDS)
     Fellow
  6. Dr. Mandeep Singh (MS)
     Fellow
- *H.N. Trivedi Polyclinic and Nursing Home:*
  1-A, Alka Society, Dairy Road,
  Mehsana-384002, Gujarat, India.
  1. Dr. Pravin H Trivedi (MS)
     Consultant Oncosurgeon
  2. Dr. Harish H Trivedi (MS)
     Consultant ENT surgeon
  3. Dr. Saroj P Trivedi (MD)
     Consultant Anaesthesiologist
  4. Dr. Nirali N Trivedi (MD)
     Consultant Medical Oncologist and Hematologist
  5. Dr. Ruchira Trivedi (MBBS, BCCPM)
     Consultant Pain and Palliative care
- *Department of Head and Neck Cancer Surgery:*
  Narayana Multispecialty Hospital,
  Rakhiyal, Ahmedabad- 380023, Gujarat, India.
  1. Dr. Girish S Shetkar (MDS)
     Consultant Head Neck Surgeon
  2. Dr. Meeta Agarwala (MD, FRCA)
     Consultant Anaesthesiologist

- *Department of Head and Neck Surgery:*
  Amrita Institute of Medical Sciences
  Cochin, Kerala, India
  1. Dr. Subramania Iyer (MS, MCh)
     Director and head of department

Contents

Concepts for Three-Dimensional Resection

1

The Compartment Surgical Approach

The entire anatomical compartment containing tumor is removed instead of removing tumor with one cm margin. The compartment is defined on the basis of anatomy of the site and pattern of tumor spread.

Treatment algorithms are continuously evolving in the era of multimodality treatment. There are two major approaches that define treatment of head–neck cancer (Fig. 1.1). The conventional approach of surgery with adjuvant treatment has been in practice since long and can be used for any stage of disease. The newer nonsurgical organ preservation approach is best suited for relatively early disease and moderately advanced stage disease. It is also necessary to remember that salvage surgery still remains an essential part of nonsurgical approach.

The new surgical technologies (laser, robot) and improved reconstructive techniques have reduced the procedure-related morbidity to a significant extent. *It is essential to understand that the oncological principle of achieving negative margins in all direction still forms the basis of any surgical treatment. It is the most important prognostic factor that can influence the outcome.* To achieve negative margins at depth (the 3rd dimension) is the most challenging and limiting factor in improving local control rate. This book proposes a novel surgical concept – compartment resection – to consistently achieve negative margins for soft tissues in depth (3-D).

Figures 1.2, 1.3, 1.4, and 1.5 show the difference in concept between conventional and this novel approach. In conventional surgical approach, dissection starts from mucosa and moves out to clear involved soft tissues. This is also called in-to-out approach (Fig. 1.2a). There is potential of leaving some disease behind for large and deeply infiltrative tumors with this approach (Fig. 1.2b). The surgeon always worries about injuring neurovascular bundle at depth, and this may restrict wide clearance in deeper areas like the infratemporal fossa (ITF) and tongue base. The final result also varies with the skill level of the operating surgeon.

The concept of compartment resection is described in Figs. 1.3, 1.4, and 1.5. It can also be called an anatomical resection approach or out-to-in approach. The aim of this procedure is to remove the entire anatomical compartment in which the tumor is contained. The compartments are defined based on the anatomy of the particular subsite and pattern of disease spread (Fig. 1.4). The principle is to remove the entire involved soft tissue from its farthest attachment at base (Fig. 1.5). The entire tissue is mobilized from its base after ligating the neurovascular bundle at the entry point in the compartment. The resection then proceeds in anterior direction (out to in) through soft tissues to end with mucosal cuts. The tumor can be palpated in front of the soft tissue cuts during the entire procedure, ensuring satisfactory negative margins at depth. There are numerous advantages of performing surgery this way. The entire involved soft tissue is removed from its origin–insertion, and hence the chance of positive margin is negligible. The neurovascular bundle is ligated upfront at the start of the procedure, and hence bleeding is always under control. The dissection is always in anatomical facial plane away from tumor margin and hence eliminates errors of personel judgement regarding tumor spread. This enables one to achieve negative margins in 3-D in a consistent manner.

The head and neck region has a multidimensional anatomy with a number of structures interwoven in a complex manner. The new concept is attractive, but the feasibility of such radical surgical approach needs proper understanding of the anatomy and pattern of spread of the disease. The tumor initially spreads within the facial barrier, and this fact can be utilized to formulate various compartments for various head and neck subsites (Figs. 1.4 and 1.5). This is not a *supra-radical* surgical approach, but a *selective radical* approach by understanding the anatomy of the region and pathology of the tumor.

This chapter essentially proposes a concept of compartment surgery to achieve negative margins in 3-D. This concept will be elaborated in each chapter in relevant fashion. It is best suited to address moderately advanced and really advanced lesions.

N. Trivedi, *Atlas of Head and Neck Cancer Surgery: The Compartment Surgery for Resection in 3-D*,
DOI 10.1007/978-81-322-2050-3_1, © Springer India 2015

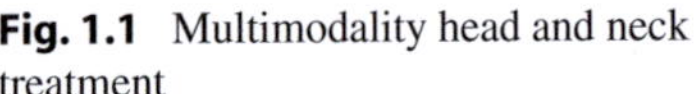

Fig. 1.1 Multimodality head and neck treatment

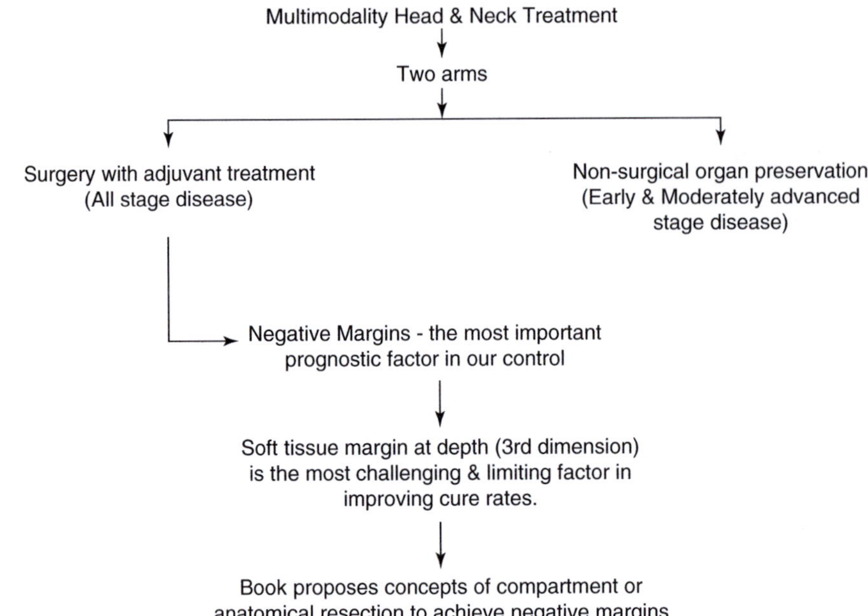

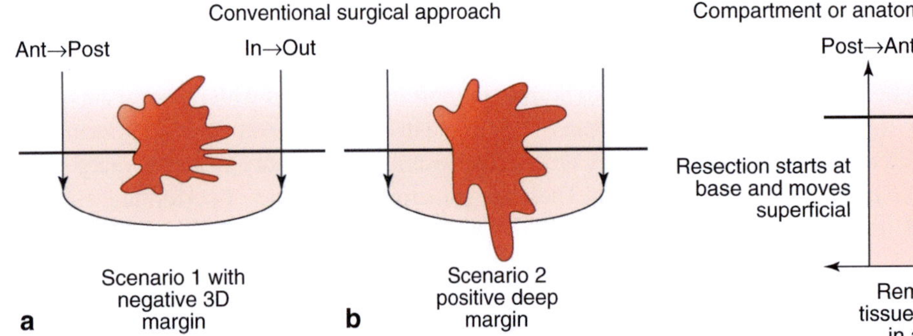

Fig. 1.2 Conventional surgical approach

Fig. 1.3 Compartment or anatomical or posterior to anterior approach

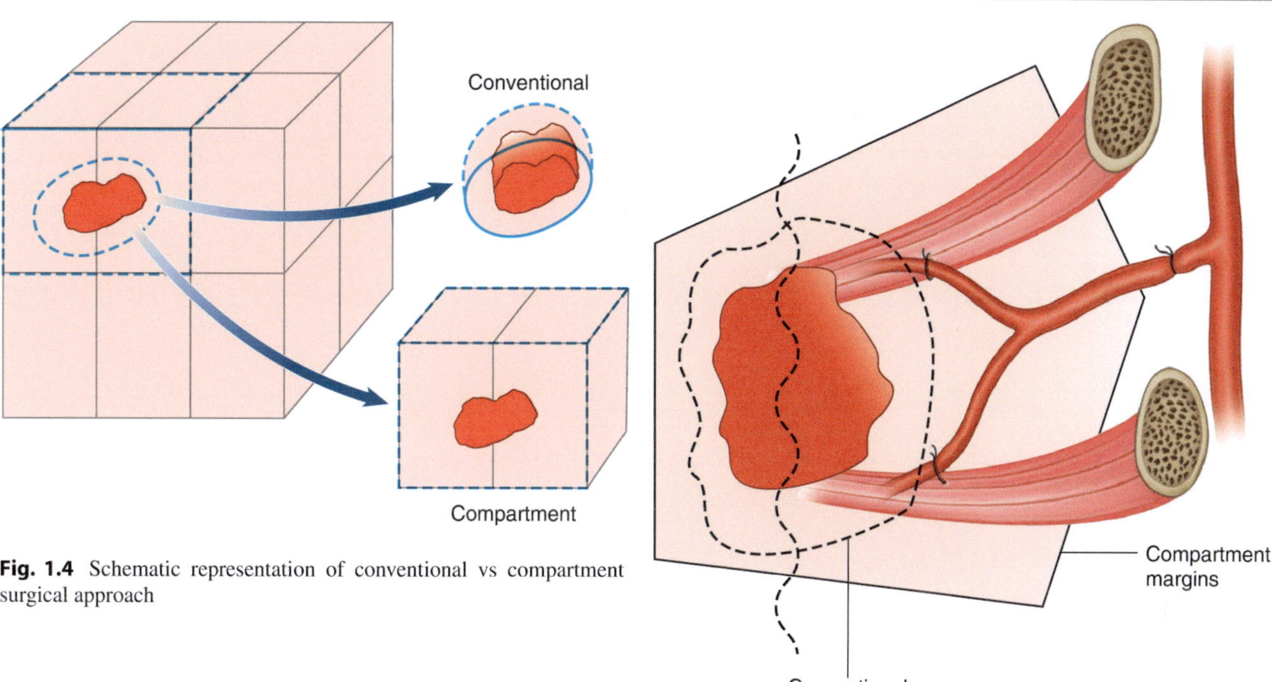

Fig. 1.4 Schematic representation of conventional vs compartment surgical approach

Fig. 1.5 Schematic representation of the technical aspect of performing compartment surgery in the head and neck region

2 Common Head and Neck Procedures

This chapter contains surgical procedures that are routine in head and neck surgery. These are basic procedures that are generally performed by residents and fellows.

Few important points are discussed for each of the procedure.

1. Lymph node biopsy
2. Tracheostomy
3. Submandibular gland excision
4. Secondary tracheoesophageal puncture
5. Sentinel node biopsy

Lymph Node Biopsy

This section demonstrates the surgical procedure to do lymph node biopsy for level II lymph node.

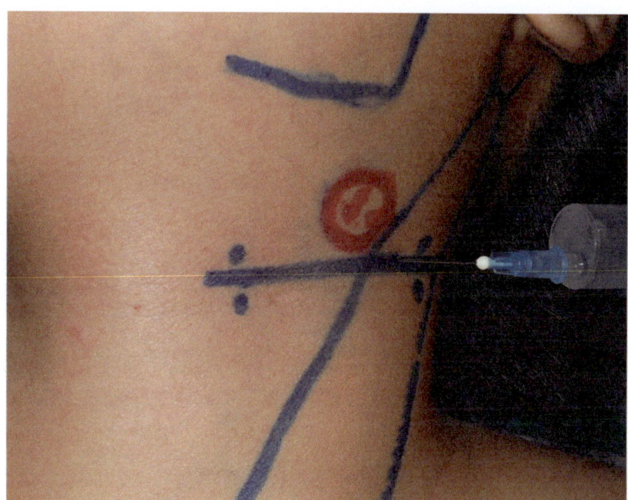

Fig. 2.1 Incision is marked for the procedure. The surface marking is showing lymph node in relation to the sternocleidomastoid (SCM) muscle and angle of mandible. The infiltration of adrenaline in line of incision reduces bleeding during skin incision

N. Trivedi, *Atlas of Head and Neck Cancer Surgery: The Compartment Surgery for Resection in 3-D*, DOI 10.1007/978-81-322-2050-3_2, © Springer India 2015

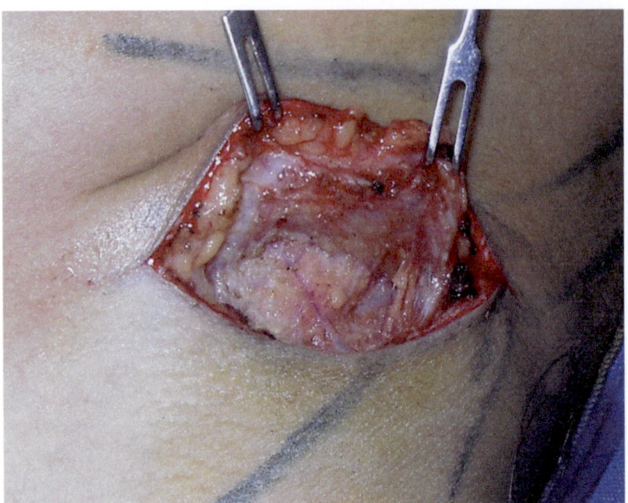

Fig. 2.2 The flaps are raised in the subplatysmal plane. It is advisable to perform this procedure in general anesthesia when the node is deep and near the internal jugular vein (IJV). Some level V nodes can be removed in local anesthesia

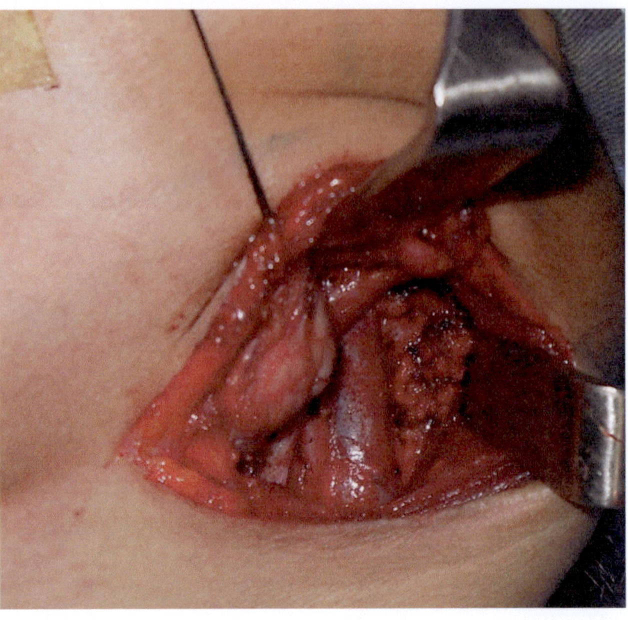

Fig. 2.4 The level II lymph node area is exposed after identifying the IJV and spinal accessory nerve. The large node is removed for evaluation

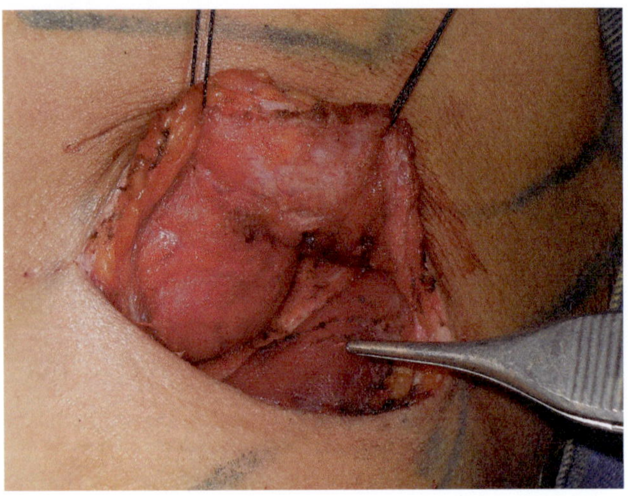

Fig. 2.3 The photograph shows exposed SCM muscle, posterior belly of digastric and submandibular gland

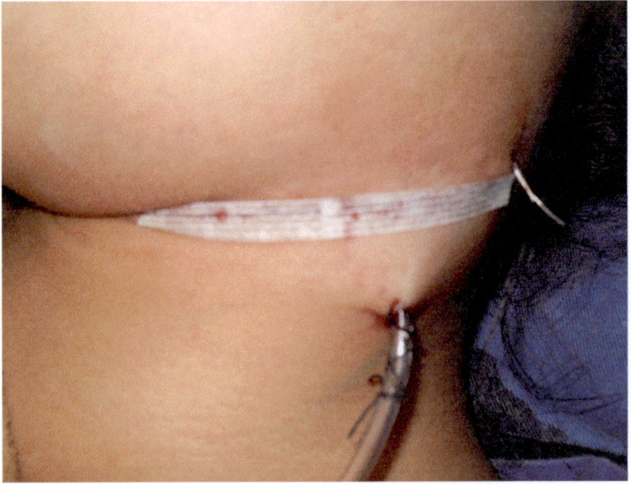

Fig. 2.5 The wound is closed in layers after drain insertion. The drain is optional and depends upon the extent of dissection performed

Tracheostomy

Tracheostomy is a life-saving procedure, and all doctors should be able to perform it in a safe way. It is relatively simple if surgical principles are observed all throughout. This procedure can result in life-threatening complications in case due care is not taken. The procedure can be performed under local anesthesia in emergency or can be performed in an intubated patient in a planned setup.

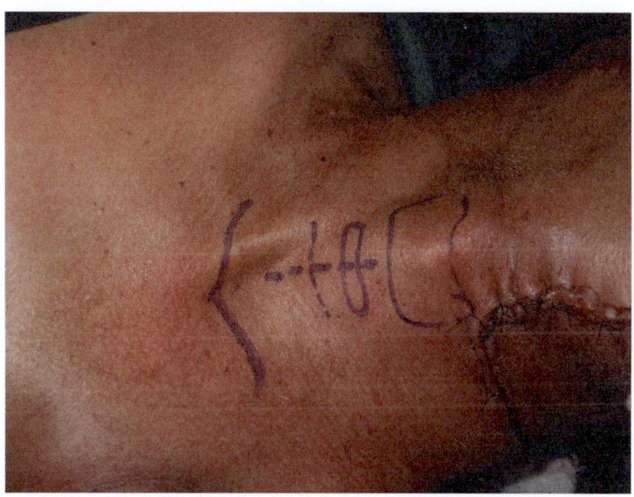

Fig. 2.6 Surface marking for incision. The most important aspect of this procedure is to stay strictly in midline. The incision is generally placed midway between the cricoid cartilage and suprasternal notch in midline. The vertical incision is used in emergency, and horizontal incision is better for cosmesis and used in planned setup. One must not compromise on exposure by using very small incision

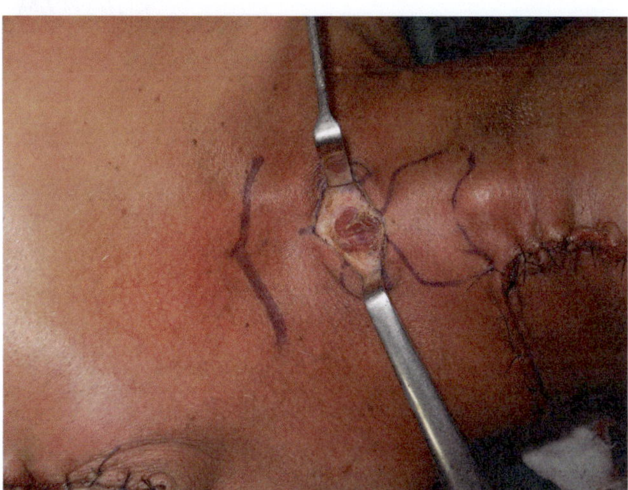

Fig. 2.7 The vertical incision is placed for about 2 cm. It is essential to put the neck in maximum extension before starting the procedure so the trachea comes as anterior as possible. It is also a good practice to palpate for the subclavian artery before the procedure as it can arch higher in some cases and one needs to be careful about avoiding it

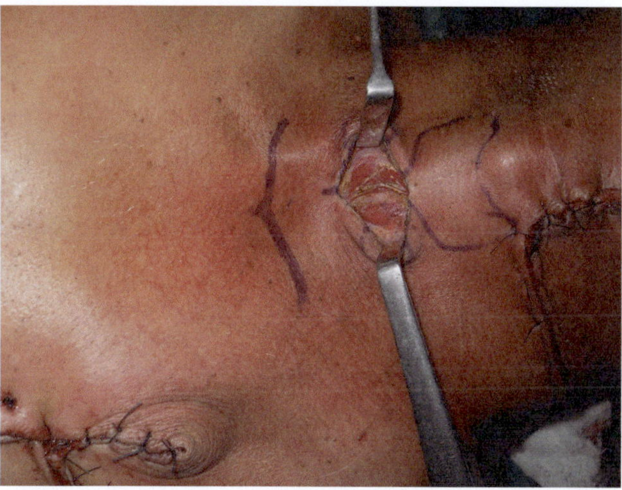

Fig. 2.8 The deep fascia over strap muscle is divided in the midline. The strap muscles are separated from each other in the midline. It helps to continuously palpate the trachea to have an idea about the midline. One may have to ligate the anterior jugular vein on either side in some cases, but care must be taken to secure them or they can cause bleeding later on

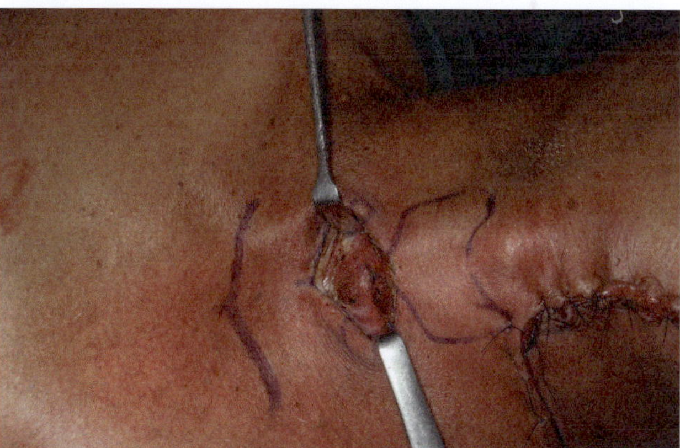

Fig. 2.9 The strap muscles are retracted laterally to expose the thyroid gland. One must be careful in avoiding injury to the capsule and gland or it can lead to persistent ooze

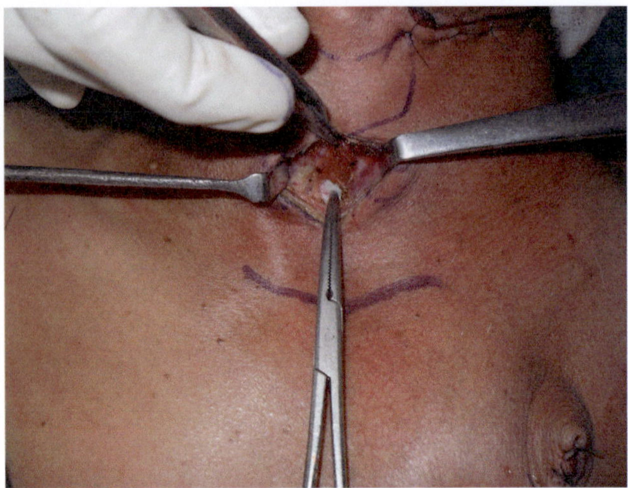

Fig. 2.10 The thyroid gland is mobilized upwards to expose the trachea. A thyroid hook is used to retract the thyroid upwards

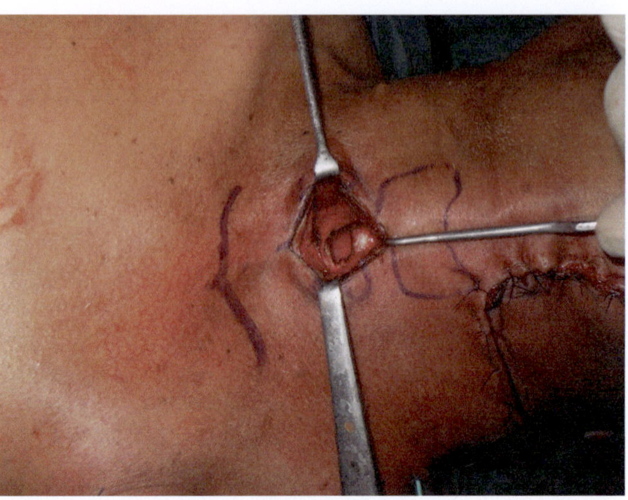

Fig. 2.12 The window is made in the trachea at the second tracheal ring level. One can also have crisscross incision on the trachea instead. It is advisable to confirm that it is the trachea only by inserting a syringe and withdrawing air bubbles before putting the incision

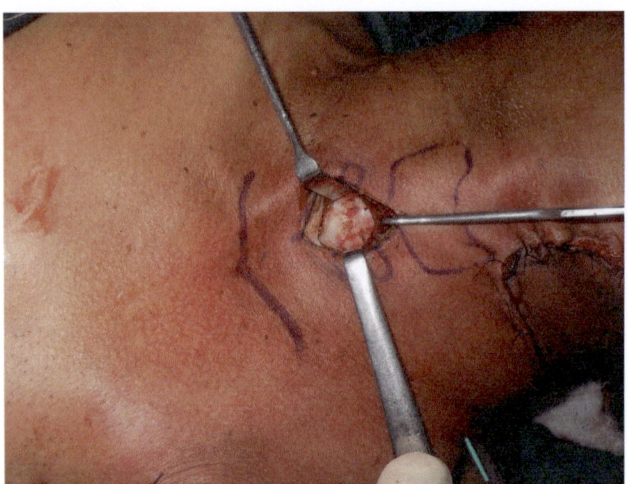

Fig. 2.11 The trachea is completely exposed and pre-tracheal fascia is separated to avoid small bleeding while making a window in the trachea

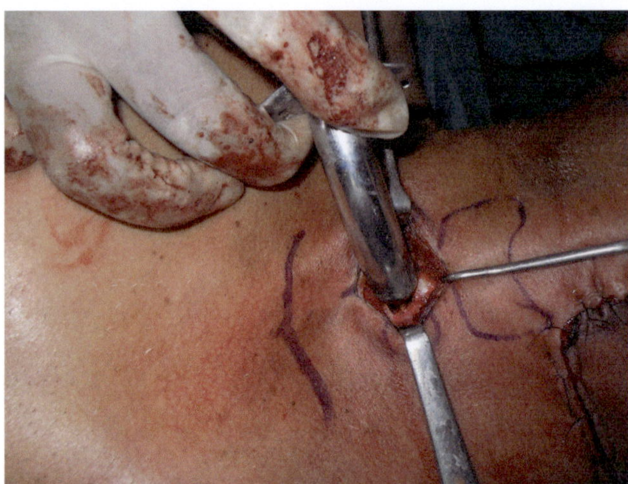

Fig. 2.13 The metal tracheostomy tube is inserted from lateral aspect of tracheostome and then rotated so that it is in trachea. One must not remove the retractors till it is confirmed that the tube is in the trachea

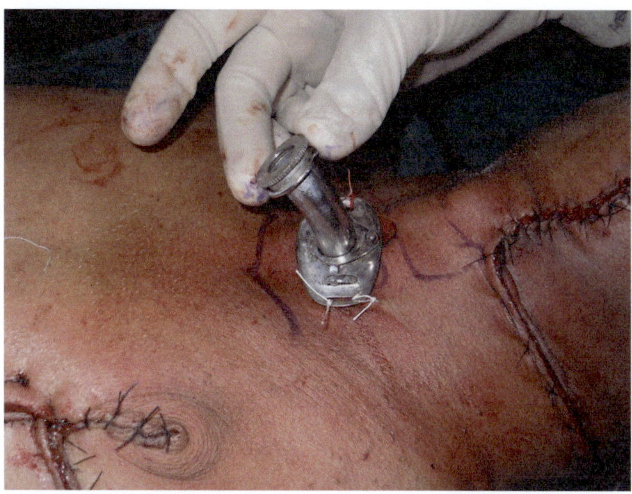

Fig. 2.14 The inner cannula is placed and locked for metal tracheostomy. It is also very important that the assistant holds the tracheostomy in place till sutures are placed as violent cough can throw the tube out if left unattended

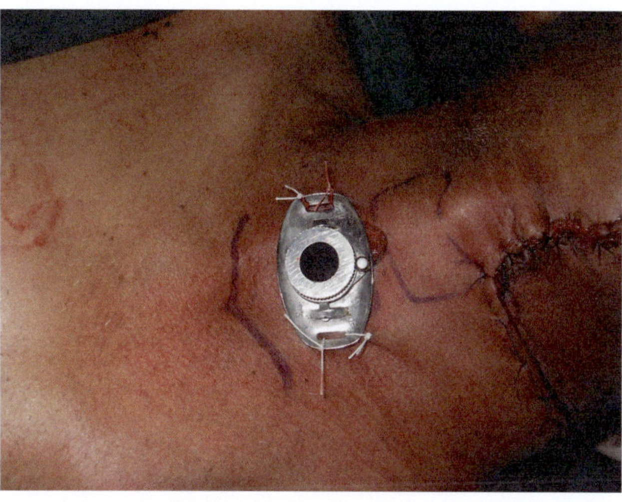

Fig. 2.15 The tube is in position. The aftercare of tracheostomy with frequent suctioning and use of moist gauze piece to cover the stoma is an equally important step. It is essential to pay necessary attention in postoperative care

Submandibular Gland Excision

This procedure demonstrates the removal of submandibular salivary gland neoplasm. This procedure is also performed to remove chronically enlarged gland due to stone obstruction. The inflammatory adhesions make this procedure more tricky in such cases.

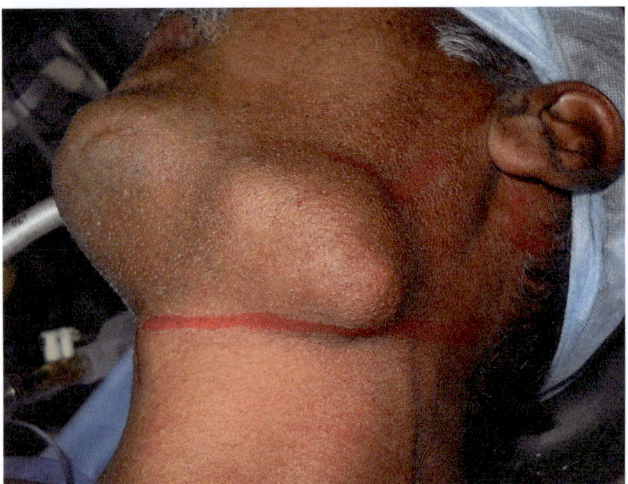

Fig. 2.16 The transverse incision is planned for removal of submandibular gland neoplasm. The incision is placed at least 2–3 cm below the mandible to prevent injury to the marginal branch of the facial nerve

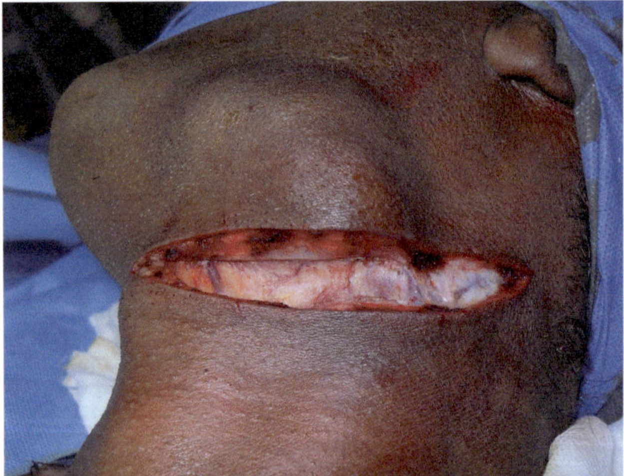

Fig. 2.17 The incision is placed and platysma is divided

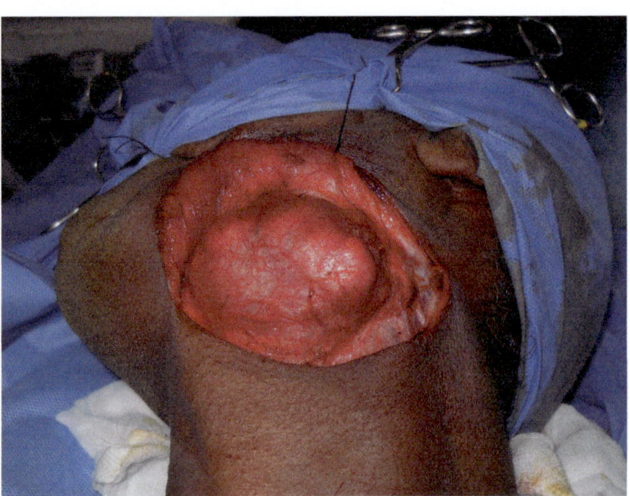

Fig. 2.18 The upper flap is raised in the subplatysmal plane. There are two methods to raise the upper flap. The facial nerve runs deep to the deep fascia of the submandibular gland. One can raise the flap in the deeper plane below the deep fascia to prevent injury to marginal branch of facial nerve. This method doesn't require exposing and identifying the nerve and is used in benign cases. In malignent neoplasm, we prefer to raise the flap in subplatysmal plane. Dividing the deep facia to expose the marginal nerve and isolating it from facial vessels and LNS

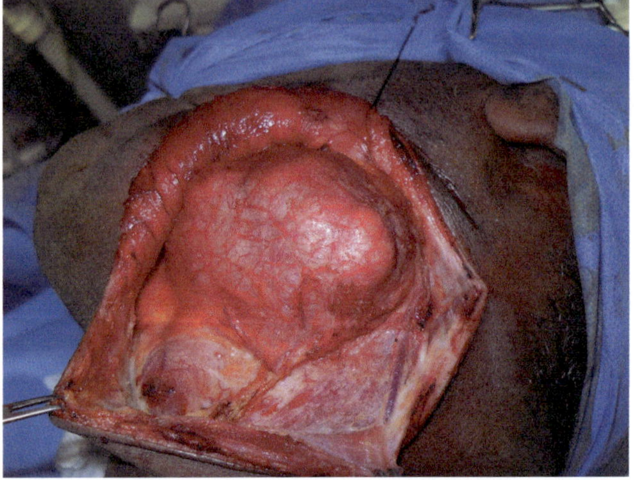

Fig. 2.19 The lower flap is raised to identify digastric muscle in entire length

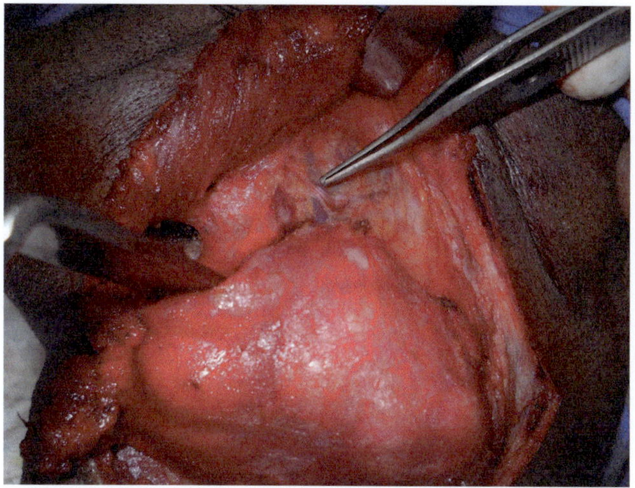

Fig. 2.20 The marginal nerve is dissected out just above the facial vessels. The vessels are ligated below the nerve and then lifted upwards to secure the nerve

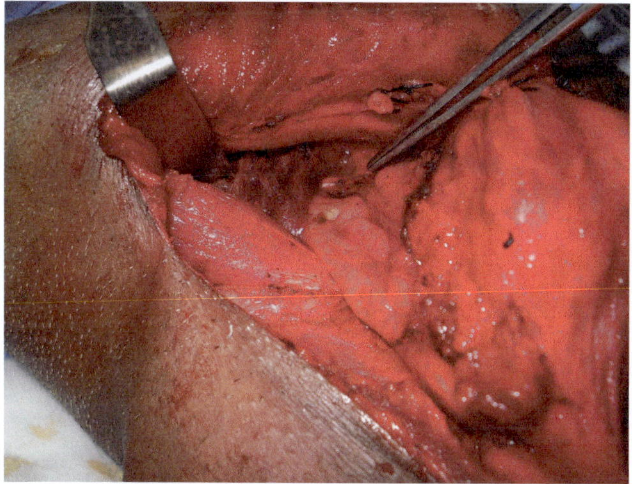

Fig. 2.21 The dissection moves forward to clear the deep portion of the gland below the mylohyoid muscle. The muscle is retracted anteriorly to expose the lingual nerve and duct. The position of the lingual nerve is demonstrated in the photograph

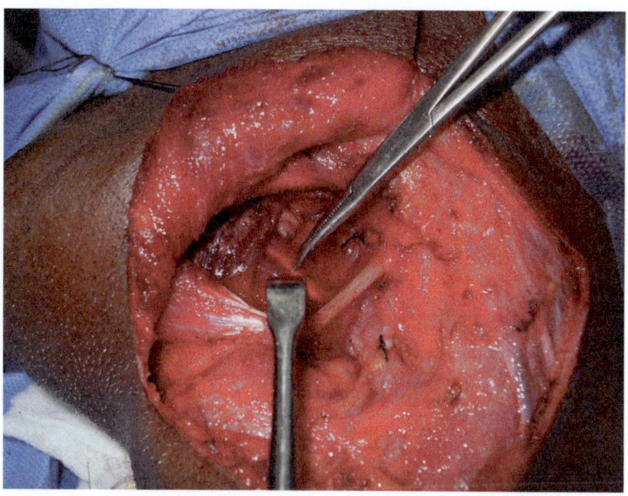

Fig. 2.22 The hypoglossal nerve is situated below the fascia in the floor and can be preserved without breaching the fascia. There are small veins in this area and I prefer to secure them before sectioning them

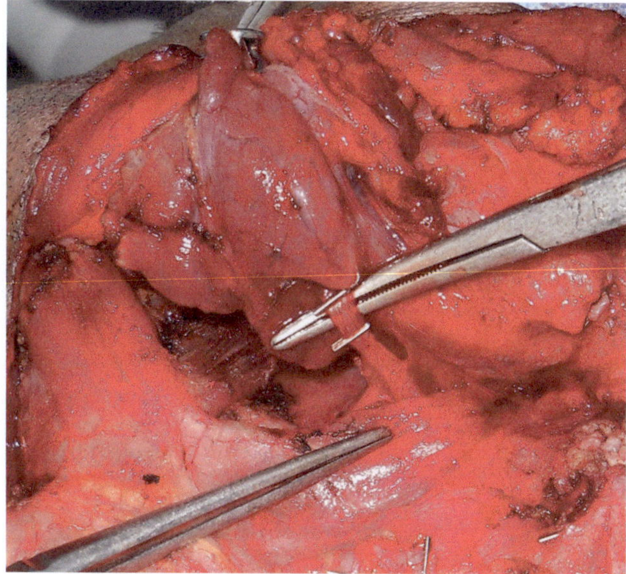

Fig. 2.23 The gland is mobilized to expose the facial artery just above the posterior belly of the digastric muscle. The vessel is secured to remove the gland

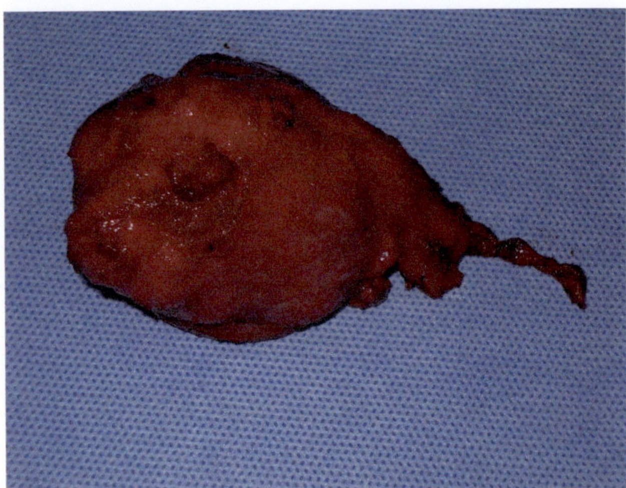

Fig. 2.24 While removing malignent neoplasm, it is advisable to remove complete gland with intact facia surrounding it. One also needs to perform selective neck dissection in such cases. The wounds are closed over drains, and the patient can be discharged on the same or next day

Secondary Tracheoesophageal Puncture (TEP)

The conventional way of performing secondary TEP is quite complicated, and we have devised a simple method to perform this procedure. This procedure is performed using curved intestinal clamps and can be performed in an outpatient clinic.

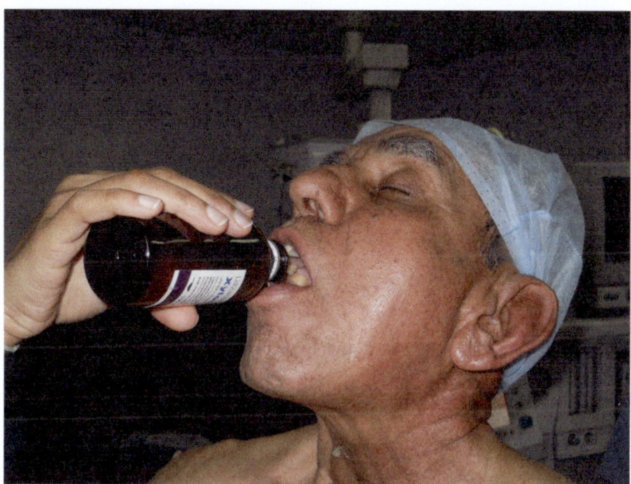

Fig. 2.25 The patient is prepared for procedure. The patient is asked to keep xylocaine viscus 4.1. In oral cavity for ten minutes

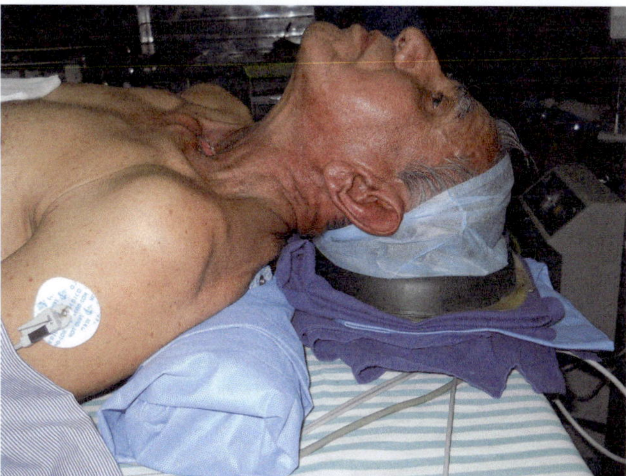

Fig. 2.26 It is advisable to achieve as much extension as possible for this procedure

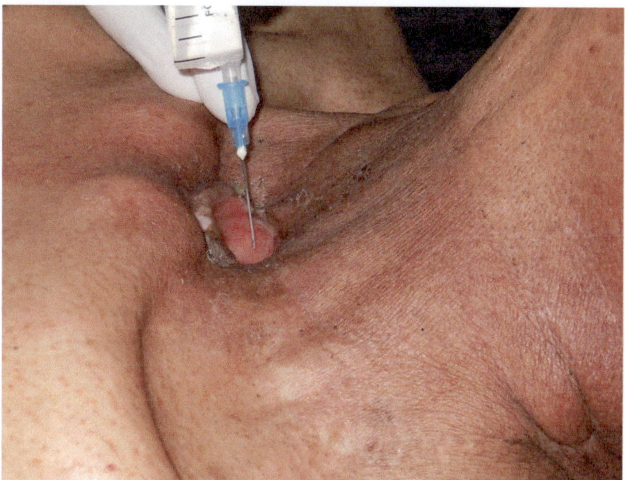

Fig. 2.27 Local anesthetic is infiltrated in the posterior wall of the trachea

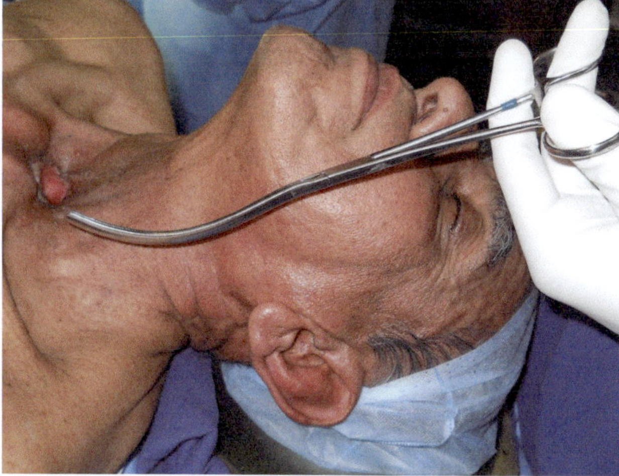

Fig. 2.28 This is an intestinal occluding clamp used by surgeons for intestinal anastomosis. Its natural curvature is in accordance with the oral and pharyngeal cavity. It is inserted softly through the oral cavity and the tip reaches the posterior wall of the trachea where it can be felt

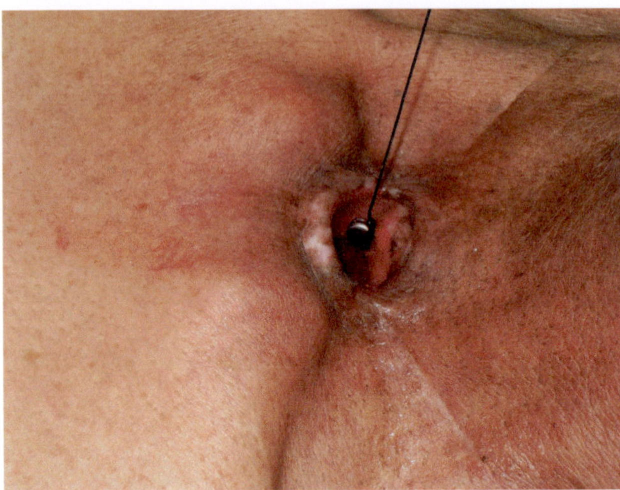

Fig. 2.29 A small incision is placed in posterior wall of trachea about 1 cm below tracheo-dermal junction to bring the tip out in cavity. A thick silk thread is tied at the tip

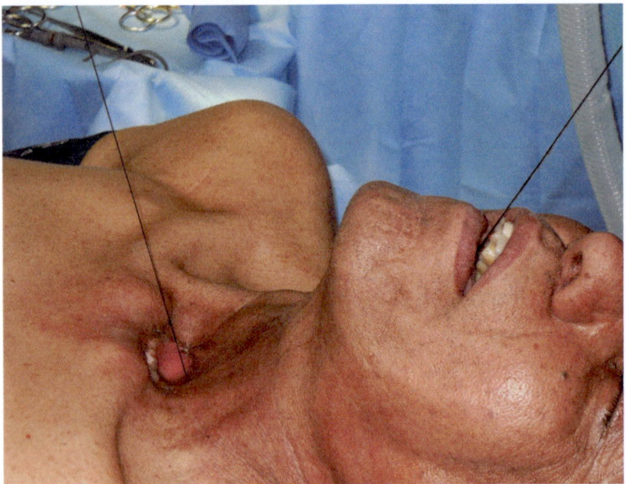

Fig. 2.30 The forceps along with the thread is pulled out from the oral cavity

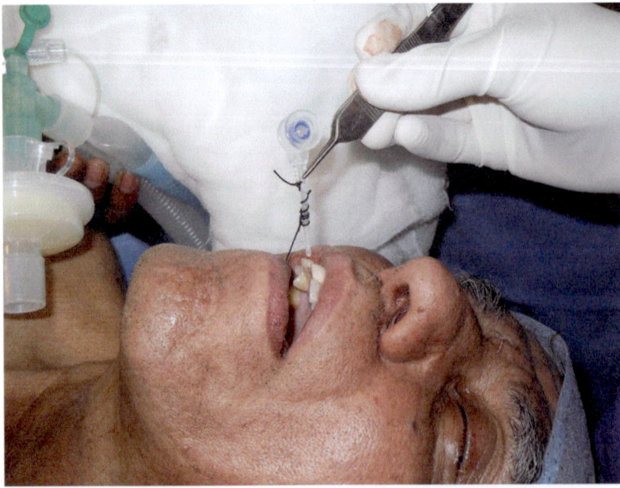

Fig. 2.31 The voice prosthesis is tied to the oral end of the thread

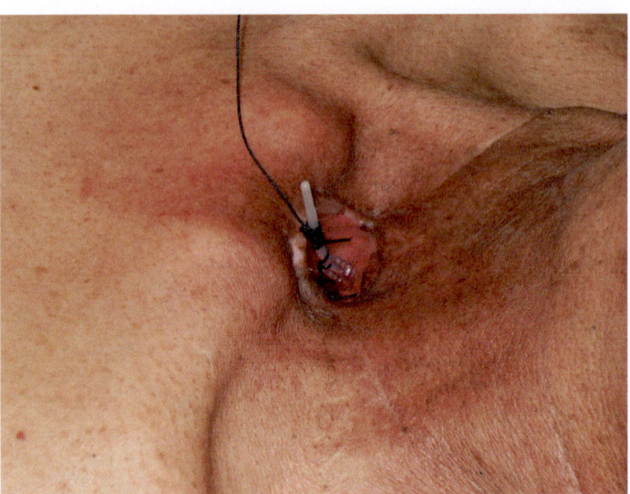

Fig. 2.32 The thread is pulled into the tracheal opening to bring the prosthesis into position. One must be careful in delivering the prosthesis to the trachea to avoid injury to the posterior wall

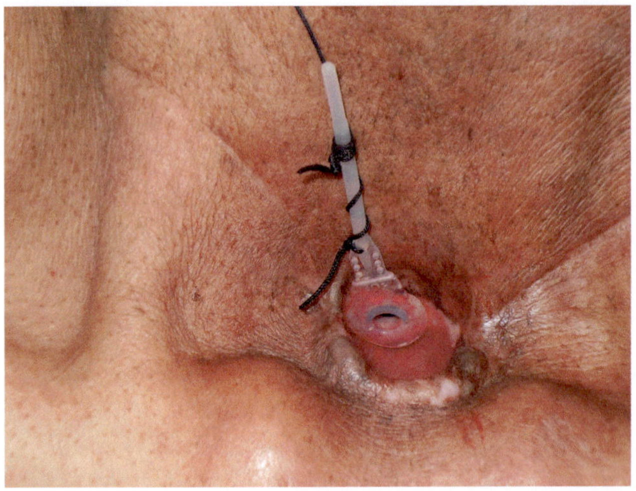

Fig. 2.33 The prosthesis snugly fits into the posterior wall of the trachea and the thread is separated from it. The procedure can be completed in a short time in the office setup without any special requirements. There are no major complications noticed with this procedure in our 5 years of experience, and we prefer this approach over the conventional approach

Sentinel Lymph Node Biopsy

Sentinel lymphnode biopsy is a standard procedure in detecting metastasis in cancer of breast and malignant melanoma. It is still in the conceptual stage for head–neck squamous cancers. This section demonstrates the surgical procedure to identify and remove sentinel lymph node.

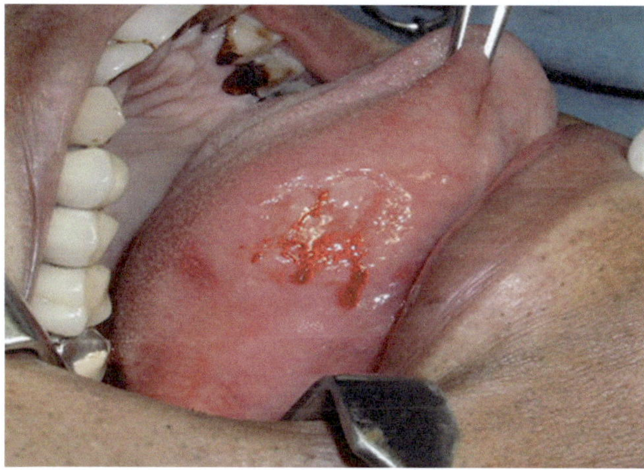

Fig. 2.34 Patient with early tongue cancer. This procedure is performed in patients with early cancer with no neck involvement

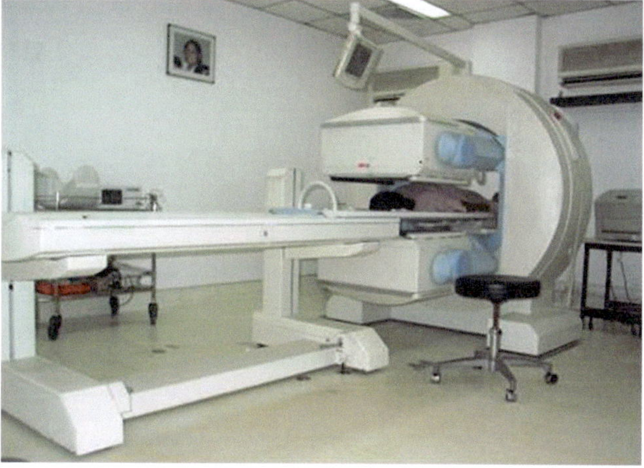

Fig. 2.36 Setup of gamma camera. The patient is placed on a table in the same way as on an operation table to have accuracy in marking of the node

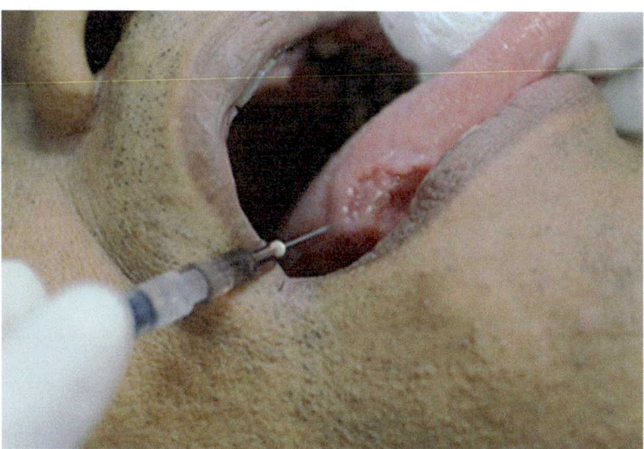

Fig. 2.35 The Tc_{99m}-labeled filtered sulfur colloid is inserted all around the tumor. It is a standard practice to use radioactive infiltration and gamma camera to identify the sentinel node. Use of blue dye alone is now not considered standard of care

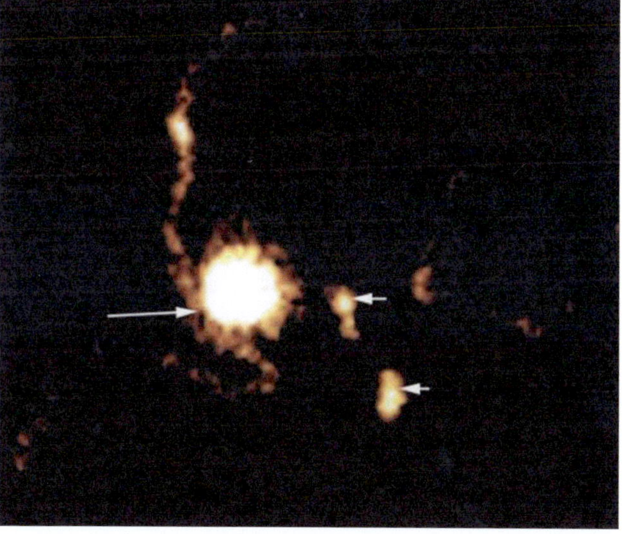

Fig. 2.37 This is a continuous procedure and these are images that you get on monitor. The large mass is primary and the small images are sentinel nodes. These nodes are marked on skin by use of a gamma pointer. The patient is shifted to the operation theater to complete the procedure

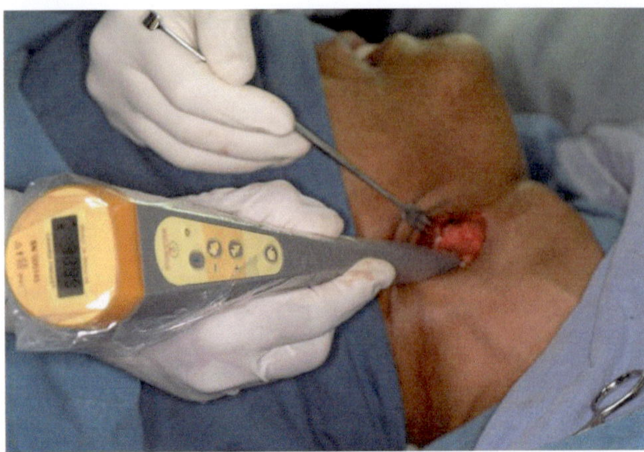

Fig. 2.38 A small 2 cm incision is placed on the skin mark to identify the sentinel nodes. The hand-helled gamma camera will help in idntifying the sentinel lymph nodes. These nodes are examined with frozen section, and formal neck dissection is carried out in case metastasis is detected. These nodes are further examined by step sectioning (later), and second stage neck dissection is advised if occult metastasis is identified

3 Tumors of the Thyroid and Parathyroid

Thyroid

Surgical Anatomy and Pathology

Thyroid surgery is one of the more commonly performed head–neck surgical procedures. It is performed for a wide variety of indications ranging from benign neoplasm of thyroid to malignant tumors. Thyroidectomy is also performed by clinicians practicing in different setups with varying resources. Though it is a relatively simple procedure, it has the potential to cause life-threatening complications. Appropriate exposure, understanding of the anatomy of recurrent laryngeal nerve and parathyroid gland, and the ability to secure hemostasis in a relatively narrow space are key in obtaining a successful outcome.

Figure 3.1 demonstrates the schematic anatomy of the thyroid and parathyroid gland. The relation of the recurrent laryngeal nerve to the inferior thyroid artery and parathyroid gland forms the backbone for surgical safety. The inferior thyroid artery most of the time passes over the recurrent laryngeal nerve and divides into multiple branches. It is essential to locate the recurrent laryngeal nerve first and then ligate the terminal branches of the inferior thyroid gland close to the gland where it enters the gland. The parathyroid gland should be preserved with its blood supply.

Figure 3.2 demonstrates algorithm for management of thyroid diseases.

- Hemithyroidectomy
  1. Unilateral benign lesions
  2. Well-differentiated malignant thyroids less than 1 cm size
- Total Thyroidectomy
  1. Bilateral large benign lesions
  2. Malignant lesions (>1 cm)

Indications for sub-total and near total thyroidectomy are rare in current day practice.

This chapter focuses on the technical aspects of performing thyroid surgeries.

A. Thyroidectomy
B. Thyroidectomy with tracheal resection
C. Thyroidectomy with sternotomy for retrosternal goiter

N. Trivedi, *Atlas of Head and Neck Cancer Surgery: The Compartment Surgery for Resection in 3-D*, DOI 10.1007/978-81-322-2050-3_3, © Springer India 2015

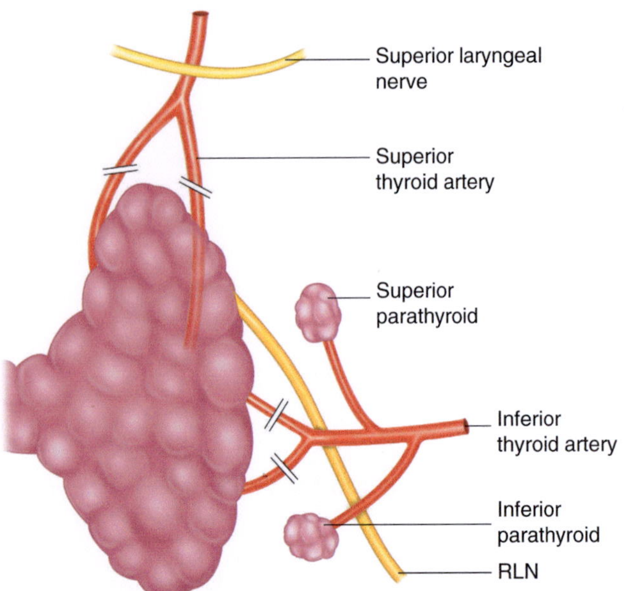

Fig. 3.1 Anatomy for thyroid surgery

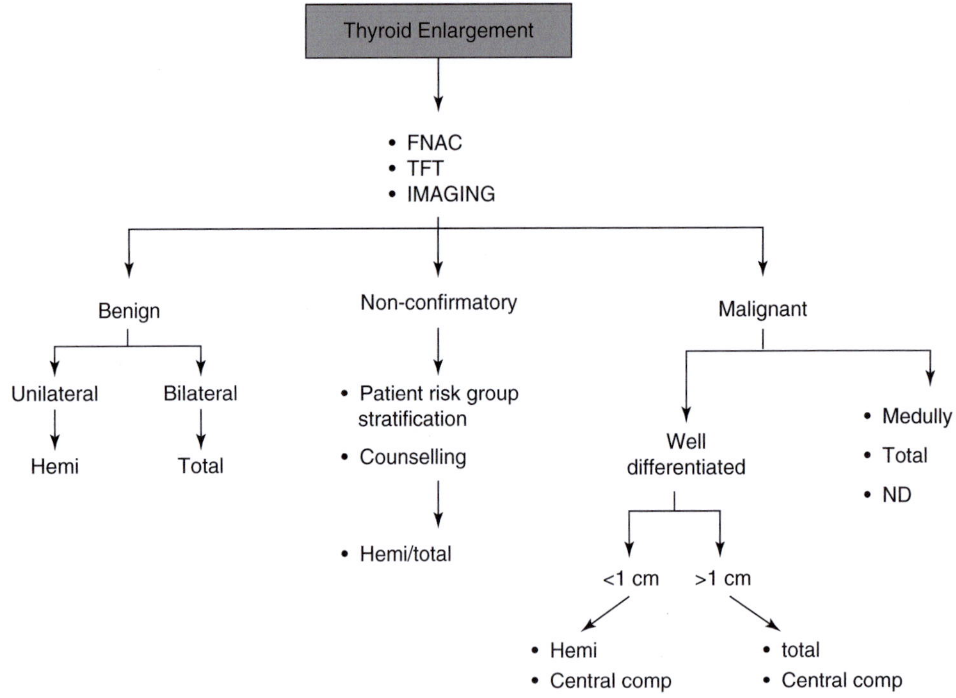

Fig. 3.2 Algorithm for management of thyroid diseases

Thyroidectomy

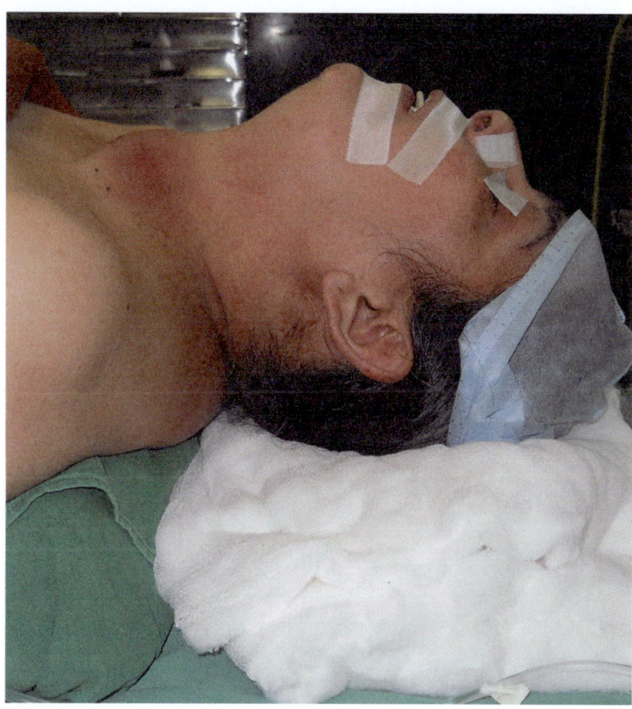

Fig. 3.3 Demonstrates the position of the patient for any thyroid procedure. It is essential to achieve as much neck extension as possible with the use of a shoulder bag and head ring

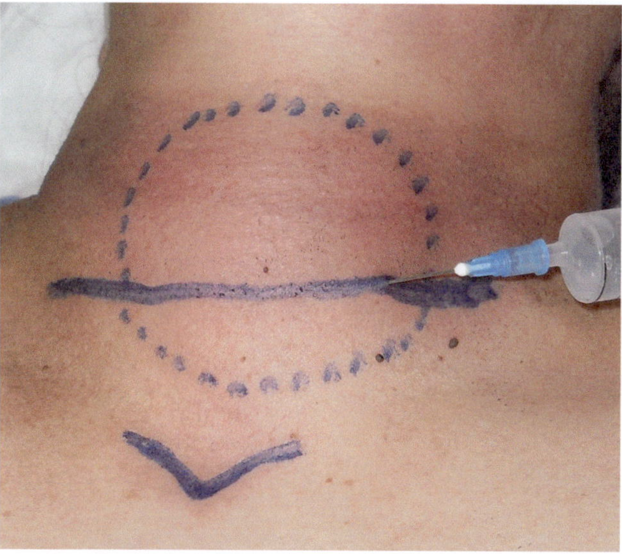

Fig. 3.4 Demonstrates surface marking for the incision. Transverse lower cervical incision about 2 cm above the suprasternal notch is preferred for thyroid surgeries. This gives better exposure, avoids the need for retraction of the lower flap, and provides better cosmesis. Infiltration of xylocaine–adrenaline solution 10 min before the start of the procedure helps in achieving better hemostasis while raising flaps

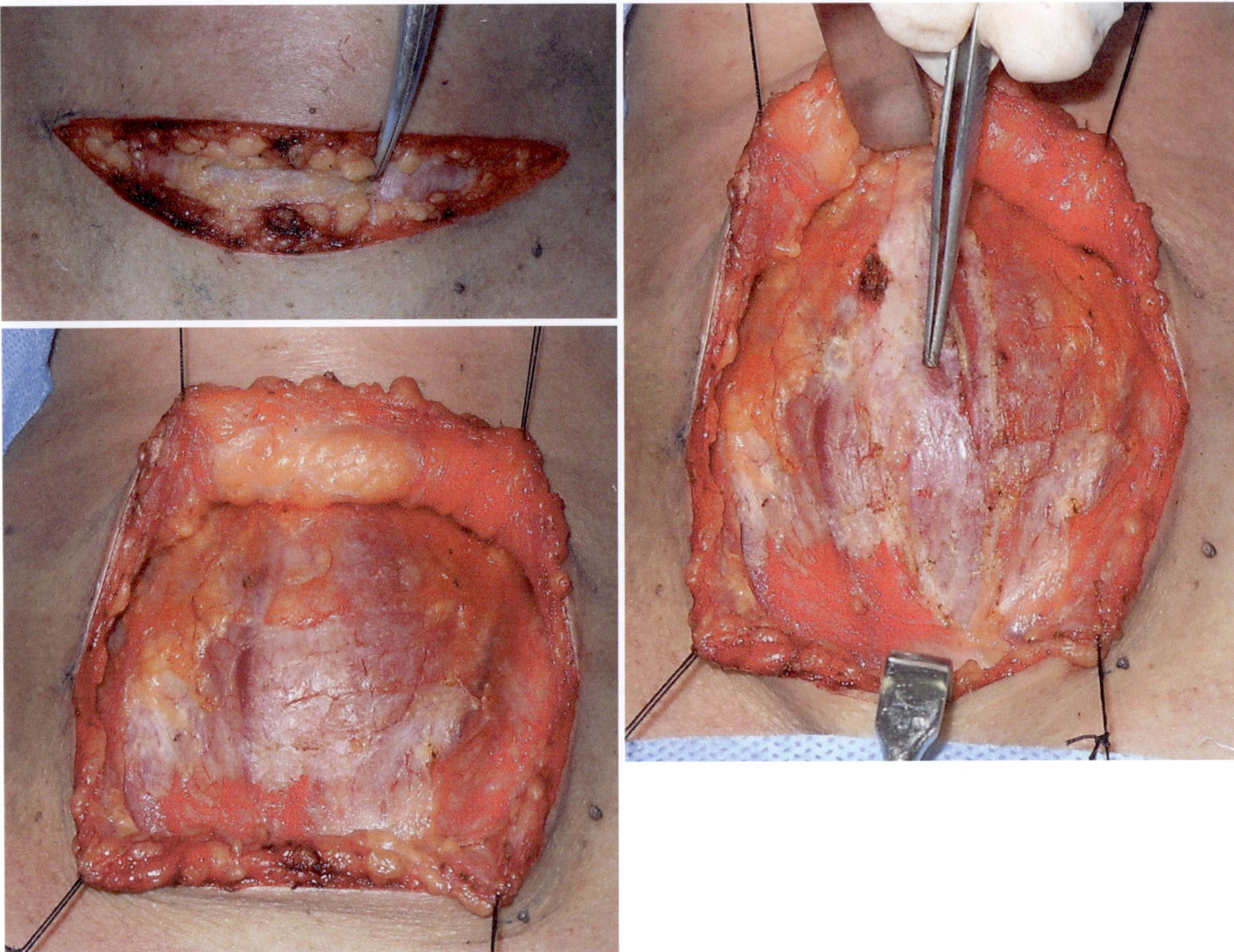

Figs. 3.5, 3.6, and 3.7 Demonstrates the anatomy of the platysma in the anterior neck. The platysma is absent in the midline in the lower neck, and it is advisable to incise the platysma on the lateral aspect to find the subplatysmal plane and raise the entire upper flap in the same plane (Fig. 3.6). Deep fascia above the strap muscle is divided in the midline to expose and separate the strap muscle from either side (Fig. 3.7)

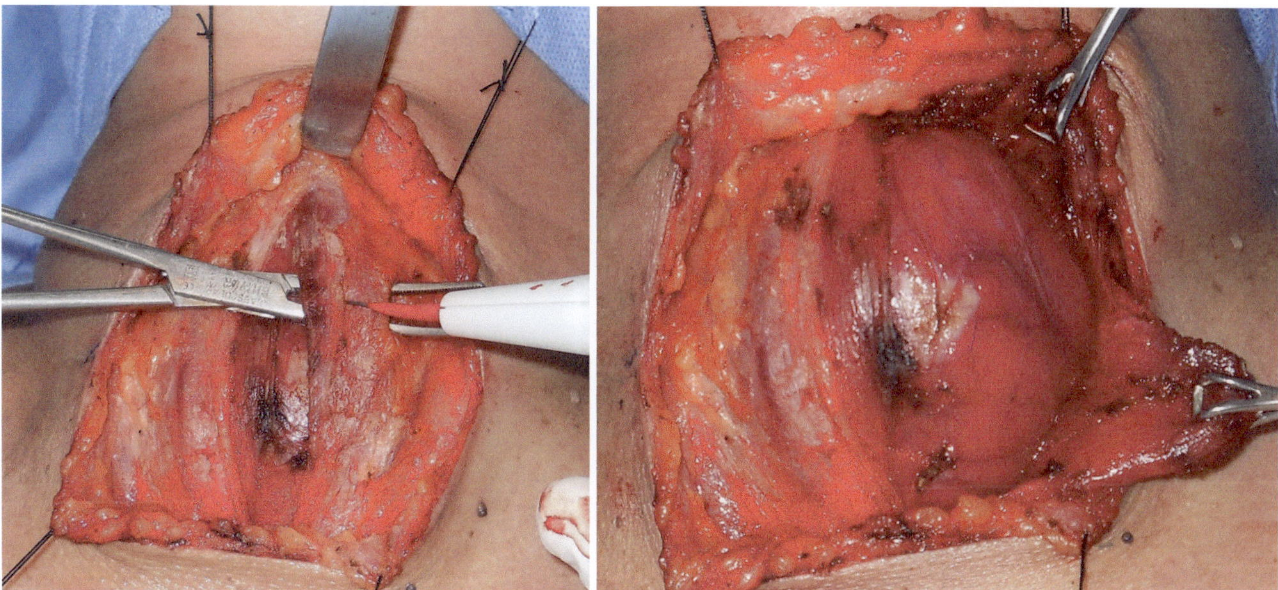

Figs. 3.8 and 3.9 Demonstrates the division of strap muscles to expose the thyroid gland. Sectioning of the strap muscle is advisable for larger and more vascular thyroid lesions and for surgeons in training period. This approach allows better exposure for dissection of the recurrent laryngeal nerve (RLN) and parathyroid glands. Muscle should be cut as high as possible to preserve its nerve supply. Care should be taken not to damage small veins on the surface of the thyroid gland while retracting the strap muscle and exposing gland (Fig. 3.9). The middle thyroid vein is secured first while mobilizing the thyroid gland

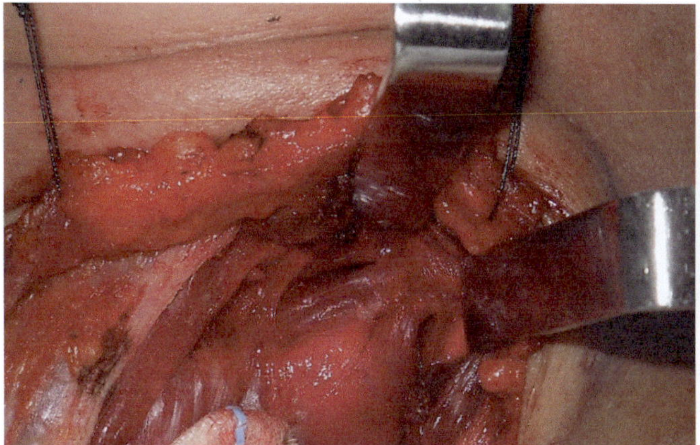

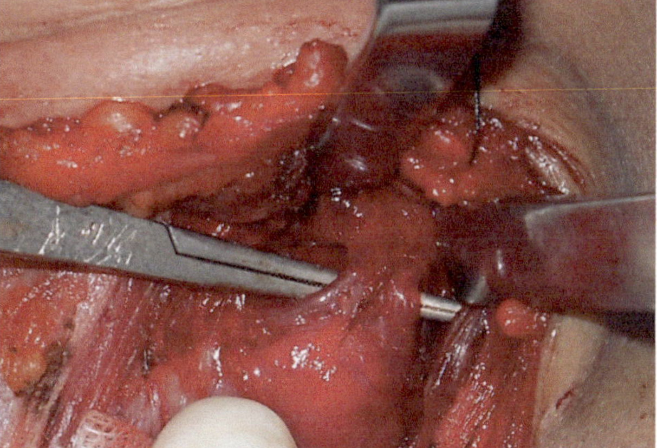

Figs. 3.10 and 3.11 Demonstrates the position of the superior thyroid pedicle in relation to the thyroid gland. This is one of the important steps for this procedure, and proper exposure to this area is essential to secure hemostasis. Two retractors are placed to expose the medial and lateral aspects of the superior thyroid pedicle. Fig. 8a shows the anterior and posterior branch of this pedicle running on the surface of the thyroid gland. The pedicle should be ligated as close to the thyroid gland as possible to avoid injury to the external laryngeal nerve. I prefer not to dissect the external laryngeal nerve and stay close to thyroid gland to avoid injuring it (Fig. 3.11)

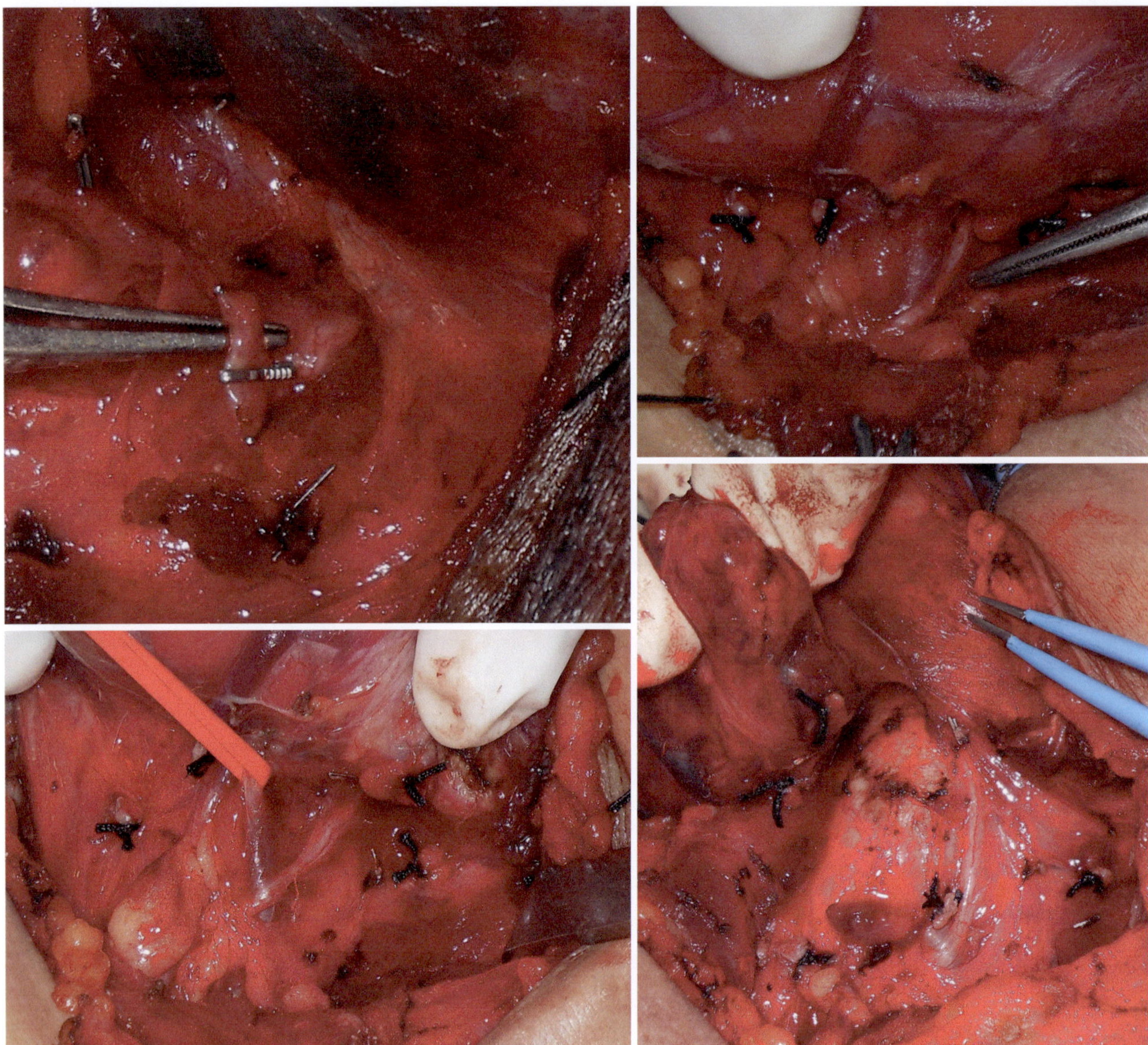

Figs. 3.12, 3.13, 3.14, and 3.15 Demonstrate the anatomy of the RLN in relation to the inferior thyroid artery and parathyroid glands. Fig. 3.12 shows the recurrent laryngeal nerve passing below the inferior thyroid artery which is the usual anatomy in this region. Fig. 3.13 shows variation of this anatomy where the RLN passes above the inferior thyroid artery. One needs to identify this relation before ligating the inferior thyroid artery. It is always advisable to ligate branches of the inferior thyroid artery after it crosses the RLN to prevent injuring the nerve. Figs. 3.14 and 3.15 show the inferior parathyroid gland with separate blood supply from the inferior thyroid artery. It is essential to preserve the parathyroid gland with its blood supply. Ligating only those branches of the inferior thyroid artery that enters the thyroid gland (near the thyroid gland) ensures preservation of functioning parathyroid gland

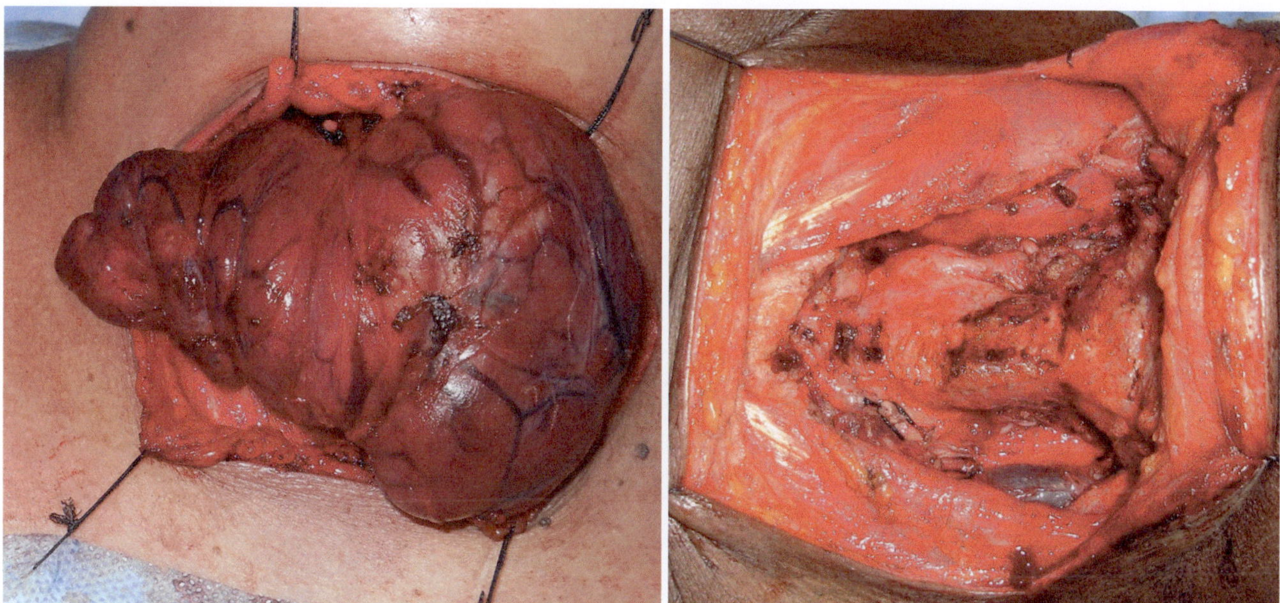

Figs. 3.16 and 3.17 Demonstrate completed total thyroidectomy. Strap muscles are sutured back to its original position. Appropriate drains are kept and closure is done. It is also advisable to remove the shoulder bag and keep neck in flexion for 10 min to check for hemostasis before starting wound closure

Thyroidectomy with Tracheal Resection

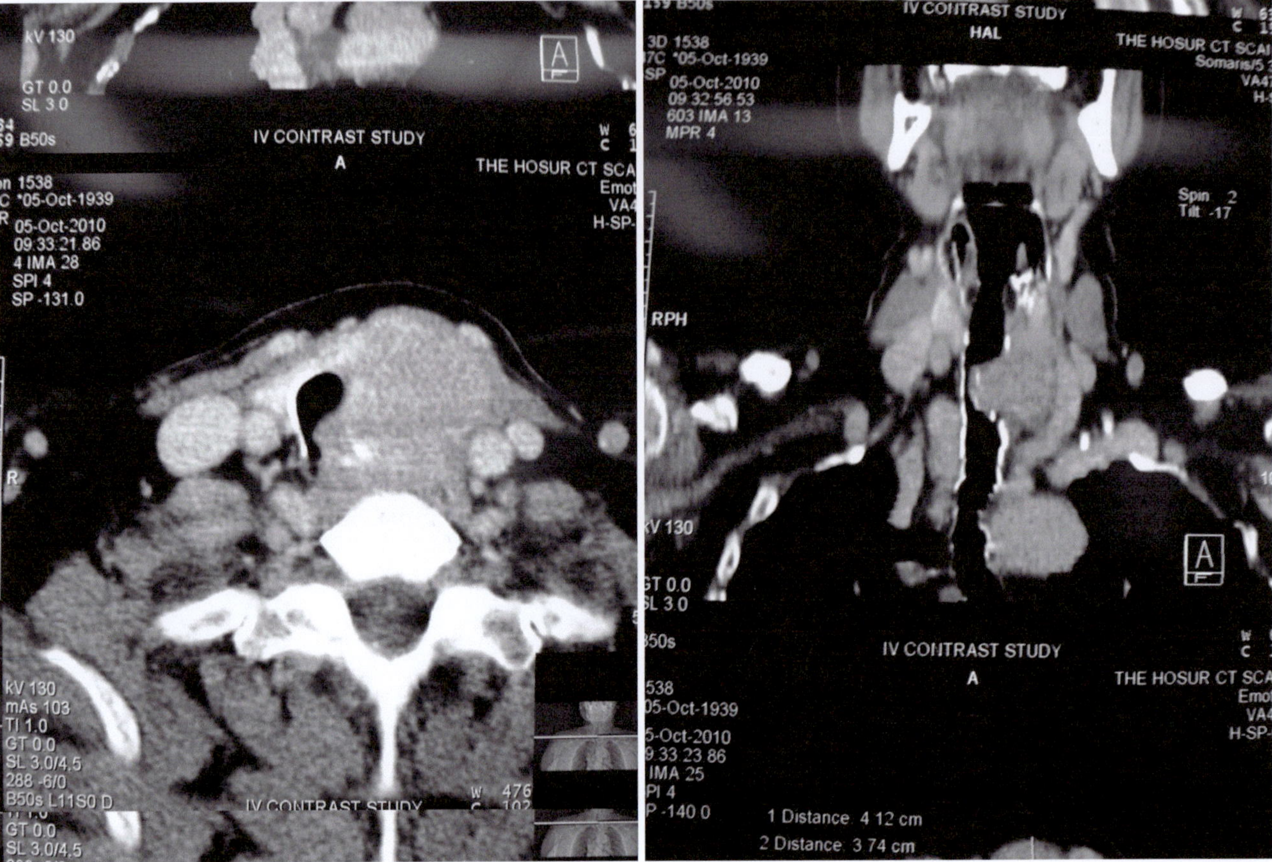

Figs. 3.18 and 3.19 Show computed tomography scan (CT scan) images of a patient of papillary carcinoma thyroid infiltrating the trachea. The left lobe of the thyroid is enlarged and has infiltrated the tracheal wall and entered into the lumen. It is very important to evaluate the level of this infiltration in relation to the cricoid cartilage. This CT scan image shows that tumor doesn't involve the cricoid cartilage and first tracheal ring. This implies that we can have adequate margin of the trachea above and below without having to resect the cricoid cartilage. In case the cricoid cartilage is involved, total laryngectomy needs to be performed. Another important fact is the extent of tracheal involvement. Around 5–6 tracheal rings can be resected without much impact on tracheal anastomosis. Tumor infiltrating more length of the trachea needs more careful planning and may need extensive mobilization of the trachea or alternative method of reconstruction

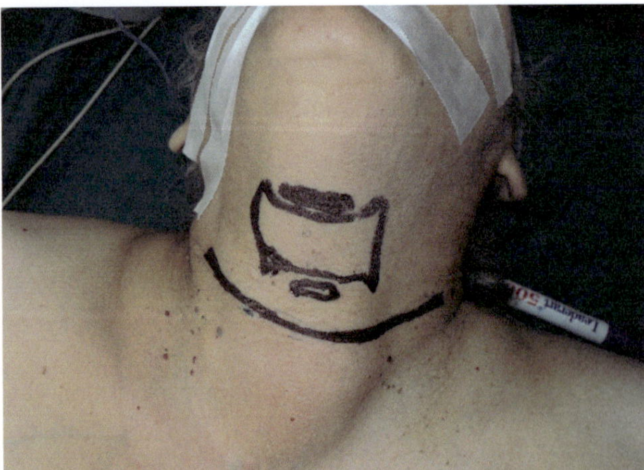

Fig. 3.20 Shows surface marking of the thyroid and cricoid cartilage and planned incision site

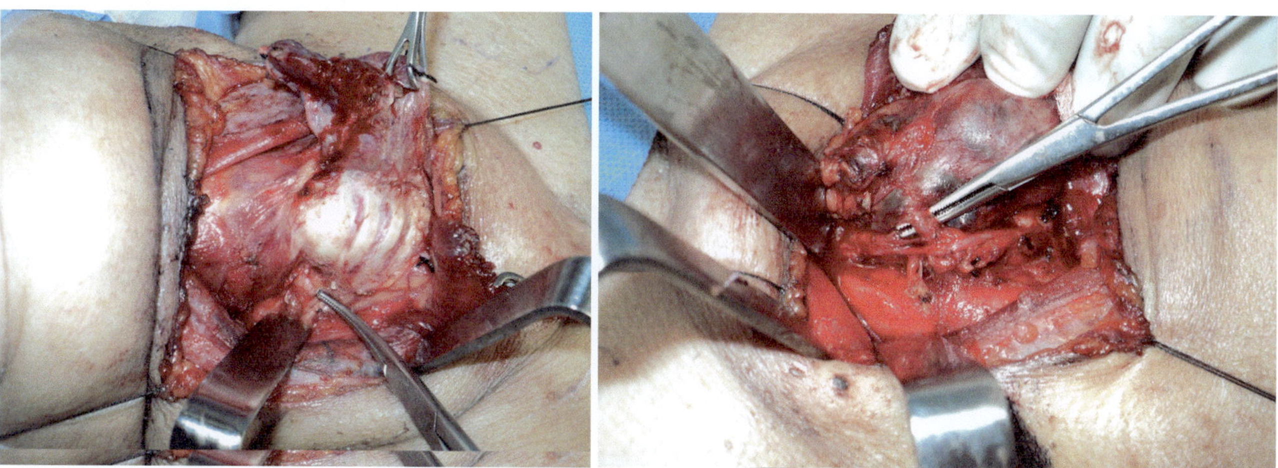

Figs. 3.21 and 3.22 Shows dissection of the recurrent laryngeal nerve and inferior thyroid artery as described in the previous section of this chapter

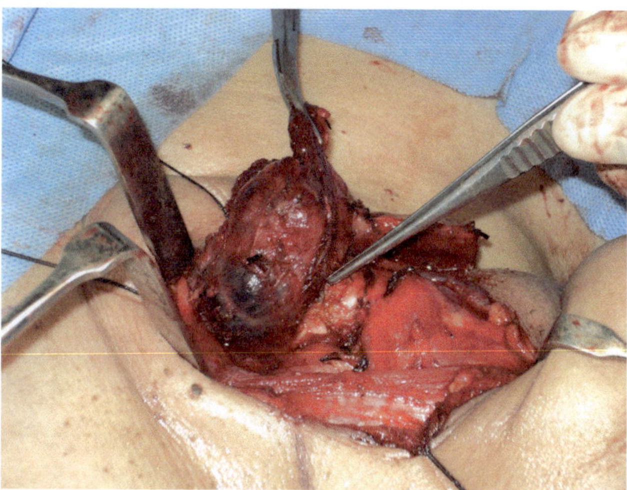

Fig. 3.23 Demonstrates the area where the tumor is entering the trachea. The thyroid needs to be dissected from all other attachments before tracheal resection is started. The tumor may involve the esophagus on many occasions, but it can be freed by just removing muscles of the esophageal wall. Mucosal continuity is preserved with this type of dissection. The tracheal resection area is marked first. It is important to arrange all the suture material, endotracheal tube with its connection and suction tube before beginning tracheal resection

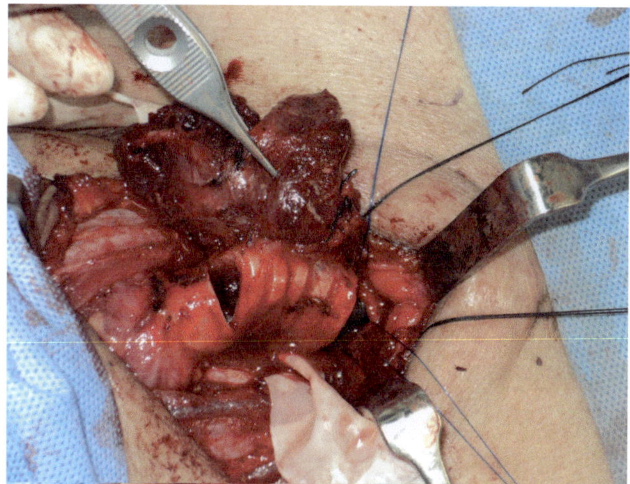

Fig. 3.24 Demonstrates tracheal cuts. I prefer to put the lower tracheal cut before the upper cut. It is important to secure the lower end of the free trachea with prolene sutures or it can go down in mediastinum (Fig. 3.24). Once the lower cut is made, disease extent in the trachea can be assessed and the upper cut can be planned. At this time, a new endotracheal tube can be placed into the lower trachea (as is done for laryngectomy) after withdrawing the existing tube. It is very important not to withdraw the tube completely and to keep it just at the vocal cord level. This will enable us to put the tube back after completion of anastomosis. Alternatively, one can work with the same endotracheal tube in place and suture around it as demonstrated in this case

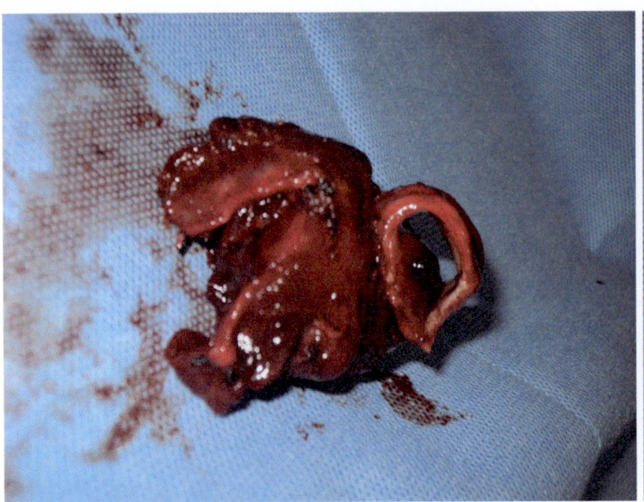

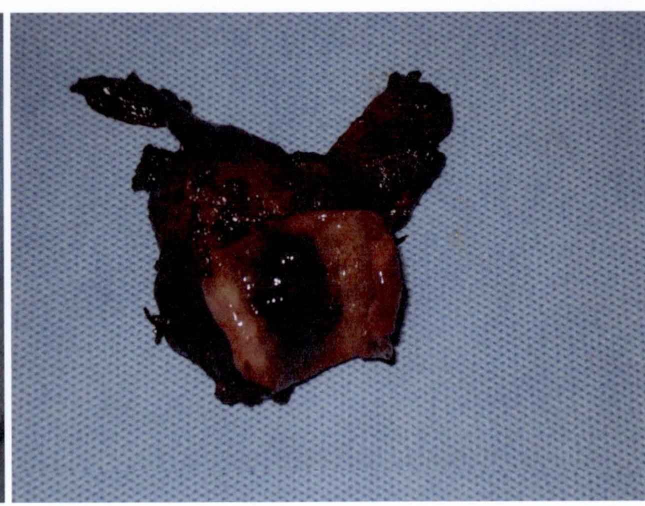

Figs. 3.25 and 3.26 Shows the resected specimen with adequate margins

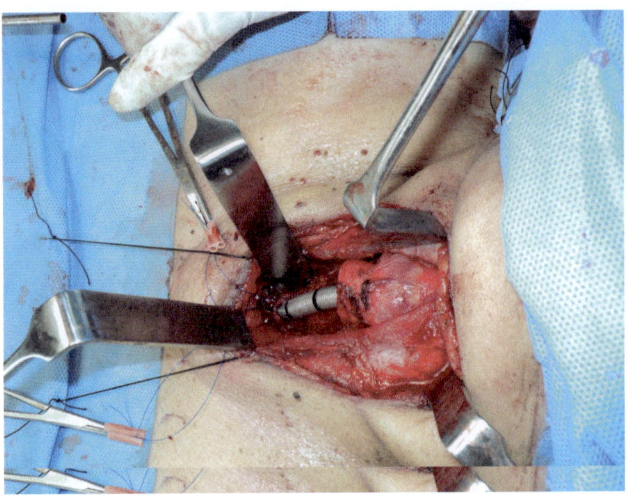

Fig. 3.27 The photogaph shows two cut ends of the trachea after removing the specimen. This figure demonstrates that gap is significant in most of the cases not to allow direct closure of two ends without tension. It is preferred to mobilize both the upper and lower ends of the trachea before beginning the anastomosis

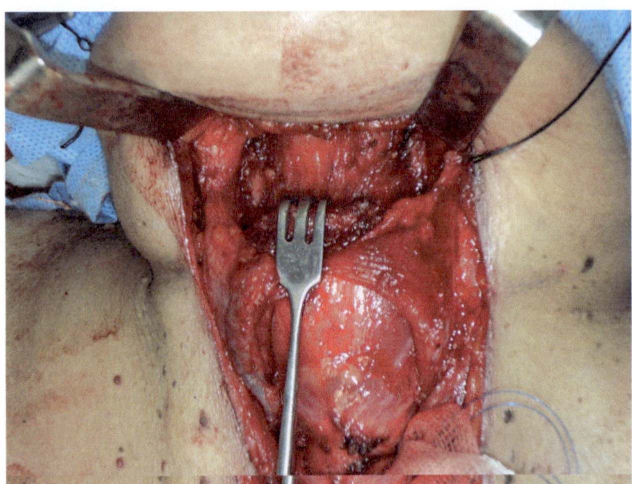

Fig. 3.28 The photogaph shows the technique to mobilize the upper half. This technique is similar to what we do in laryngectomy to expose the vallecula region. Suprahyoid muscles are released from the hyoid bone. This will help us to drop down the hyoid–thyroid cartilage unit and gain about 3–5 cm extra length

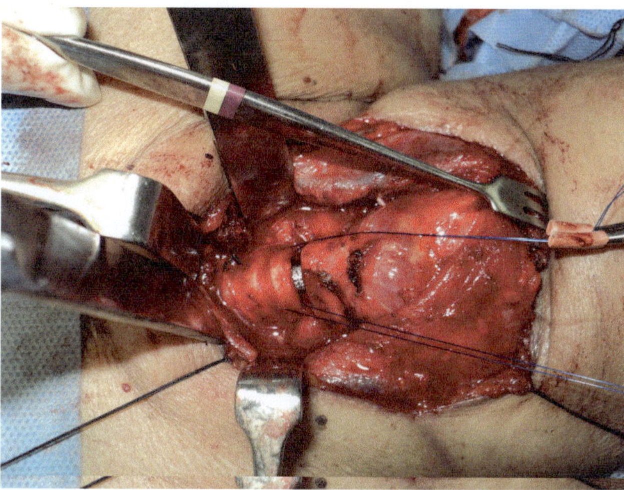

Fig. 3.29 Shows mobilization of the lower trachea. It is very important to preserve the blood supply of the trachea by not disturbing the lateral blood supply to the trachea and keeping the perichondrium intact. Both ends should be mobilized enough to have tension-free repair

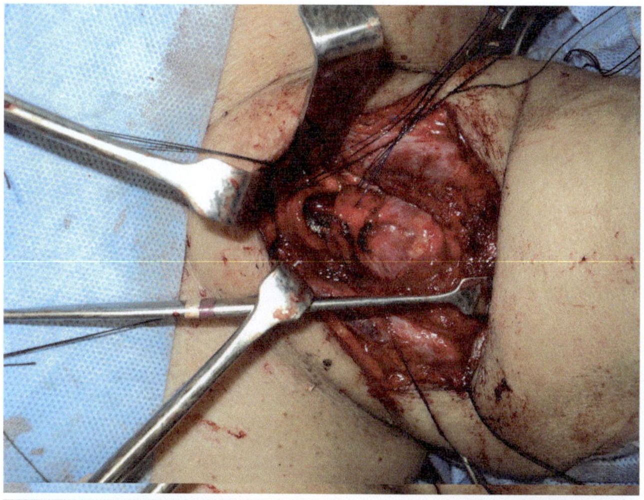

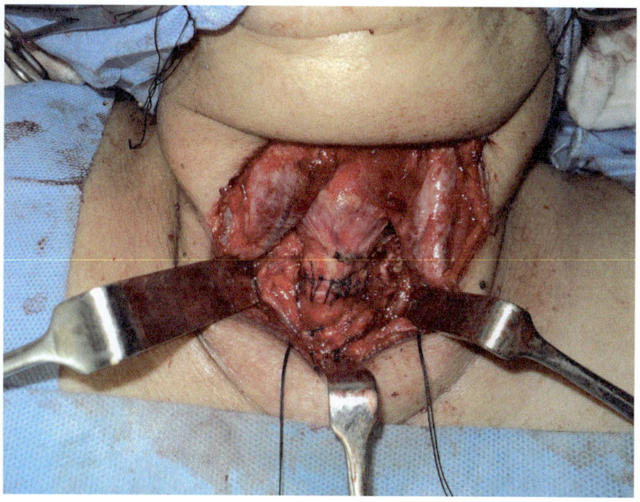

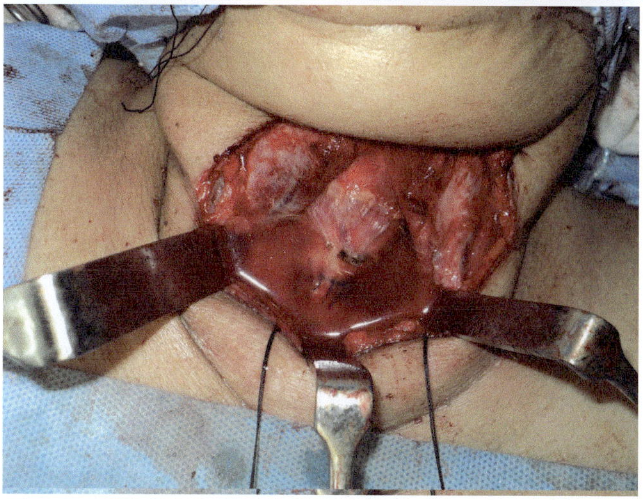

Figs. 3.30, 3.31, and 3.32 Demonstrates technical concepts in suturing of the trachea. Stay sutures with prolene are taken on the lateral aspect of the trachea. The posterior wall of the trachea is sutured first. It is preferable to keep the knots outside of the tracheal lumen to prevent granulation tissue. If a separate endotracheal tube was inserted through the lower tracheal stoma earlier, it needs to come out now. The tube which was kept at the level of the vocal cord can be guided into the lower trachea. Anterior wall suturing is completed once posterior wall sutures are taken (Fig. 3.31). Completeness of suturing is checked by filling the cavity with water and looking for air leak (Fig. 3.32)

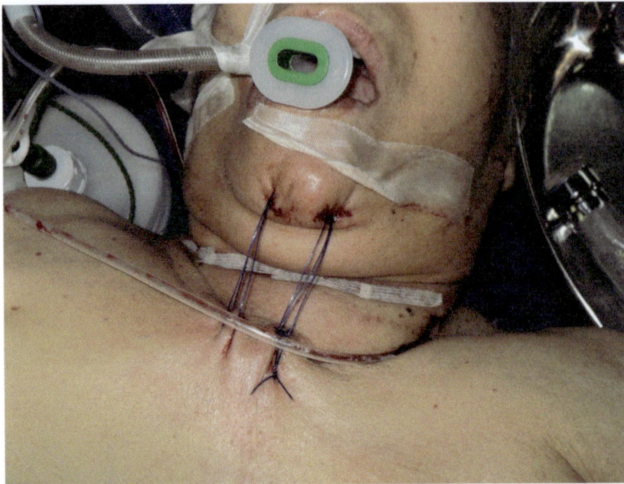

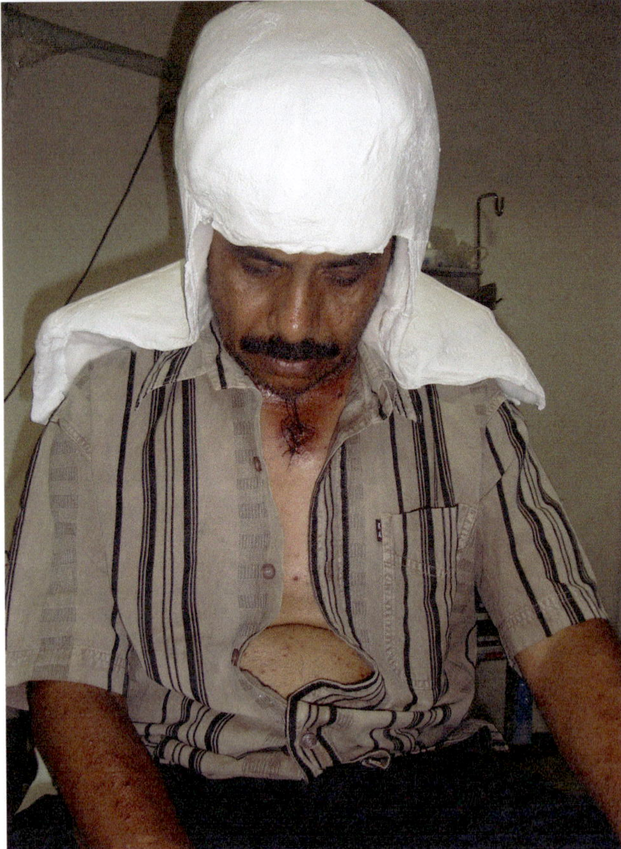

Figs. 3.33 and 3.34 Show the postoperative position of the patient. This is very important in avoiding sudden extension of the neck that can result in shearing of tracheal anastomosis. We prefer to keep this suturing for around 3 weeks. The headgear shown in Fig. 3.34 is very heavy and not commonly used now. In case of accident leading to shearing of tracheal anastomosis, one should open the wound and try to secure the lower end of the trachea and airway. Patient can be taken to the theater and managed accordingly

Thyroidectomy with Sternotomy for Retrosternal Goiter

The majority of retrosternal goiters can be removed from the neck by subcapsular dissection. Very few actually require sternotomy. It is important to keep a thoracic surgeon informed before planning any case with retrosternal extension. Very obese patients or patients with limited neck mobility can have problems while operating through only neck incision. I prefer to perform sternotomy when the scan shows the tumor in close proximity with large mediastinal vessels or during operation when the tumor is not getting mobilized easily. Injuring major blood vessels in the mediastinum can be a life-threatening complication, and one should not hesitate in performing sternotomy when in doubt.

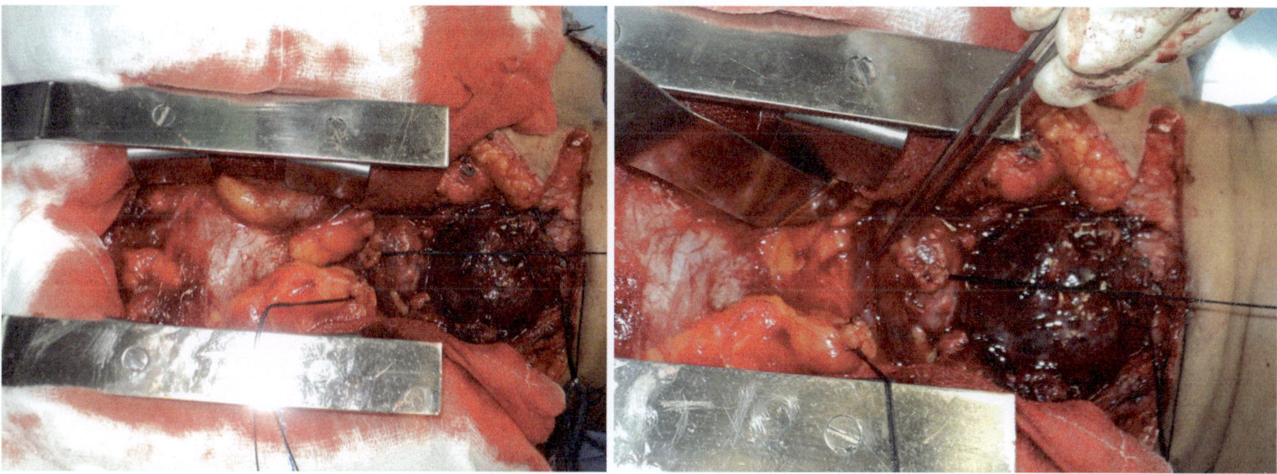

Figs. 3.35 and 3.36 Shows exposure after sternotomy. Enlarged thyroid gland can be seen in close proximity of neck vessels

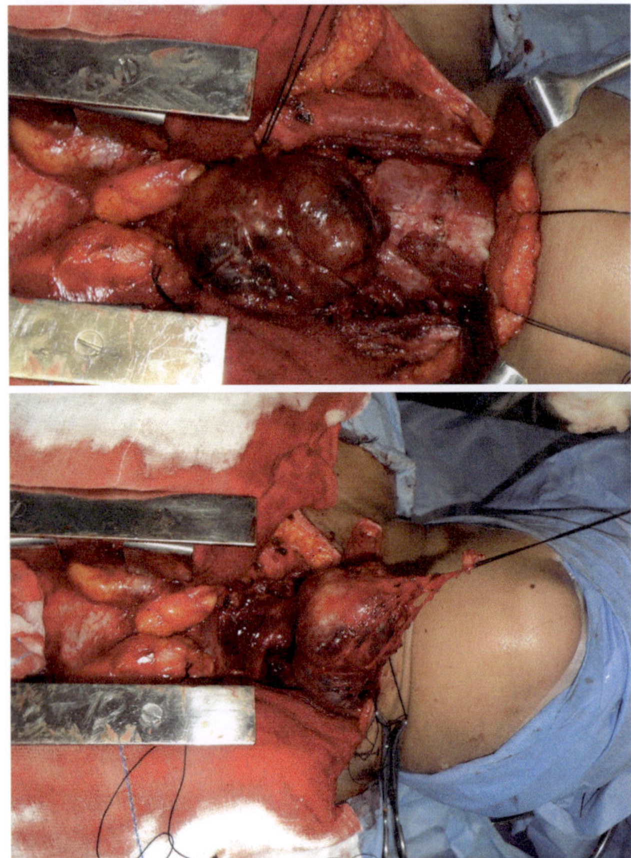

Figs. 3.37 and 3.38 Show the gland mobilized from the mediastinum preserving the thoracic vessels

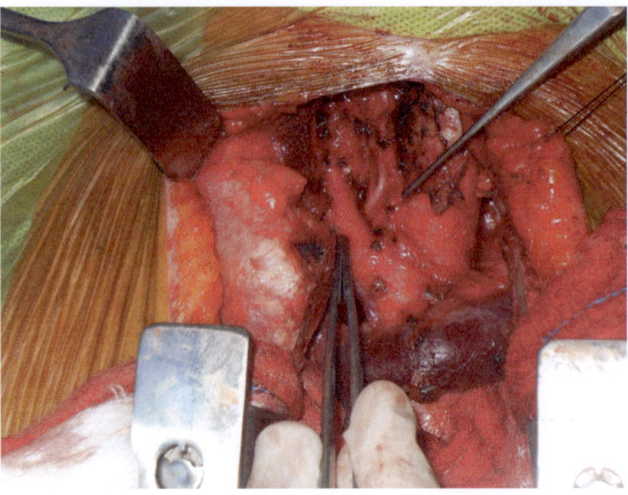

Fig. 3.39 Shows recurrent laryngeal nerve coming from the back of the carotid artery

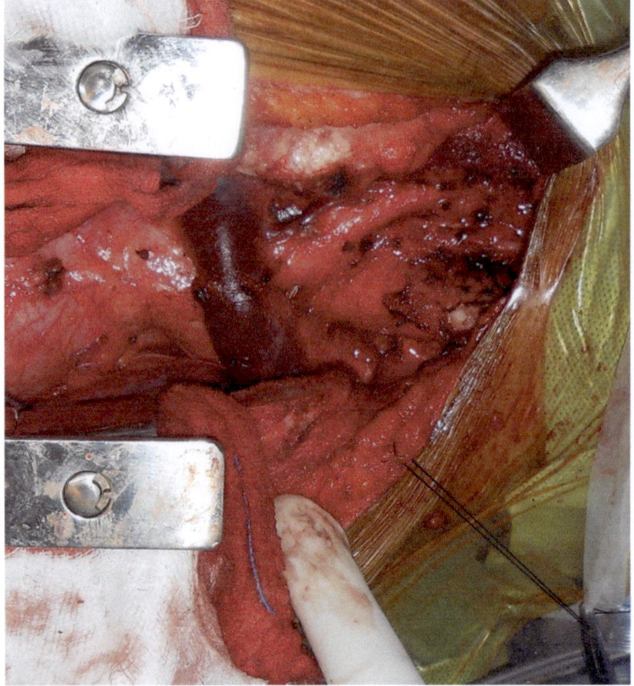

Fig. 3.40 Shows the thyroid bed after completion of thyroidectomy

Parathyroid

Introduction

Parathyroid surgery is one of the most interesting and challenging procedure in head an neck region. Localization of the involved parathyroid gland is the main challenge. After adequate surgery, results are dramatic and improvement in patient's condition is immense. The essence of parathyroid surgery is appropriate planning and accurate localization of parathyroid glands.

Indications

1. Parathyroid adenoma
2. Parathyroid hyperplasia
3. Parathyroid carcinoma

Only one parathyroid gland is normally enlarged in parathyroid adenoma and carcinoma. Incidence of parathyroid carcinoma is extremely rare (1 %). In both these indications, removal of the involved gland is sufficient. The treatment approach for parathyroid hyperplasia is different from the above conditions. One has to localize all four glands and remove 3 and ½ glands. Alternatively, one can remove all four glands and re-implant half (1/2) of one gland in neck muscle or in the forearm.

Diagnosis and Localization of the Parathyroid

Parathyroid glands secrete parathormone (PTH) which plays an integral part in regulating calcium metabolism. Essential diagnosis of hyperparathyroidism can be obtained by elevated serum calcium and PTH level. Systemic symptoms and signs with X-ray findings can be of additional help. The key lies in identifying the cause of hyperparathyroidism. Carcinoma is very rare and cannot be diagnosed preoperatively unless metastatic. Ultrasound findings of enlarged single parathyroid gland can establish diagnosis of parathyroid adenoma. Absence of a single enlarged gland or enlargement of multiple enlarged glands on ultrasound suggests diagnosis of parathyroid hyperplasia.

Sestamibi scan can be of great help in localizing the parathyroid gland. Tc99m sestamibi is absorbed faster by a hyperfunctioning parathyroid gland than by a normal parathyroid gland. It is the investigation of choice but not a must before routine parathyroid surgery. Ultrasound in experienced hand can be equally effective in localizing normally placed parathyroid glands. Scan is strongly recommended in case of any absence of significant finding on ultrasound or performing re-do surgery after the first failed attempt. It is also the only way to locate ectopic parathyroid glands. Scan is also ideal before performing minimally invasive parathyroid surgery.

Parathyroid Adenoma

It is relatively easy to identify enlarged parathyroid adenoma. It is very difficult to identify parathyroid glands in case of hyperplasia. They look similar to other fibrofatty tissue or lymph nodes in this region. Various methods are described like shape, size, color, and weight of the removed structure to identify it as parathyroid gland. One simple way to confirm your intraoperative judgment is to send the removed structure for frozen section examination. Confirmation of the structure as parathyroid gland is enough for us to proceed. We prefer to remove all four glands and re-implant half gland in sternocleidomastoid muscle. The parathyroid gland can be meshed into small slices and re-implanted into muscle (alternatively in the forearm). Intraoperative quick PTH assay if available is the most accurate way in establishing adequacy of procedure. Fall of PTH to <50 % of preoperative value after procedure is confirmatory of the removal of the involved gland.

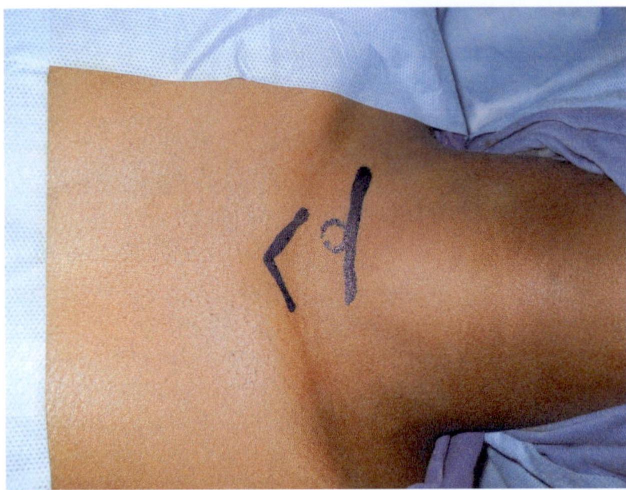

Fig. 3.41 Shows surface marking for localized right superior parathyroid adenoma. A small incision of about 2 cm in size can be used for this procedure. It is important to be sure of the location of the adenoma in order to use a small incision. If not sure or for hyperplasia, one needs to use conventional thyroidectomy incision and explore all four glands

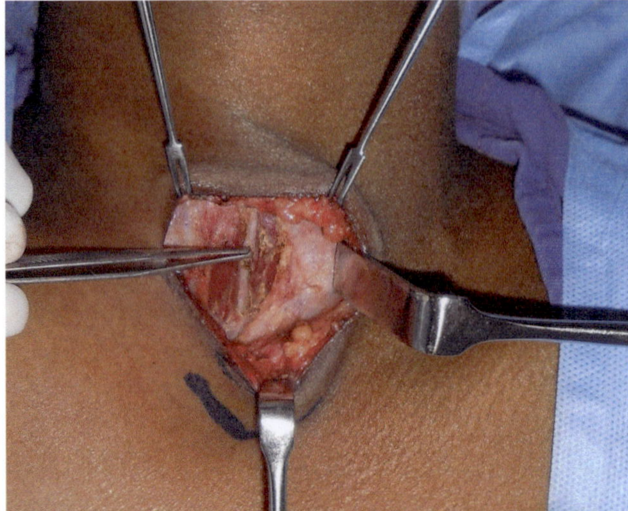

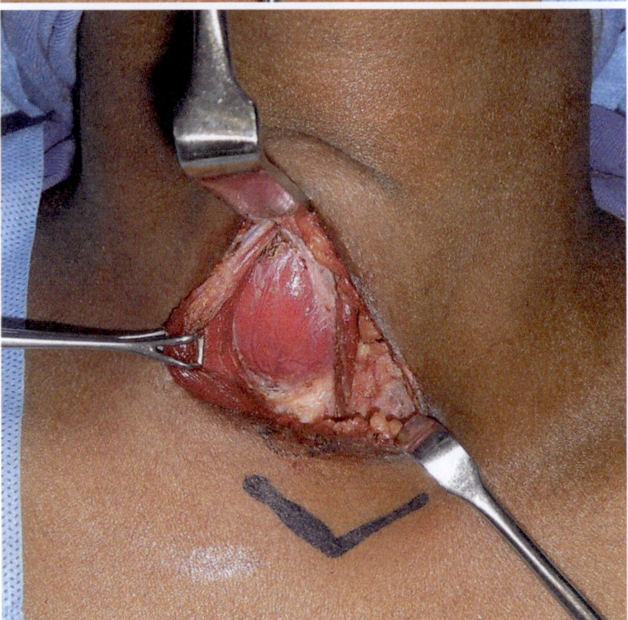

Figs. 3.42 and 3.43 Show standard steps to expose the thyroid gland. Deep cervical fascia is split from midline, and strap muscle is retracted laterally to expose the lobe of the thyroid gland

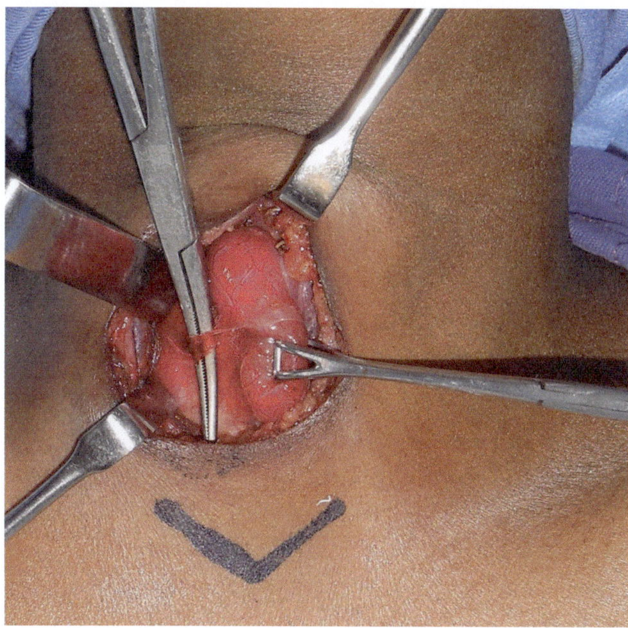

Fig. 3.44 Shows ligation of the middle thyroid vein to expose the recurrent laryngeal nerve and inferior thyroid artery

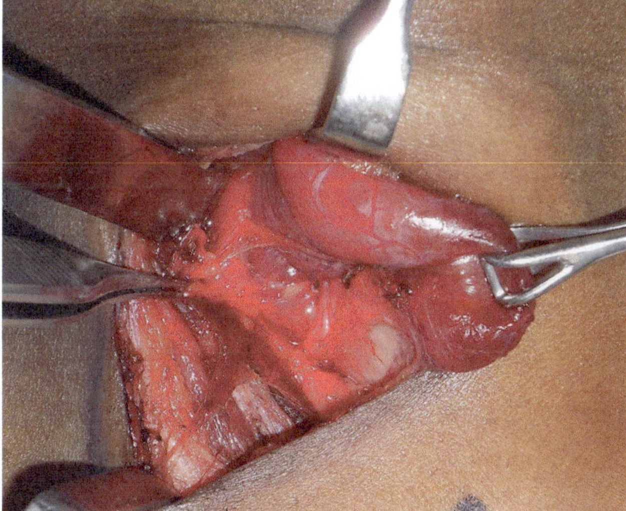

Fig. 3.45 Shows exposed recurrent laryngeal nerve

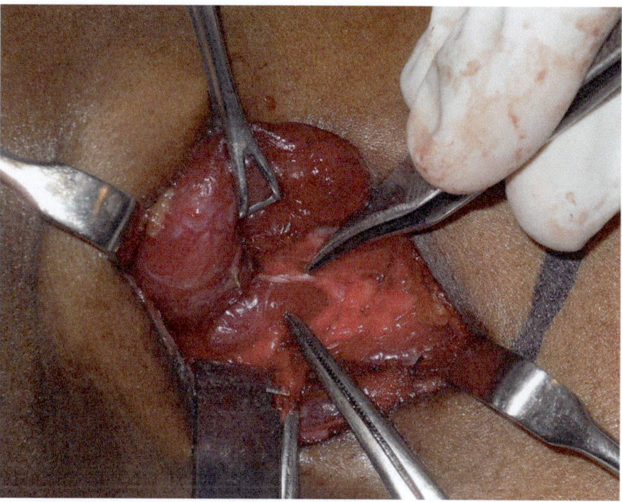

Fig. 3.46 Shows parathyroid adenoma in relation to the recurrent laryngeal nerve. This adenoma is situated posterior to the nerve and hence comes from the superior gland

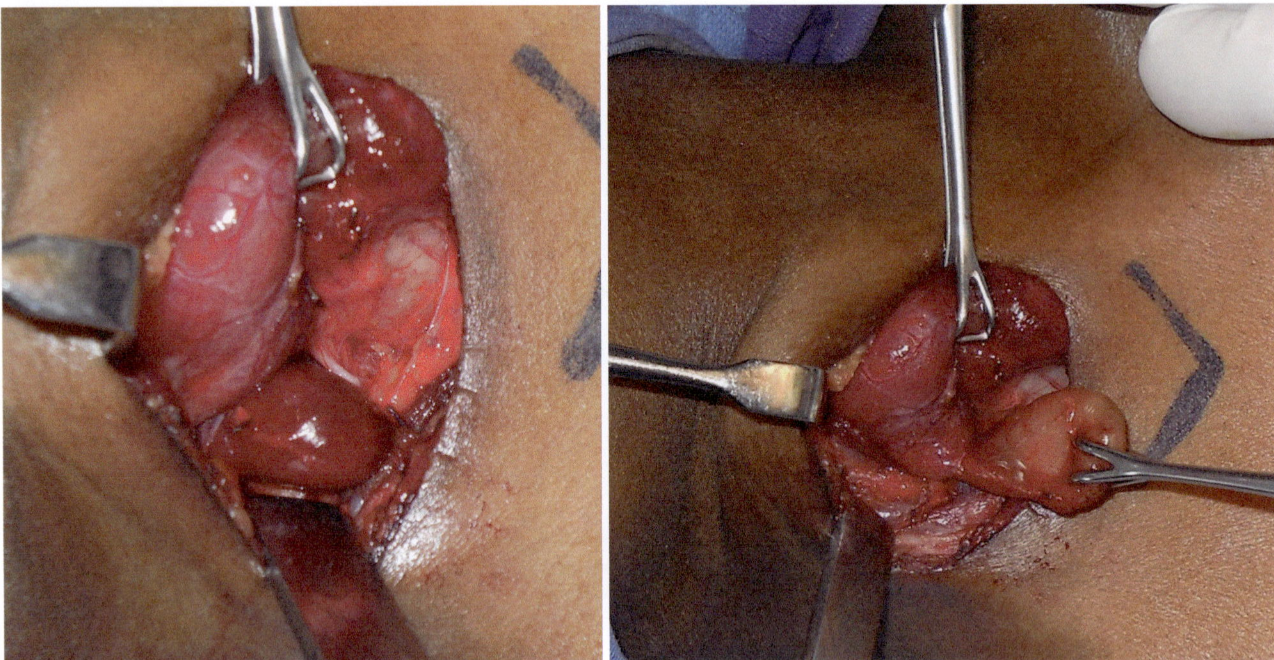

Figs. 3.47 and 3.48 Show the removal of adenoma preserving the nerve

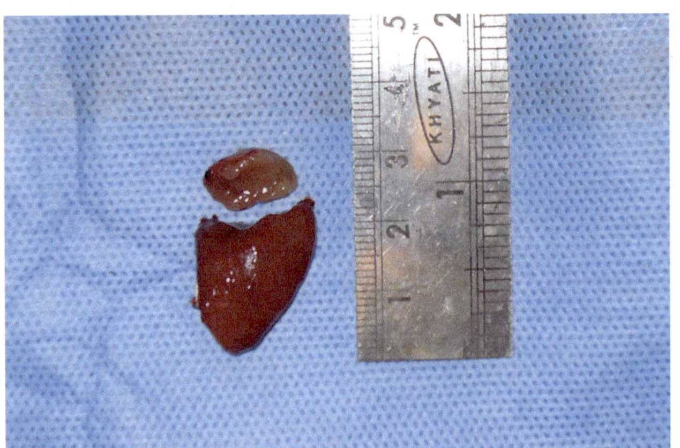

Fig. 3.49 Shows the removed parathyroid gland

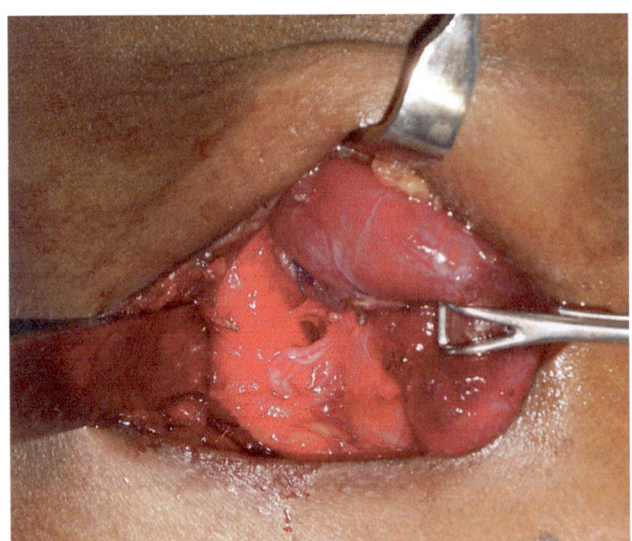

Fig. 3.50 Shows intact recurrent laryngeal nerve

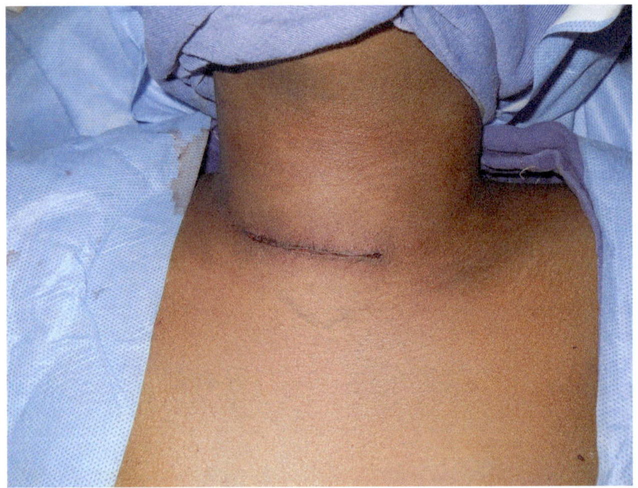

Fig. 3.51 Shows the final picture after closure of the wound

Parathyroid Carcinoma

It is extremely rare to come across a case of parathyroid carcinoma and almost impossible to diagnosis it preoperatively. Basic laboratory values are relatively more raised for carcinoma compared to adenoma and symptoms of patient are more pronounced. These are just some findings which may help you confirm your intraoperative suspicion of carcinoma.

Diagnosis of carcinoma is essentially an intraoperative diagnosis if the gland is hard and adherent to surrounding structures, surgeon must suspect it to be a case of carcinoma. It is important for the surgeon to have suspicion with the above findings as extent and approach to surgery with carcinoma is completely different from that of adenoma and recurrence is very difficult to salvage (multifocal).

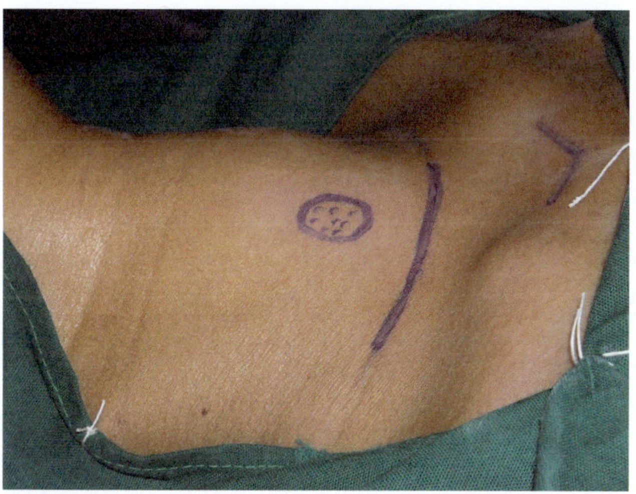

Fig. 3.52 Shows surface marking for surgery

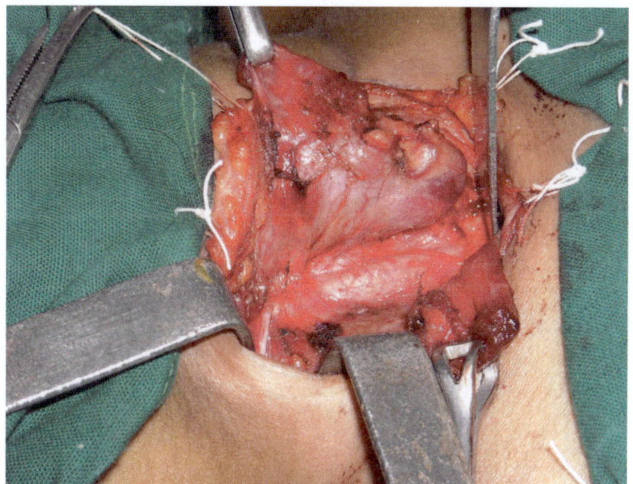

Fig. 3.54 Shows exposed carotid artery separated from the thyroid and parathyroid

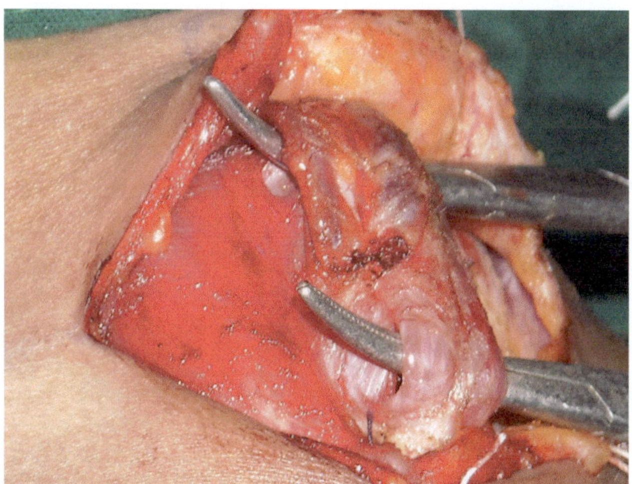

Fig. 3.53 Shows exposed strap muscle. Surgery for carcinoma includes the removal of the parathyroid gland with thyroid lobe and strap muscles if involved. It is recommended to remove all involved structures including recurrent laryngeal nerve to prevent multifocal recurrence

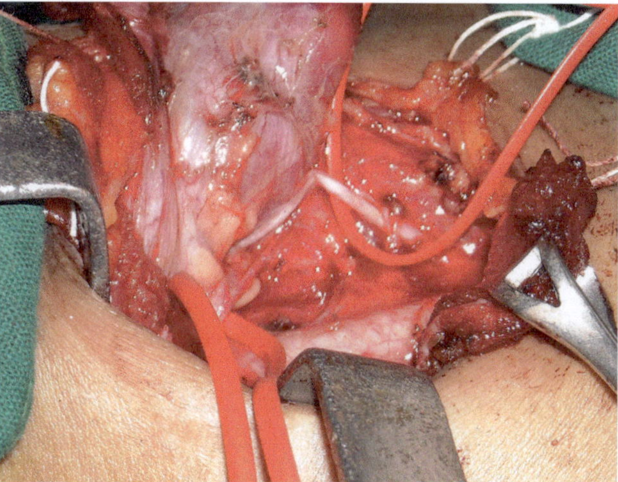

Fig. 3.55 Shows dissected recurrent laryngeal nerve

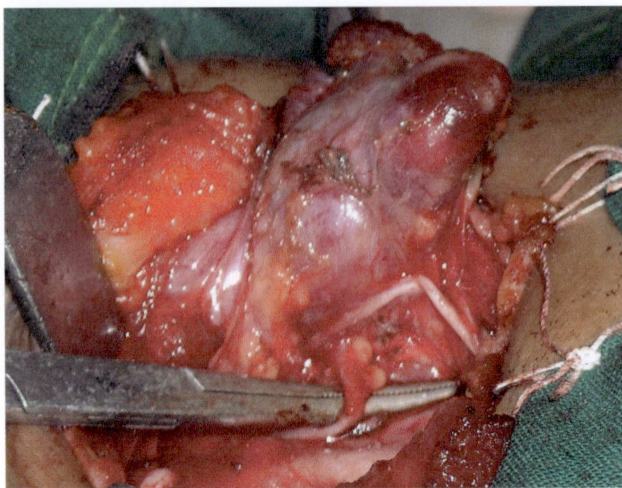

Fig. 3.56 Shows recurrent laryngeal nerve, inferior thyroid artery, and enlarged parathyroid gland. The nerve was free and could be separated from the gland

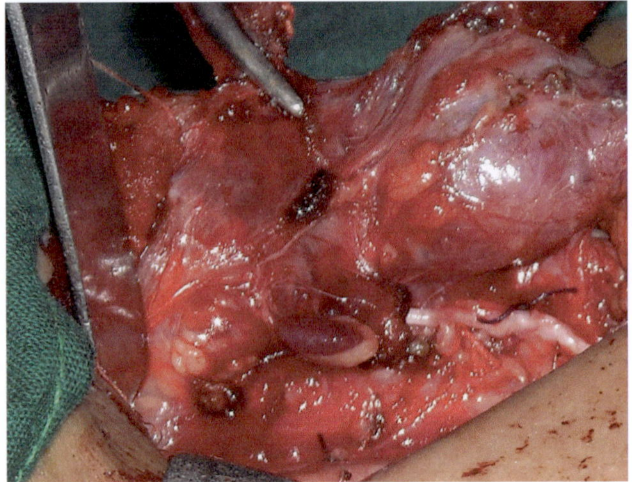

Fig. 3.57 Shows ligated inferior thyroid artery, recurrent nerve, and superior and enlarged inferior parathyroid gland

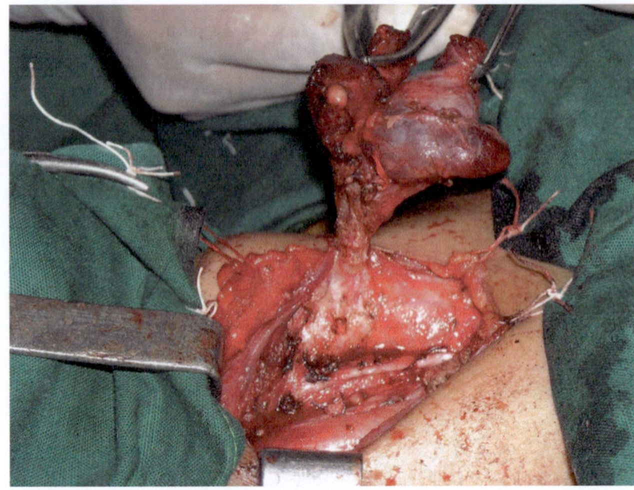

Fig. 3.58 Shows completed surgery. Hemithyroidectomy with removal of involved strap muscle and parathyroid gland was performed with no residual disease

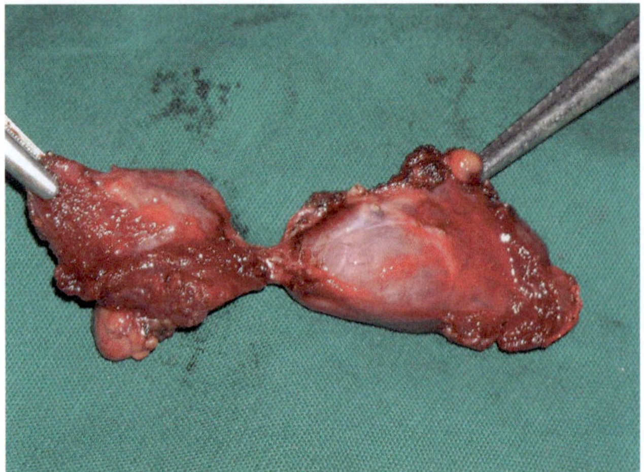

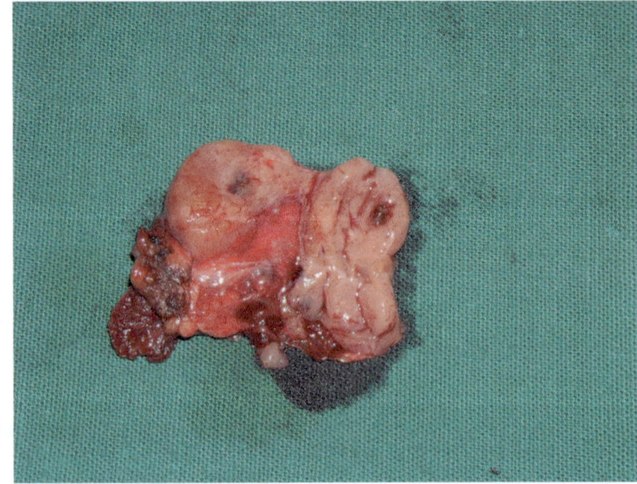

Figs. 3.59 and 3.60 Show the removed specimen with intact capsule

Thyroglossal Cyst

Sistrunk procedure is performed for thyroglossal cyst. Thyroglossal cyst is a developmental anomaly of the thyroid track and is due to non-fusion of some part of the track during development. It can be seen in any part of the track but is seen most commonly in the infrahyoid region. It moves on protrusion of tongue and with swallowing. Removal of the entire track with cyst and central portion of the hyoid bone is essential in preventing recurrence. Many patients present with a fistula instead of a cyst. This can be the result of inadequate removal of the cyst track or infection in the cyst.

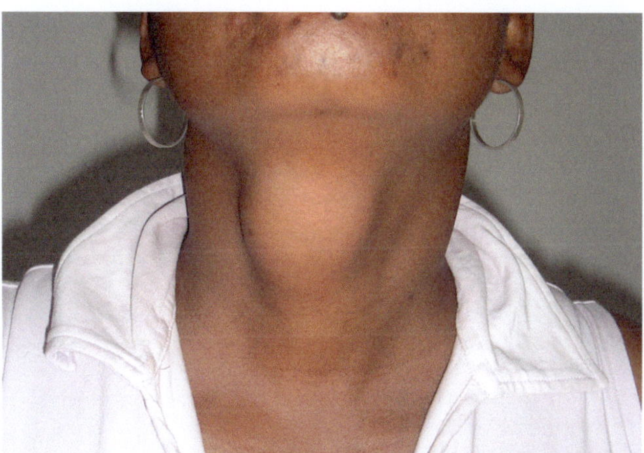

Fig. 3.61 Demonstrates clinical picture of thyroglossal cyst

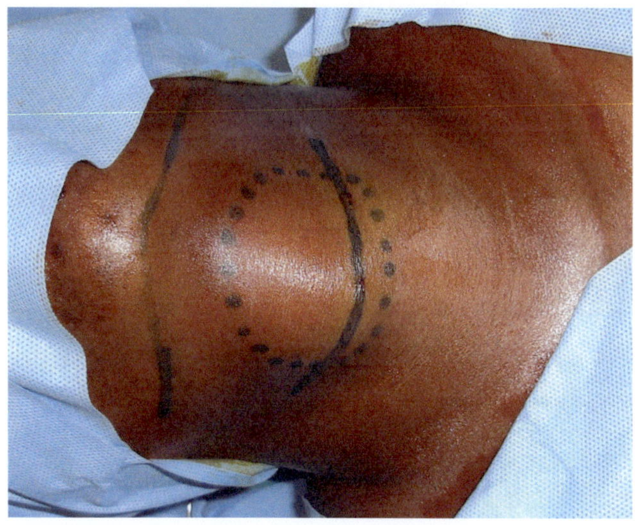

Fig. 3.62 Shows surface marking for this procedure. Incision is placed slightly higher than normal thyroidectomy incision

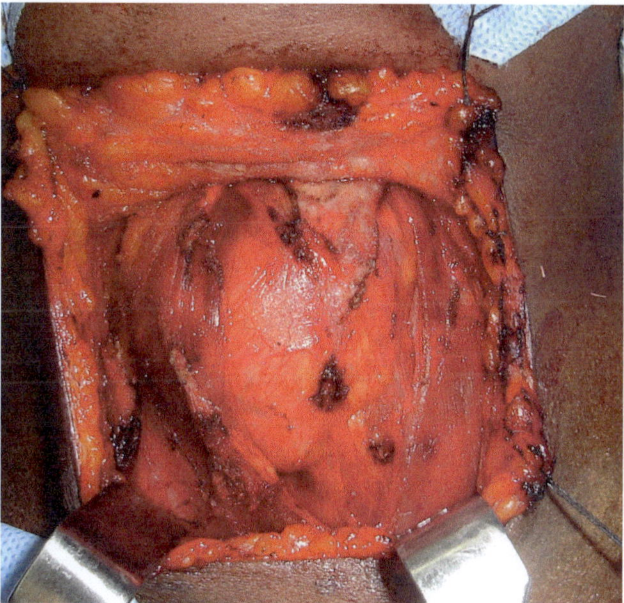

Fig. 3.63 Shows exposed thyroglossal cyst. Flaps are raised in subplatysmal plane and strap muscles are separated from the midline

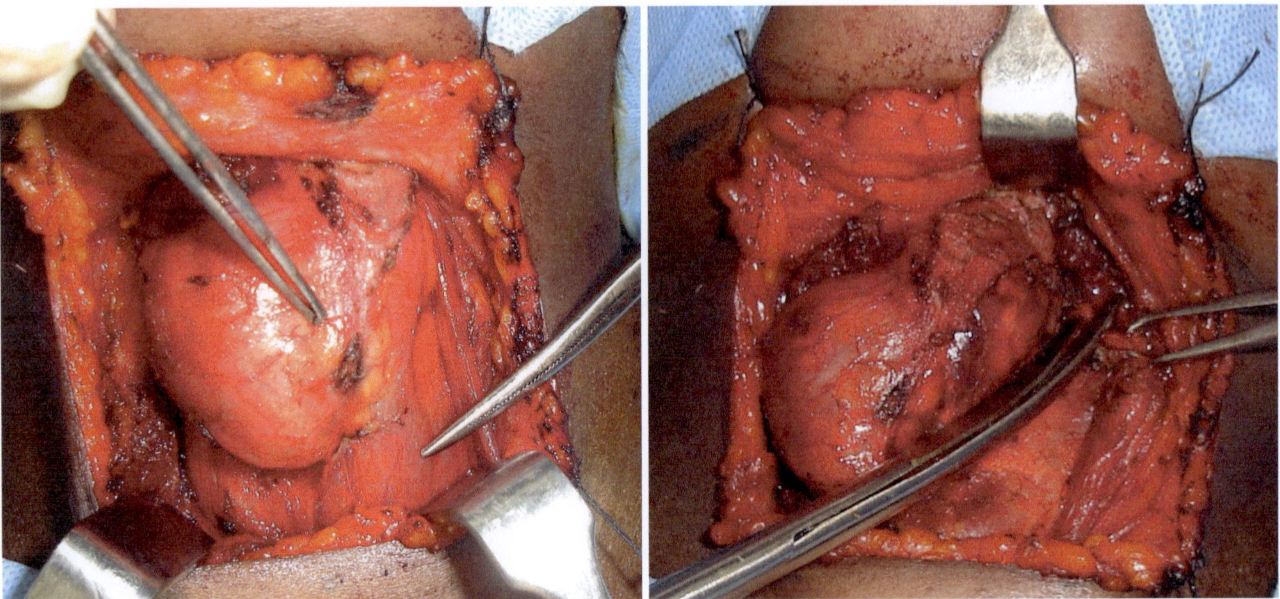

Figs. 3.64 and 3.65 Shows thyroglossal cyst is separate from the thyroid gland. The cyst is separated all around, and the central portion of the hyoid bone is exposed. Heavy scissors is used to cut the central portion of the hyoid bone (Fig. 3.65)

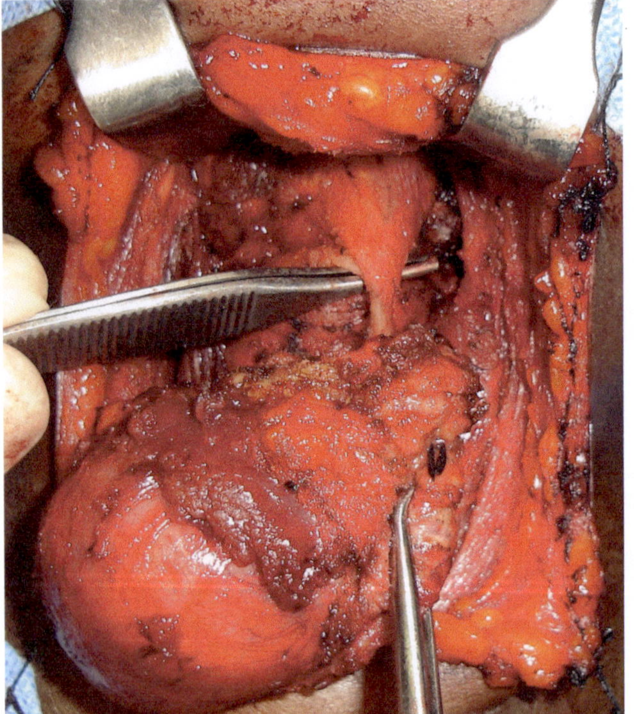

Fig. 3.66 Shows the track extending to the base of the tongue after dropping down the hyoid bone. This track is ligated at the base of the tongue region, and specimen is removed

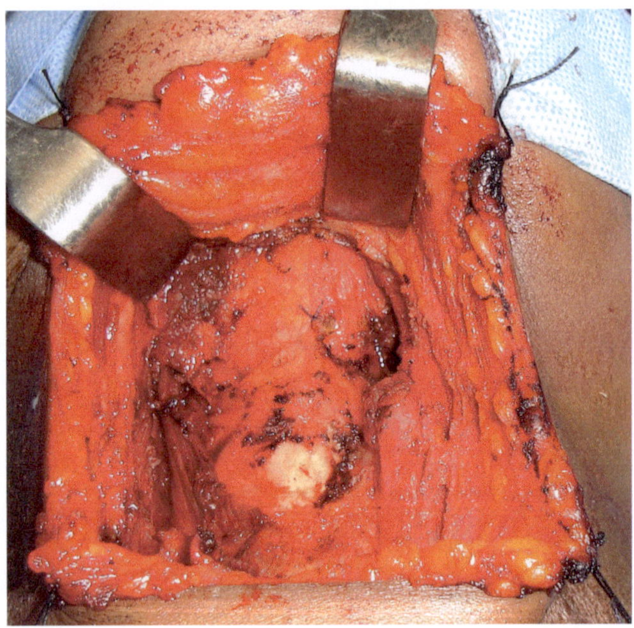

Fig. 3.67 Demonstrates completed procedure

4 Tumors of the Parotid

Surgical Anatomy and Pathology

Parotid gland surgery is interesting because the facial nerve traverses through its substance. The entire procedure revolves around removing the tumor while preserving branches of the facial nerve. Figure 4.1 shows the schematic anatomy of the facial nerve. The nerve comes out of the stylomastoid tunnel and enters the gland. It can be identified anterior to posterior most fibers of digastric muscle that is inserted on mastoid. Identification of the tragal pointer and digastric tendon serves as a guide to facial nerve. The nerve divides into two main trunks which further divide into five branches. These branches run through the gland and become more and more superficial in the periphery. The terminal parts of the branches run deep to the buccinator muscle in the subcutaneous plane. The braches to eye and angle of mouth are most important in terms of functions.

The parotid neoplasm can be classified as benign and malignant lesions (Fig. 4.2). The malignant ones are further subdivided into low-, intermediate-, and high-grade lesions. The surgical extent remains the same for all these lesions, and the aim is to remove the entire lesion with cuff of normal tissue all around. If nerve function is normal in the preoperative phase, it is possible to preserve it in the postoperative phase in majority of cases. Salivary gland pathology is complex, and it is not always feasible to establish exact diagnosis before surgery. The fine-needle cytology is advisable in every case, and this can be helpful in counseling of the patient regarding management of the facial nerve. The operative procedure remains unchanged irrespective of pathology.

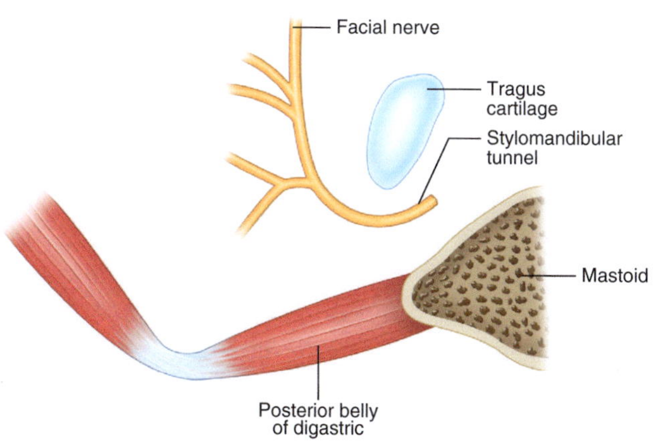

Fig. 4.1 Schematic representation of facial nerve anatomy

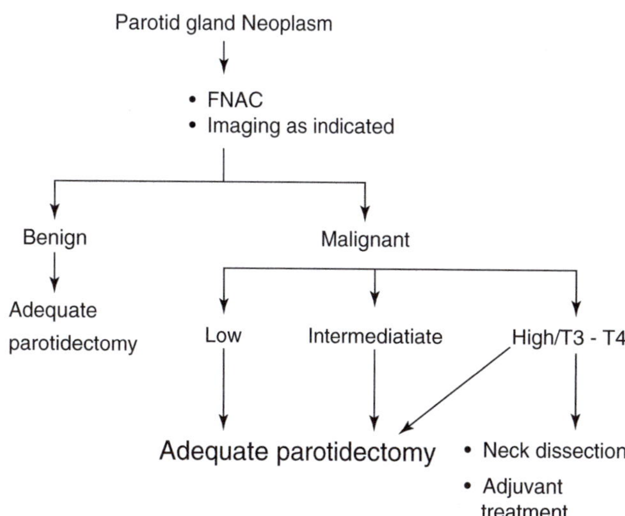

Fig. 4.2 Treatment algorithm

N. Trivedi, *Atlas of Head and Neck Cancer Surgery: The Compartment Surgery for Resection in 3-D*, DOI 10.1007/978-81-322-2050-3_4, © Springer India 2015

Surgical Concepts

- Removal of lesion with cuff of normal tissue around is called adequate parotidectomy and is current standard of care for parotid neoplasm. This is performed irrespective of pathology.
- The margin on the nerve is often positive in the pathology report, and it is not possible to have cuff of normal tissue on this margin. If the capsule of the tumor is intact, this is considered negative margin, and intraoperative decision by the surgeon is considered adequate in deciding adjuvant treatment.
- In the case of nerve involvement, the nerve must be sacrificed. It is not advisable to leave behind gross residual disease on the nerve. One can consider leaving behind microscopic disease in some low-grade malignancies.
- The nerve must be repaired by interposition nerve graft if resected.
- Neck dissection is performed for node-positive lesions only. Some surgeons advocate performing selective neck dissection for high-grade neoplasm. Some surgeons also advocate frozen section of sampled lymph node in level II area.
- Radiotherapy is reserved for high-grade neoplasm, neck node-positive case, large lesions (T3 and T4), and recurrent malignant neoplasm.
- An inappropriately operated parotid case poses a difficult challenge. Re-exploration is considered only if there is reasonable doubt about previous surgery, biopsy suggests grossly inadequate previous surgery, and imaging studies reveal residual lesion.

Superficial Lobe Parotid Lesion

This procedure demonstrates adequate parotidectomy for superficial lobe parotid tumor.

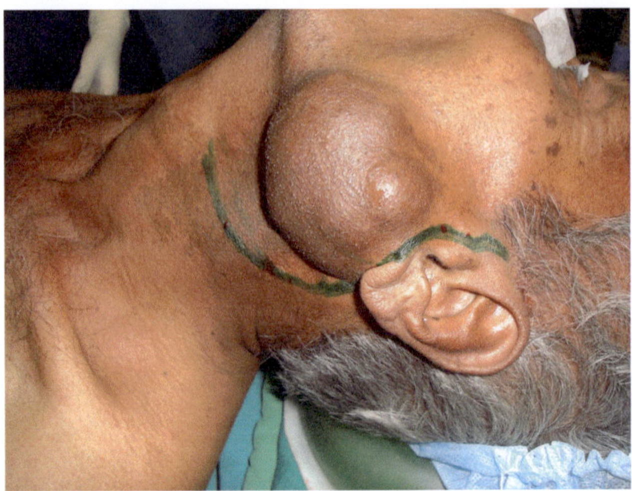

Fig. 4.3 Patient with parotid swelling. The incision is marked in "s" shape. It is important to have a gentle wide curve for the postauricular part to avoid tip necrosis

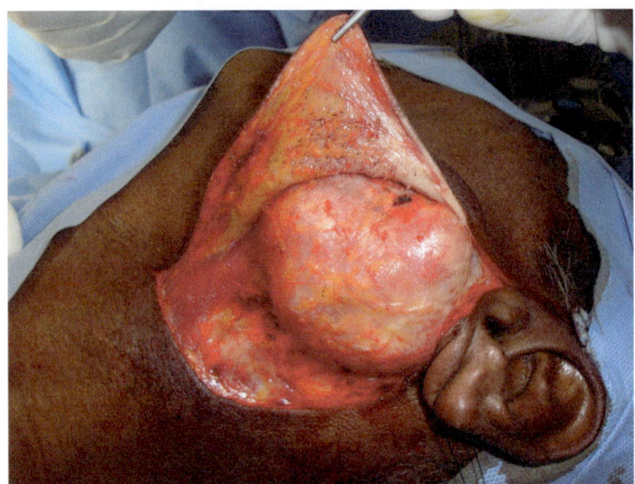

Fig. 4.4 Flap is raised in subcutaneous plane. Branches of fascial nerve become superficial in periphery and hence this area should be carefully dissected

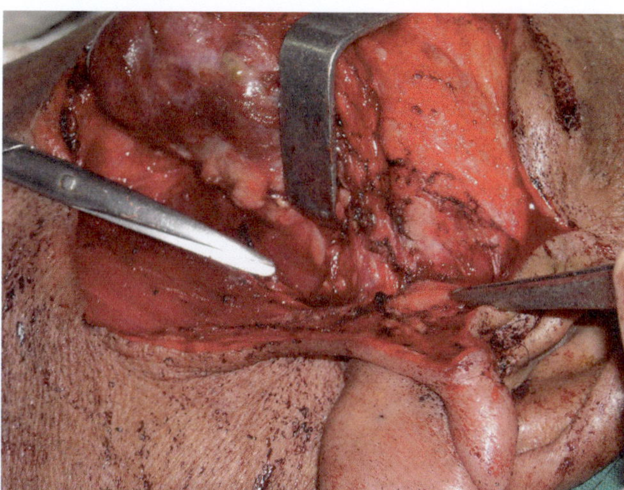

Fig. 4.5 The photograph shows posterior belly of digastric muscle and tragus cartilage. Nerve can be located in the middle of these two landmarks. There is always a small vessel just superficial to the nerve, and this can be considered as an important guide to the facial nerve

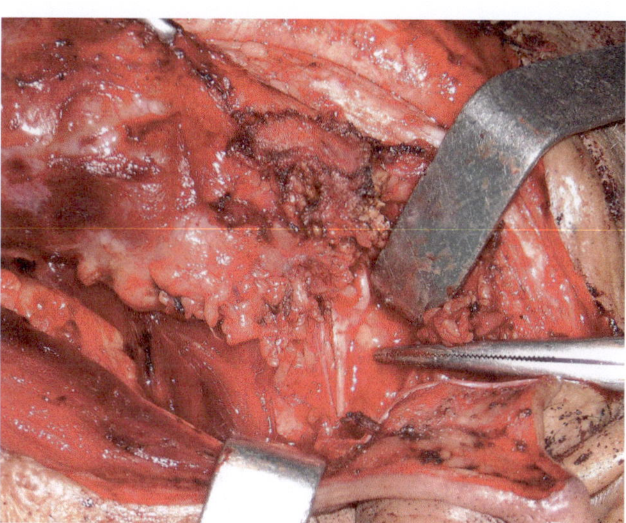

Fig. 4.6 The nerve is identified. It is mandatory to identify its bifurcation before labeling it as the facial nerve

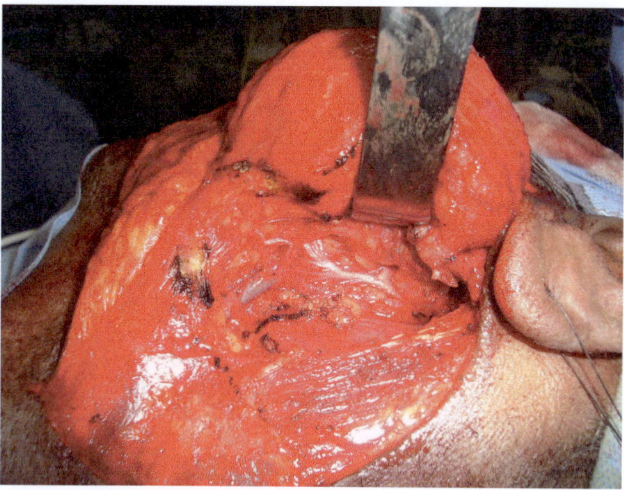

Fig. 4.7 The lesion is slowly mobilized preserving all branches of the nerve

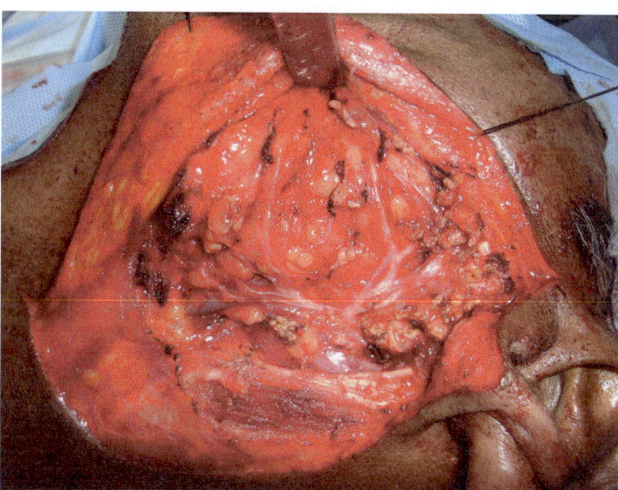

Fig. 4.8 Complete tumor removal with preserved branches of the facial nerve

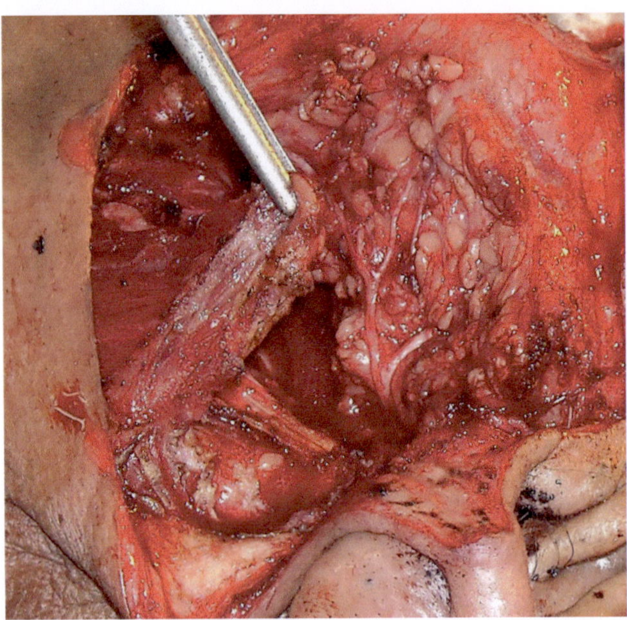

Fig. 4.9 The anterior portion of the sternocleidomastoid (SCM) can be used as local rotation flap to improve the aesthesis

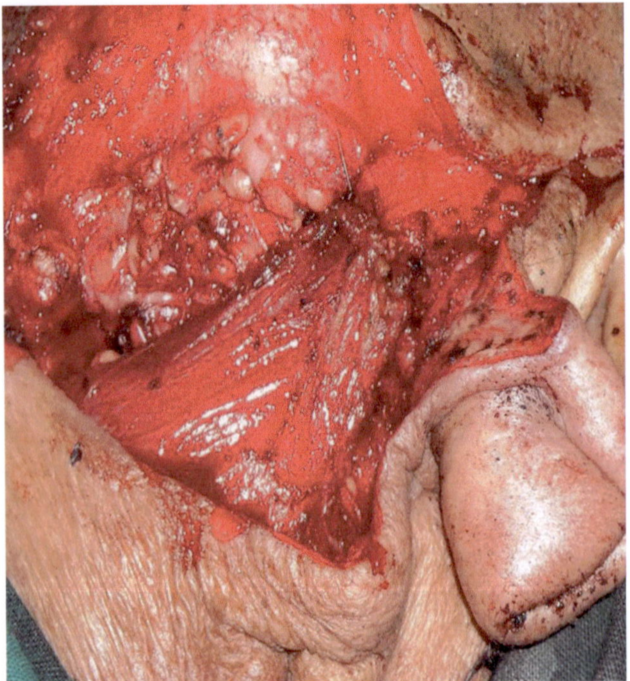

Fig. 4.10 Flap is sutured to the remaining gland

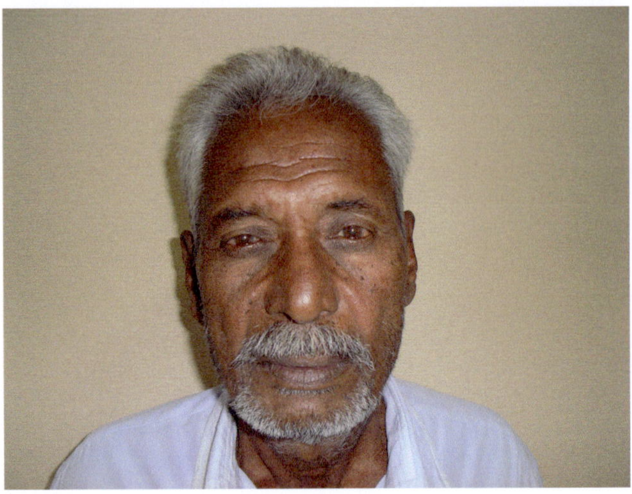

Fig. 4.11 Final outcome

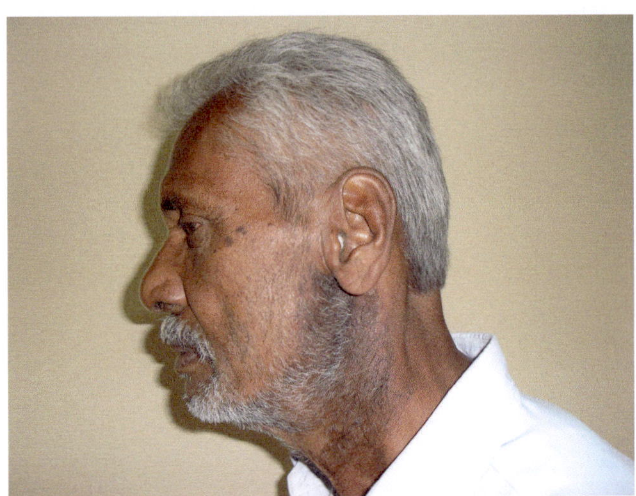

Fig. 4.12 Photograph showing side view demonstrating utility of SCM flap

Deep Lobe Tumor

This procedure demonstrates removal of the deep lobe parotid tumor.

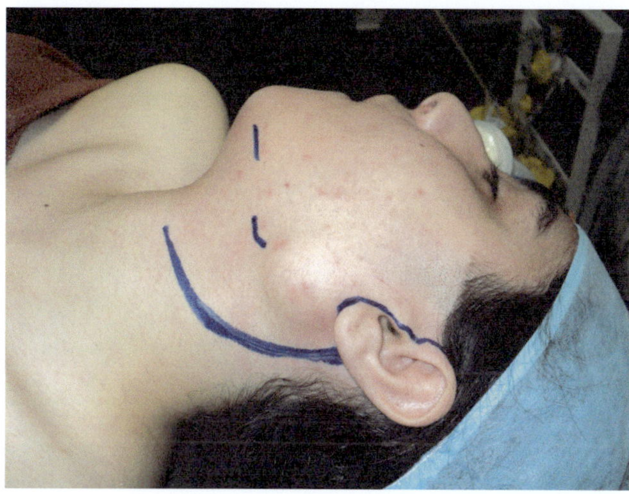

Fig. 4.13 Incision for parotidectomy

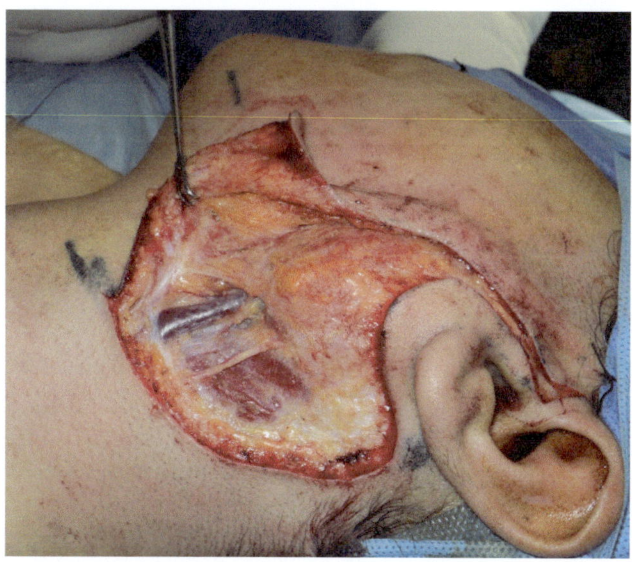

Fig. 4.14 Flap being raised

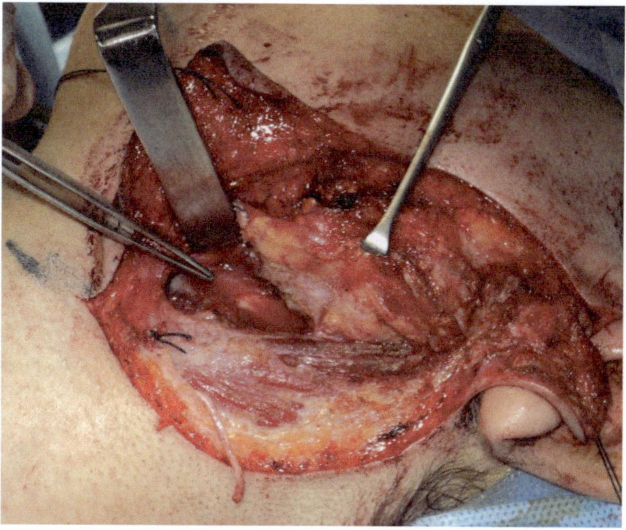

Fig. 4.15 Exposed posterior belly of the digastric muscle

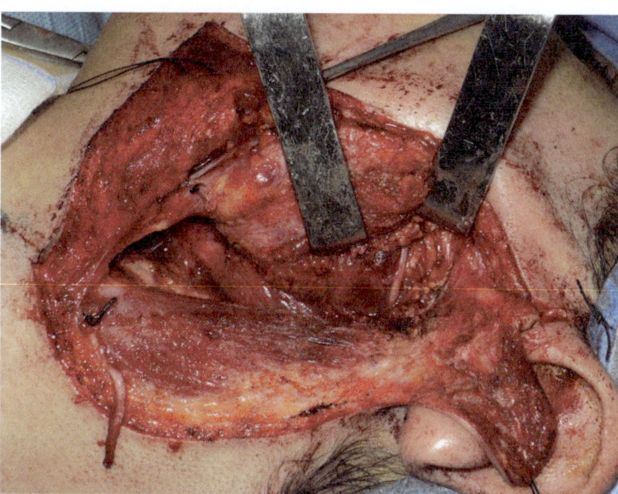

Fig. 4.16 Identification of the facial nerve trunk. The tumor is pushing the nerve anteriorly

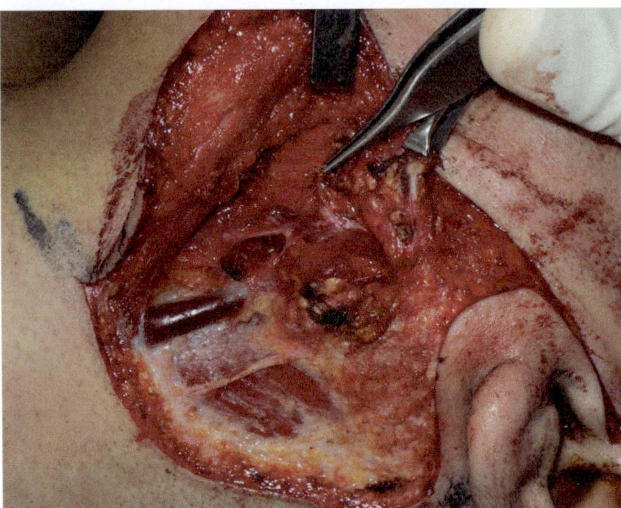

Fig. 4.17 In the case of recurrent parotid lesions where it is difficult to identify main trunk due to fibrosis, identification of peripheral branches of facial nerve serves as a good guide in tracing main trunk

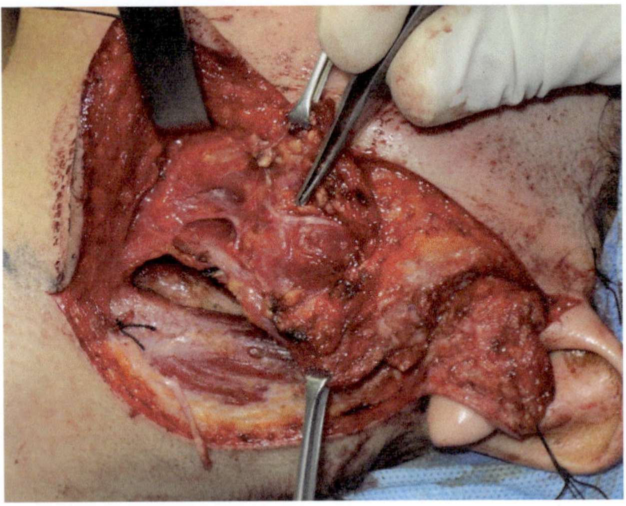

Fig. 4.18 The peripheral nerve is traced proximally in retrograde manner. The lesion is located deep to nerve branches

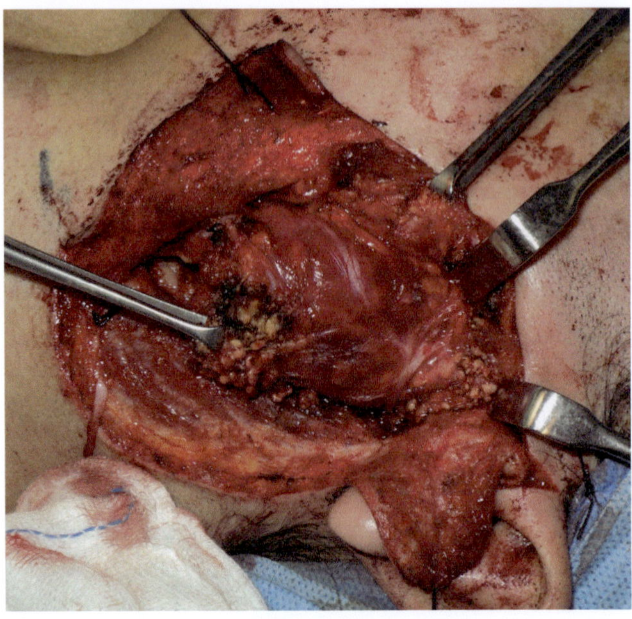

Fig. 4.19 The superficial lobe is separated completely to expose the nerve branches and lesion underneath. One should plan to remove this tumor between two branches of the facial nerve that is located farthest apart

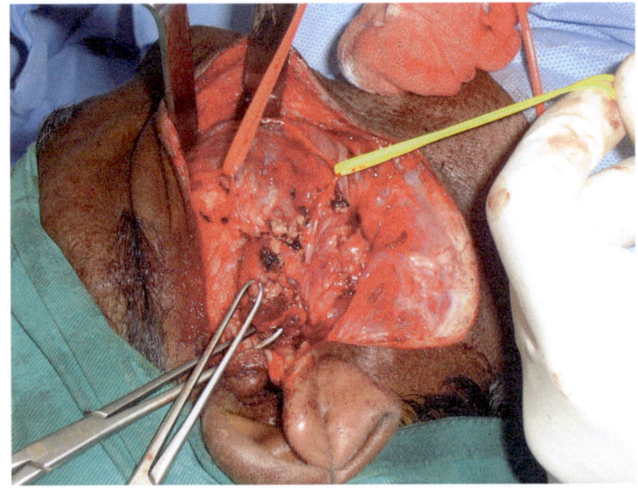

Fig. 4.20 The nerve branches are separated apart with great care not to tear them. The assistant must be advised not to pull these branches in haste

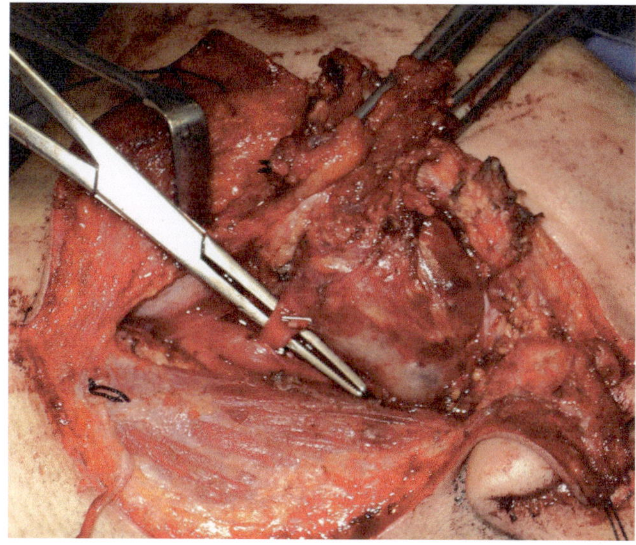

Fig. 4.21 The external carotid artery is identified and secured

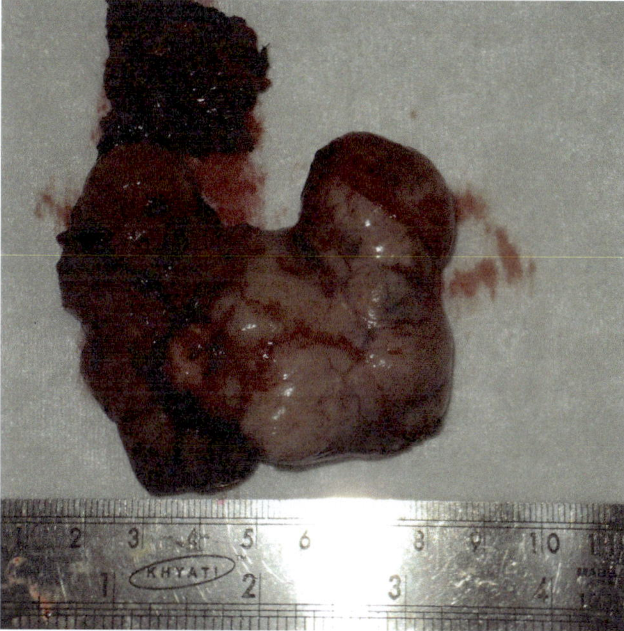

Fig. 4.22 Complete removal of the lesion with intact capsule

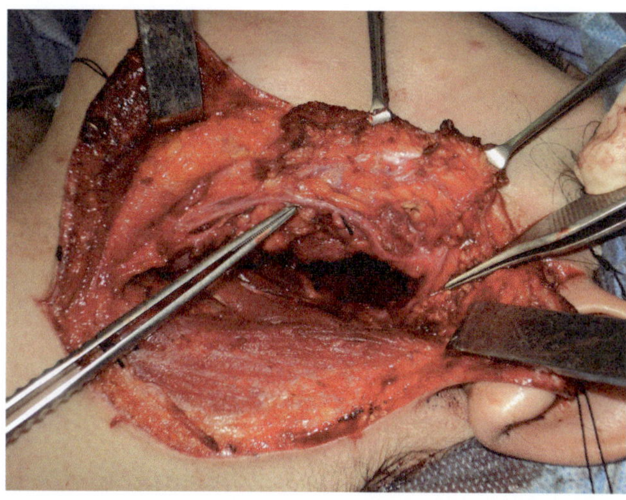

Fig. 4.23 The photograph is showing intact branches of facial nerve and cavity created by removal of tumor

Advanced Stage Parotid Tumor

This procedure demonstrates removal of advanced stage parotid tumor and facial nerve reconstruction.

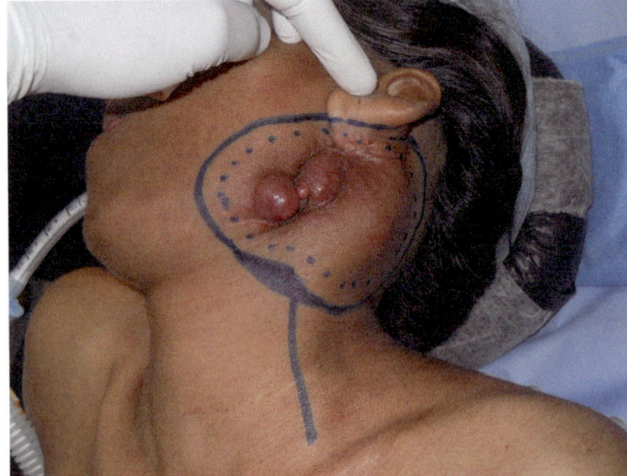

Fig. 4.24 Patient with advanced lesion

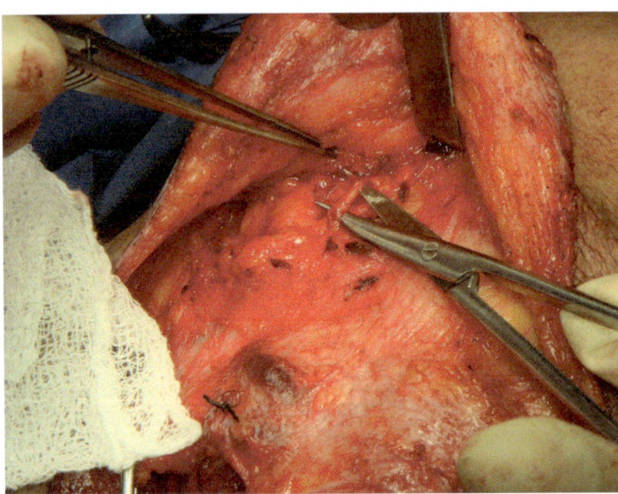

Fig. 4.25 Identification of the peripheral branch of the facial nerve

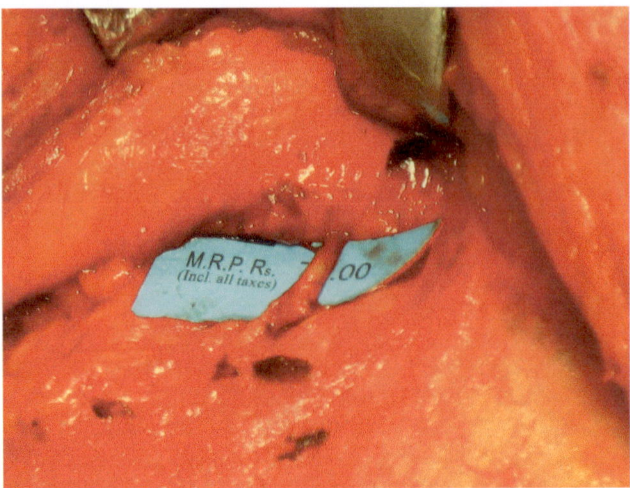

Fig. 4.26 Isolation of the peripheral branch

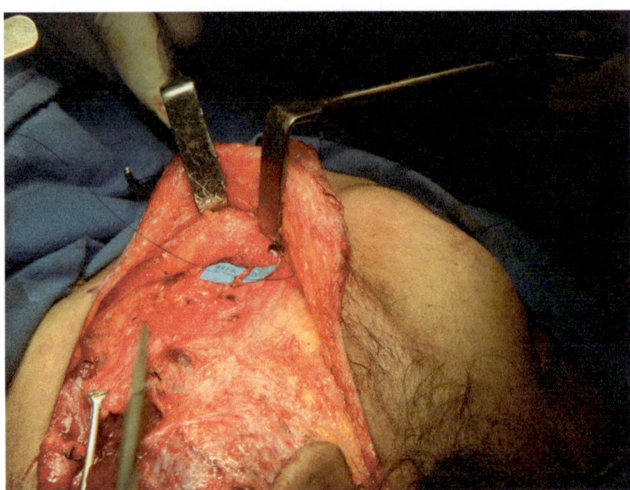

Fig. 4.27 Tagging of this branch with ethilon stitch before cutting it

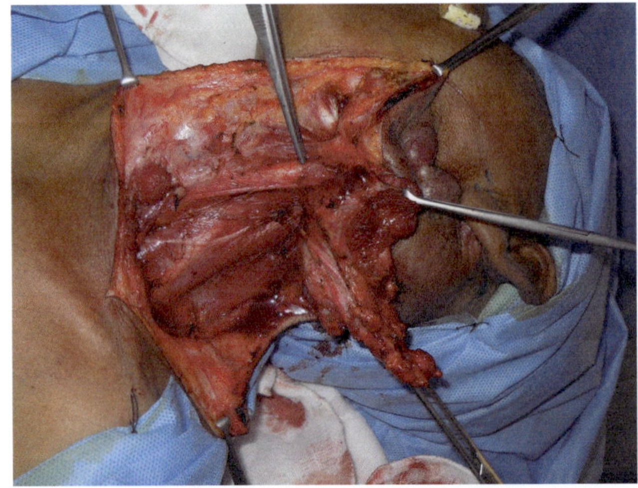

Fig. 4.28 Removal of lesion. The carotid vessels are dissected and secured early in operation

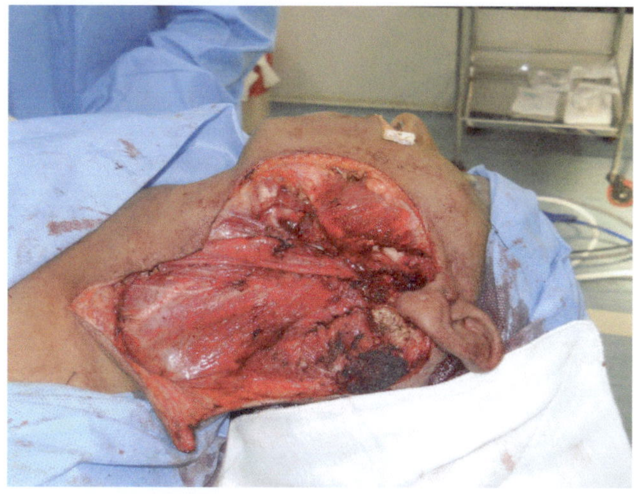

Fig. 4.29 Complete removal of the tumor with all branches of the nerve sacrificed. The trunk is identified at the proximal end, and all peripheral branches are tagged at the distal end

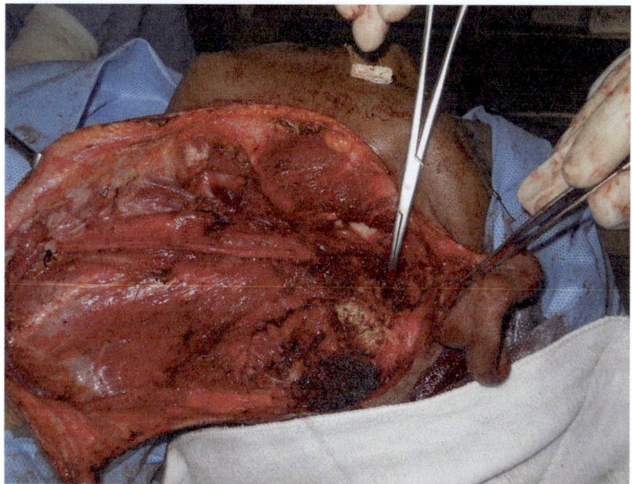

Fig. 4.30 Photograph showing proximal stump of the nerve

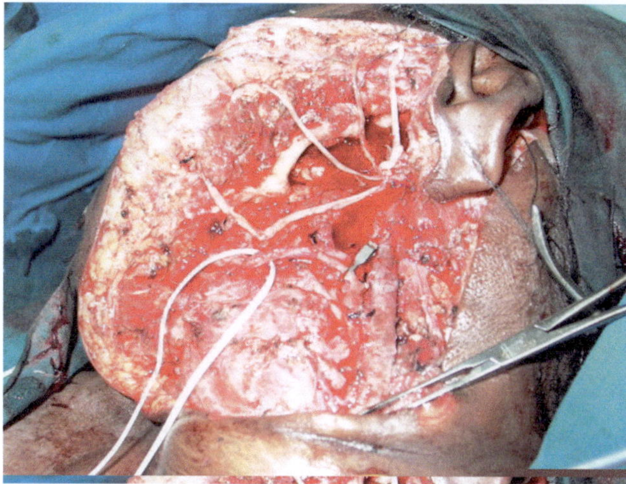

Fig. 4.31 Sural nerve grafting for all major branches. The principle is to anastomose major branches first and then the smaller ones. It is advisable to perform this anastomosis under microscope

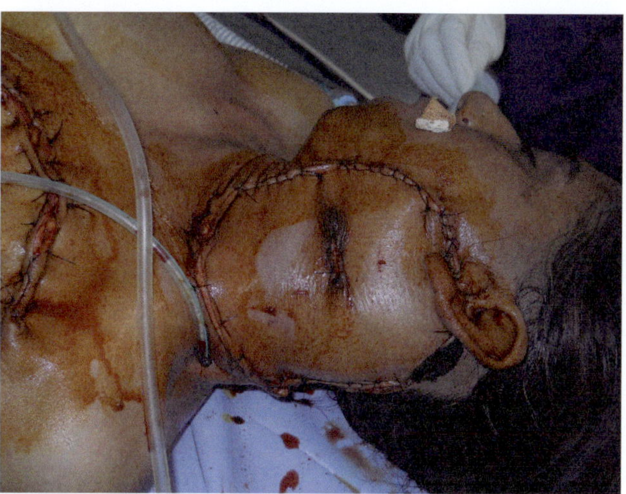

Fig. 4.32 Reconstruction with pectoralis major myocutaneous (PMMC) flap

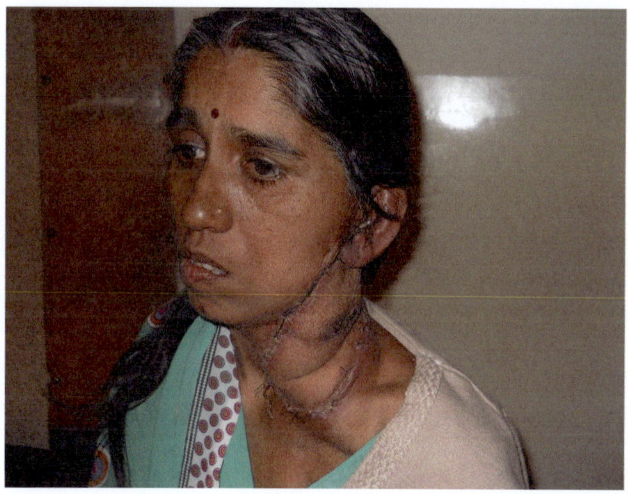

Fig. 4.33 Postoperative picture after 2 weeks of surgery

Very Advanced Parotid Tumor

This procedure demonstrates removal of very advanced parotid tumor with placement of brachytherapy catheters to address residual disease.

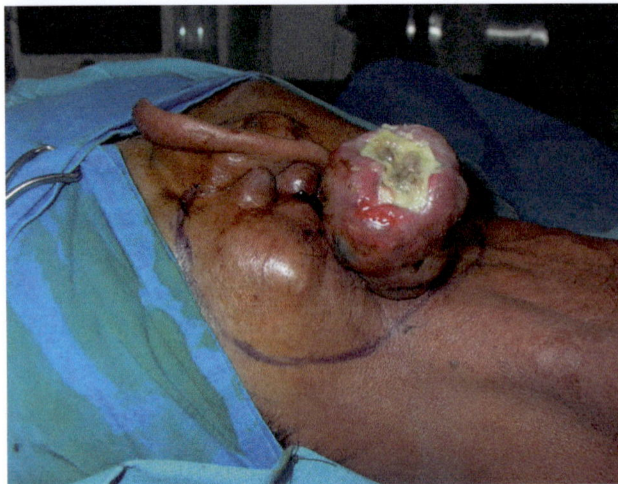

Fig. 4.34 Very advanced disease with involvement of temporal bone

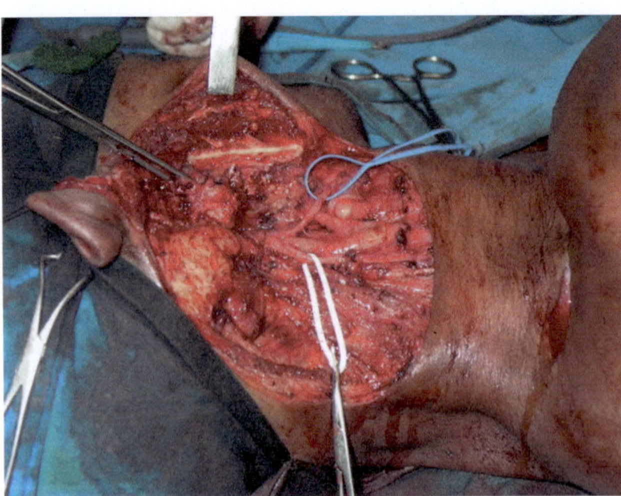

Fig. 4.35 Resection of lesion. It is important to note that carotid vessels are separated and controlled all throughout the procedure

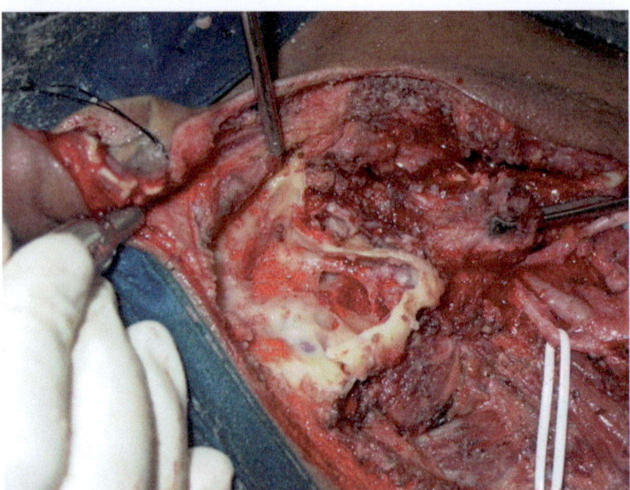

Fig. 4.36 Exposed temporal bone lesion

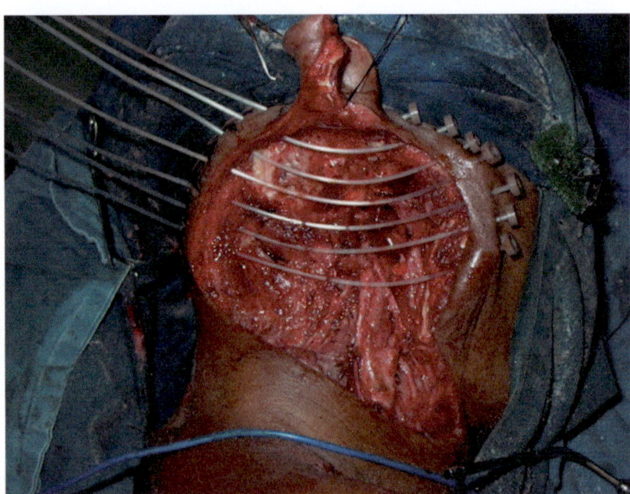

Fig. 4.37 Placement of brachytherapy catheter to address residual lesion. With advent of intensity-modulated radiation therapy (IMRT), the use of brachytherapy has become limited, but we still use it for cases where there is gross residual disease left. These patients are in miserable state and we have a policy to attempt surgical clearance with aggressive adjuvant therapy. This provides the best care to the patient in this situation

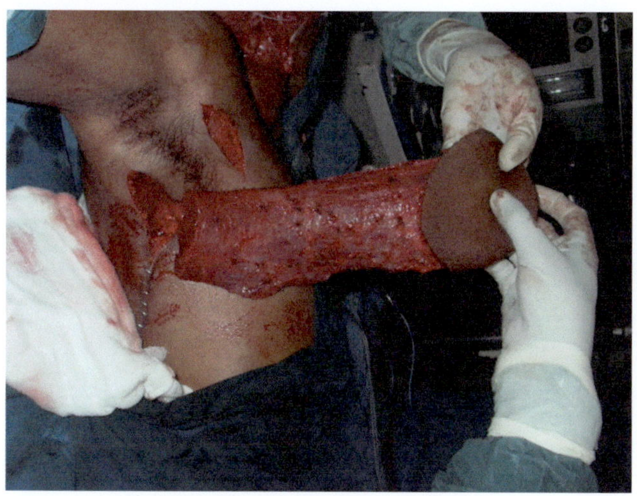

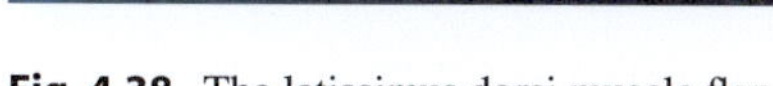

Fig. 4.38 The latissimus dorsi muscle flap

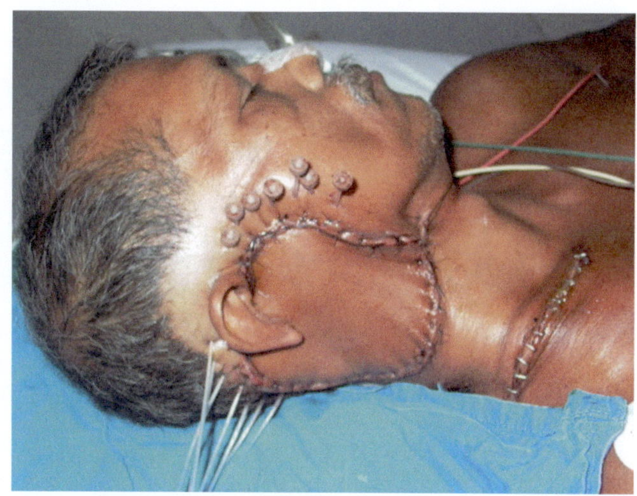

Fig. 4.39 Photograph showing final outcome

Facial Nerve Sheath Tumor

This procedure demonstrates removal of facial nerve sheath tumor which is very rare. The lesion was located at a point where the nerve exits the stylomandibular canal.

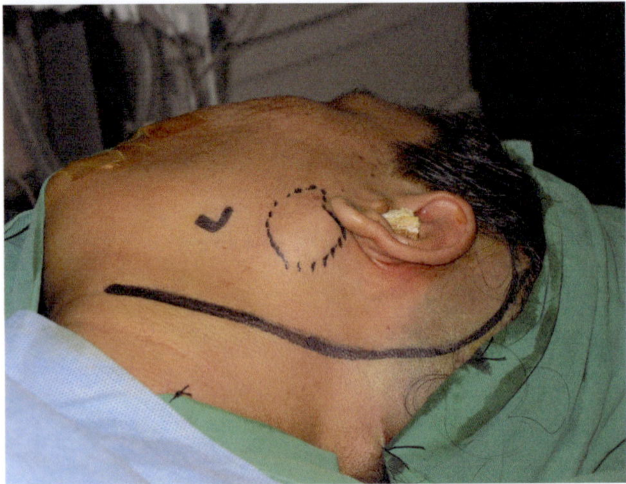

Fig. 4.40 Postauricular incision to expose the mastoid process

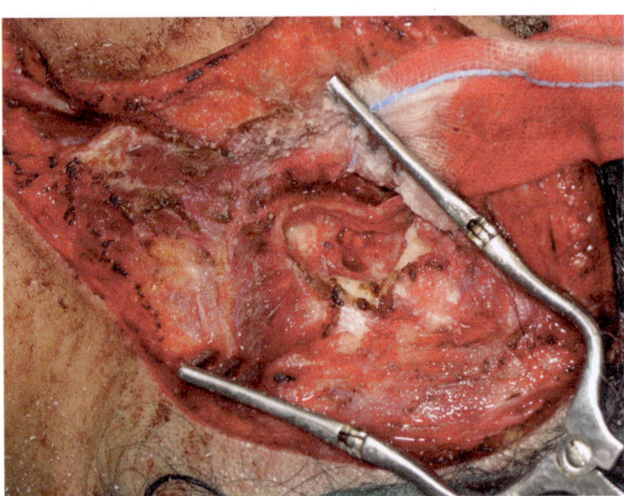

Fig. 4.41 The mastoid cavity is drilled to expose the facial nerve

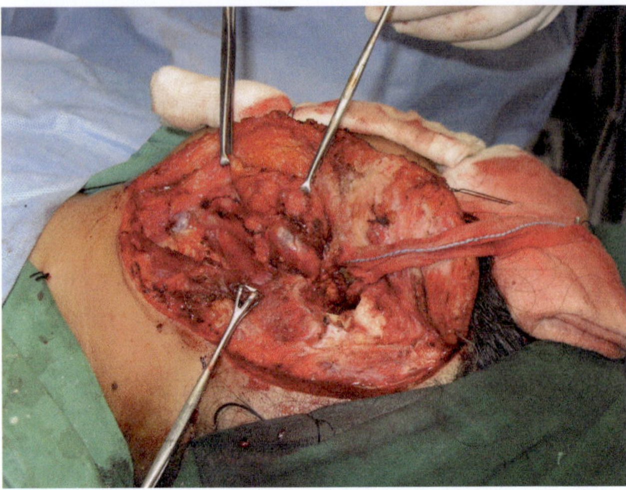

Fig. 4.42 The schwannoma is exposed in entire length

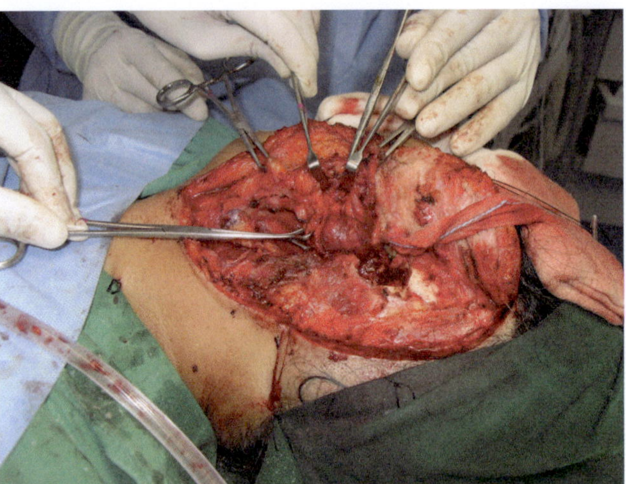

Fig. 4.43 The lesion is mobilized all around

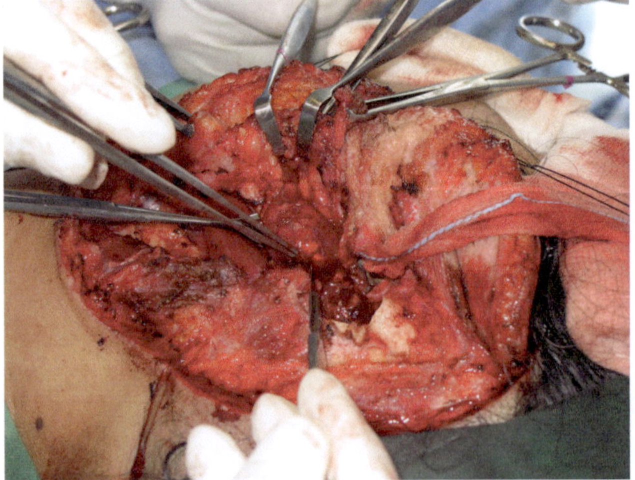

Fig. 4.44 The schwannoma is being removed. We performed a subcapsular dissection to preserve the peripheral fibers of the facial nerve with the hope that nerve function may recover. This is an experimental approach for nerve sheath tumors and part of a study protocol at our institute

Large Deep Lobe Parotid Tumor

Mandibulotomy is rarely necessary to address parotid tumors, but it may become necessary for certain large or recurrent malignant neoplasms extending into pre-styloid parapharynx compartment.

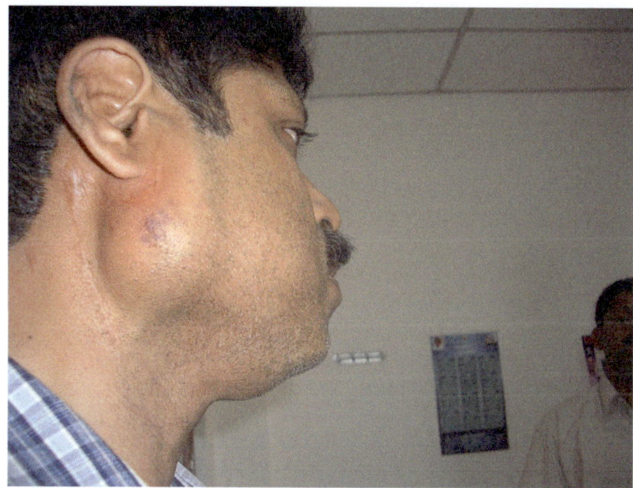

Fig. 4.45 Recurrent parotid neoplasm

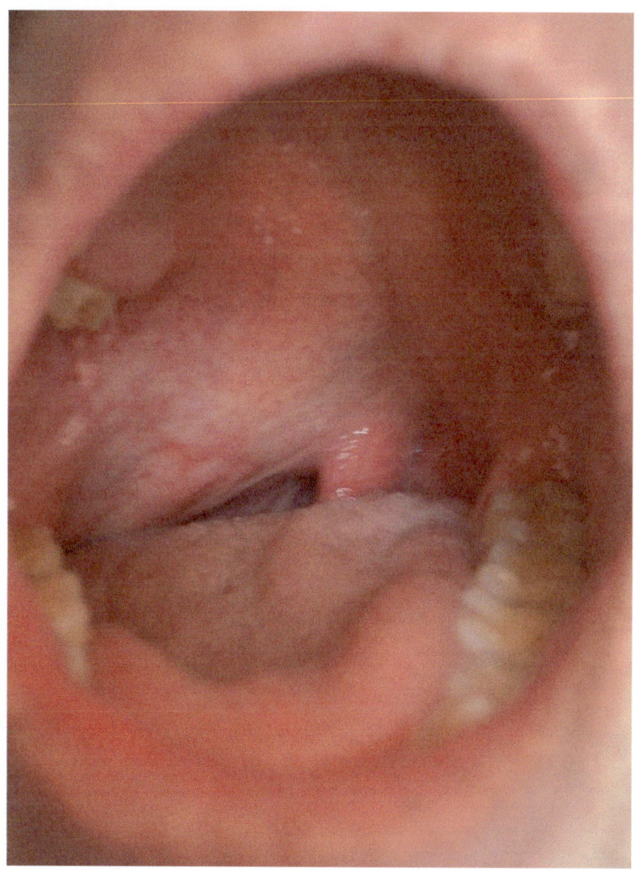

Fig. 4.46 Large intraoral bulge showing involvement of deep lobe in pre-styloid compartment

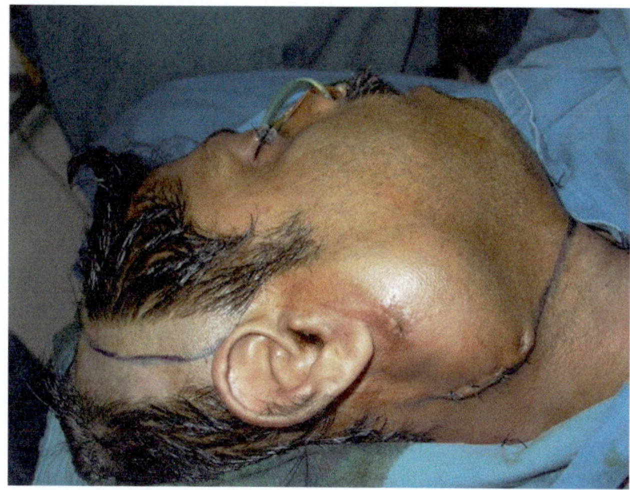

Fig. 4.47 Planned incision for mandibulotomy. The scalp incision is demonstrated for planning of temporalis sling for eye rehabilitation

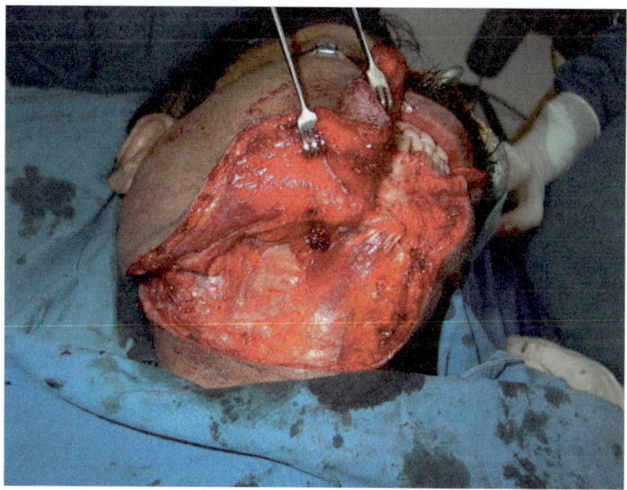

Fig. 4.48 Cheek flap is being raised

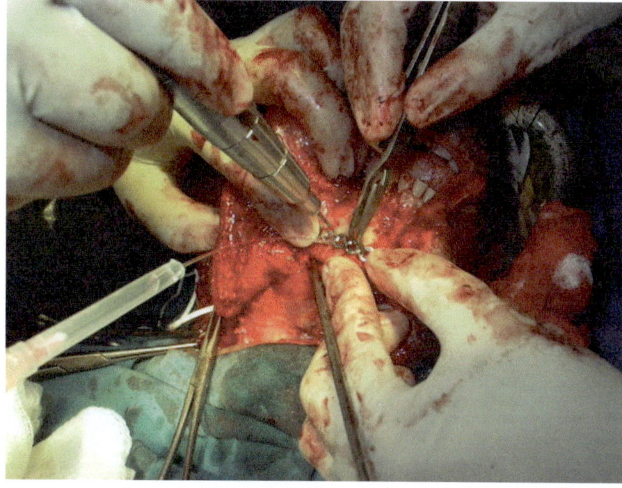

Fig. 4.49 Pre-plating for mandibulotomy cut

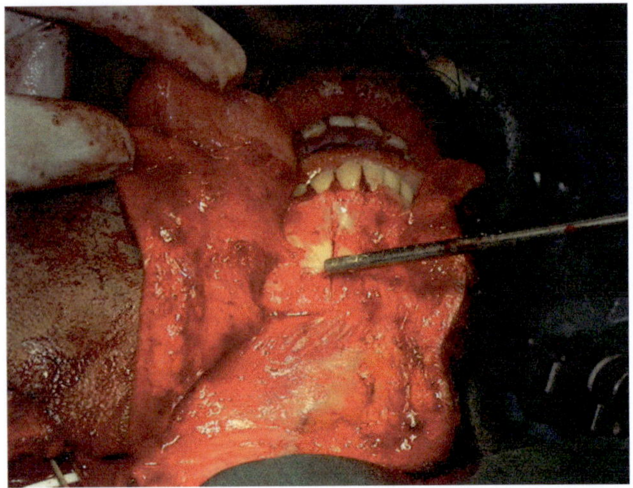

Fig. 4.50 The mandibulotomy is performed in the parasymphysis region

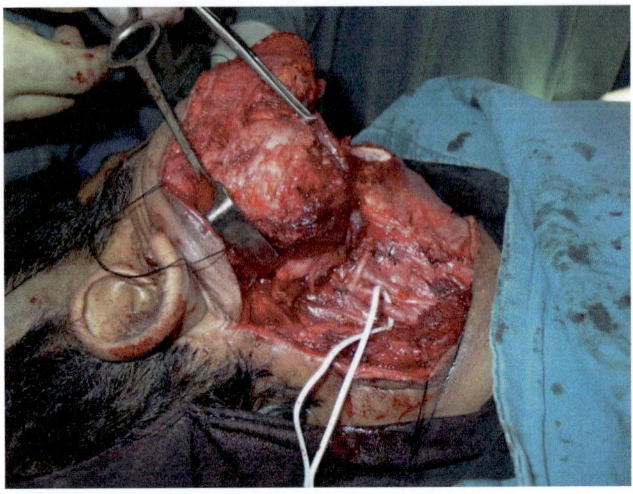

Fig. 4.52 The carotid vessels are secured before addressing the tumor

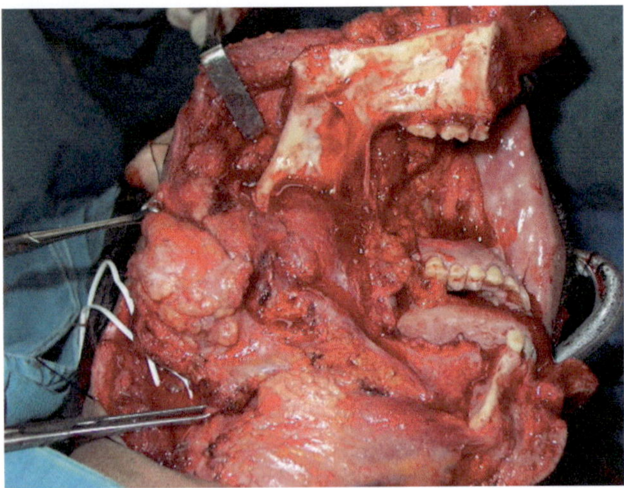

Fig. 4.51 The mandible is mobilized laterally to expose the tumor

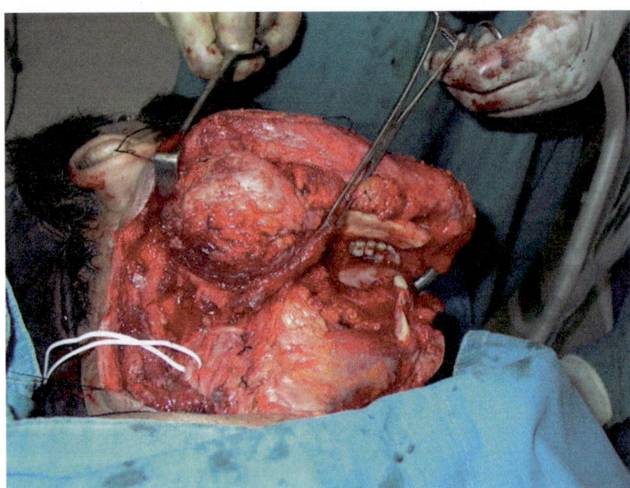

Fig. 4.53 Tumor being removed

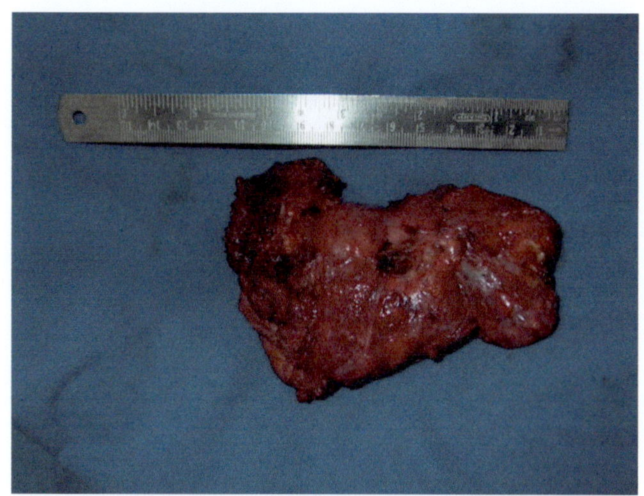

Fig. 4.54 The specimen

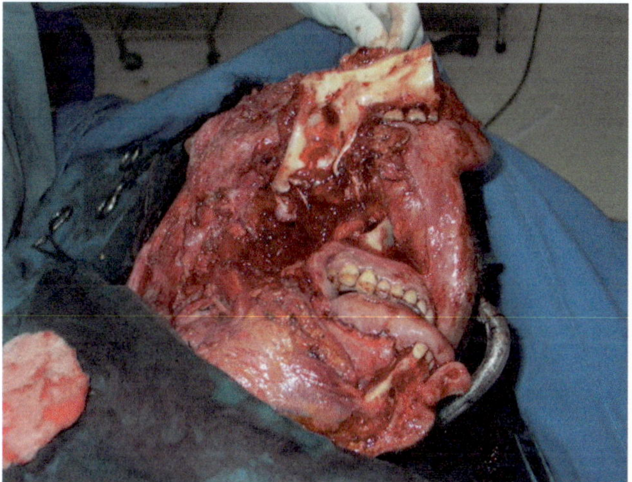

Fig. 4.55 The postoperative photograph showing complete removal of the tumor

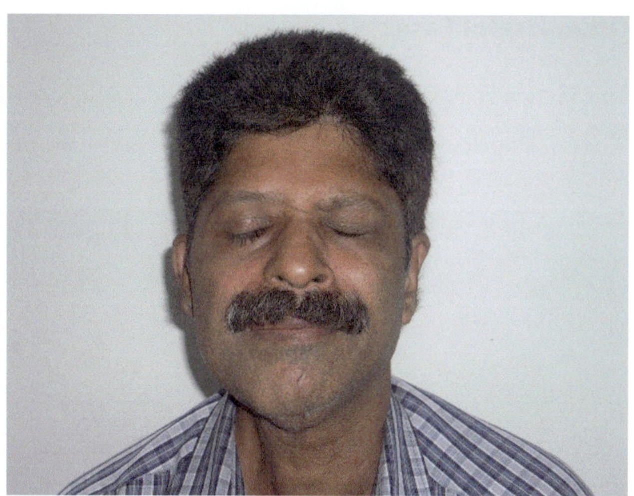

Fig. 4.56 The long-term outcome

Other Useful Cases

This section demonstrates two useful tips to address uncommon scenario.

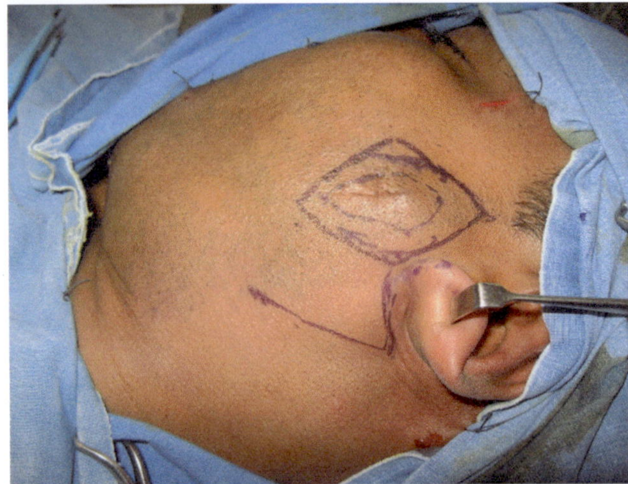

Fig. 4.57 The parotid tumor involving limited skin

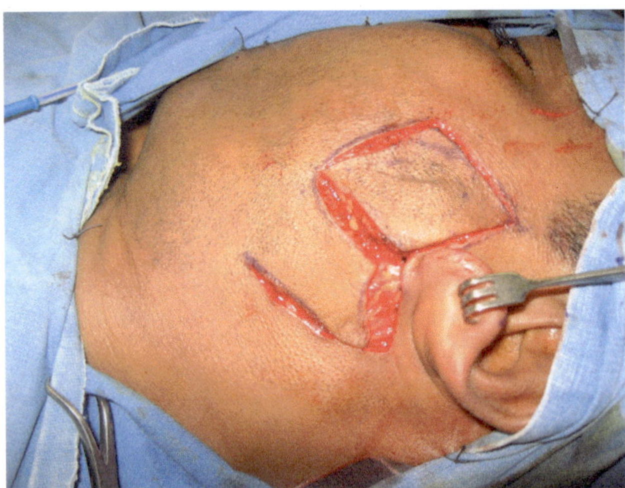

Fig. 4.58 The incision is planned in a way that reconstruction can be achieved with local flap

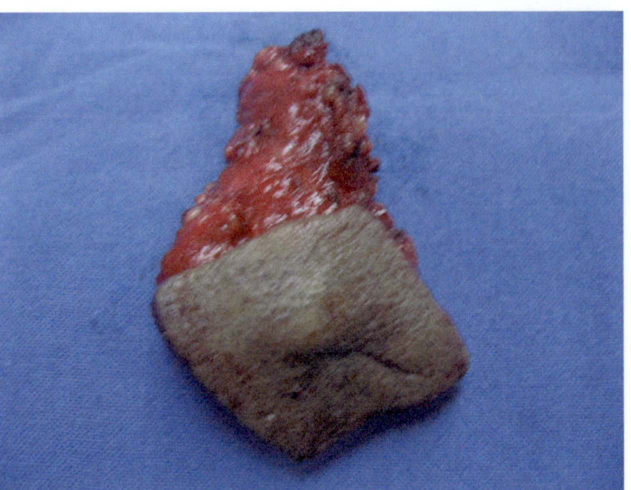

Fig. 4.59 Resected specimen

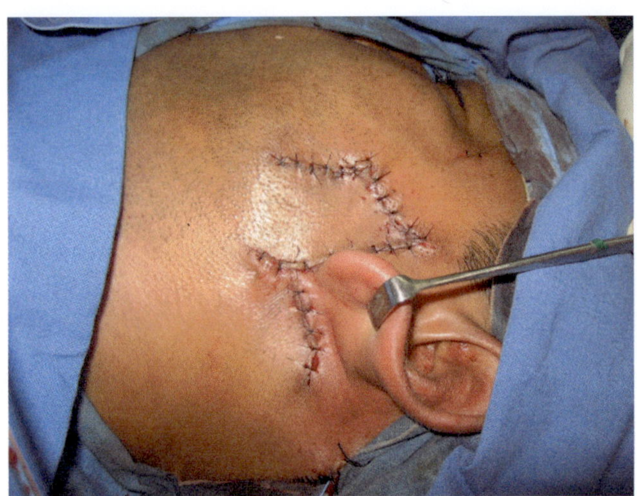

Fig. 4.60 Photograph showing tension-free closure

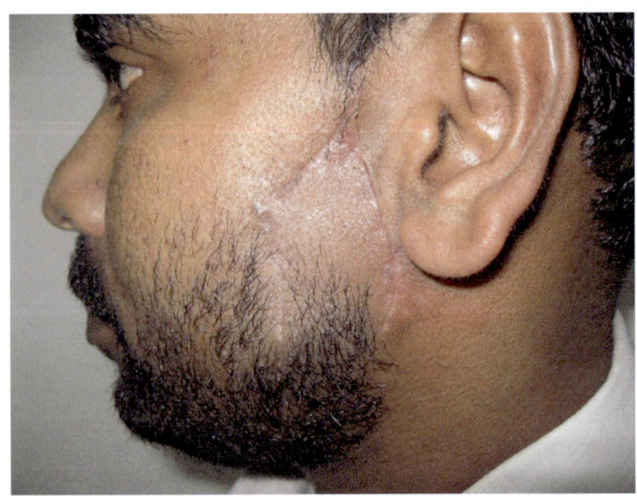

Fig. 4.61 Long-term outcome

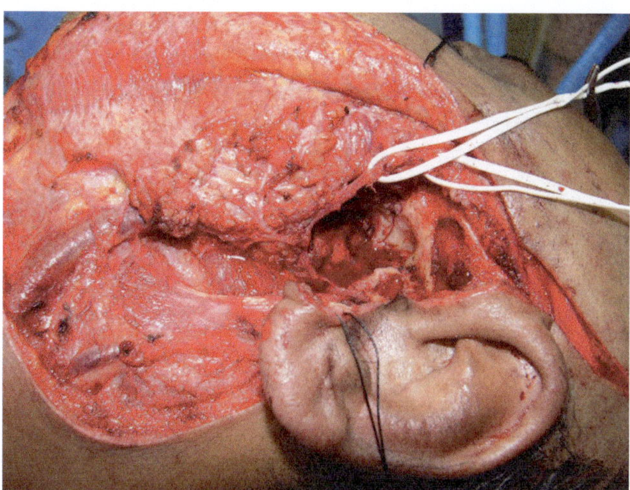

Fig. 4.62 A case involving parotidectomy with resection of the external auditory canal

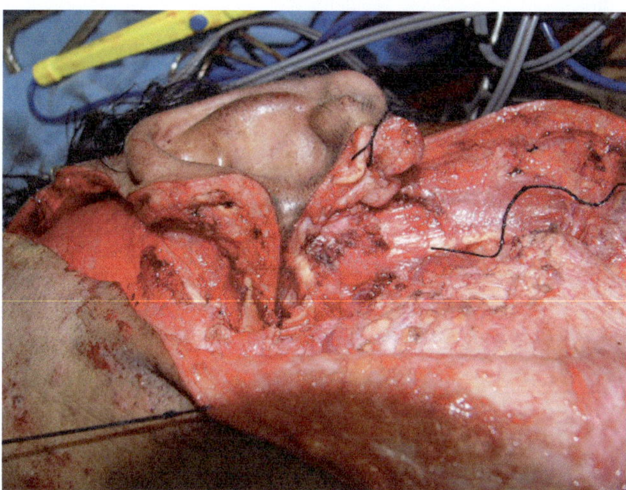

Fig. 4.63 The canal needs to be reconstructed to maintain hearing

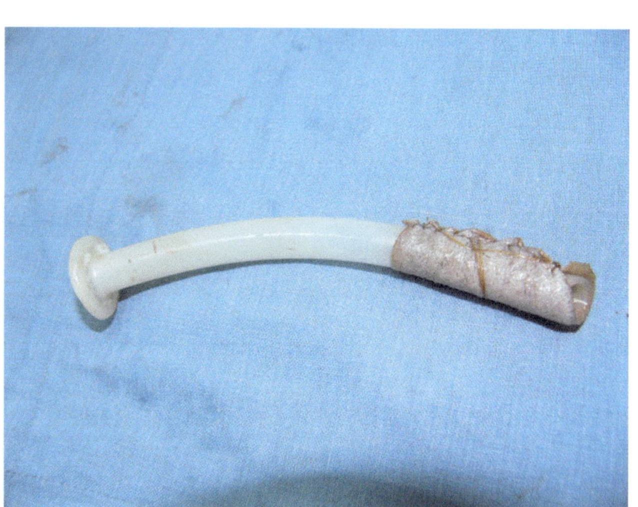

Fig. 4.64 Split-thickness graft (STG) is wrapped around a stent that can be inserted to form the canal

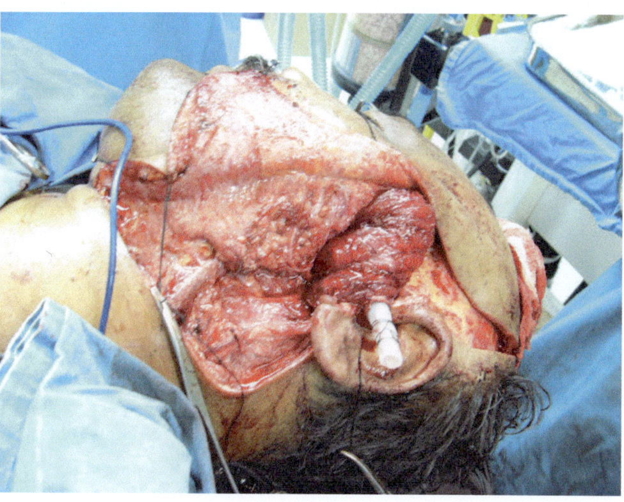

Fig. 4.65 Temporalis muscle is wrapped to fill the mastoid cavity and tube is placed in the auditory canal

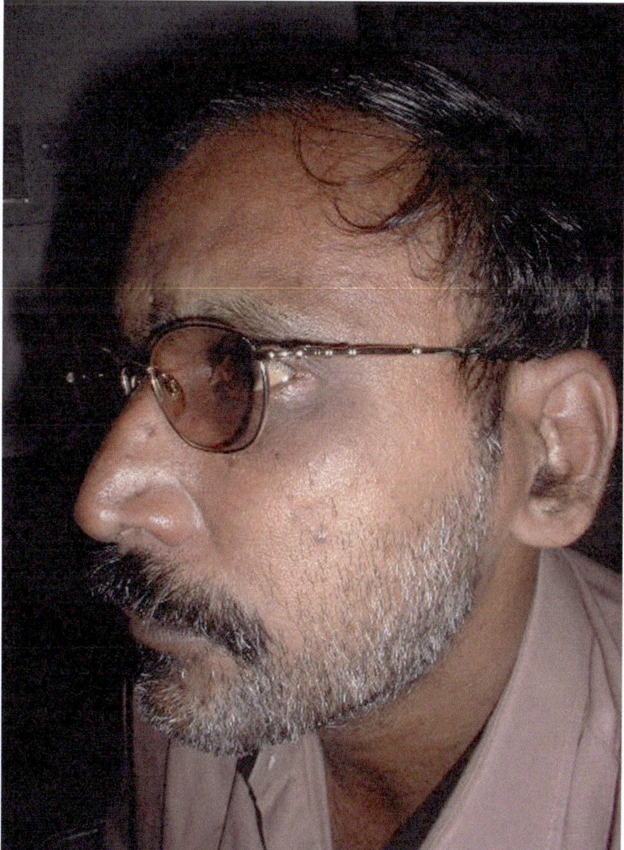

Fig. 4.66 Long-term outcome of the same patient

Facial Nerve Rehabilitation

The facial nerve rehabilitation is an important issue, and all surgeons who treat parotid tumors must have basic concepts about it. Figure 4.67 demonstrates algorithm for facial nerve rehabilitation. It is essential to rehabilitate eye closure immediately in case of injury to the facial nerve. This protects eye from exposure-related damage. The remaining rehabilitation can be managed according to the situation demonstrated in the algorithm.

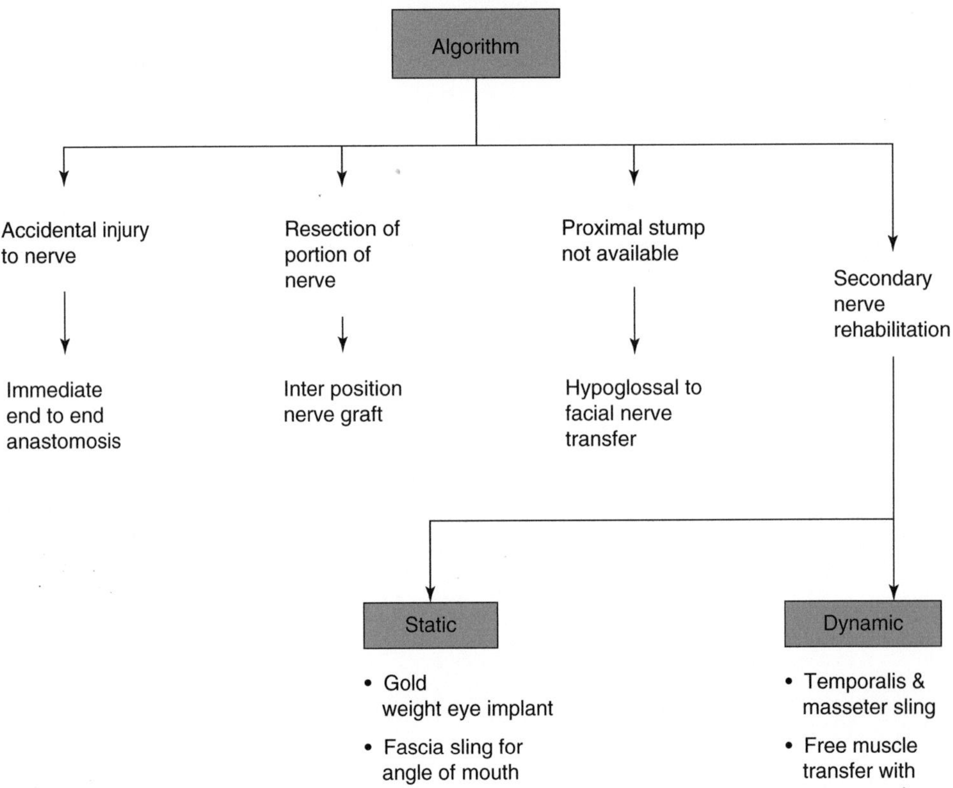

Fig. 4.67 Facial nerve rehabilitation for parotid surgery

5 Disease of the Neck

Surgical Anatomy and Pathology

The neck node remains the most important prognostic factor for head and neck cancer, and its management is of paramount importance. The neck nodes can be classified into five levels (Fig. 5.1). Level I is subdivided into IA (submental) and IB (submandibular). Levels II, III, and IV are deep cervical nodes along with internal jugular vein. Level II is further divided into IIA (anterior to spinal accessory) and IIB (posterior to spinal accessory). Levels III and IV are lower cervical nodes. Level V is situated posterior to the sternocleidomastoid muscle. It is further subdivided into VA (anterior to spinal accessory) and VB (posterior to spinal accessory).

Figure 5.2 demonstrates the algorithm for neck management for head–neck squamous cell carcinoma. The treatment approach has constantly been changing over the past few years and becoming more and more selective. This shift from radical neck dissection (RND) to modified neck dissection (MND) and to selective neck dissection (SND) has helped in improving the morbidity profile after the surgical procedure. This selective approach is based on better understanding of the spread of disease to the neck. Salvage neck dissection still remains a challenge and can lead to major postoperative complications like bleeding and wound breakdown. The concept of supra-selective neck dissection is becoming popular in salvage setting where selective removal of the involved lymph node (involved level with one level above and below) is considered adequate. The oral cavity generally drains into level I to III while tongue and floor of mouth (FOM) drains into level IV as well. The primary nodal basin for the larynx and pharynx is level II to IV. The level V nodes are addressed only in case of involvement of level IV or V.

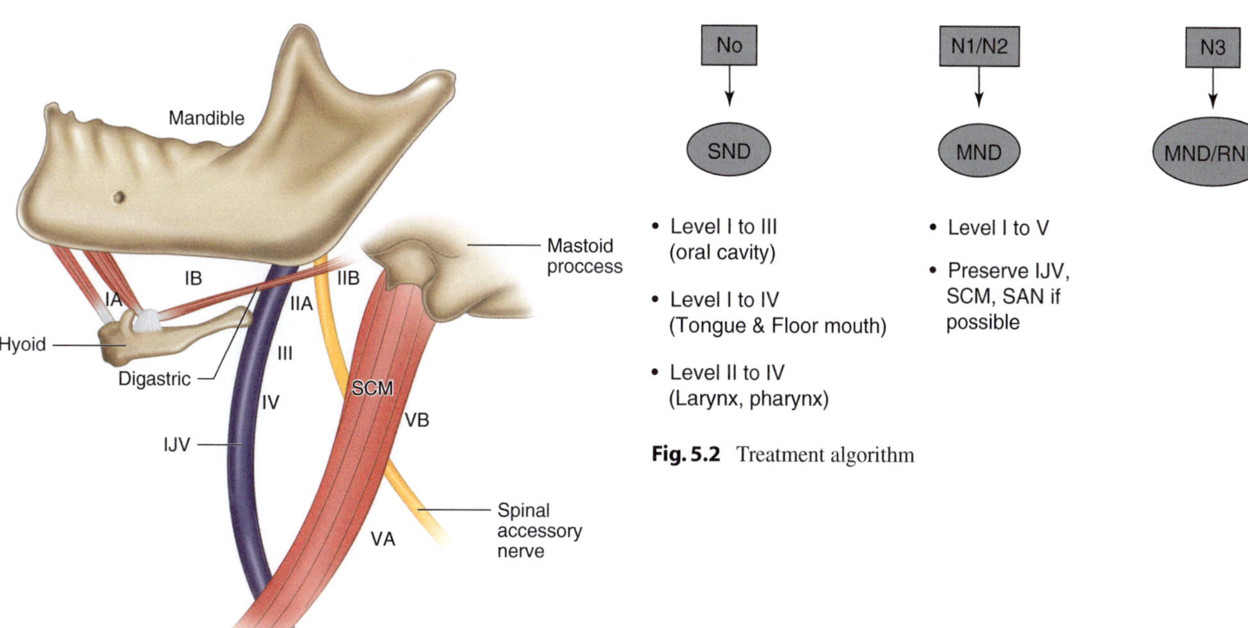

Fig. 5.1 Levels of neck

Fig. 5.2 Treatment algorithm

N. Trivedi, *Atlas of Head and Neck Cancer Surgery: The Compartment Surgery for Resection in 3-D*,
DOI 10.1007/978-81-322-2050-3_5, © Springer India 2015

Surgical Concepts

- The treatment approach is becoming more selective with better understanding of nodal drainage patterns.
- SND is the most commonly performed operation for N0 neck. It is also becoming acceptable for multiple node-positive patients (N+) where lower level nodes are not involved. These patients must receive adjuvant radiotherapy.
- MND is commonly performed for N+ neck where nodes involve level III to V. The spinal accessory nerve, internal jugular vein, and sternocleidomastoid (SCM) muscle are preserved as far as possible.
- RND is generally reserved for N3 node involving surrounding structures.
- The concept is to do minimal dissection as far as possible to salvage neck to avoid undue complications.

Selective and Modified Neck Dissection

This procedure demonstrates SND and MND removing level I to IV lymph nodes.

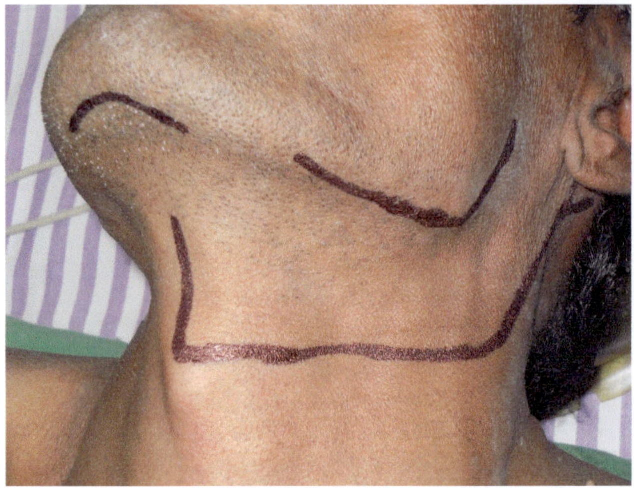

Fig. 5.3 Upper transverse cervical incision. The vertical incision in submental area can be restricted based upon surgeons comfort

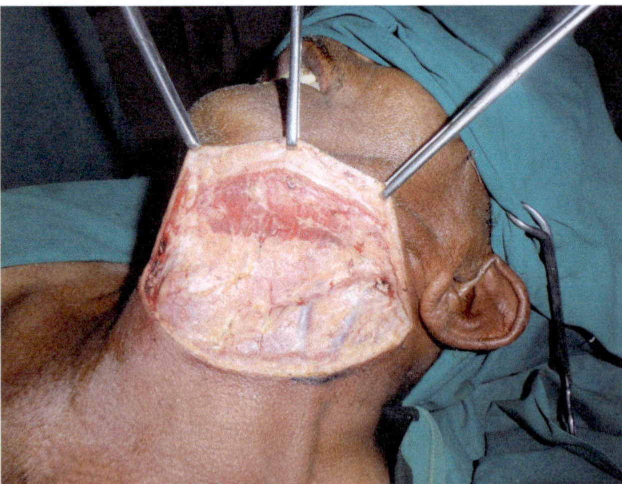

Fig. 5.4 Upper flap is raised in subplatysmal plane. In case of large matted node, platysma can be left attached to node and flap can be raised in subcutaneous plane

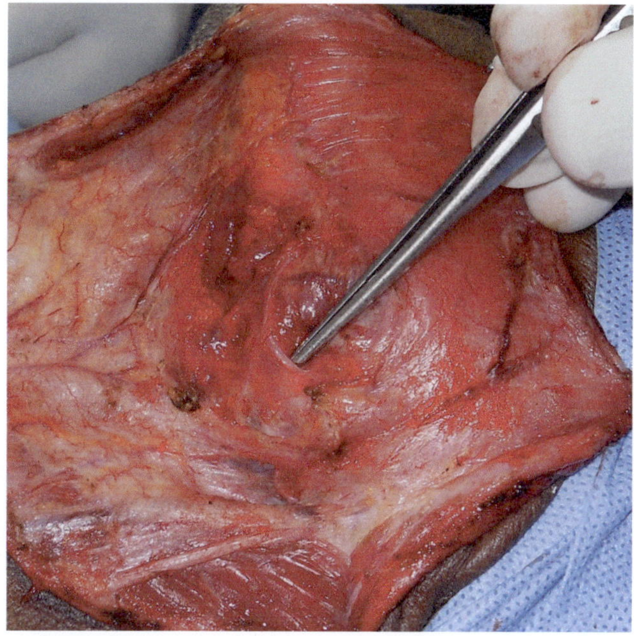

Fig. 5.5 Identification of marginal mandibular nerve. This nerve runs in deep fascia and can be exposed by opening the deep fascia near angle of mandible. For malignant case, one can raise flap in sub-platysmal plane and gradually dissect marginal nerve from deep fascia. The facial nodes are removed with specimen. For benign case, the flap can be raised deep to deep facia while removing submandinular gland completly without exposing the nerve and thereby preserving it. The facial nodes are left behind with this approach which is inappropriate for oral cancers

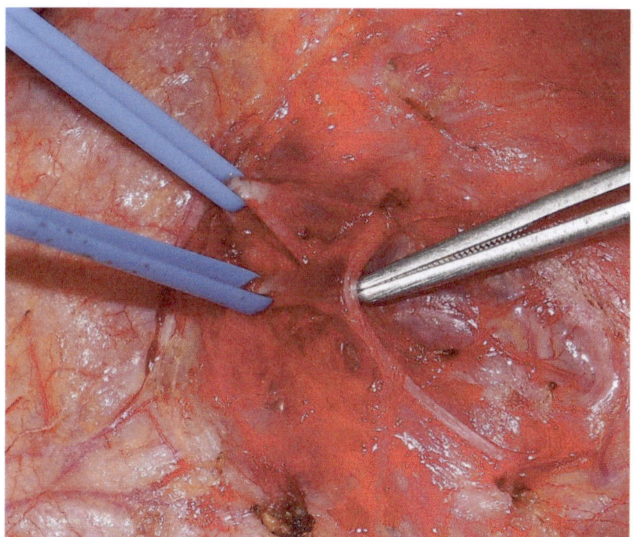

Fig. 5.6 Identification of facial vessels below the nerve. They are ligated and then lifted up to preserve marginal nerve

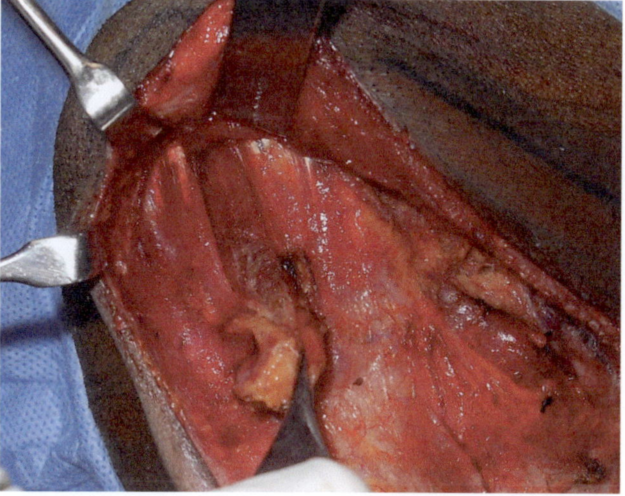

Fig. 5.7 The photograph shows clearance of level IA both belly of digastric muscle is exposed fully to remove all tissue from mandible to hyoid

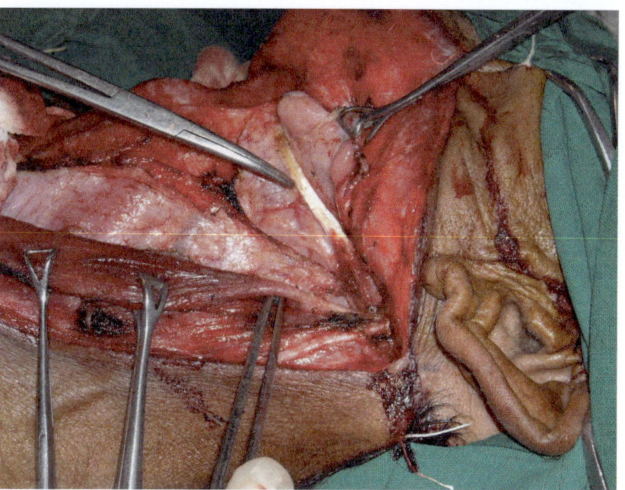

Fig. 5.8 The next step is to expose the posterior belly of the digastric tendon. This is a very important step as this clearly defines the anatomy of the neck. The facial vein is the only structure that runs above it and can be ligated. All other important vascular structures run deep to this muscle

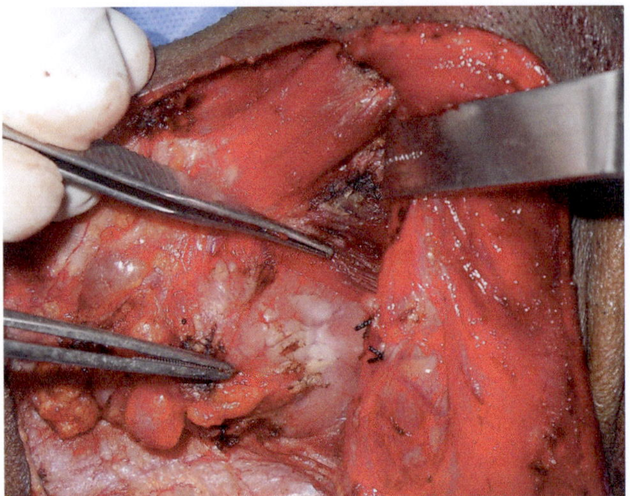

Fig. 5.9 Exposure of mylohyoid muscle while removing submandibular gland. There are small veins in this area that need proper hemostasis

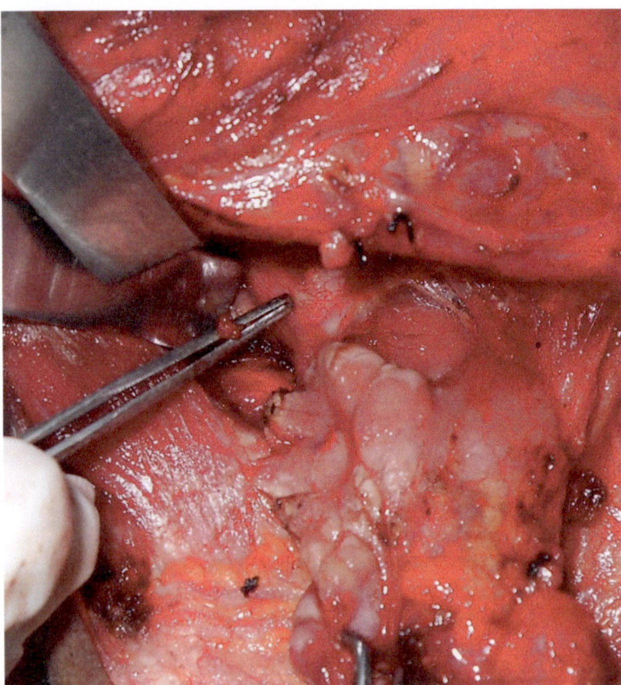

Fig. 5.10 Exposing the lingual nerve that is tethered to deep portion of gland. This band contains small vessels and release of this band frees the lingual nerve

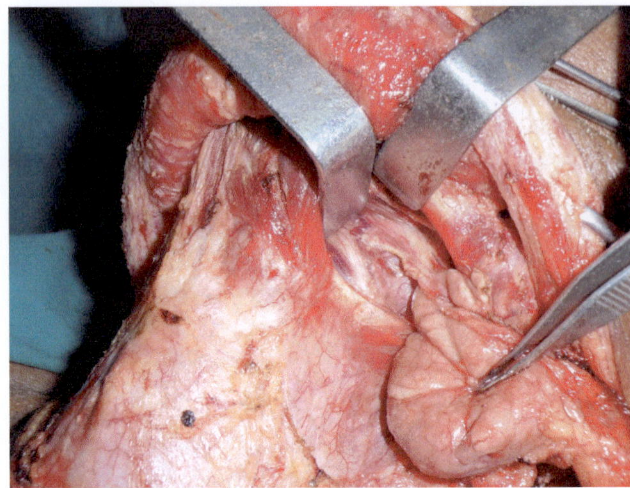

Fig. 5.11 Both the hypoglossal and lingual nerves are seen in this photograph. The hypoglossal nerve is in the floor of the gland and runs deep to fascia

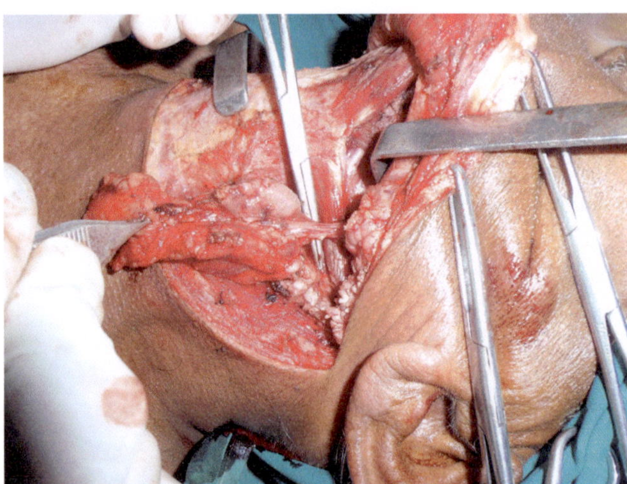

Fig. 5.12 Isolation of facial artery that enters in the gland just above the posterior belly of digastric near angle of mandible

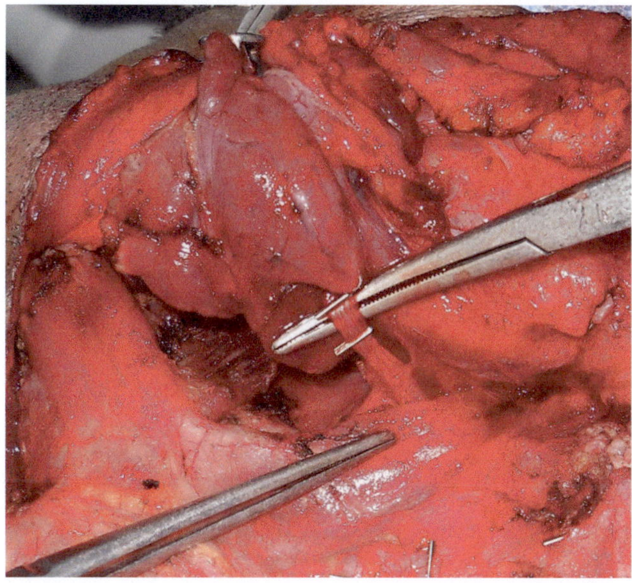

Fig. 5.13 The facial artery is ligated and gland along with facial node is removed

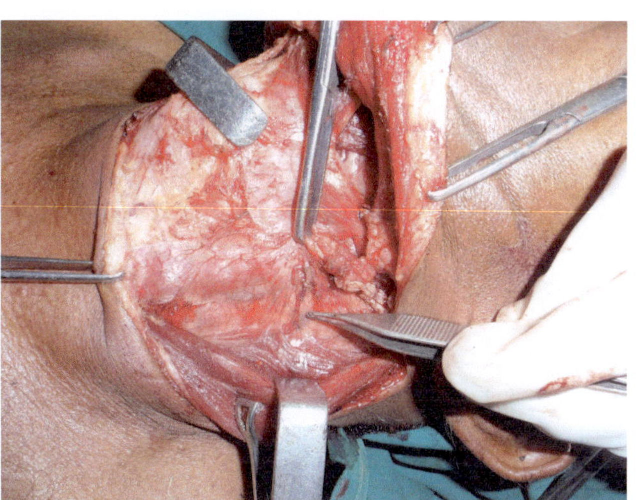

Fig. 5.14 The dissection starts to clear level II nodes. The first step is to identify spinal accessory nerve. The SCM muscle is retracted backward. Key is to stay right on muscle taking all fascia anteriorly. There is a small blood vessel just above the nerve, and this can serve as a guide to the nerve

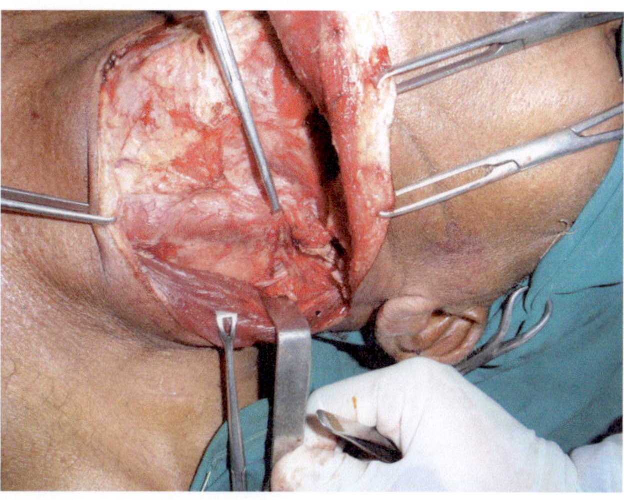

Fig. 5.15 The nerve is exposed. It is advisable to use bipolar cautery in this region

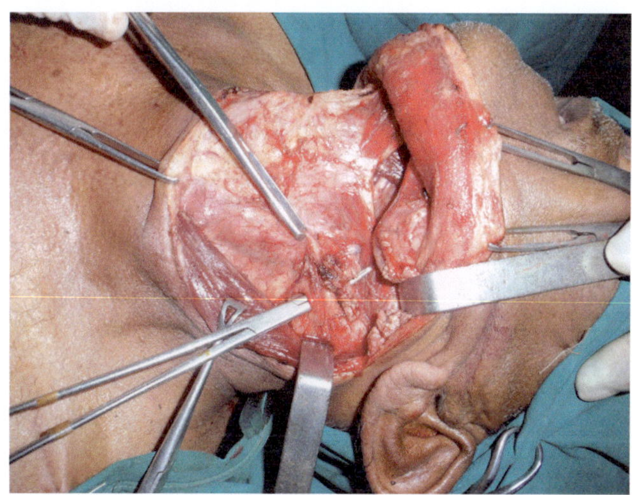

Fig. 5.16 Lymph nodes and surroundings tissues are dissected out at level 2A and 2B

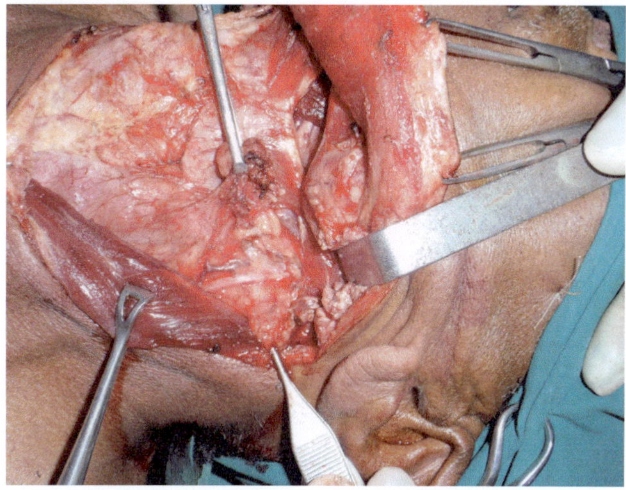

Fig. 5.17 The nerve is exposed in its entire length

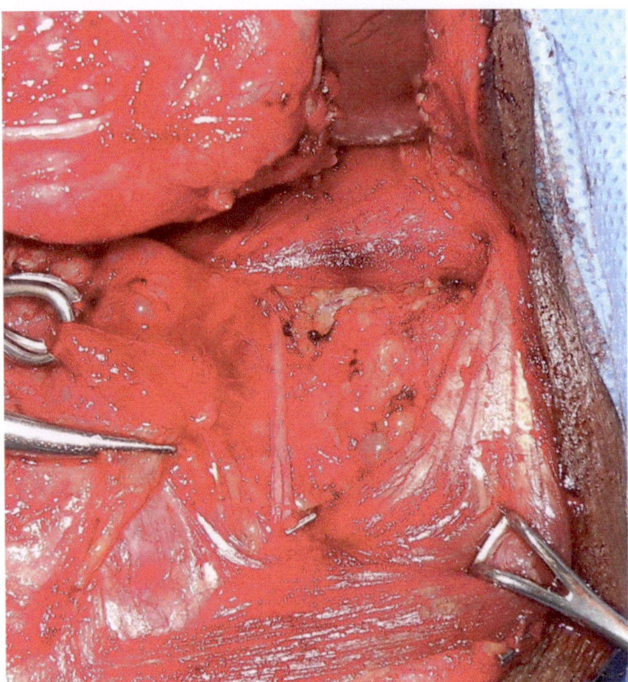

Fig. 5.18 The anatomy of level II nodes. The nerve divides it into level A and B. Clearance of level IIB is important and should be carried out by exposing digastric and SCM muscle till mastoid process

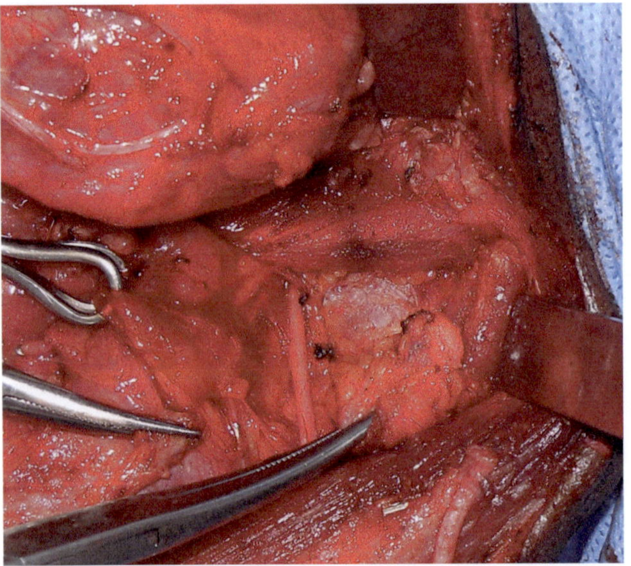

Fig. 5.19 The level IIB clearance. The posterior occipital artery can be encountered here sometimes and can be ligated

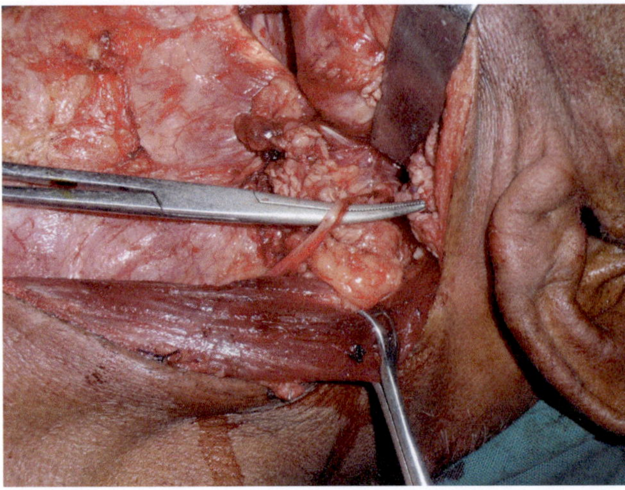

Fig. 5.20 The IIB nodes are mobilized under the nerve to IIA compartment. This isolates and secures the nerve. It is important to minimize handling of the nerve during this entire procedure. Skin incision till mastoid process significantly enhances the exposure and aids in this process

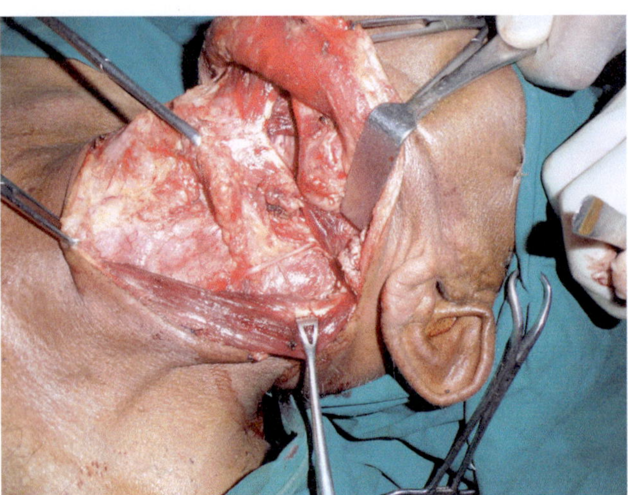

Fig. 5.21 The level II and III nodes are being mobilized. The cervical roots serve as a guide to posterior dissection, and posterior boundary of SCM is the posterior limit of this dissection

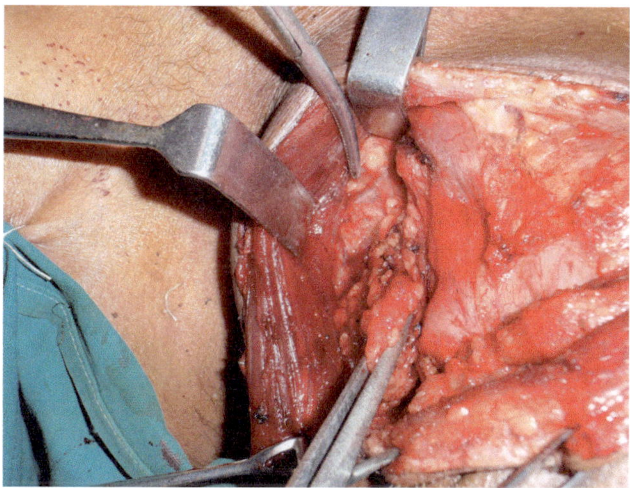

Fig. 5.22 Clearance of level IV. It is easy to perform this process if one stands on the head end and the assistant retracts the SCM laterally. The omohyoid muscle can be transected to gain better exposure to this area. The photograph demonstrates exposed transverse cervical vessels which are the lower limit of dissection. It is also prudent to secure chyle leak if encountered. One must look for leak before closure of the wound

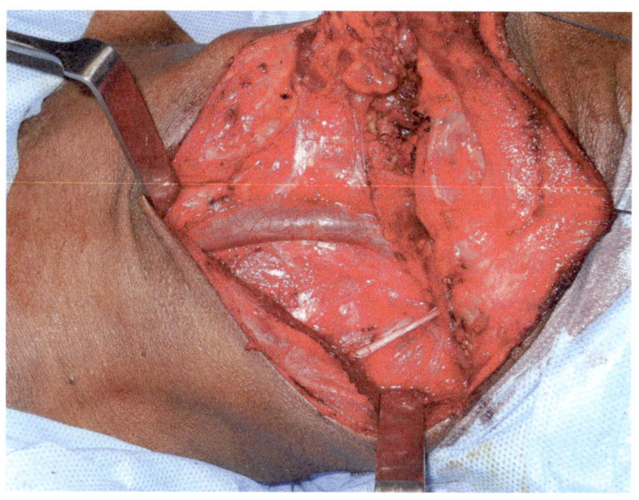

Fig. 5.23 The fascia over the internal jugular vein (IJV) is being removed along with the specimen

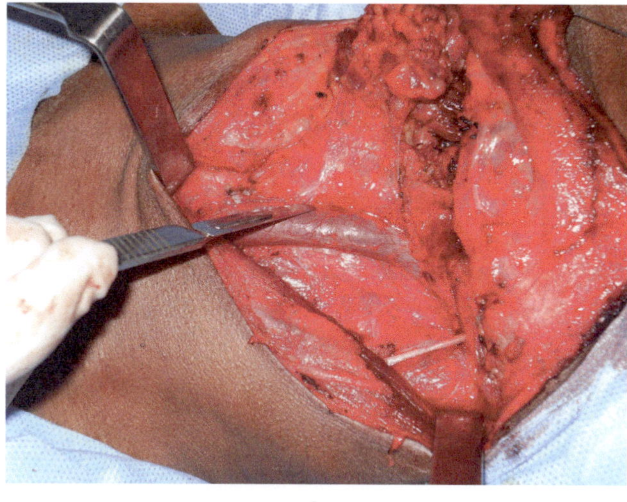

Fig. 5.24 Knife dissection is ideal for this portion

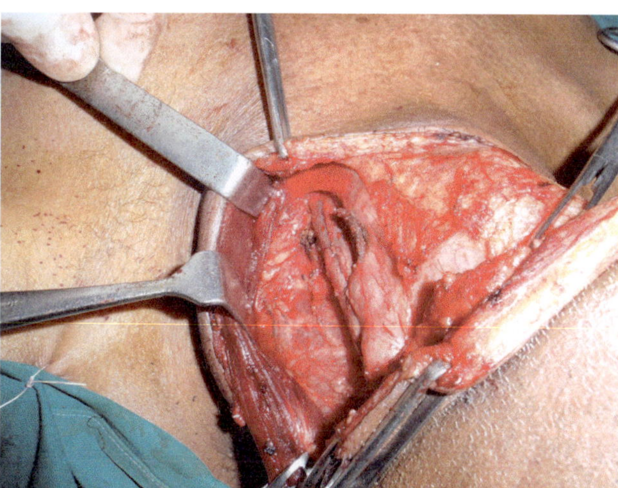

Fig. 5.25 Clearance of level IV

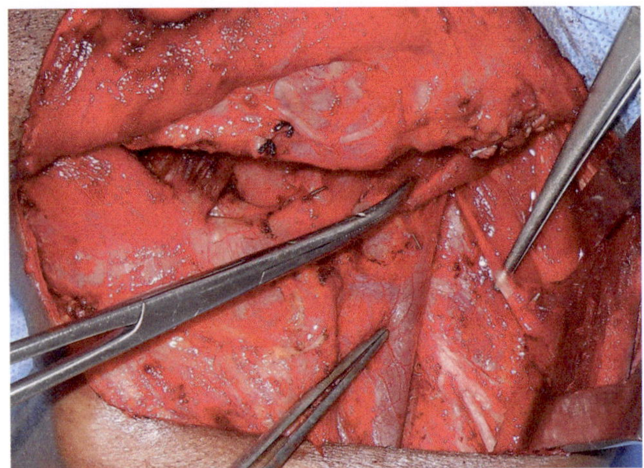

Fig. 5.26 Clearance of level II and III with preservation of all structures

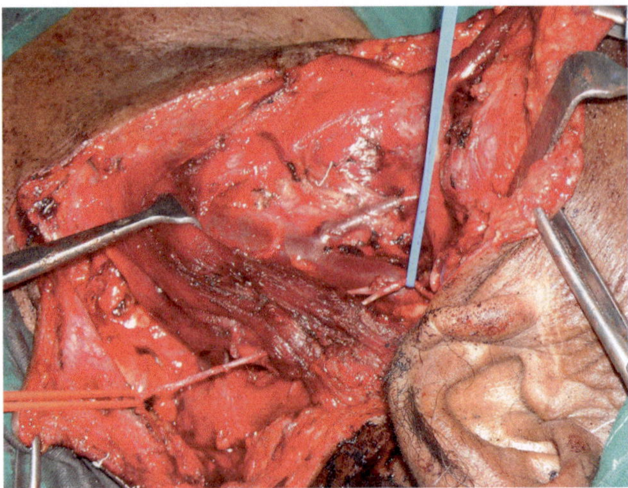

Fig. 5.27 Preserved spinal accessory nerve in its entire length after a modified neck dissection. All the steps remain the same as described before. Level V dissection starts by raising the posterior flap till the trapezius muscle. The nerve can be identified either at its lower end while entering in trapezius muscle or where it exits from the SCM. Once identified, it is dissected and preserved in entire length. The lymph nodes along with tissues present in the space formed by omohyoid muscle below, trapezius muscle posteriorly and prevertebral fascia above, are removed. It is tunneled below the SCM and removed along with the remaining lymph node tissue dissected earlier

Radical Neck Dissection

This procedure demonstrates the case of RND for a matted nodal mass.

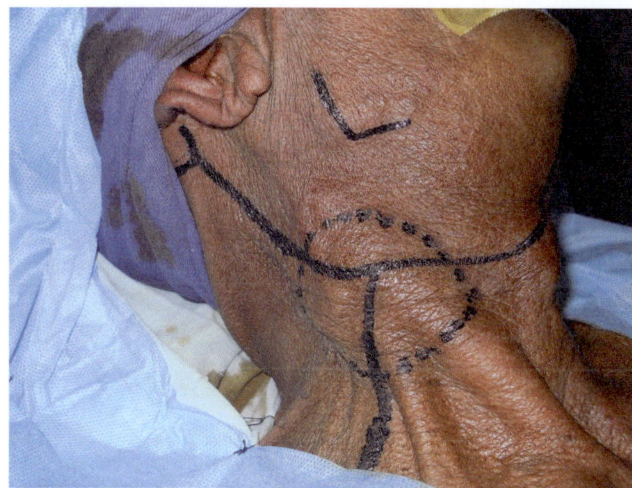

Fig. 5.28 The case of a matted neck node infiltrating the SCM and skin

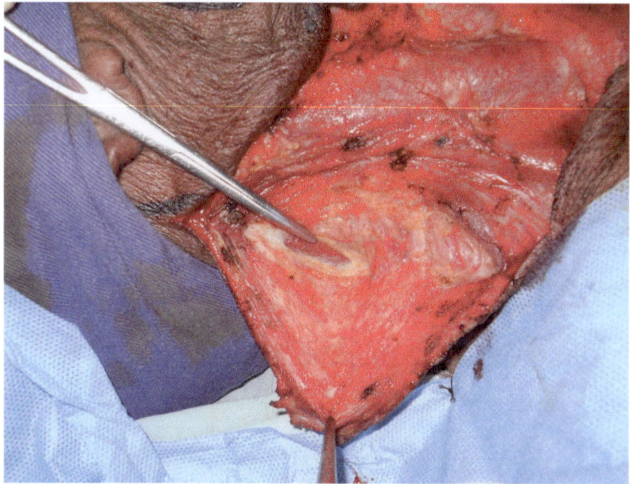

Fig. 5.29 Posterior flap is raised to expose the trapezius muscle

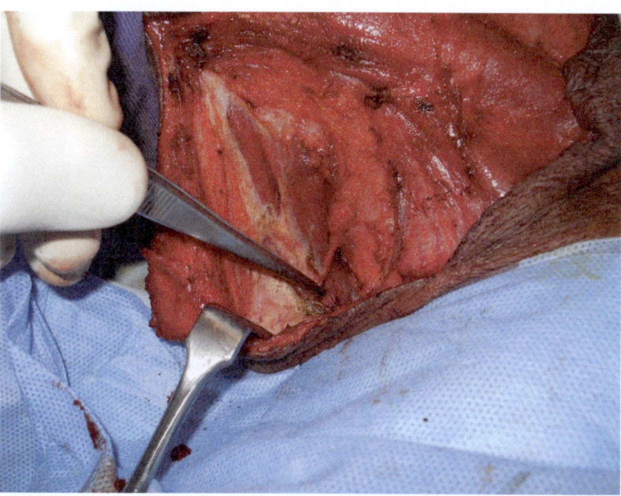

Fig. 5.30 Identification of the spinal accessory nerve. The nerve can be sacrificed early as there is no chance of saving it in this case

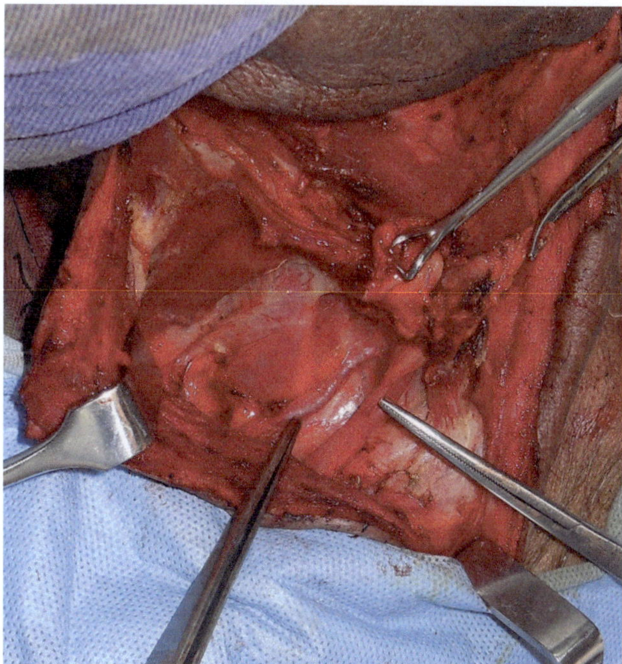

Fig. 5.31 The transverse cervical vessels and omohyoid muscle demonstrating clearance of level V nodes

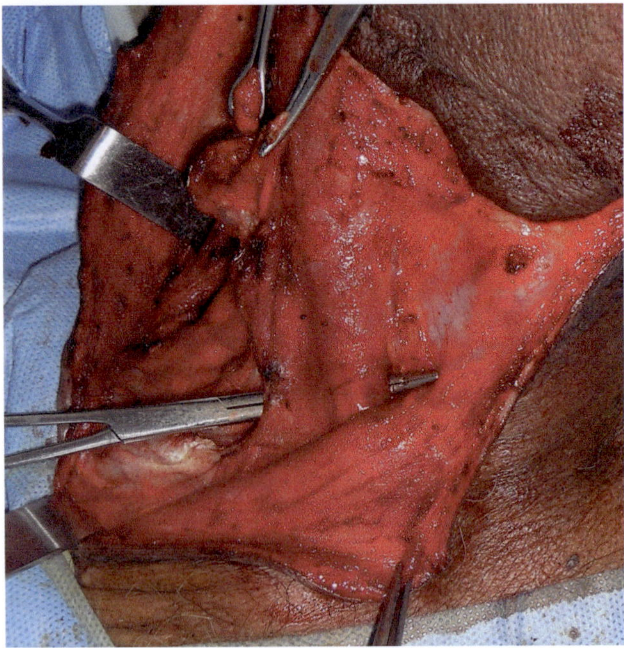

Fig. 5.32 The SCM is transacted at the lower end

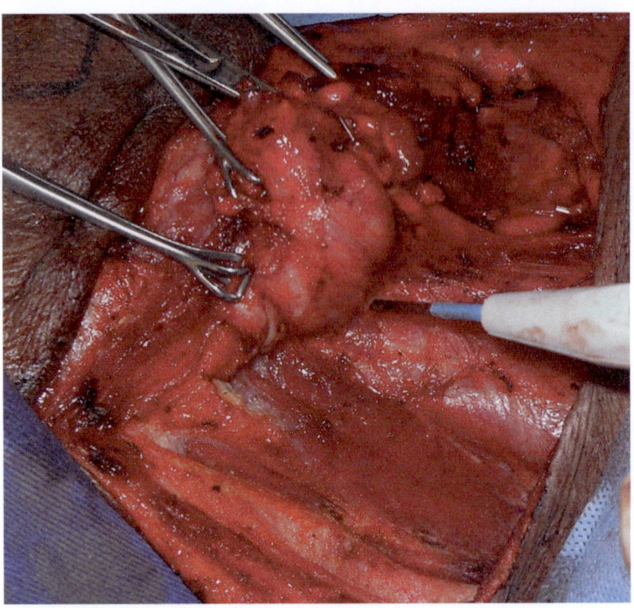

Fig. 5.34 Lifting of the mass above the prevertebral fascia. This is an important factor in predicting operability of the mass. The clinical examination with assessment of mobility remains the most important guiding factor for predicting complete removal of tumor

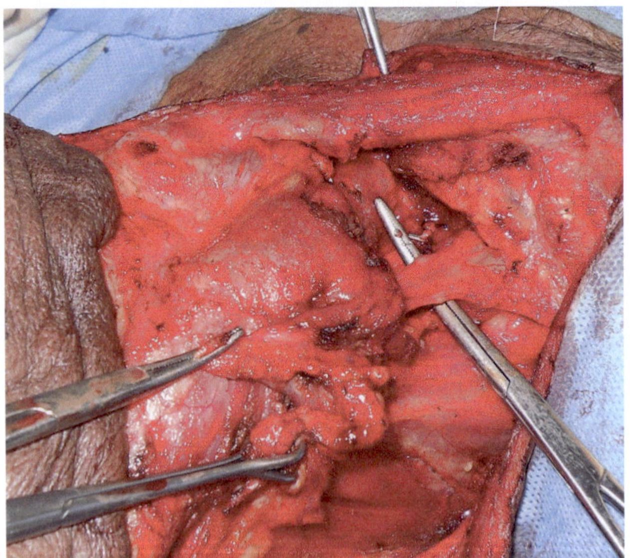

Fig. 5.33 The lower end of the IJV that is thrombosed and has become band like. Always transfix the lower end of the IJV to prevent slipping of ligature in the postoperative period

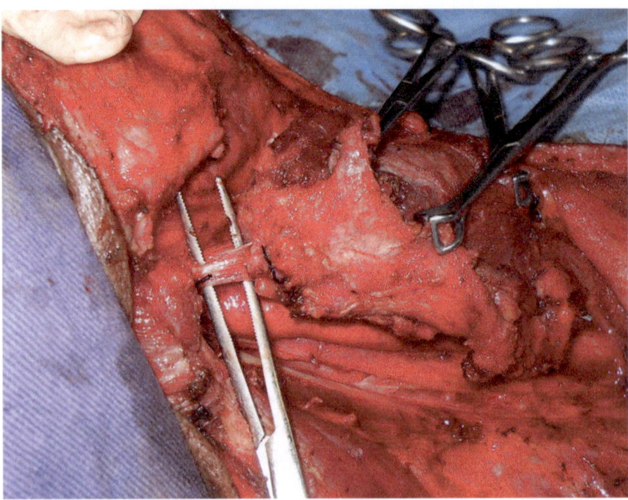

Fig. 5.35 Identification and ligation of the upper end of the IJV. The upper end of the vein can be identified in majority of cases and the posterior belly of digastric serves as guide in its identification. In rare occasions when this cannot be found, it can be transected and area can be packed. The pack can be removed after 2–3 days and bleeding would have ceased in majority of instances

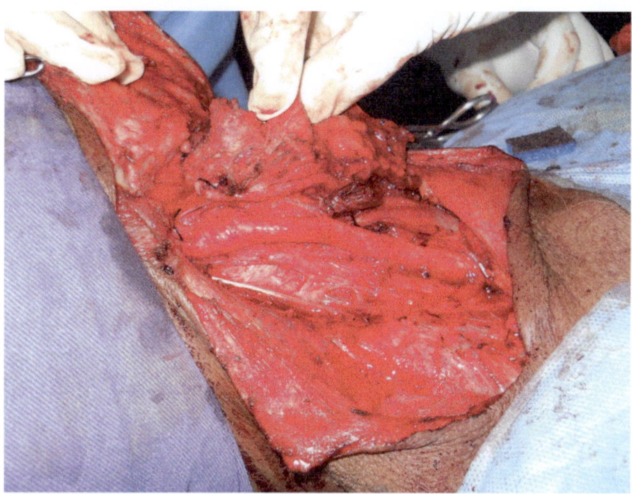

Fig. 5.36 The node is being freed from the vagus and carotid artery. In large mass, the external carotid artery can be sacrificed to achieve satisfactory clearance

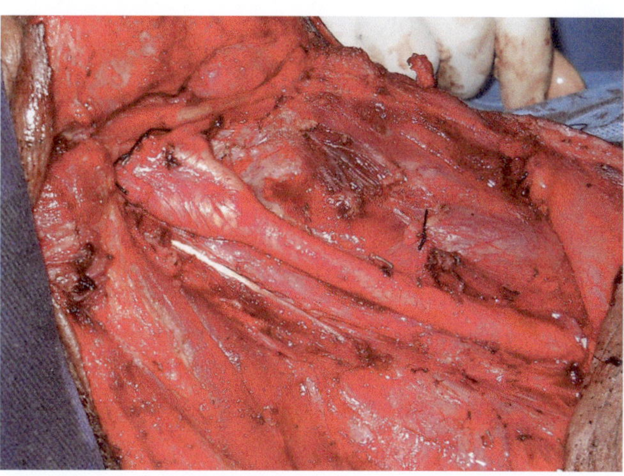

Fig. 5.37 Photograph showing complete clearance. The reconstruction was done with PMMC flap

Extended Neck Dissection

This procedure demonstrates resection of carotid artery along with matted mass and saphenous venous grafting to maintain continuity of intracranial blood flow. This can be performed in selected cases of otherwise healthy young patient where the primary tumor is under control, there is no distant metastasis, and the prevertebral fascia is free.

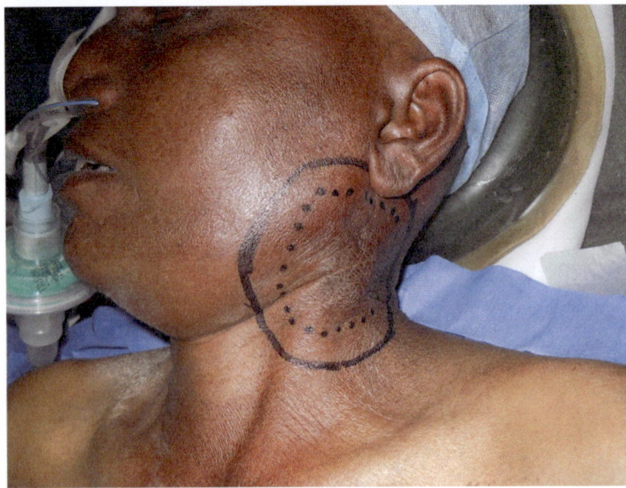

Fig. 5.38 Case with nodal mass involving carotid artery. The conventional teaching is that if the mass is involving carotid more than 270°, it cannot be separated. This may change in the case of post-radiated salvage neck dissection

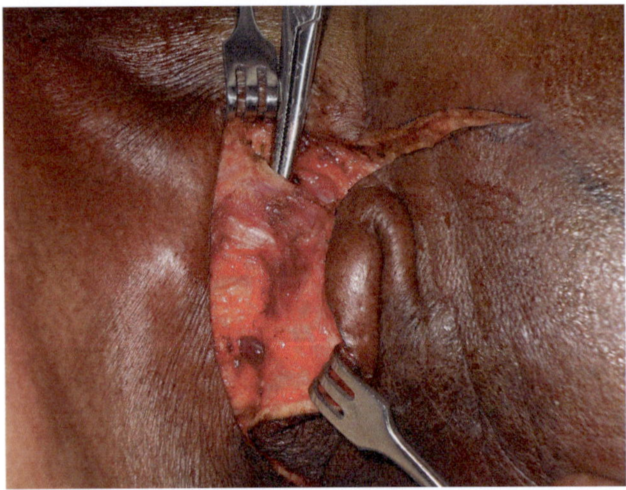

Fig. 5.39 Exposure of the lower end of the SCM and its division

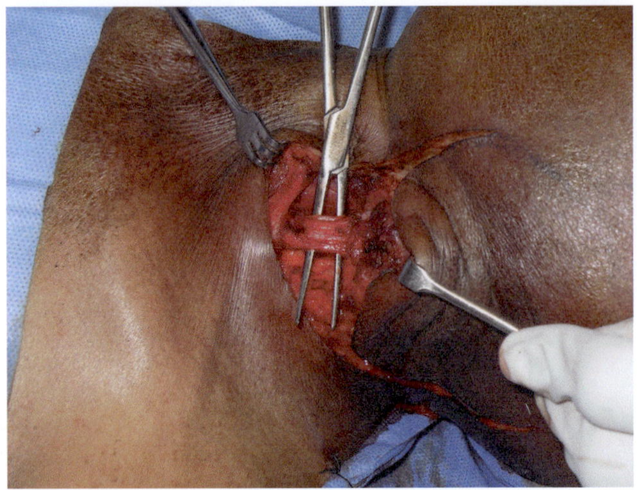

Fig. 5.40 Identifying the IJV and ligating it

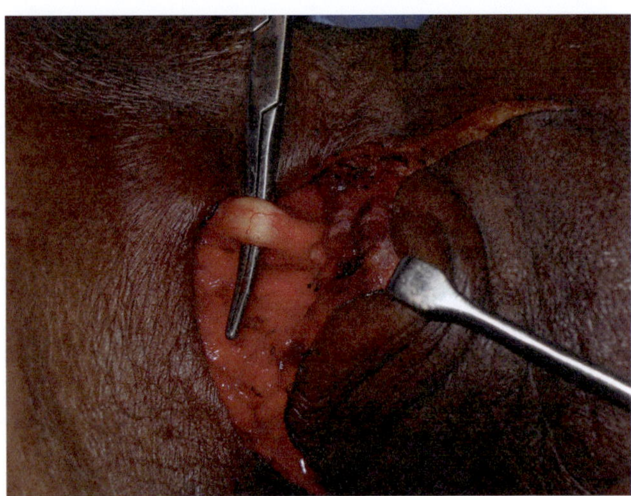

Fig. 5.41 Exposing the common carotid artery in the lower end. This should be the first step in the procedure. This helps in controlling bleeding in case of emergency

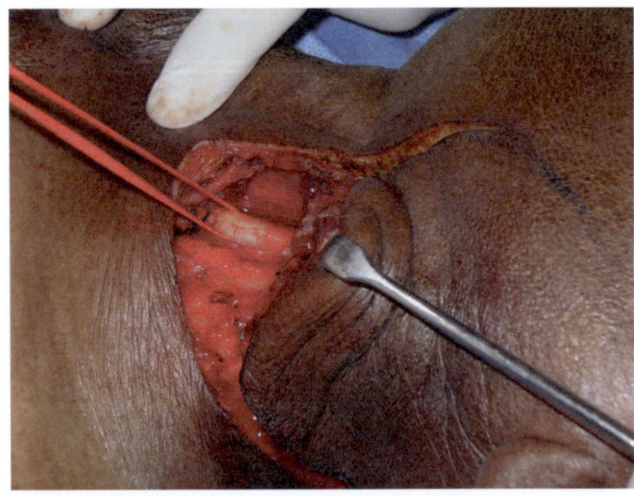

Fig. 5.42 The carotid vessel is slinged and isolated

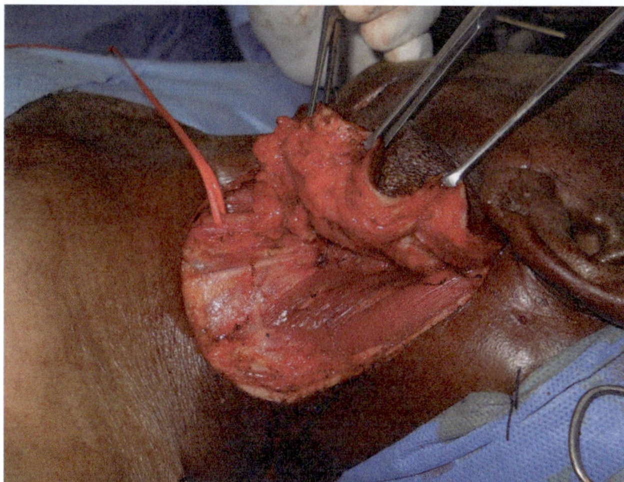

Fig. 5.43 The mass being mobilized from prevertebral fascia

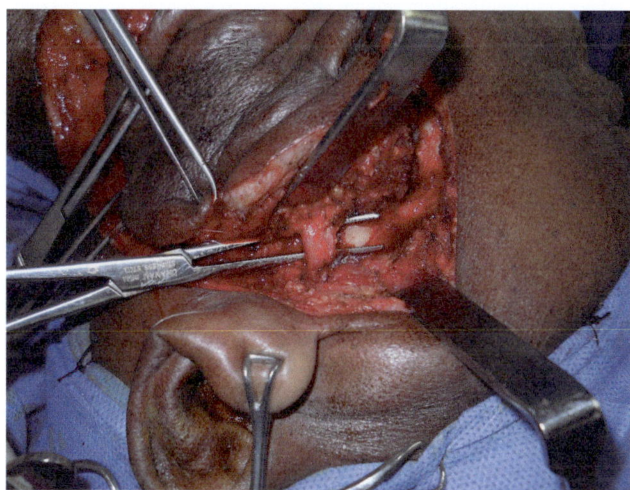

Fig. 5.44 Identification of the upper end of the external carotid vessel. This is ligated where it enters the deep lobe of the parotid gland

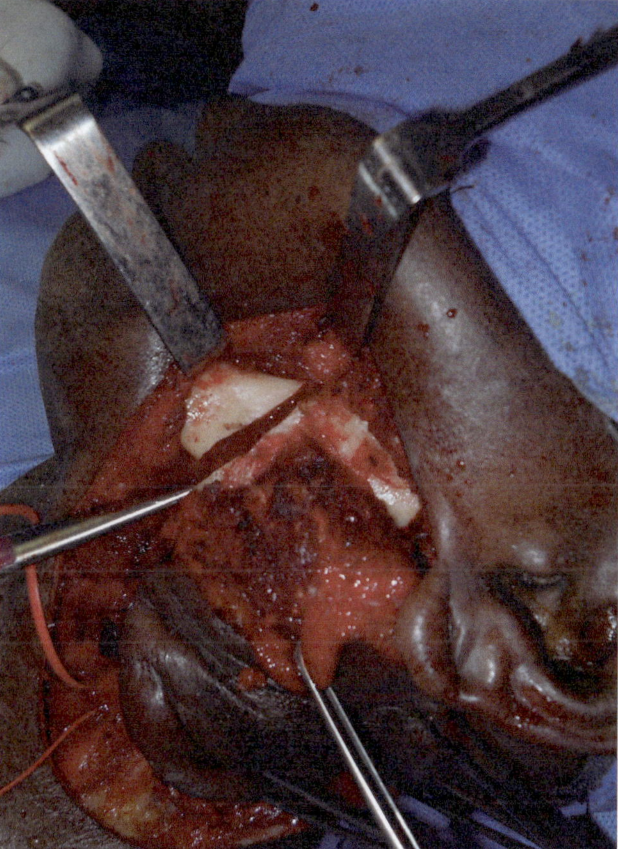

Fig. 5.45 The lesion involves the lower end of the mandible, and reverse marginal resection is being performed

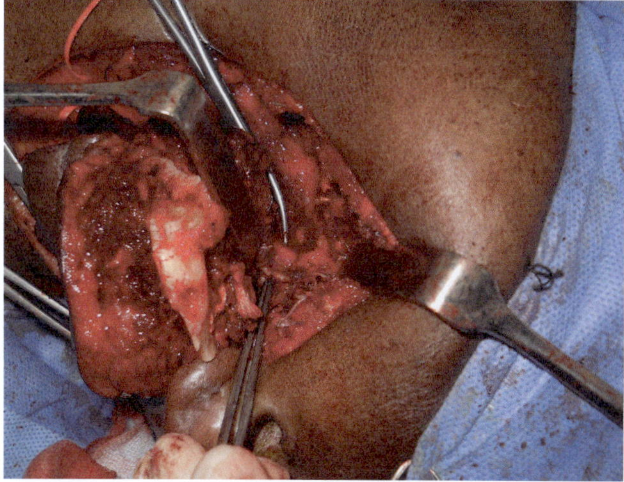

Fig. 5.46 The styloid process with attached muscles. The internal carotid artery is deep to styloid process and deep to fascia. Careful dissection in this area can expose the internal carotid artery

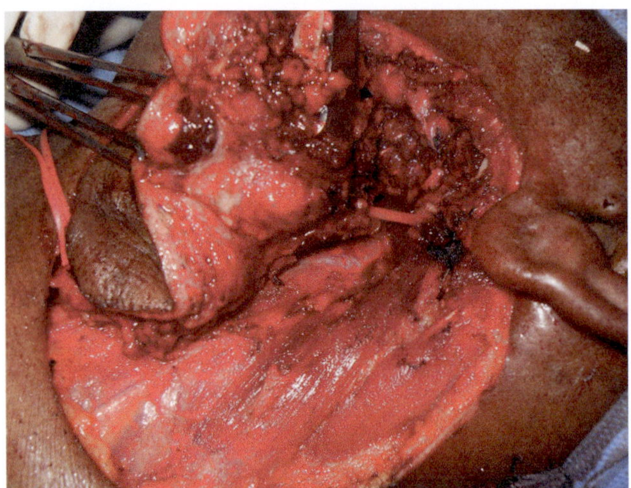

Fig. 5.47 Exposed internal carotid artery. It is important to expose a longer segment of ICA to provide adequate space for vascular anastomosis at upper end

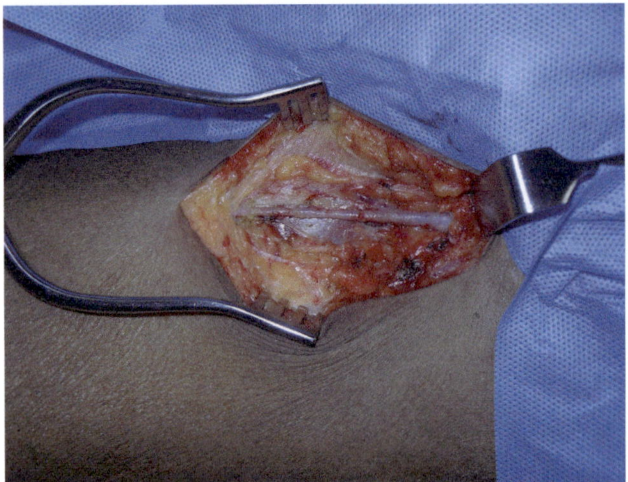

Fig. 5.48 The saphenous vein being isolated

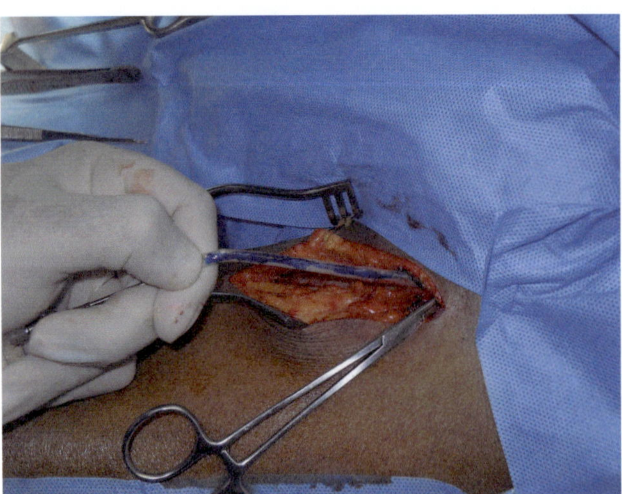

Fig. 5.49 The vein is ink marked for orientation and removed

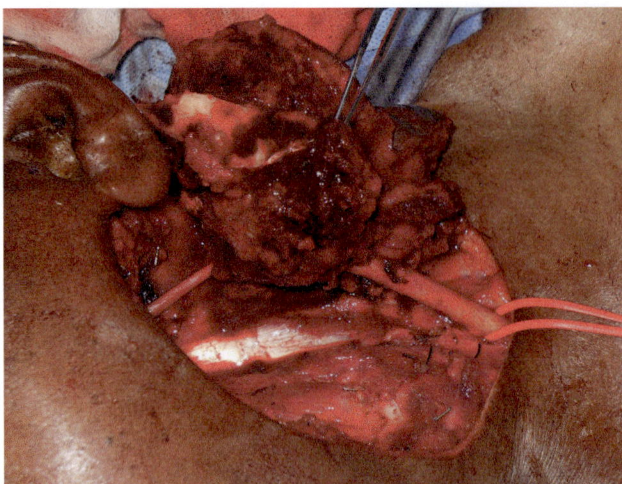

Fig. 5.50 The lesion is completely free from all around including prevertebral fascia. All peripheral branches of the external carotid vessel are ligated. This dissection is ready for the vascular surgeon to come and perform interposition venous graft. The vein graft is preferred over synthetic graft because asymmetry in caliber of common carotid and internal carotid artery can be better adjusted with vein graft

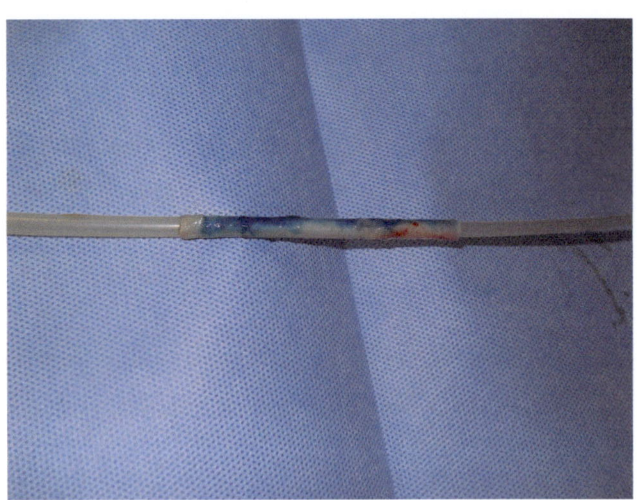

Fig. 5.51 The graft is placed over shunt

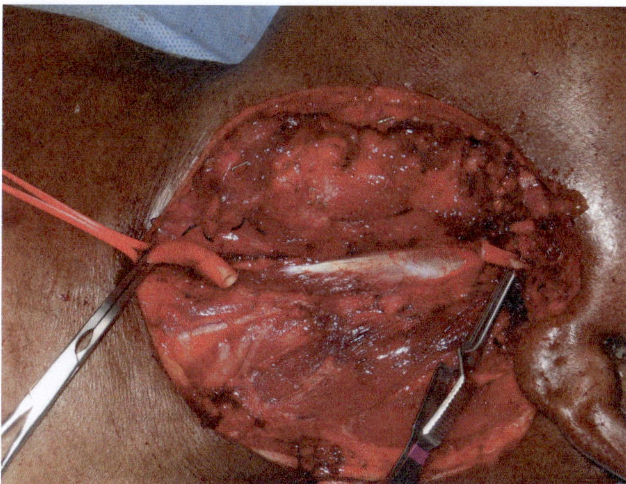

Fig. 5.52 The tumor is removed after applying vascular clamps to both ends of cardio artery

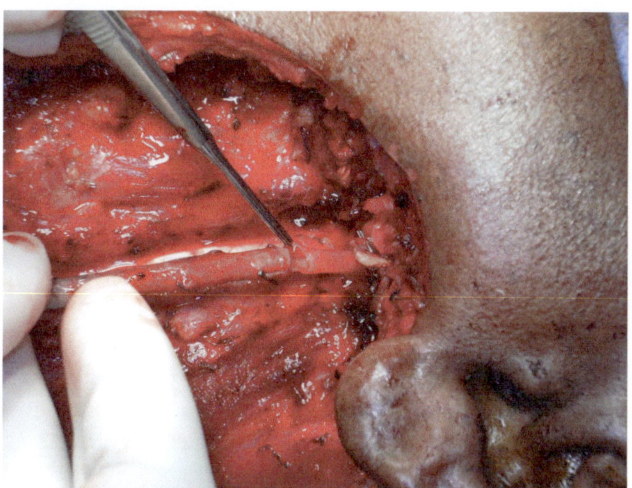

Fig. 5.53 The shunt is placed in the upper end of the carotid vessel

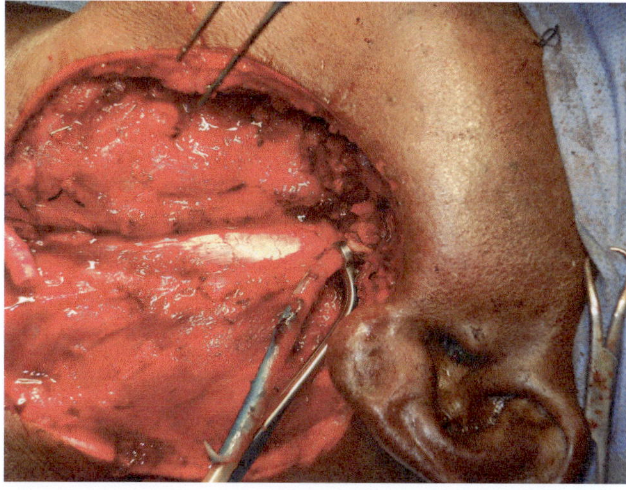

Fig. 5.54 The shunt is in the upper end of vessel and carotid clamps are applied over it

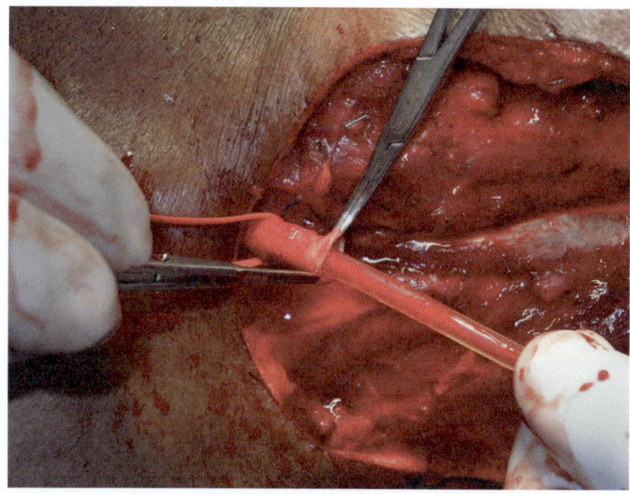

Fig. 5.55 The stent being guided in the lower end of the carotid in similar way

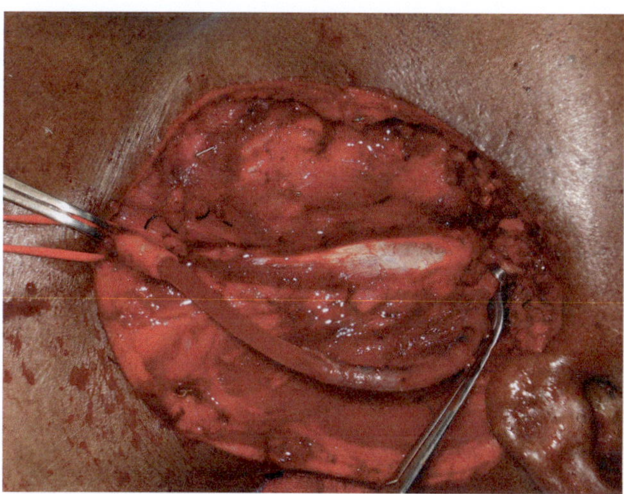

Fig. 5.56 Stent with vein graft in situ with blood flow restored. This process takes approximately 2–3 min and the anesthetist is asked to keep systolic pressure high and give anticoagulants during this time

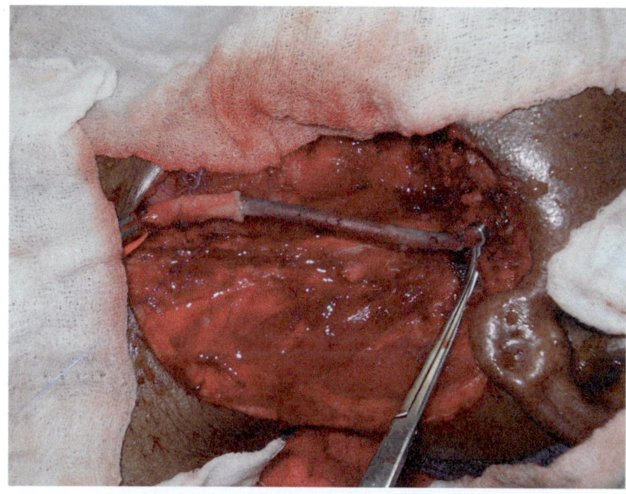

Fig. 5.57 The upper and lower anastomosis is completed

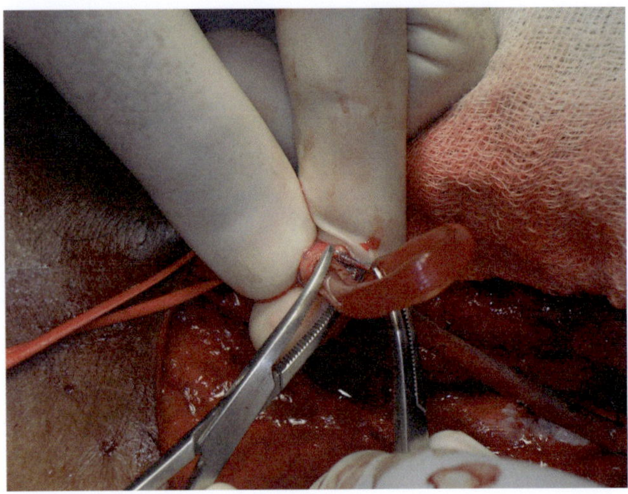

Fig. 5.58 The stent is being removed from the lower end where the stitches were left slightly loose

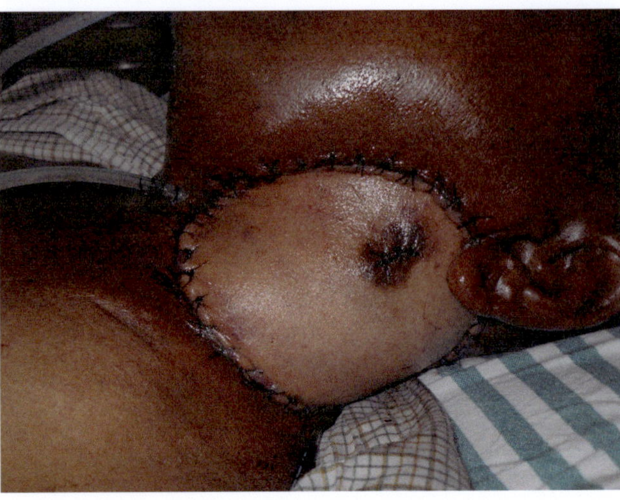

Fig. 5.61 The flap closure. It is important to adjust lie of flap to avoid twisting of pedicle. This is particularly important while inserting flap in neck

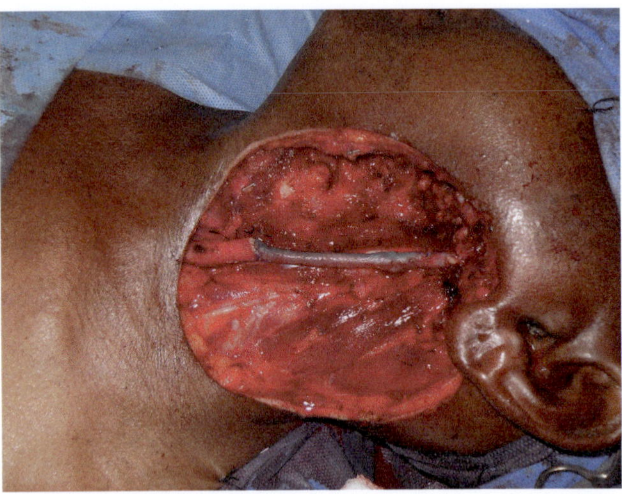

Fig. 5.59 The stitches are tied tighty, anastomosis is complete and functioning. The patient is administered intravenous anticoagulants for a few days in the postoperative phase

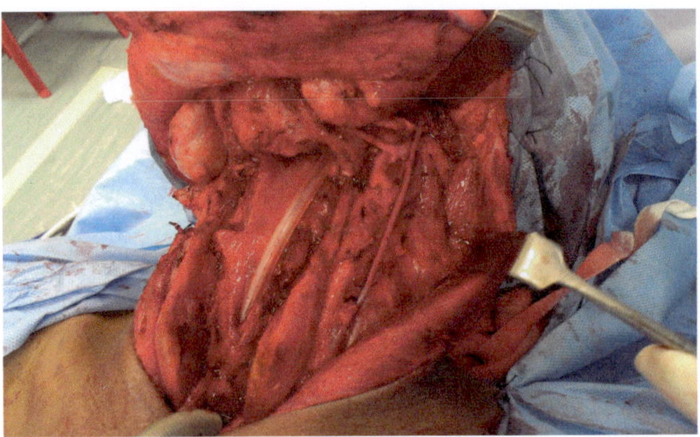

Fig. 5.62 This is a case of bilateral neck nodes infiltrating the bilateral IJV. This is a challenging problem and morbidity and mortality is high in these cases. The conventional approach is to perform one side of the neck first and then wait for 3 weeks before performing on another side. We prefer to put interposition venous graft on either side provided both ends of the IJV are available for anastomosis. It is still advisable to do this in staged manner in case venous graft fails. This photograph shows one sided vein is reconstructed with venous graft

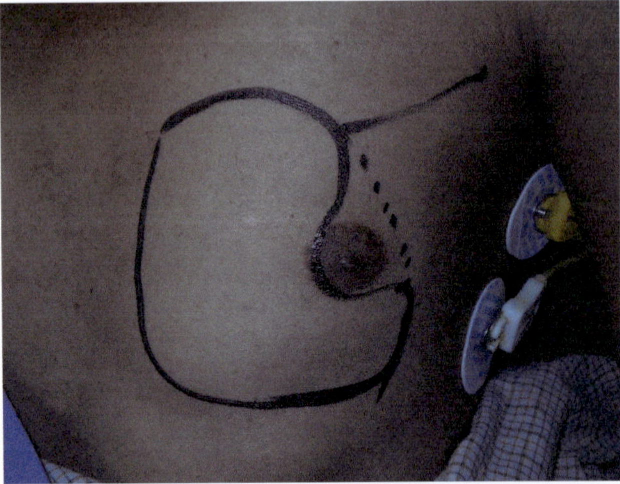

Fig. 5.60 Proposed pectoralis major myocutaneous (PMMC) flap

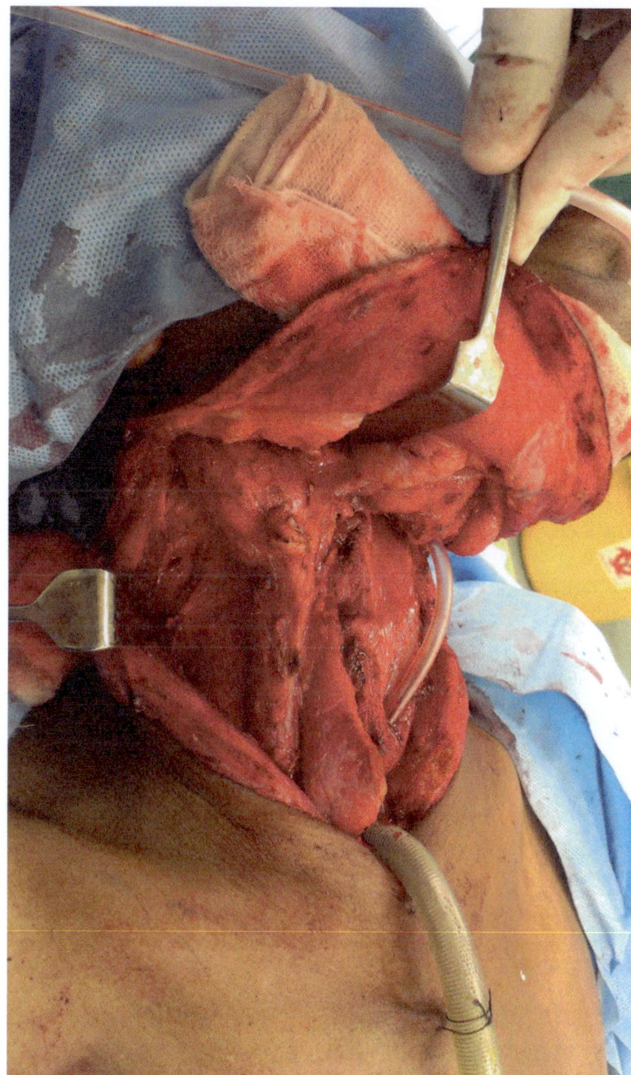

Fig. 5.63 This photo shows a neck node on the other side that is infiltrating the vein. This should be addressed after 3 weeks of first surgery to avoid facial congestion. We prefer to put venous graft to this side as well. The most important and limiting factor is the availability of the upper end of the IJV for anastomosis. This is ideal for level III nodes where adequate length of the upper end of the IJV is available

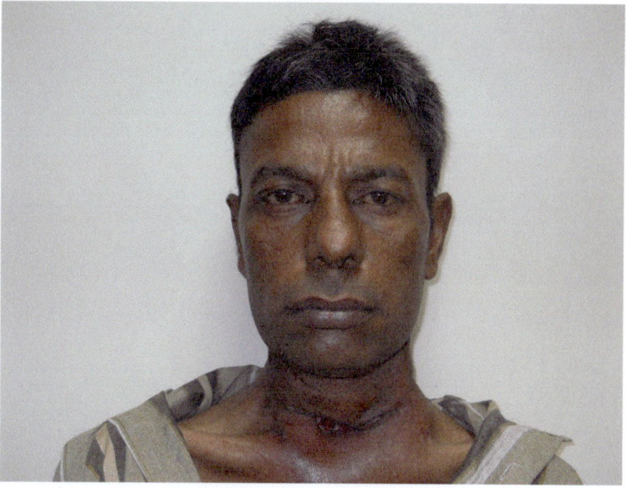

Fig. 5.64 The patient after complete surgical treatment without any significant facial edema

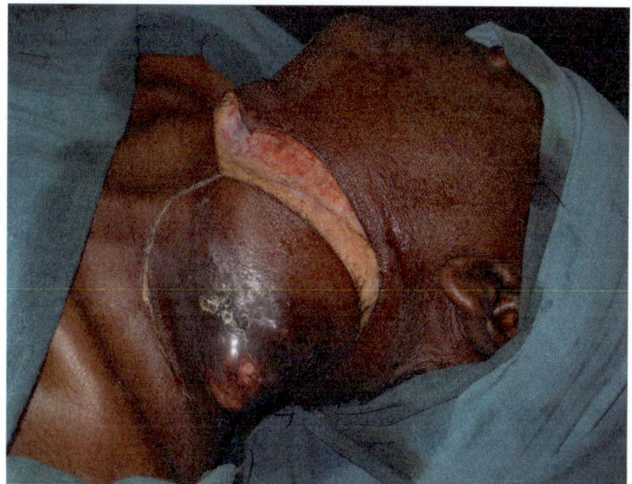

Fig. 5.65 This photograph shows neck mass that is infiltrating carotid vessels. It is not necessary always to bypass carotid artery if it is infiltrated, and it can be ligated in select cases. The preoperative assessment of adequacy of contralateral brain circulation is necessary in such situation. The standard method is to perform balloon occlusion test and check for neurological adequacy. It is also advisable to evaluate computed tomography scan (CT scan) of the brain to see if anterior and posterior communicating vessels are present. If this is established, one can safely resect carotid without reconstructing it

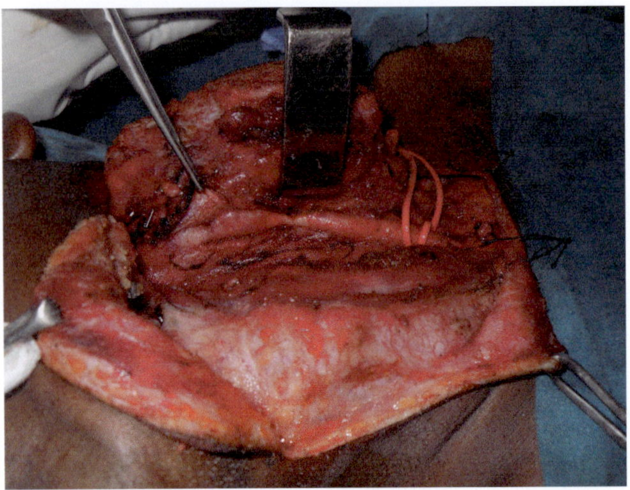

Fig. 5.66 The photograph shows that the tumor is infiltrating carotid artery in 360°. It is generally not possible to free the carotid when mass is infiltrating more than 270°

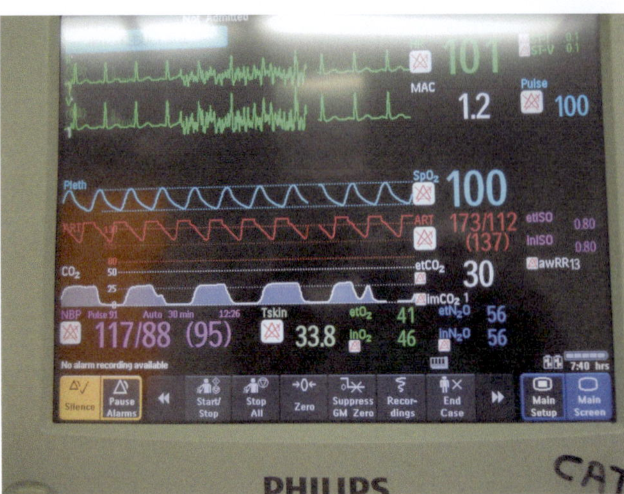

Fig. 5.68 If pressure is about 70–80 mmHg, the contralateral circulation is considered adequate. This has proved correct in all instances in our experience

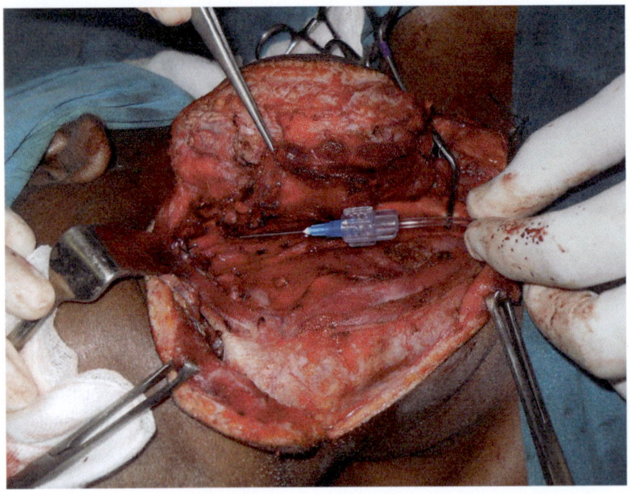

Fig. 5.67 This is a simple intraoperative test to check adequacy of contralateral circulation. After mobilizing all other aspects, the proximal common carotid is clamped. A fine needle is inserted in the distal internal carotid artery, and this is connected to the arterial pressure monitoring system

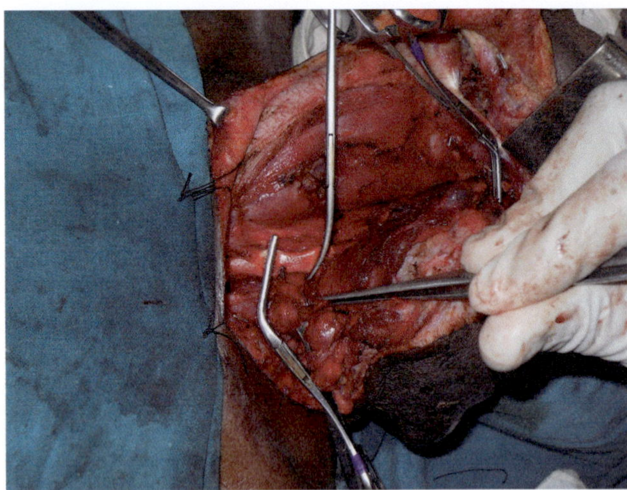

Fig. 5.69 The carotid artery is clamped and ligated at the lower end. It is advisable to transfix both ends to have secure hemostasis

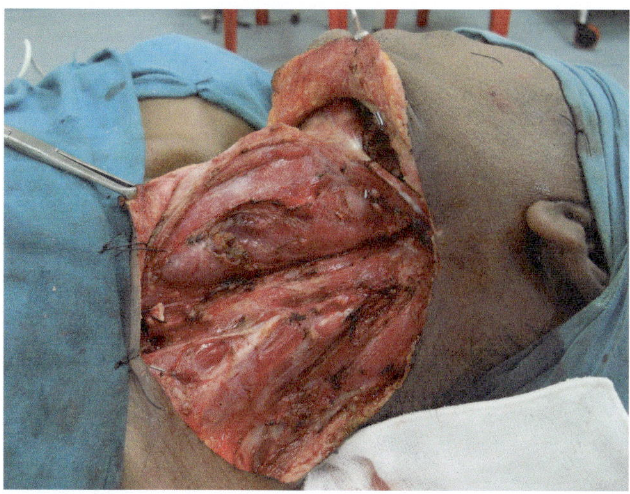

Fig. 5.70 The mass is removed completely without any residual disease

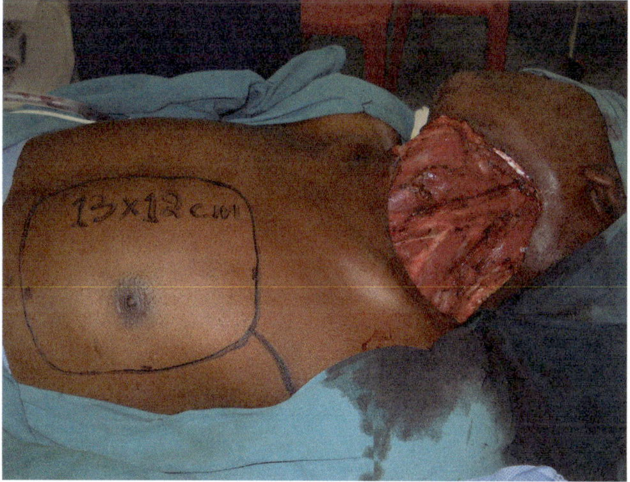

Fig. 5.71 The reconstruction is planned with the PMMC flap

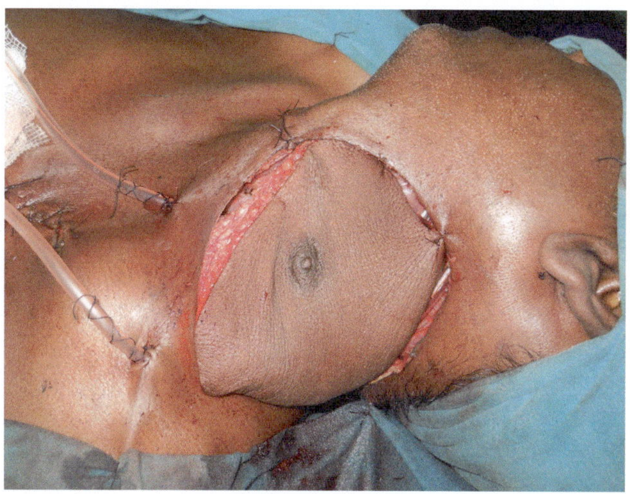

Fig. 5.72 The flap is inserted in the defect. One has to be careful not to overtwist the muscle and cause venous congestion that can actually cause flap loss

Tumors of the Parapharyngeal Space

6

Surgical Anatomy and Pathology

The parapharyngeal space is an imaginary space situated lateral to the pharyngeal tube containing vital neurovascular bundles. It is an inverse triangle where the base is formed by base of skull, while apex is formed by hyoid bone. This space is strategically situated in the head and neck as tumor starting from the pharyngeal mucosa spreads laterally and this space proves as a barrier to deep spread. Isolation of the tumor base early in this space makes clearance easy and complete at depth. Figure 6.1 demonstrates the important neurovascular bundles that traverse this space. It essentially contains the carotid artery and branches of external carotid artery and internal jugular vein. Various cranial nerves run along and across this space. Ligation of branches of the external carotid artery and parapharyngeal venous plexus exposes the parapharyngeal space.

Figure 6.2 demonstrates cross-sectional anatomy of the parapharyngeal space. The band connecting the styloid process and pterygoid plate divides this space into an anterior pre-styloid compartment and a posterior post-styloid compartment. The pre-styloid space contains the deep lobe of the parotid, minor salivary gland, parapharyngeal fat pad, and few lymph nodes. The post-styloid compartment contains the carotid sheath and cervical sympathetic chain. The diagnosis of tumor in this space is essentially made by understanding the anatomy of this space. Imaging study with a CT scan or magnetic resonance imaging (MRI) classifies the lesion as a pre-styloid or post-styloid one. This provides a differential diagnosis regarding the origin of the tumor. The tumor arising from the pre-styloid compartment generally presents as an intraoral bulge and displaces the parapharyngeal fat pad posteriorly, while the post-styloid tumor presents as a lump in the neck and pushes fat anteriorly. The carotid sheath is pushed posteriorly by the pre-styloid tumor, and the stylomandibular tunnel is widened in case of deep lobe parotid lesion. For long-standing pre-styloid lesions, the posterolateral wall of the maxilla can be pushed anteriorly due to persistent pressure. The post-styloid lesions generally arise from the carotid sheath, and the carotid body tumor is one of the most common among them. This tumor originates from the carotid bulb area and splays both carotid arteries that can be clearly demonstrated in scans. The nerve sheath tumors arising from the vagus and sympathetic chain are located posterior to the carotid vessels. It is essential to remember that tissue diagnosis is not routinely required in parapharyngeal space lesions. Imaging is a primary diagnostic modality and diagnosis is based on its location and understanding of the anatomy. Fine-needle cytology (FNAC) should always be considered after confirming findings of imaging study to avoid injuring vascular lesions.

N. Trivedi, *Atlas of Head and Neck Cancer Surgery: The Compartment Surgery for Resection in 3-D*,
DOI 10.1007/978-81-322-2050-3_6, © Springer India 2015

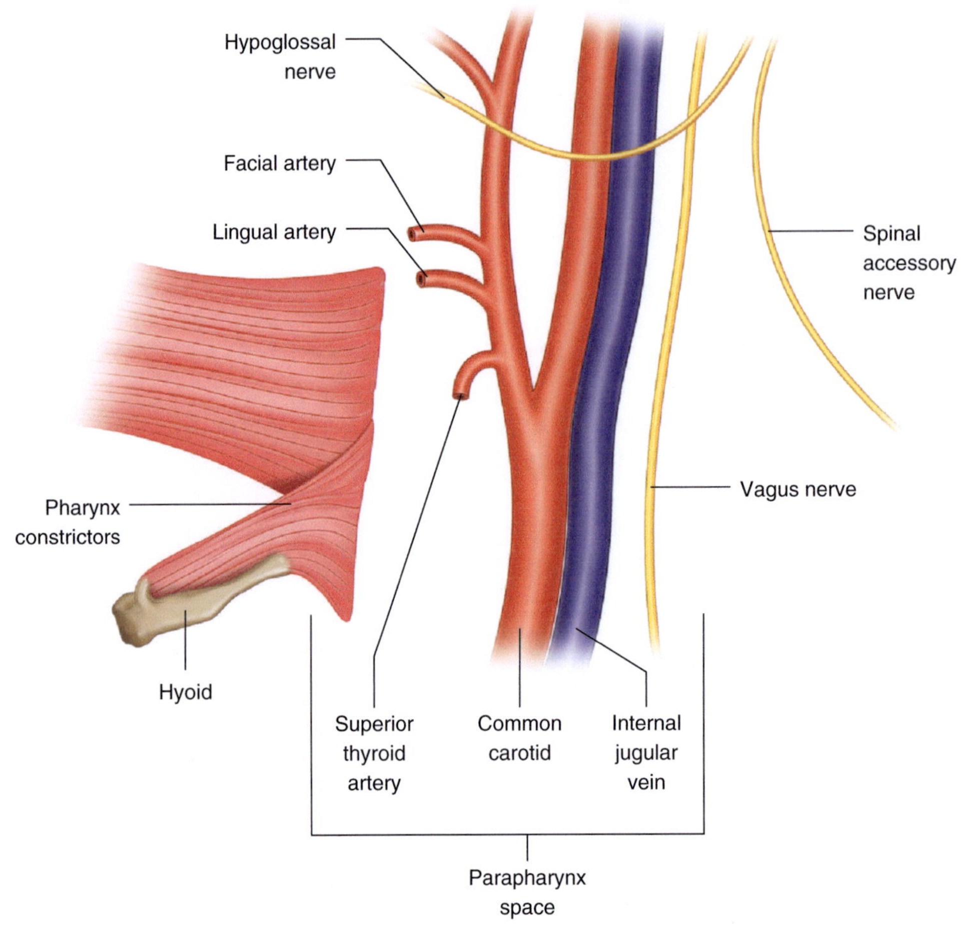

Fig. 6.1 Schematic representation of surgical anatomy

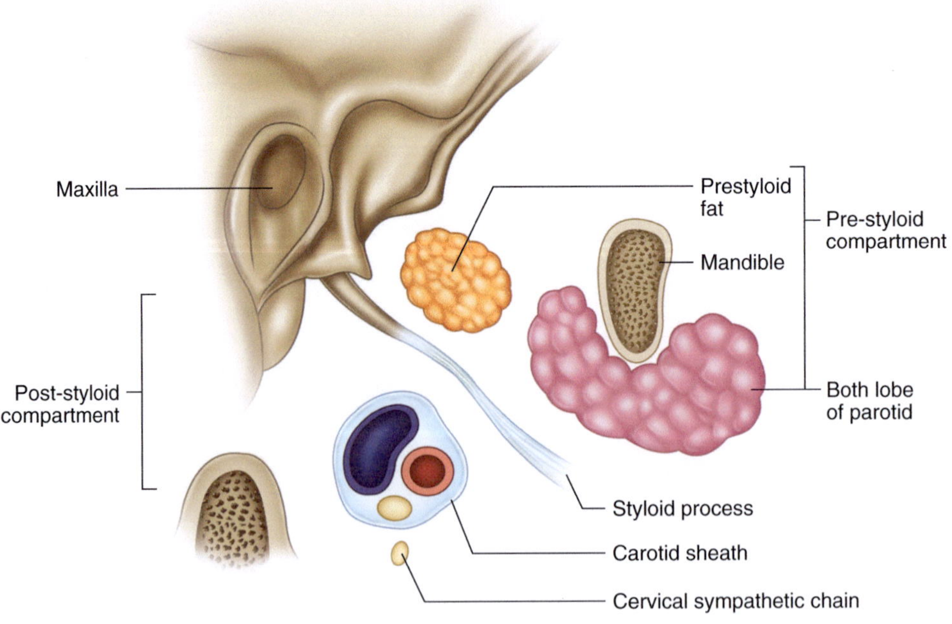

Fig. 6.2 Classification of parapharynx space

Surgical Concepts

- Diagnosis is based on imaging study. Understanding of surgical anatomy is key in identifying the origin of the lesion.
- The concept is to identify all nerves and vessels early in the surgical procedure rather than trying to focus on removing the tumor. This enables us to avoid injury to any important structure, and in the process the tumor automatically gets mobilized.
- The pre-styloid lesions generally originate from deep lobe of the parotid or minor salivary gland, and transcervical or trans-parotid surgical approaches are commonly preferred.
- The post-styloid tumors are generally approached from the transcervical route (Fig. 6.3). The conventional mandibulotomy approach for high parapharyngeal space lesions is almost obsolete in the current surgical practice. The vast majority of lesions can be removed through the neck by mobilizing the mandible anteriorly by releasing the stylomandibular ligament. Ligation of external carotid artery can expose high parapharyngeal space, and these lesions can be easily addressed.
- It is advisable to pack this space with absorbable hemostatic materials to prevent persistent postoperative bleeding.

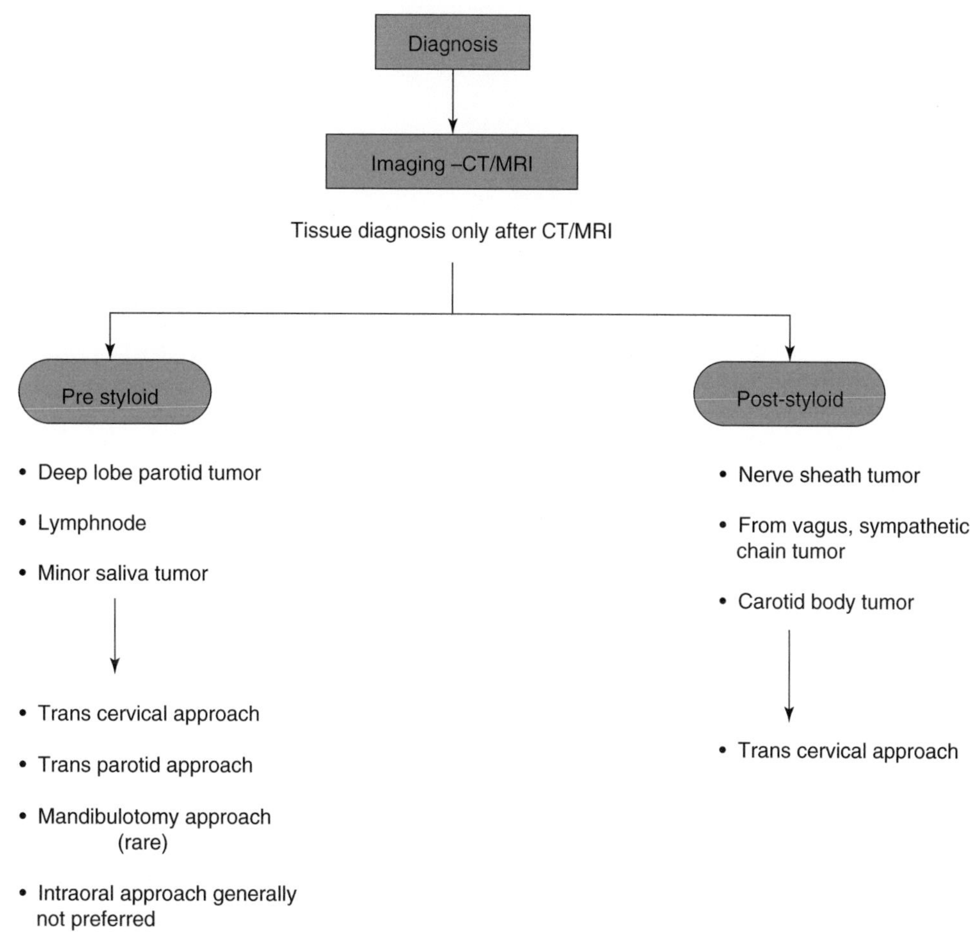

Fig. 6.3 Treatment algorithm

Post-styloid Tumor

This procedure demonstrates removal of a nerve sheath lesion arising from the cervical sympathetic chain in post-styloid space.

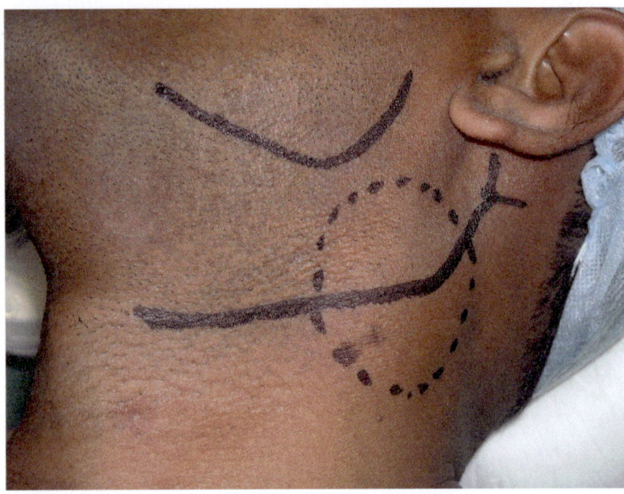

Fig. 6.4 Presentation of a patient with deep upper cervical swelling. The pre-styloid lesion generally presents with an intraoral swelling

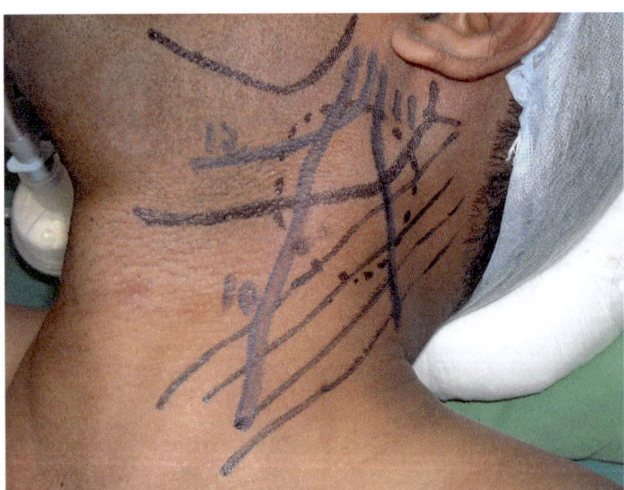

Fig. 6.5 Surface marking of cranial nerves – vagus, spinal accessory, and hypoglossal nerves

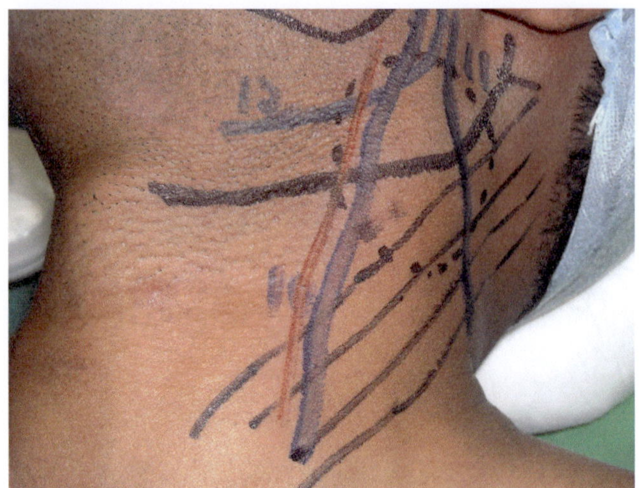

Fig. 6.6 Relation with carotid sheath

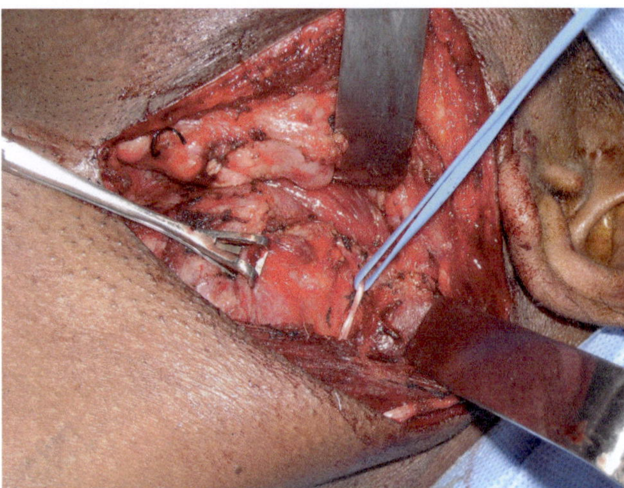

Fig. 6.7 It is advisable to remove fibro-fatty tissue at level II nodal area at an early stage to get enough space to mobilise the tumor

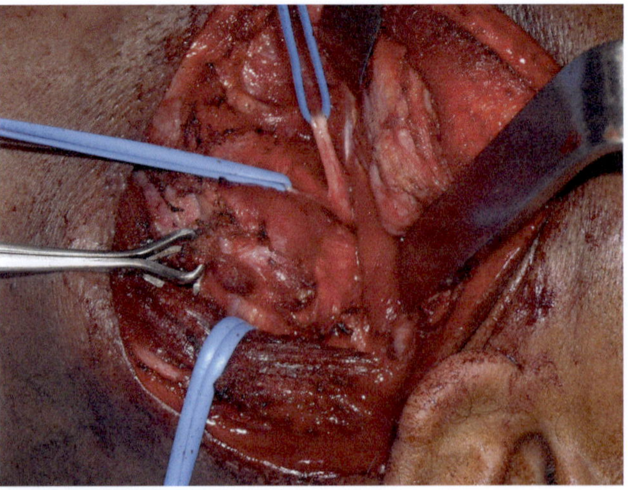

Fig. 6.8 The hypoglossal nerve with its descending branch

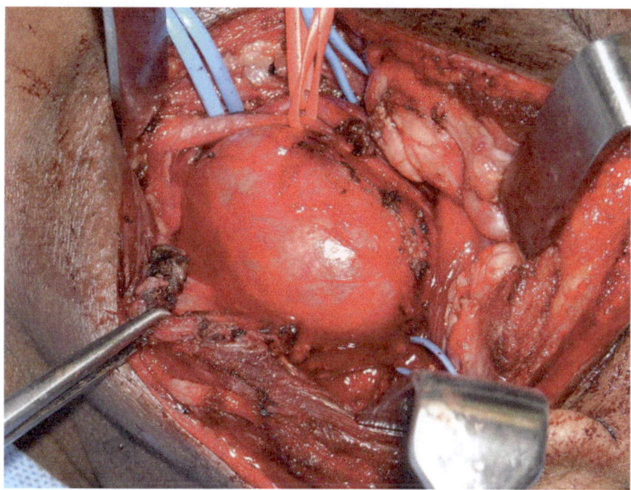

Fig. 6.9 Exposure of lesion after separating the carotid artery. It is of utmost importance to isolate all neurovascular structures before focusing attention to address the tumor. This prevents injury to important structures and the lesion gets mobilized in the process

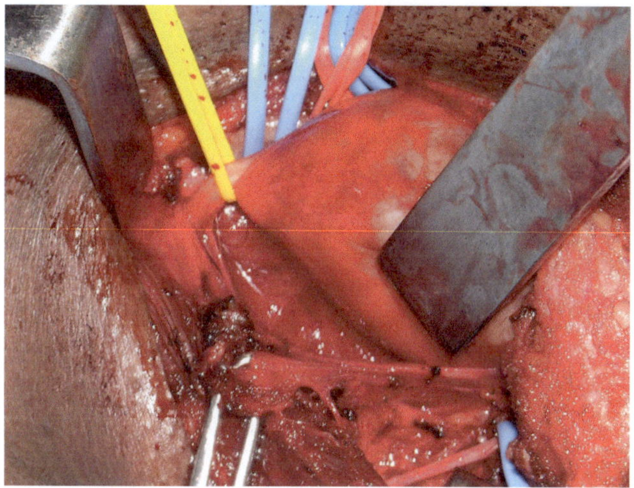

Fig. 6.10 Sympathetic nerve stump

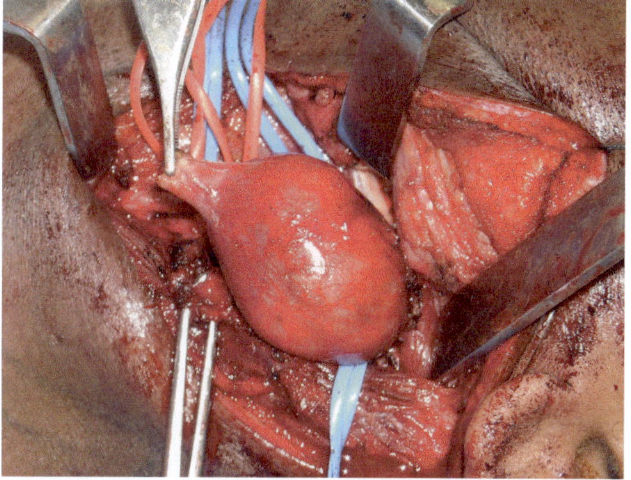

Fig. 6.11 Complete excision of lesion

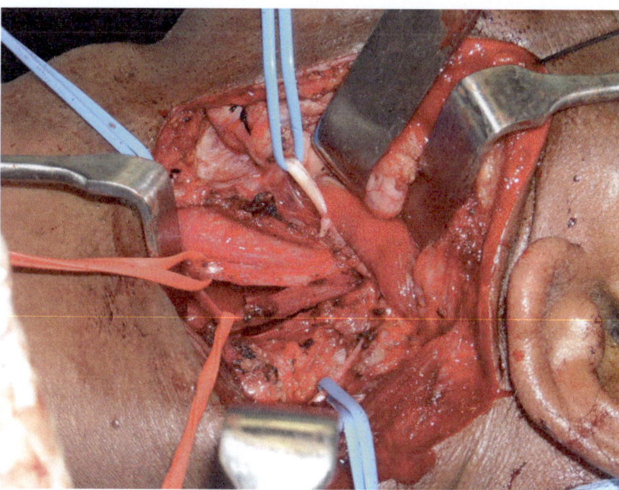

Fig. 6.12 All neurovascular structures are preserved. There may be paresis of some nerves, post-operatively and the resulting problems should be discussed with the patient before the operative procedure. These are usually self-limiting and the nerve recovers within few months

Pre-styloid Tumor

This procedure demonstrates removal of a pre-styloid minor salivary gland pleomorphic adenoma.

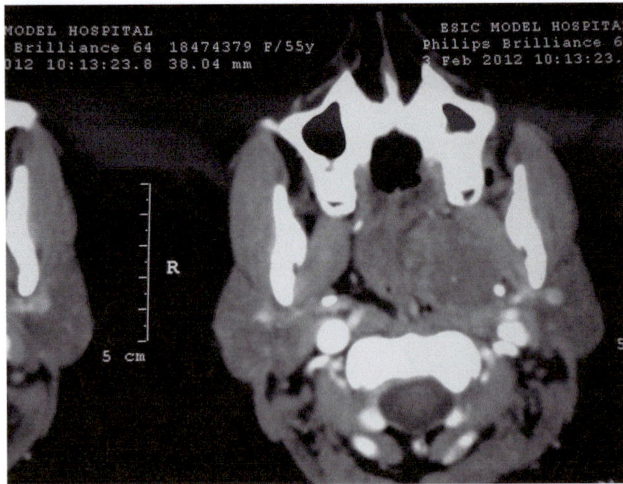

Fig. 6.13 CT scan shows pre-styloid lesion. The fat pad is pushed backwards, and the carotid vessels are posterior to the lesion. The stylomandibular tunnel is not enlarged, and there is a plane between the lesion and deep lobe of parotid gland. This favors diagnosis of minor salivary gland lesion compared to deep lobe tumor. This helps in planning the surgical approach as this lesion can be delivered by a transcervical approach rather than trans-parotid approach

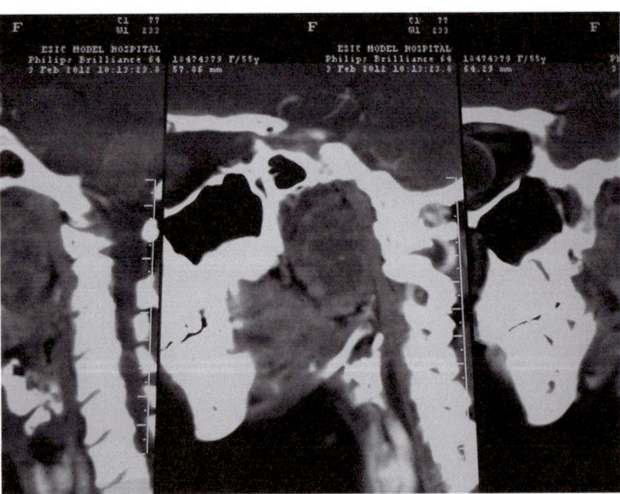

Fig. 6.14 CT scan of lesion reaching the skull base. This lesion will not present as a swelling in the neck but will present as intraoral swelling in the oropharynx area

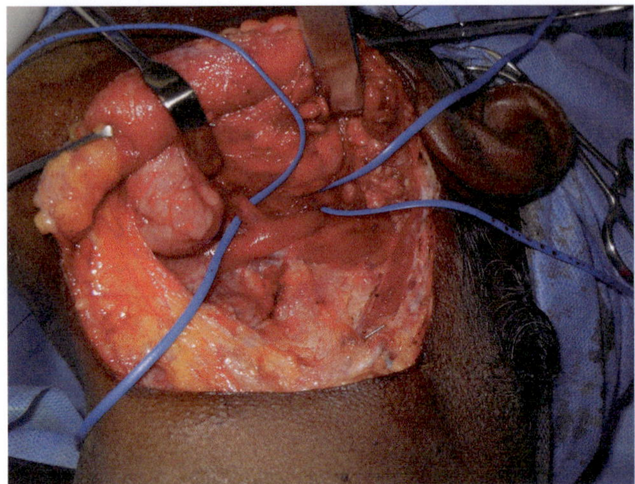

Fig. 6.15 The submandibular gland is exposed and pushed anteriorly. The facial vessel is isolated

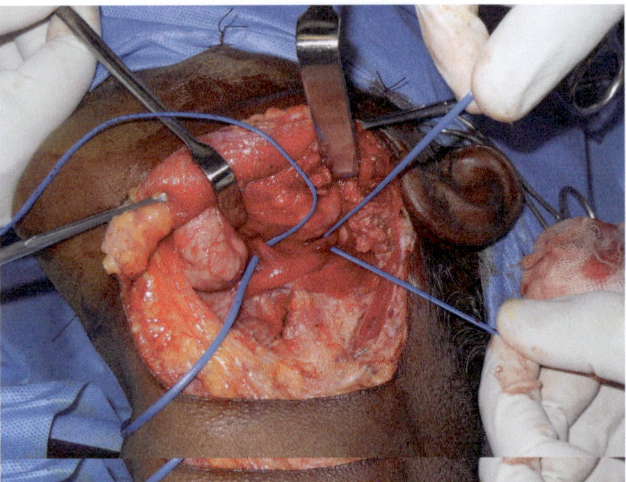

Fig. 6.16 The photograph shows exposed isolated and secured external carotid artery where it enters the deep lobe of parotid. This is an important step while dealing tumor in this area as unexpected bleeding can be easily avoided

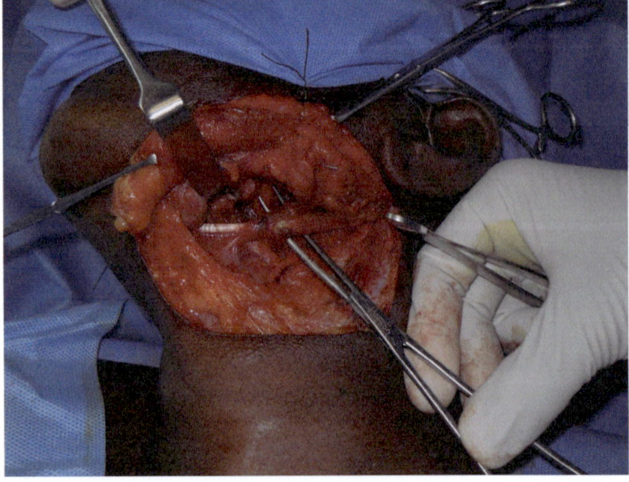

Fig. 6.17 The posterior belly of digastric is cut to gain adequate exposure

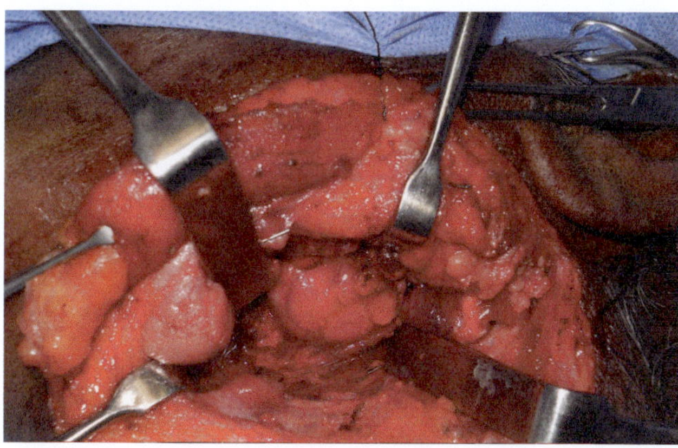

Fig. 6.18 The tumor is coming into vision

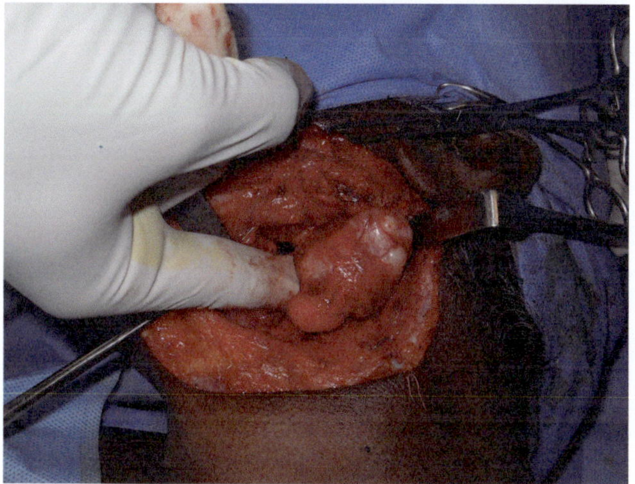

Fig. 6.19 The lesion can be mobilized easily by finger dissection. This needs to be gentle and one has to take care of adequate hemostasis

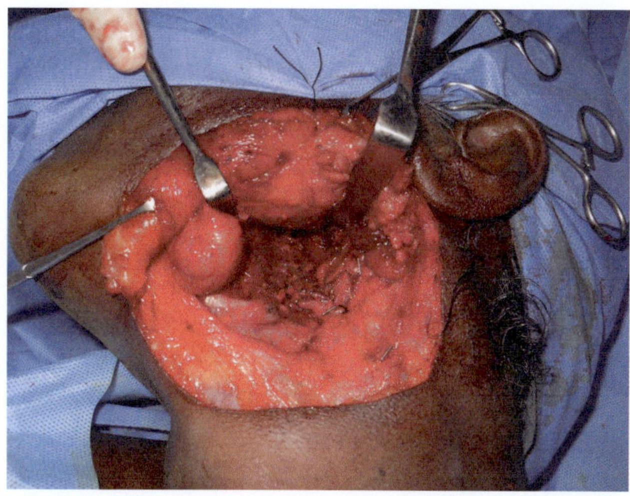

Fig. 6.20 The postoperative picture. It is important to fill the defect with absorbable hemostatic materials to prevent collection

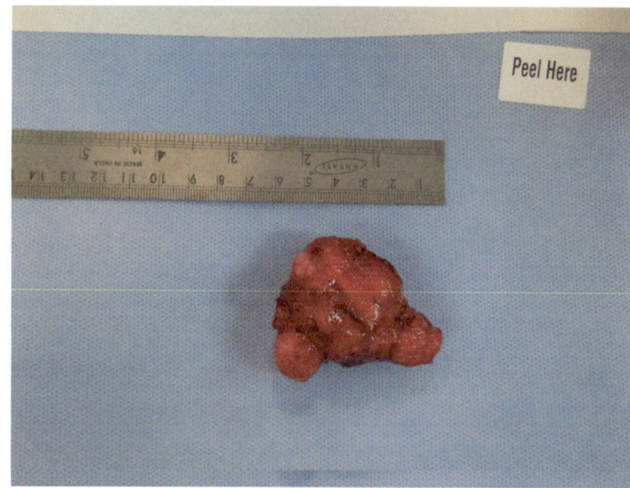

Fig. 6.21 The photograph of the specimen

The Carotid Body Tumor

This procedure demonstrates resection of the carotid body tumor.

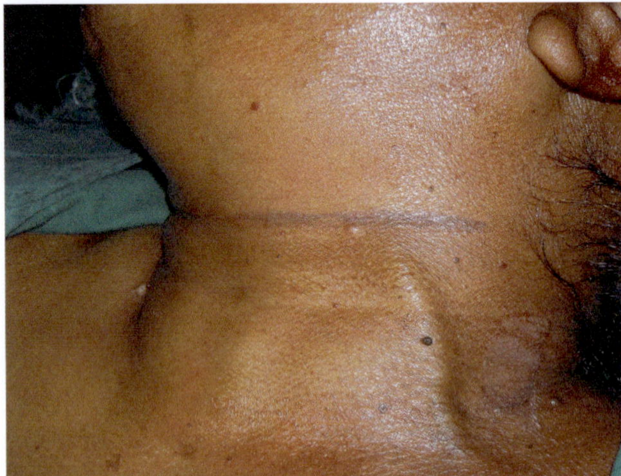

Fig. 6.22 Transverse cervical incision

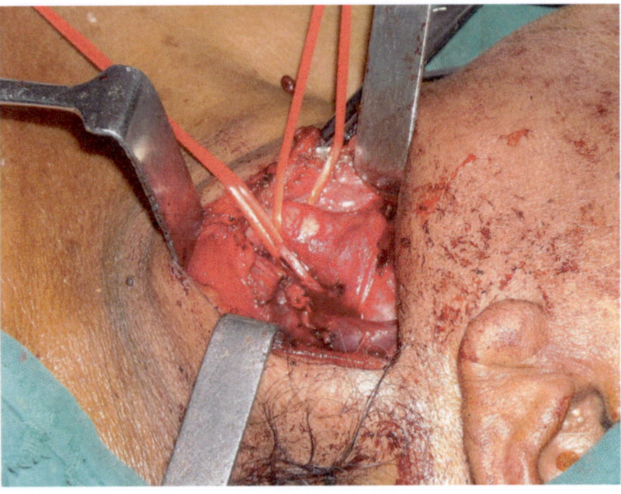

Fig. 6.23 Exposure of the spinal accessory nerve, internal jugular vein, and common carotid artery after removing tissue in level II

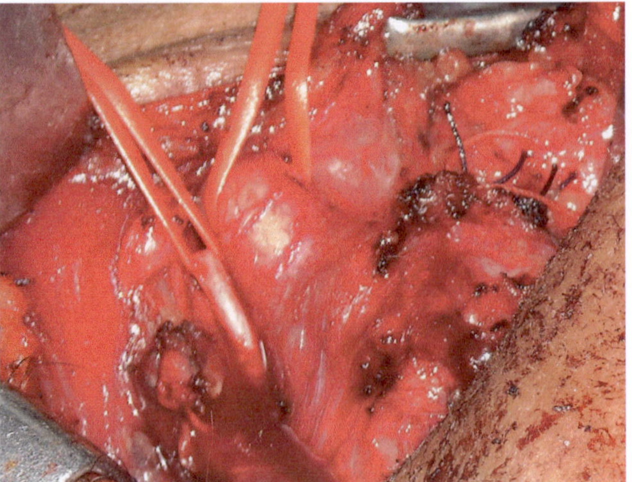

Fig. 6.24 Exposure of the vagus nerve and carotid bulb

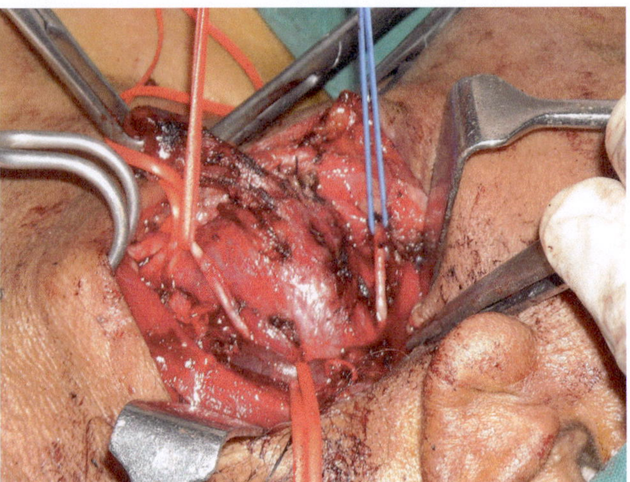

Fig. 6.25 Isolation of hypoglossal nerve. All the related nerves and vessels have been isolated. It is also advisable to identify branches of external carotid artery and ligate them at the periphery. In majority of carotid body tumors, the external carotid artery is ligated at its origin from the common carotid artery. Early ligation of its branches also helps in case of unexpected injury to major vessels. The back flow is prevented and clamping is easy

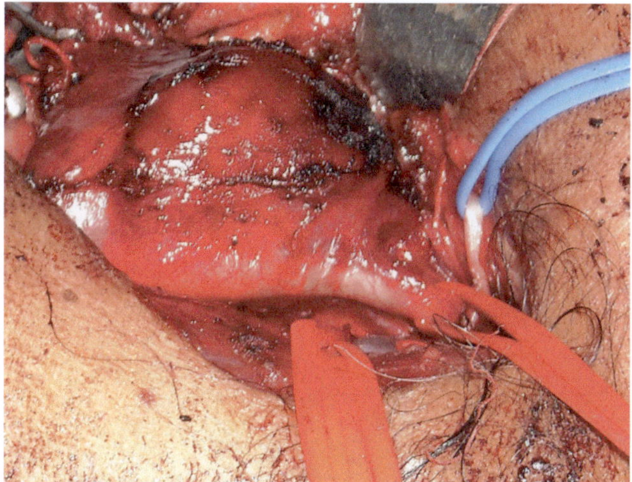

Fig. 6.26 With this manoeuvre, bottom portion of common cartoid and top portion of internal cartoid is under control. This helps in controlling the bleeding in case of an emergency

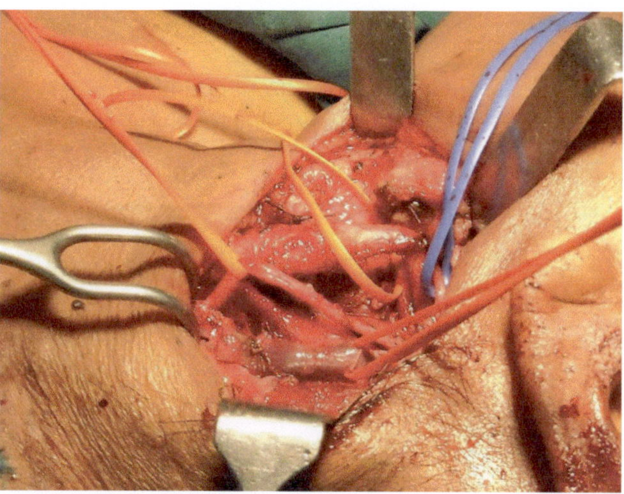

Fig. 6.28 The final picture with all structures preserved

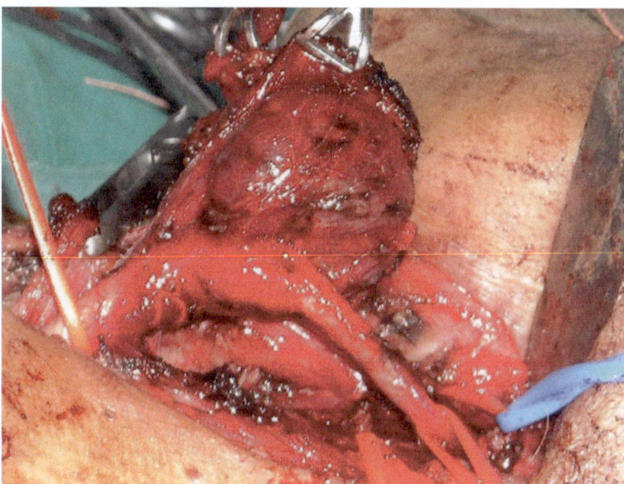

Fig. 6.27 The further dissection is carried out with bipolar cautery. The textbook description is to perform subadventitial dissection, but one can use bipolar cautery to peel off the lesion from the carotid artery. The major feeder comes in the carotid bulb area in the posteromedial aspect, and one should be very careful in dealing with this area. Ideally this area should be dealt at last after separating the tumor all around. In case of bleeding, clamps can be applied to CCA and ICA in emergency.

In case of emergency bleeding, apply the clamps and secure the bleeding. Advise the anesthetist to keep the systolic blood pressure high and administer intravenous anticoagulants to minimize intracranial hypoxia. The tumor can be removed and the small rent can be primarily sutured. If the rent is big or the vessel wall is very weak, it is advisable to either bypass the area with venous graft or synthetic graft. One may have to ligate the vessel if this is not possible. The retrograde flow from the upper end of the internal carotid vessel gives a good indication regarding adequacy of contralateral circulation

Vascular Malformation

This procedure demonstrates steps of operation for the case of low-flow malformation in the parapharyngeal space.

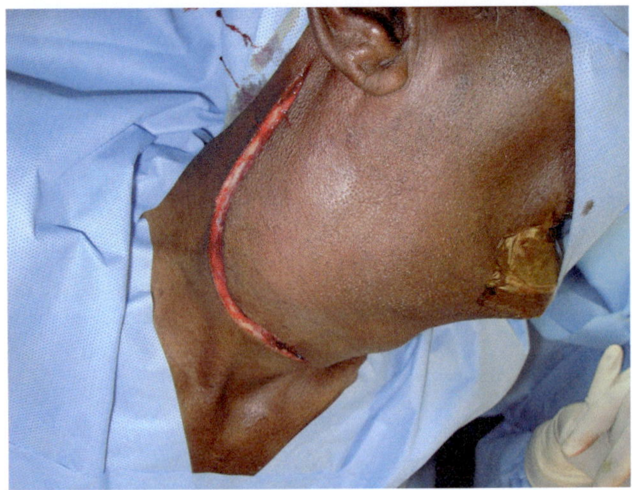

Fig. 6.29 Hockey-shaped incision for complete exposure of the neck

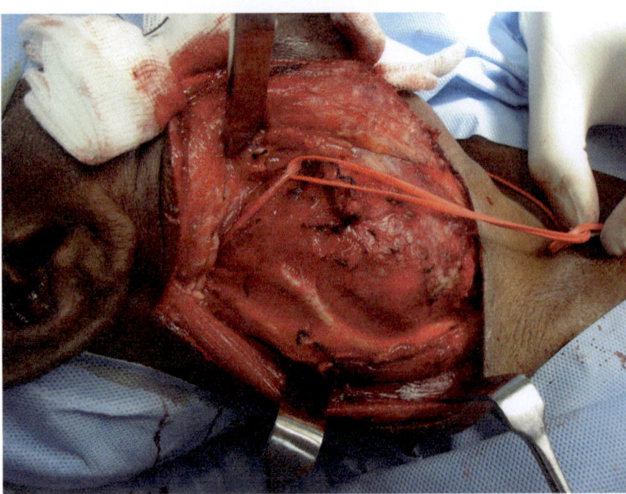

Fig. 6.31 Exposing the carotid vessels and cranial nerves before addressing the lesion

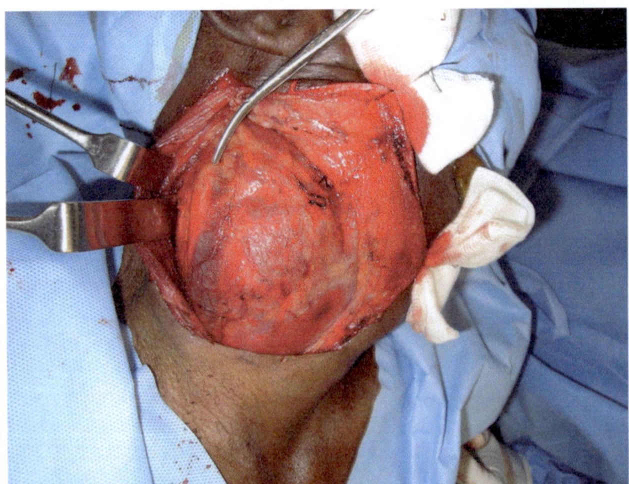

Fig. 6.30 Exposure of the lesion. The IJV is embedded in the fascia containing the lesion

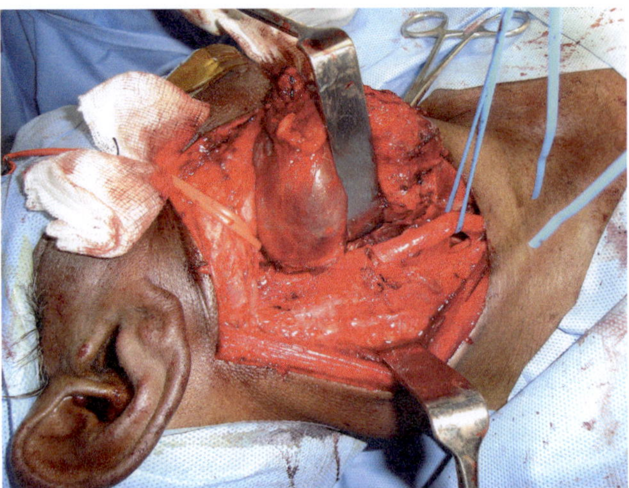

Fig. 6.32 The lesion is being isolated gradually. It is important to be gentle to avoid rupturing the lesion

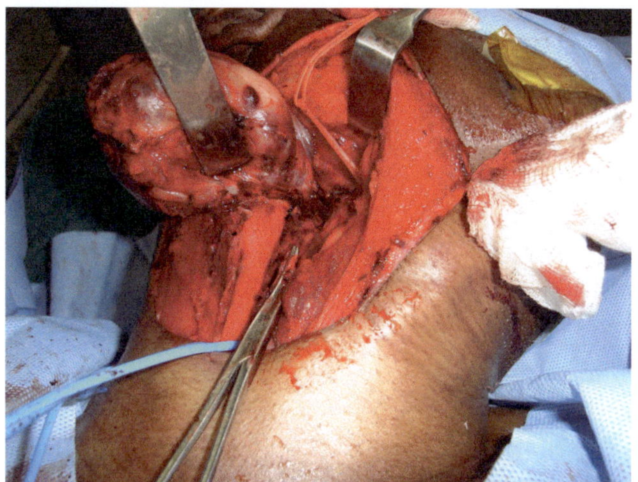

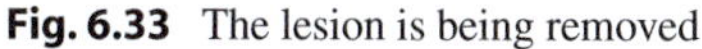

Fig. 6.33 The lesion is being removed

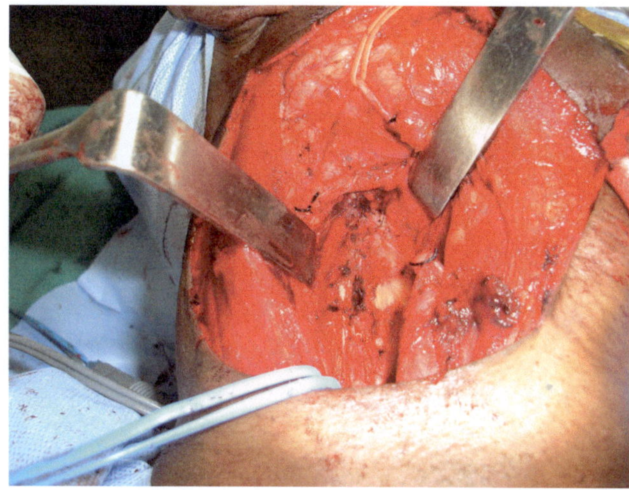

Fig. 6.34 Exposed parapharyngeal space after complete removal of lesion

7 Tumors of the Buccal Mucosa and Alveolus

Surgical Anatomy

The buccal mucosa complex essentially consists of the buccal mucosa (BM), gingivo-buccal sulcus (GBS), lower alveolus, and retromolar trigone (RMT). The buccal complex consists of four layers starting with the mucosa, buccinator muscle, subcutaneous tissue, and skin (in to out). The branches of the facial nerve run in subcutaneous tissue planes over the buccinator muscle. The average distance from mucosa to skin is approximately 1–1.5 cm, and it is very easy for infiltrating tumors to travel across and involve the outermost level. The GBS is located at the junction of the buccal mucosa reflecting over the alveolus. The cancer occurring at this site is very common in the Indian subcontinent due to the habit of tobacco chewing. The retromolar trigone has a unique anatomy with potential for tumor spread into the masticator space. The RMT is bounded below and above by the alveolar ridge, medially by the tonsil, and laterally by the buccal mucosa. It is the third dimension – the base that holds the key to the tumor spread. The mucosa lies directly on ascending ramus of the mandible. The masseter muscle lies lateral to the mandible, and the medial pterygoid muscle lies medial to the mandible with lingual and inferior alveolar nerve running through its substance. The temporalis muscle gets inserted on the coronoid process, and the lateral pterygoid muscle occupies the top half of the masticator space.

Surgical Pathology and Pattern of Infiltration

This complex can be divided into anterior region and posterior region for understanding the pattern of infiltration and planning the surgical approach. The anteriorly located tumors spread laterally to involve soft tissue and skin while posteriorly located tumors spread through the RMT to masticator space (Figs. 7.1, 7.2, and 7.3). The surgical approach remains distinctively separate for both groups of tumors.

The anteriorly located infiltrative tumors have a tendency to invade through the layers of buccal mucosa and fungate through the skin. These tumors start from mucosa and easily infiltrate the buccinator muscle. Involvement of the subcutaneous tissue is also not uncommon and seen quite early in the disease progress. It is strongly recommended to remove one layer extra to get negative margins at depth. The skin invasion is considered a sign of aggressive biology in conventional thinking, and many patients are offered only palliation. This infiltration of the skin is just due to the close proximity to the mucosa and a natural progression of disease. If adequately resected, outcome of these patients have been comparable to other advanced lesions in our experience. The GBS tumors show paramandibular spread mainly due to their location (Fig. 7.4). The actual invasion of the mandible is seen in very few cases even with large soft tissue involvement. It is technically feasible and oncologically safe to perform marginal mandibular resection if bone is not involved – the soft tissue margins need to be adequate. The alveolar tumors generally infiltrate the mandible and then spread either towards the lingual or buccal side.

The posteriorly located lesions tend to infiltrate masticator space (Fig. 7.2). The early lesions of RMT have the potential to invade the mandible, masseter, and the medial pterygoid muscle. It is essential to evaluate the involvement of these structures before planning any conservative surgery. The gross infiltration of masticator space warrants complete clearance of soft tissue in infratemporal fossa. Involvement of lateral pterygoid muscle and pterygoid plate is no longer considered contraindication for surgery. The spread of tumor to pterygomaxillary tissue is considered a relative contraindication as chance of intracranial tumor spread is relatively high.

The buccal cancer patient with history of tobacco chewing commonly presents with premalignant changes in surrounding mucosa and submucous fibrosis. These two factors have significant bearing on surgical planning. It is essential to try and include the area of premalignancy into surgical resection margin. The submucous fibrosis causes trismus that reduces the mouth opening and influences the resection approach and reconstructive options.

N. Trivedi, *Atlas of Head and Neck Cancer Surgery: The Compartment Surgery for Resection in 3-D*,
DOI 10.1007/978-81-322-2050-3_7, © Springer India 2015

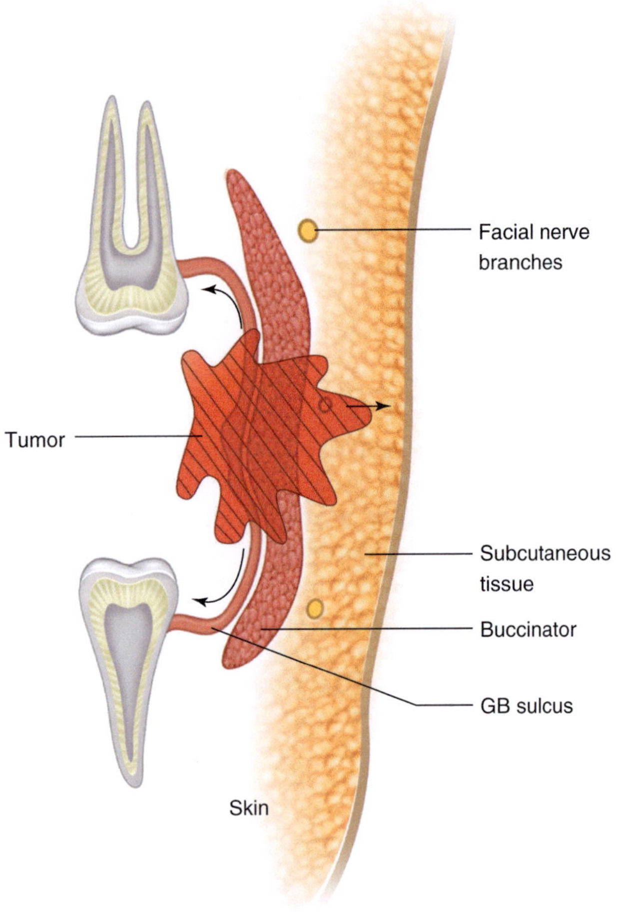

Facial nerve branches
Tumor
Subcutaneous tissue
Buccinator
GB sulcus
Skin

Fig. 7.1 Surgical anatomy and tumor spread in anterior compartment

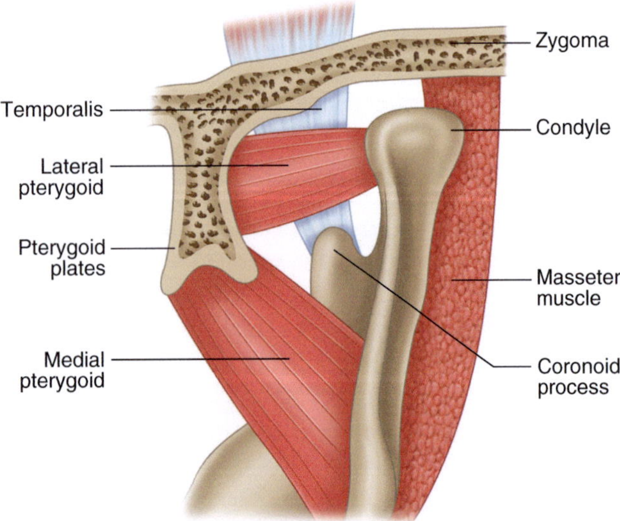

Fig. 7.2 Anatomy of masticator space and tumor spread in posterior compartment

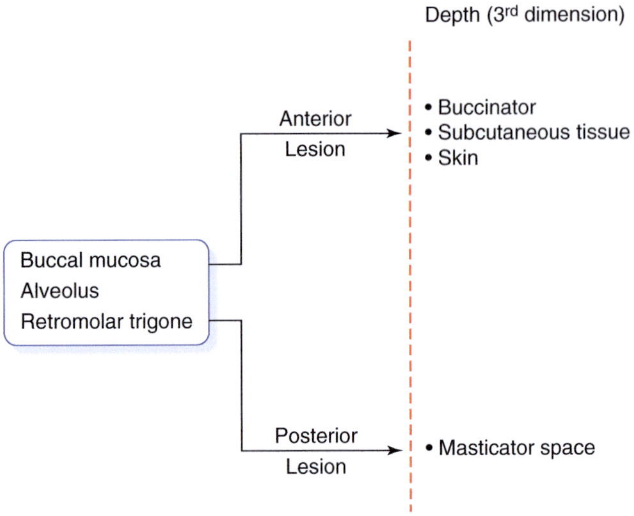

Depth (3rd dimension)

Buccal mucosa
Alveolus
Retromolar trigone

Anterior Lesion → • Buccinator • Subcutaneous tissue • Skin

Posterior Lesion → • Masticator space

Fig. 7.3 Conceptual diagram for proposed 3-D resection

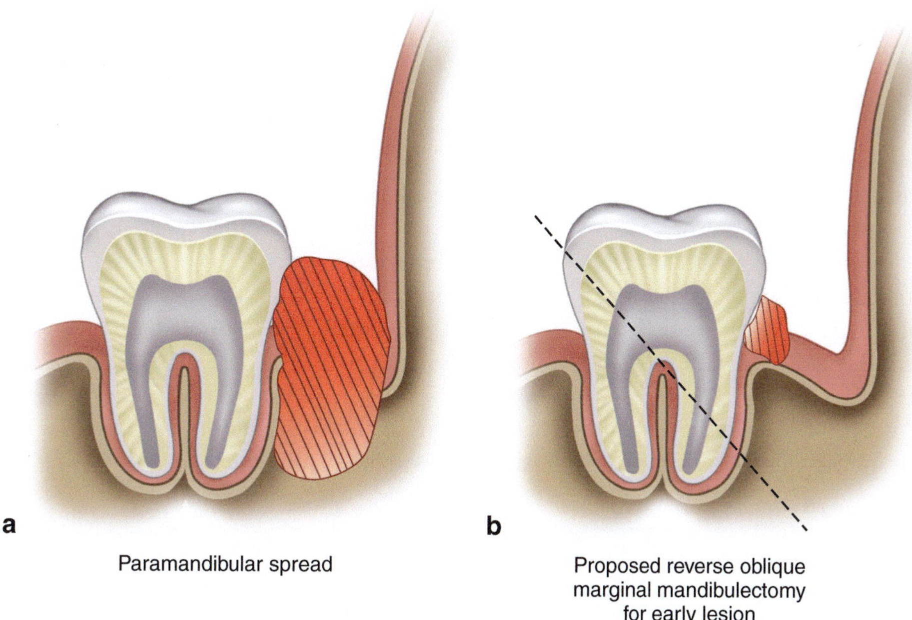

Fig. 7.4 Gingivo-buccal sulcus tumor ÷ pattern of spread

Fig. 7.5 Treatment algorithm

	Pre-cancer	T1/T2	T3/T4	T4b (ITF)
Resection	• (Wide excision) • Intra-oral	(WLE ± marginal mandibulectomy) • Lipsplit • Intra-oral	Composite resection	Composite + ITF clearance
Reconstruction	• 1° closure • Skin grafing • Buccal pad fat • Local flap	• 1° closure • STG • Buccal fat pad • Local flap 1 Infrahyoid 2 Masseter 3 Platysma • PMMC flap • Radial forearm flap	• PMMC • Anterolateral thigh flap (ALT) • Fibula flap • Combined lap	• PMMC • ALT

Surgical Concepts

- Anteriorly located, superficial lesion with adequate mouth opening can be resected through the intraoral approach. It is essential to include buccinator muscle in resection for any malignant lesion.
- Posteriorly located tumors are better approached through lip-split incision.
- It is acceptable to perform marginal mandibulectomy for early GBS cancer abutting but not invading mandible. This is particularly useful for anteriorly located lesions and for patients with minimal submucous fibrosis.
- It is advisable to perform segmental mandibular resection for more advanced lesions with paramandibular spread.
- The posteriorly located tumors with moderate to severe submucous fibrosis do better with segmental resection compared with marginal resection in terms of functional outcome.
- Tumors in the RMT region are tricky to resect, and it is better to be aggressive with these lesions. The local recurrences at skull base after conservative approach are very common and difficult to salvage.

Precancer Lesions

Approach: These lesions can be excised by intraoral approach in majority of cases. The lip split approach may be required for extensive lesions with associated fibrosis.

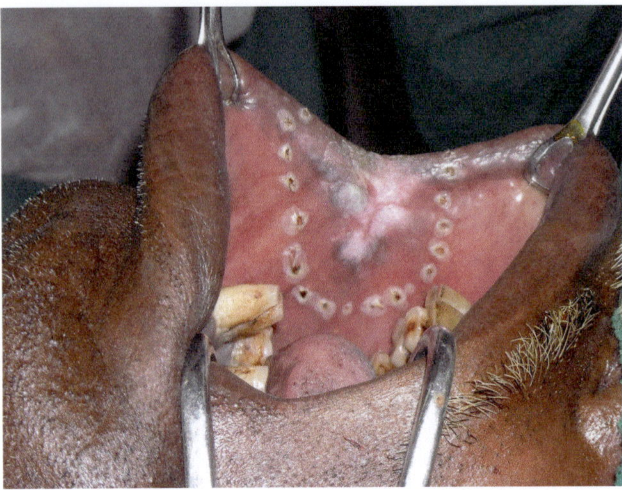

Fig. 7.6 This is a premalignant lesion involving angle of mouth and anterior buccal mucosa. It is important to include all unhealthy mucosa in resection margin. This becomes a bit difficult in certain cases where mucosa of the entire oral cavity is unhealthy, but at least the premalignant lesion needs to be resected

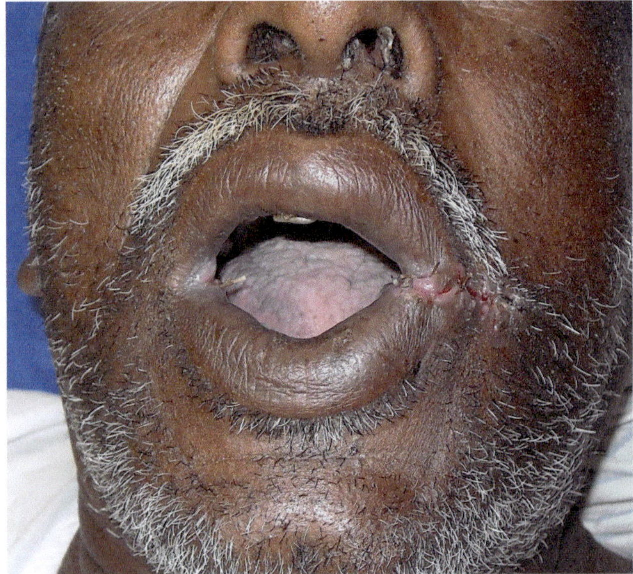

Fig. 7.8 Postoperative recovery after 1 week of surgery. Repair of angle of mouth and approximation of lip muscles are key in maintaining continence

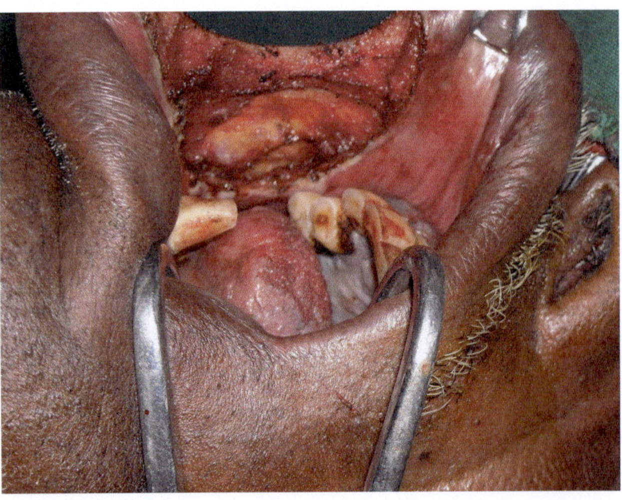

Fig. 7.7 The photograph showing extent of resection. It is better to include buccinator muscle in your resection base if lesion is a malignant one. It is sufficient to remove the mucosa and submucosa and superficial part of the buccinator muscle for purely premalignant lesion

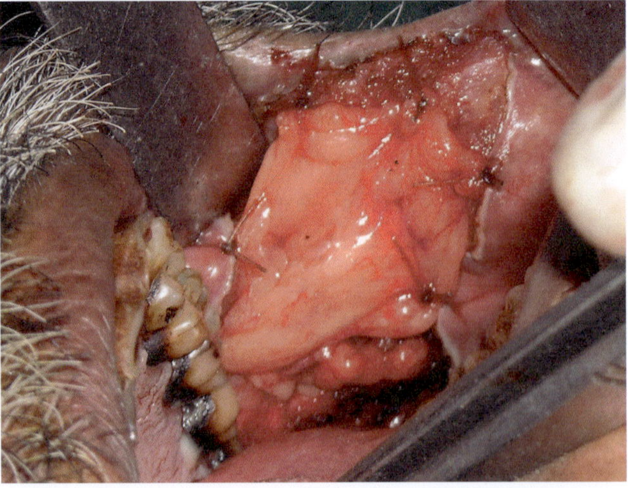

Fig. 7.9 Similar defect being repaired by buccal pad of fat. The fat pad is situated in the infratemporal fossa region and can be easily teased out to repair small buccal defects

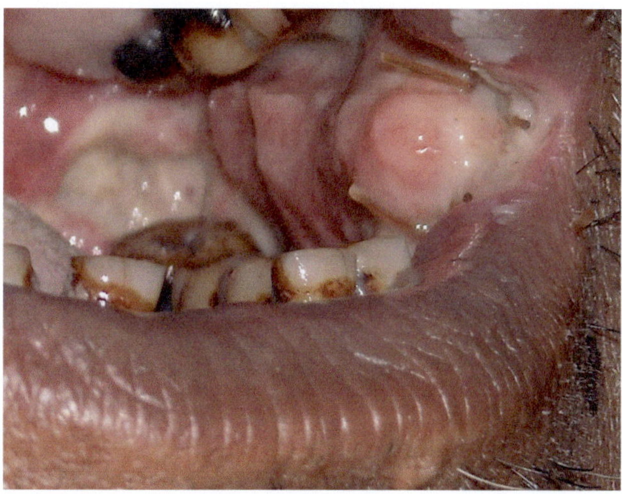

Fig. 7.10 Result after 10 days of healing

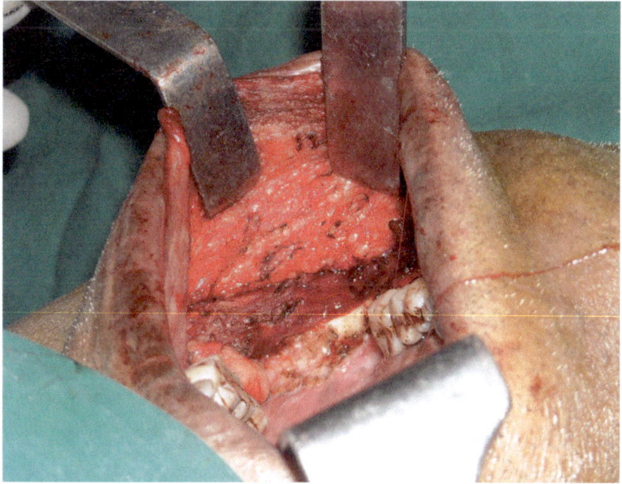

Fig. 7.11 Removal of entire buccal mucosa and buccinator muscle for extensive precancer lesion

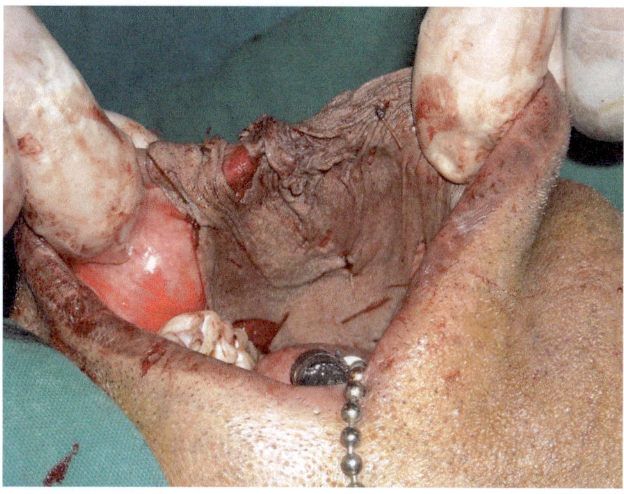

Fig. 7.12 Reconstruction with split thickness skin graft (STG). It is essential to fix the graft with bolster in cheek with through and through stitch. In majority of cases, STG gradually comes off but acts as biological dressing and improves mucolization. Trismus is a real problem with this kind of reconstruction, and it is essential to do rigorous mouth opening exercise for a period of 6–12 months

T1–T2 Lesions

Approach: Intraoral if small lesion with adequate mouth opening. Lip-split approach is preferred for large, infiltrative, or posteriorly located tumors and with associated trismus.

Intraoral Resection

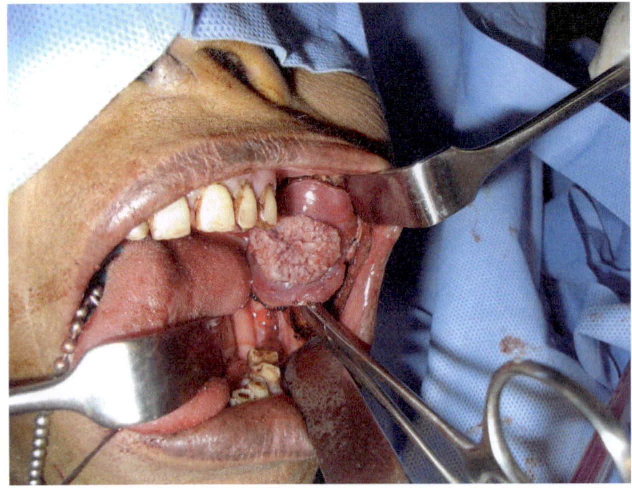

Fig. 7.13 A verrucous lesion of anterior buccal mucosa. These lesions are more exophytic than infiltrative and can be ideally approached without lip split

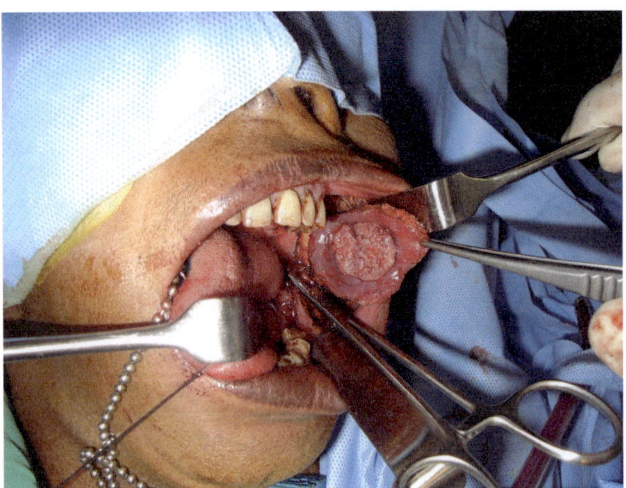

Fig. 7.14 It is advisable to include buccinator muscle in base. The branches of facial artery run across the field and securing them early in resection (below and posterior aspect) reduces bleeding. The branches of facial nerve run deep to the buccinator in subcutaneous tissue. These branches can be preserved for superficial lesions by keeping some fibers of buccinator muscle. It is our strong recommendation not to compromise on resection at depth in case of infiltrative lesion to preserve facial nerve branches

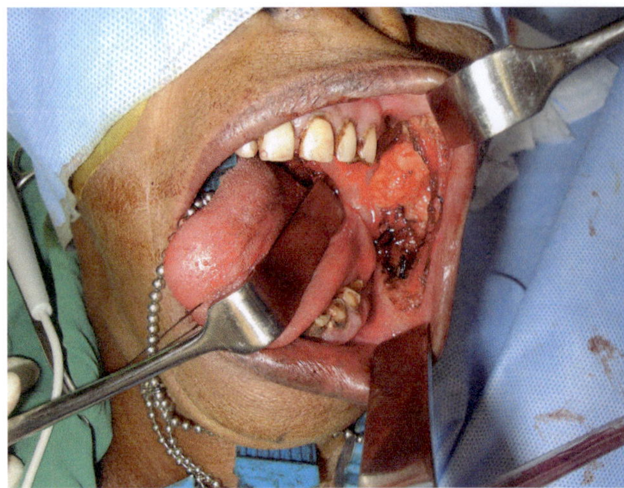

Fig. 7.15 Photograph showing ligated branches of facial artery. The subcutaneous tissue is visible in bed demonstrating removal of buccinator muscle in specimen

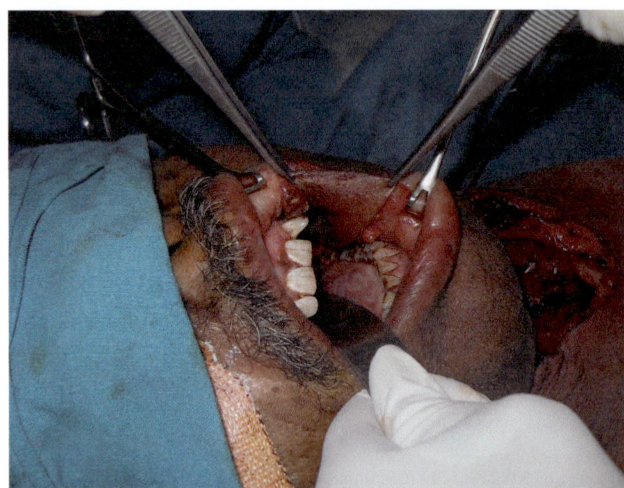

Fig. 7.16 The infrahyoid local flap being inserted for defect

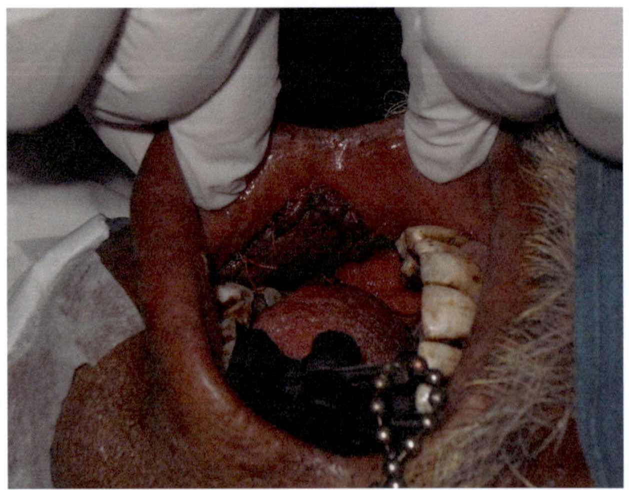

Fig. 7.17 Flap in position

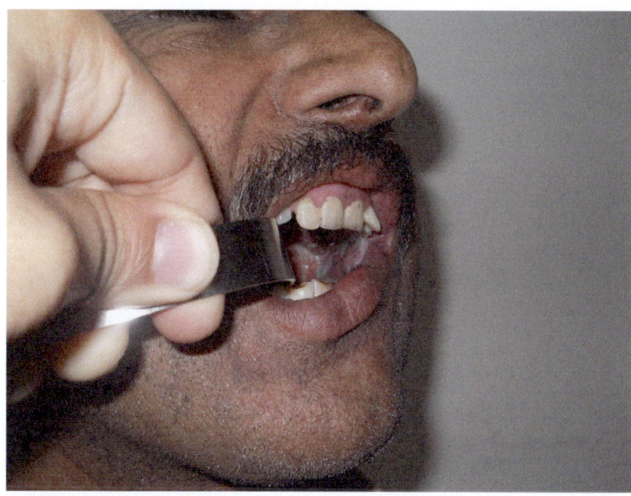

Fig. 7.18 Photograph after 1 month of procedure

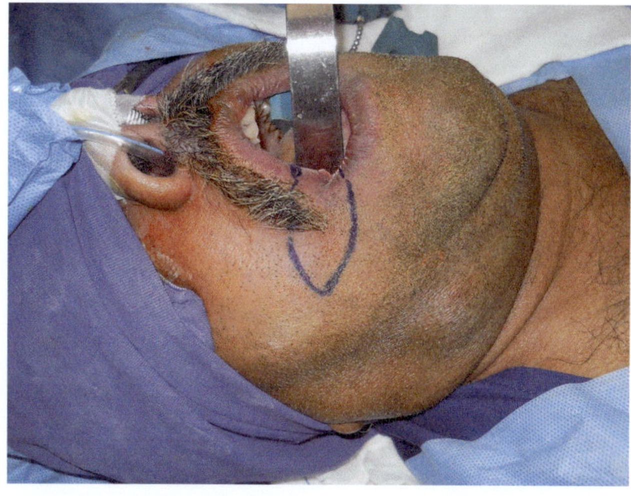

Fig. 7.21 The planning included part of the skin even though it was not obviously involved. It gives complete control of removal of base, and there is no chance of positive margin at depth

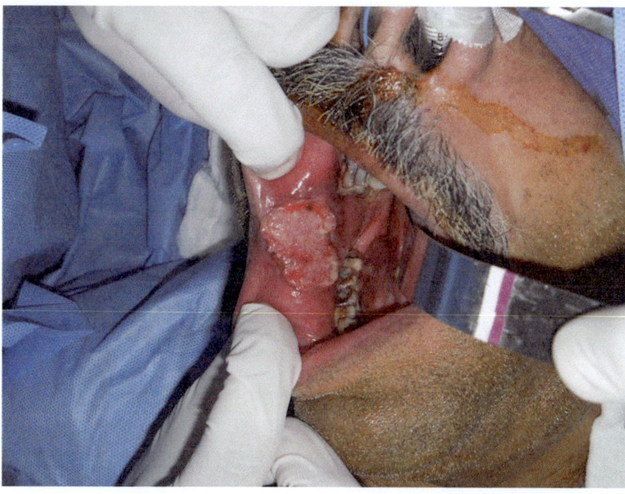

Fig. 7.19 Infiltrative lesion in anterior buccal mucosa with no trismus

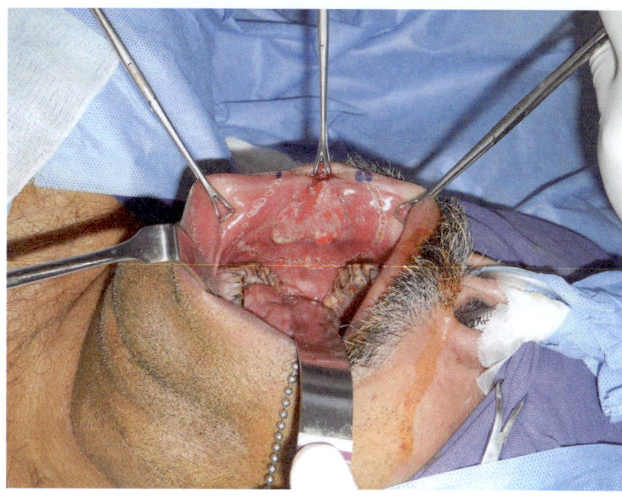

Fig. 7.22 Mucosal markings with adequate margins

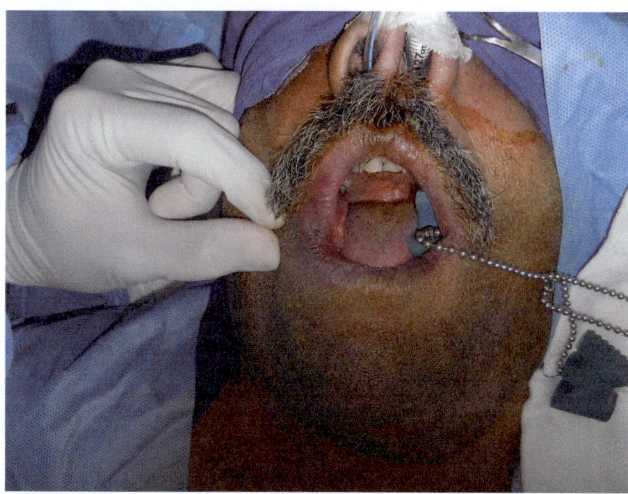

Fig. 7.20 The way to feel for involvement of subcutaneous tissue or skin

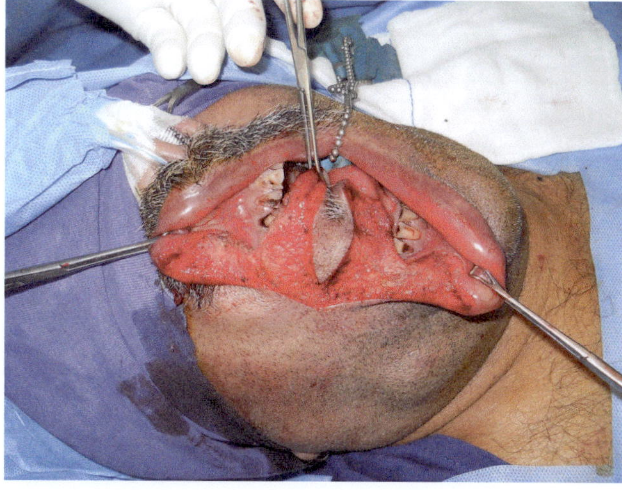

Fig. 7.23 Resection including skin

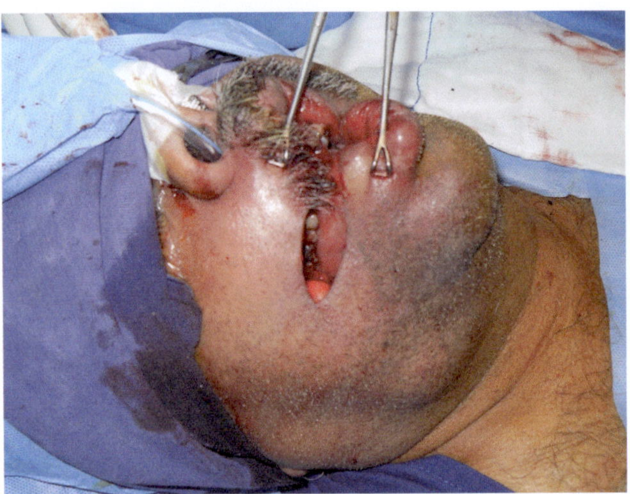

Fig. 7.24 Planned primary closure with buccal pad of fat for cover

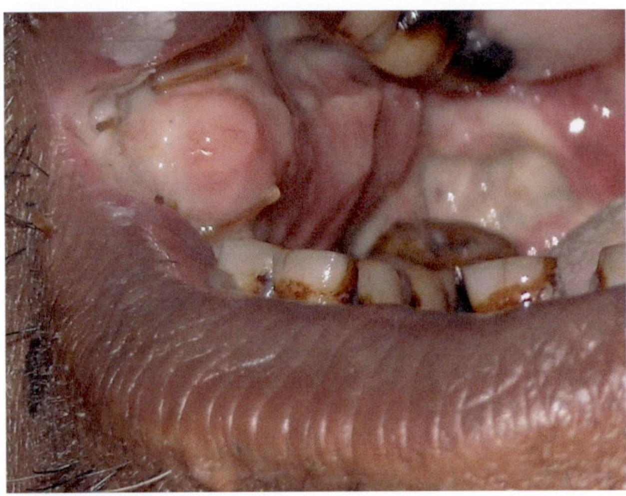

Fig. 7.25 Post-op photo showing healed buccal pad of fat. Mouth opening exercise in post-op phase remains the most important factor influencing trismus

Lip-Split Approach

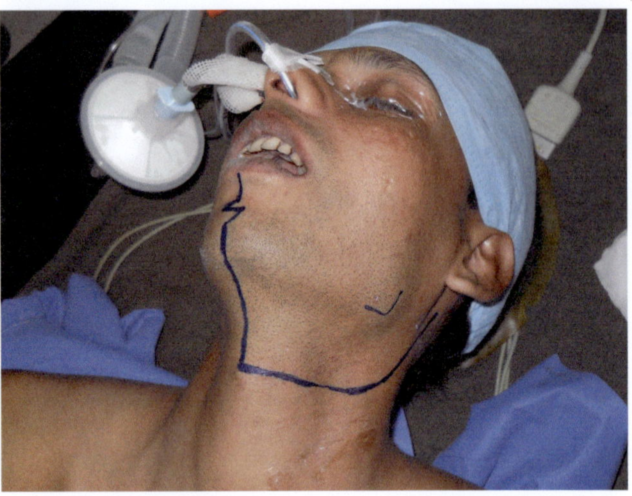

Fig. 7.26 The planned incision for midline lip split. There are various ways to mark the midline lip split, and this photo shows step ladder approach. It is just a personal preference and all approaches give equal cosmetic outcome if properly sutured

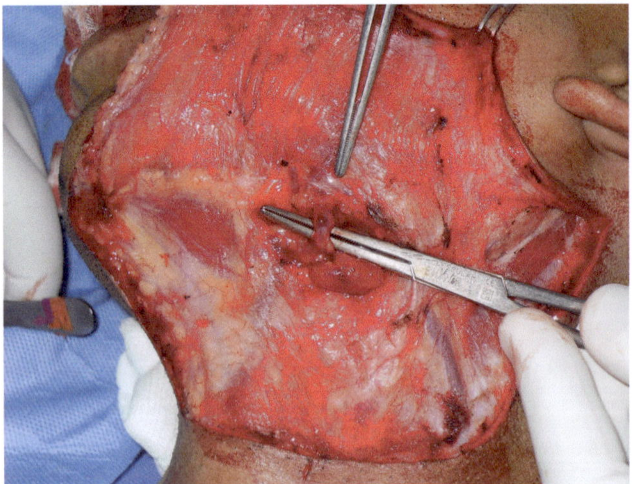

Fig. 7.27 The photograph shows relation of marginal mandibular nerve with facial artery

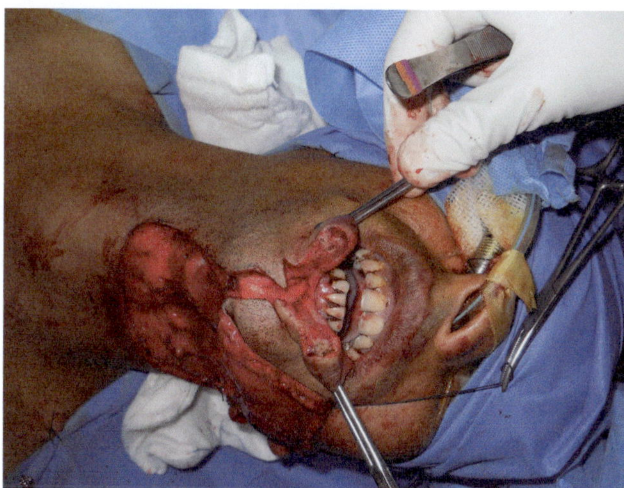

Fig. 7.28 The splitting of the lip. It is advisable to use a knife to split the lip mucosa to avoid post-op edema. The labial arteries are secured with use of electrocautery preferably with bipolar cautery

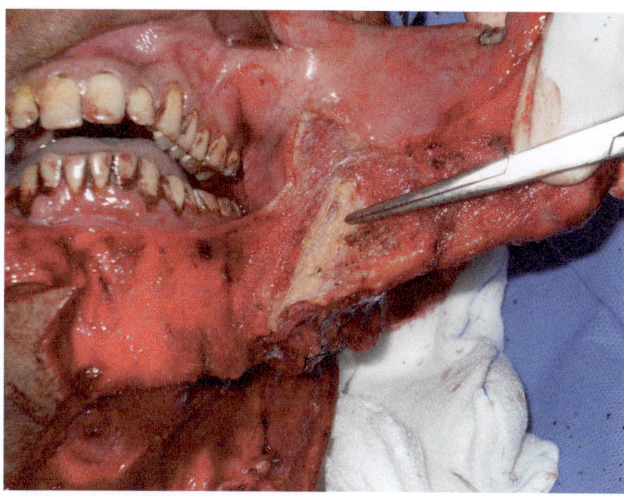

Fig. 7.31 The cheek flap is raised in subcutaneous plane deep to the buccinator muscle. The facial nerve branches are sacrificed in case if tumor is an infiltrative one and preserved if it is an exophytic one

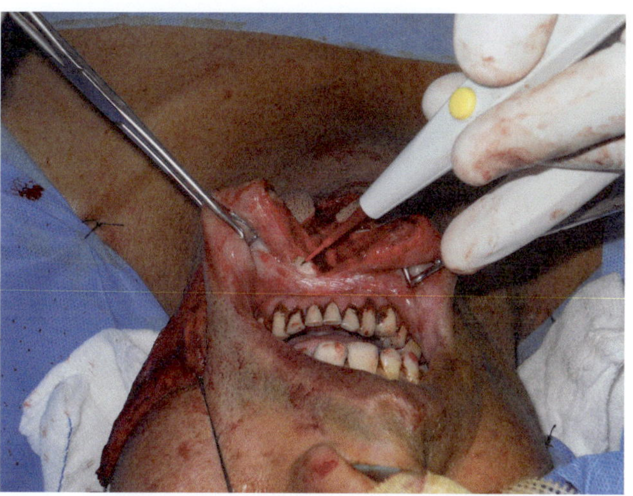

Fig. 7.29 The cheek flap is raised on the side of the lesion

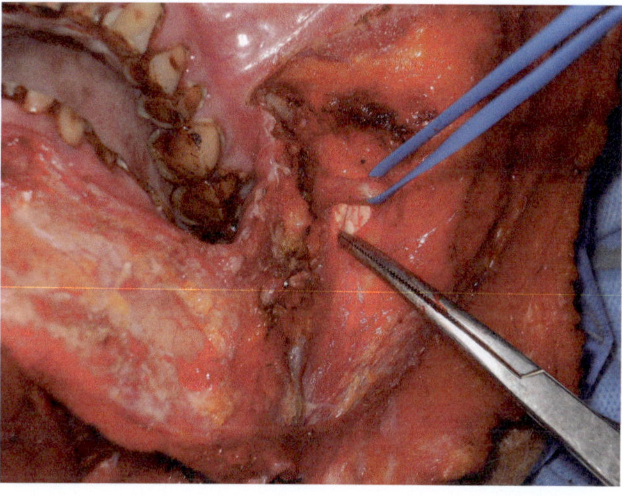

Fig. 7.32 The photo shows the masseter muscle and parotid duct. The masseter muscle is included in specimen if lesion is posteriorly located. The muscle is included in cheek flap if not involved

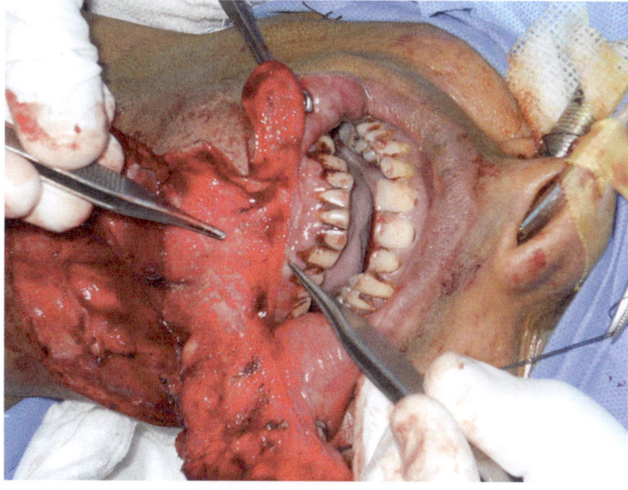

Fig. 7.30 The closure becomes easy if part of buccal mucosa is left attached to the alveolar ridge. It is also advisable to leave periosteum over mandible while raising the cheek flap

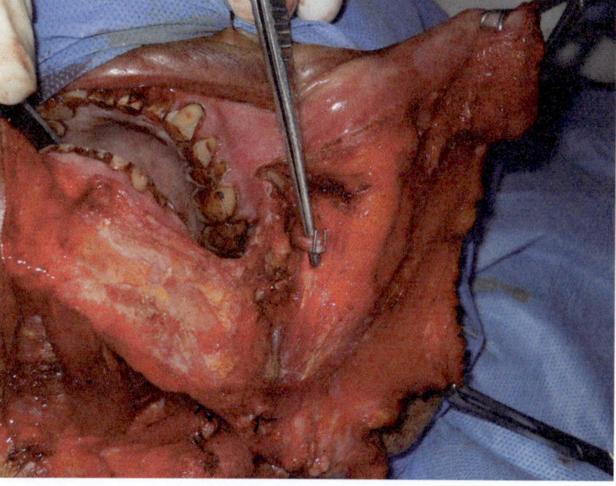

Fig. 7.33 The ligated parotid duct. It can be left untied as well but can cause parotid fistula on rare occasion

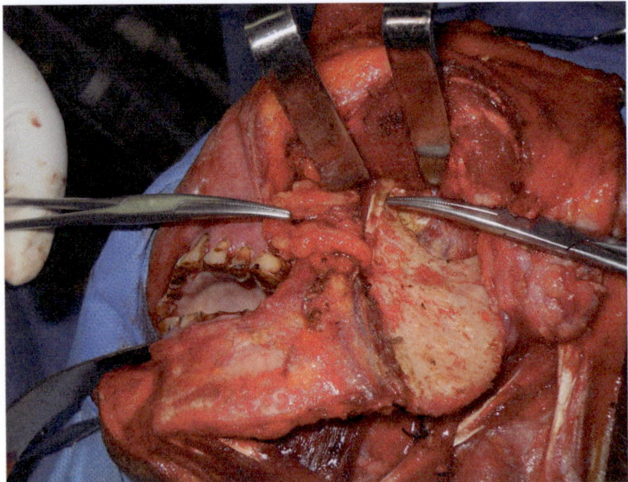

Fig. 7.34 The buccal pad of fat and insertion of temporalis muscle on coronoid process

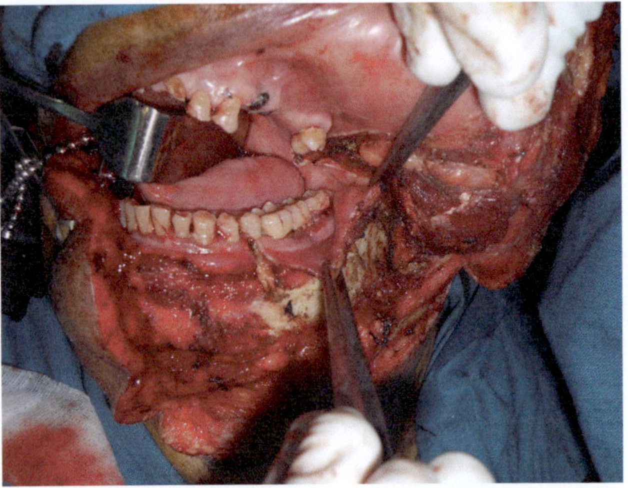

Fig. 7.35 The gingivo-buccal lesion abutting alveolus mucosa

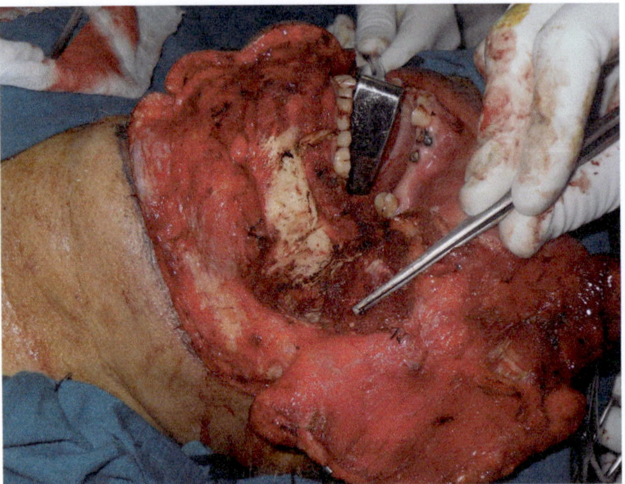

Fig. 7.36 The mandible is exposed from sigmoid notch till lateral body

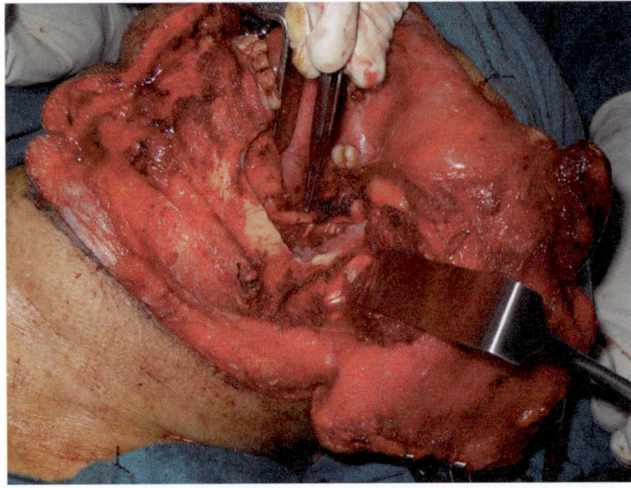

Fig. 7.37 The completed resection. The preserved lingual nerve can be seen. This is important when performing marginal mandibular resection for posterior lesion. The bone wax was applied on remaining rim to avoid continuous bleeding

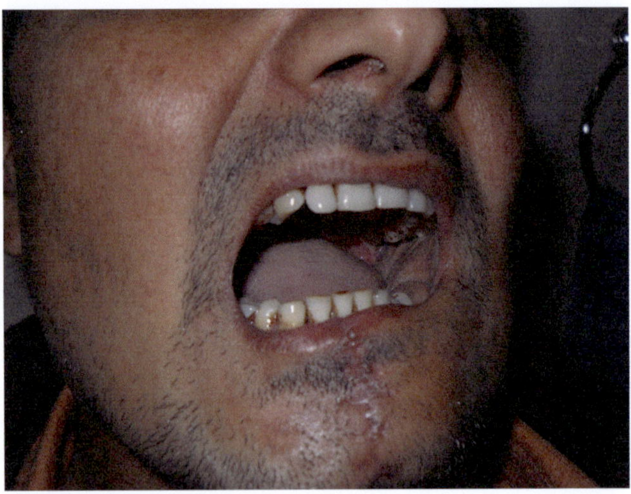

Fig. 7.38 Reconstruction with pectoralis major myocutaneous (PMMC) flap. One can notice decent mouth opening even in patient with pre-op trismus. Performing coronoidectomy and detaching masseter and medial pterygoid muscle helps in improving postoperative mouth opening

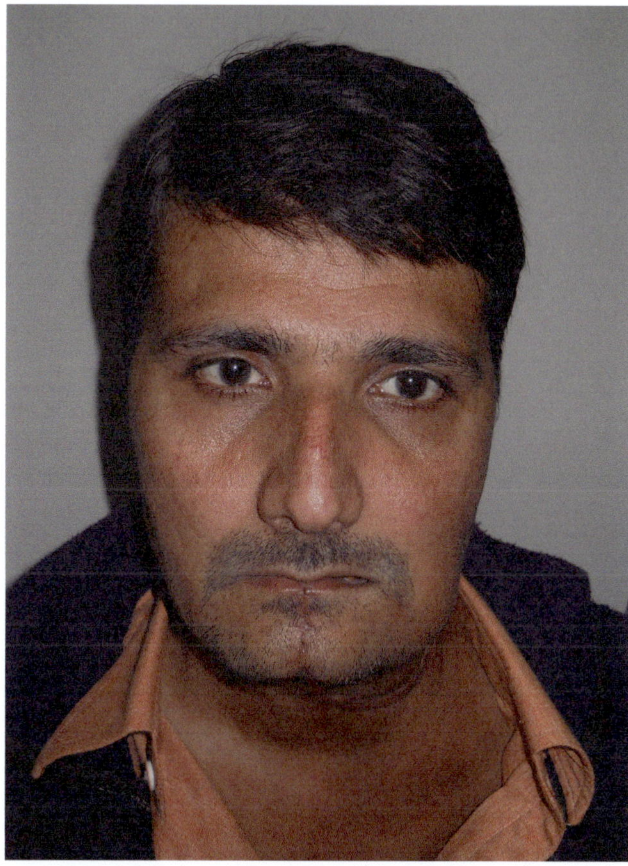

Fig. 7.39 Acceptable cosmetic outcome front view

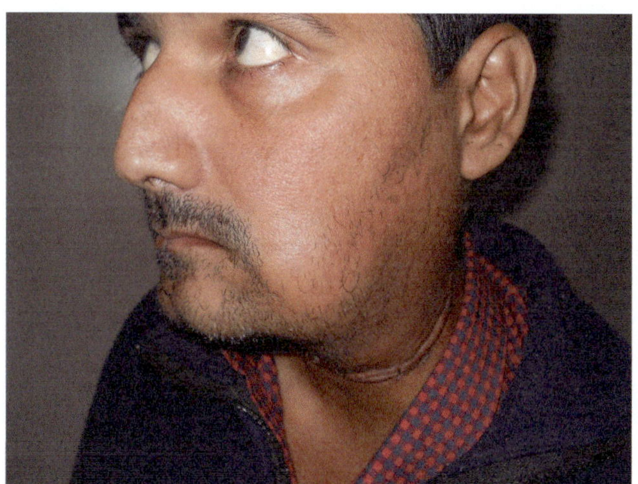

Fig. 7.40 Photograph with lateral view showing minimal bulge with PMMC flap

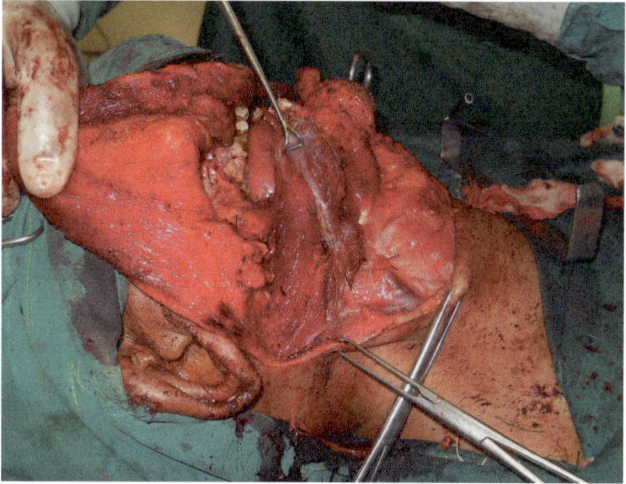

Fig. 7.41 Reconstruction with muscle only flap (SCM or PMMC)

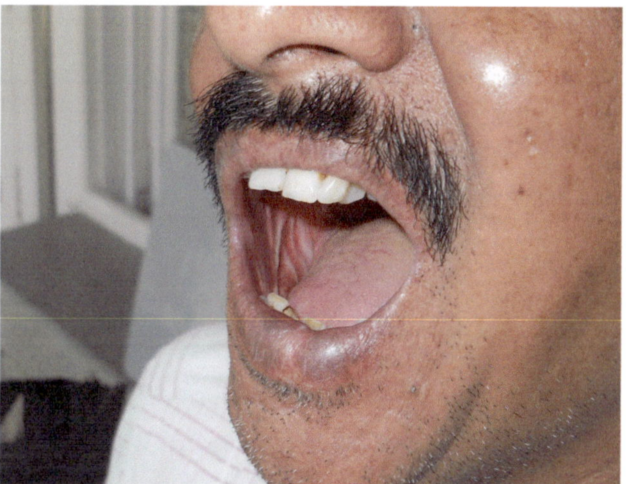

Fig. 7.42 The postoperative outcome after healing. The mucolization is faster and we prefer this flap when minimal bulk is required

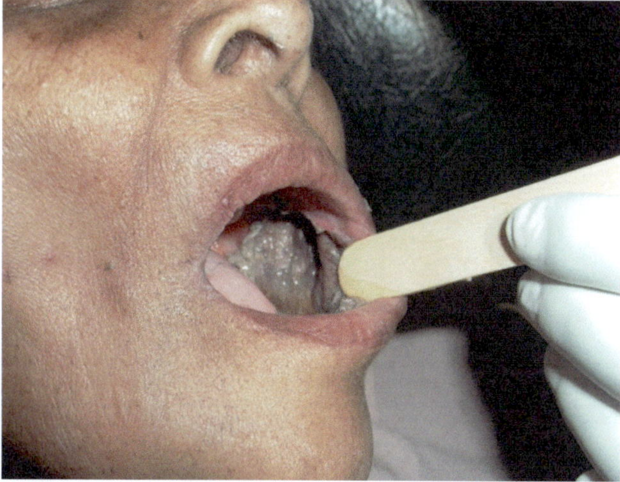

Fig. 7.43 Reconstruction with STG

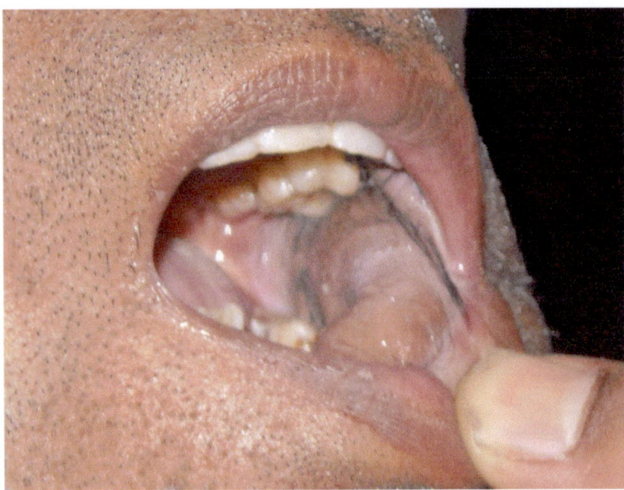

Fig. 7.44 Reconstruction with radial forearm free flap (RFFF)

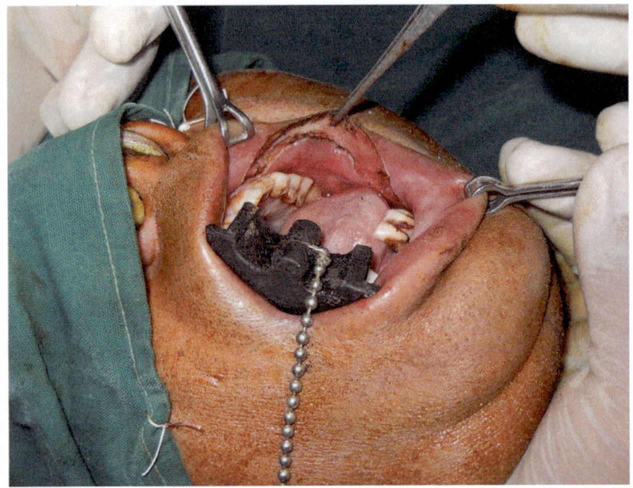

Fig. 7.45 Another lesion that is coming close to angle of mouth. The resection margin includes mucosa of angle of mouth and lip. This leads to ligation of lip vessels

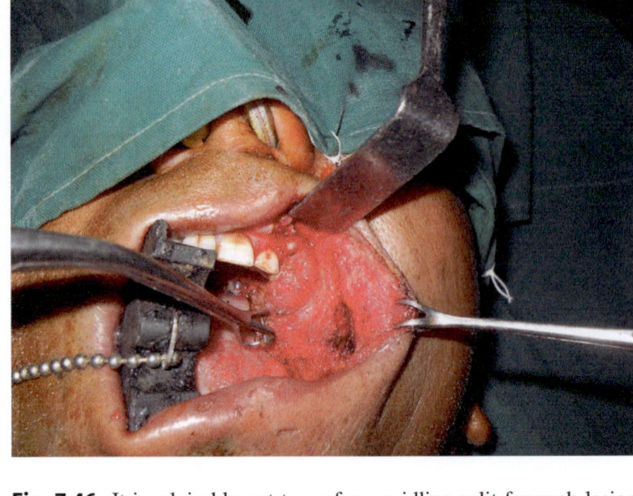

Fig. 7.46 It is advisable not to perform midline split for such lesion but to perform angle lip-split incision. This photo demonstrates mobilization of buccal mucosa away from angle of mouth

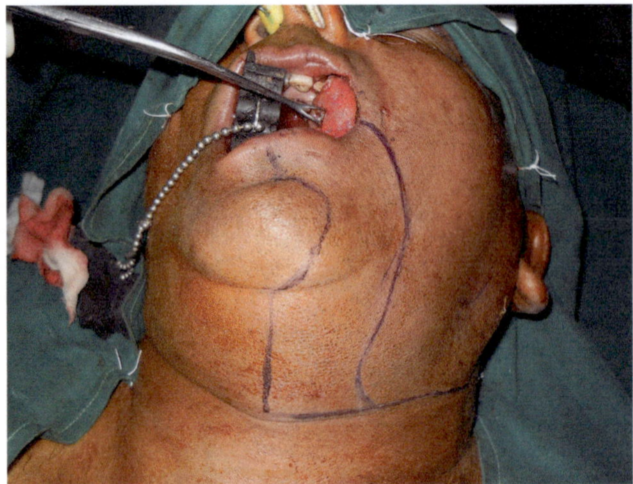

Fig. 7.47 This photo shows difference between midline and angle lip-split approach. There is a chance of necrosis of interplaced portion of lip if midline split is performed. The blood supply to the lip is from the midline, due to ligation of labial artery while resecting angle of mouth, The midline lip-split incision has the potential to damage that supply causing necrosis of the central portion of the lip

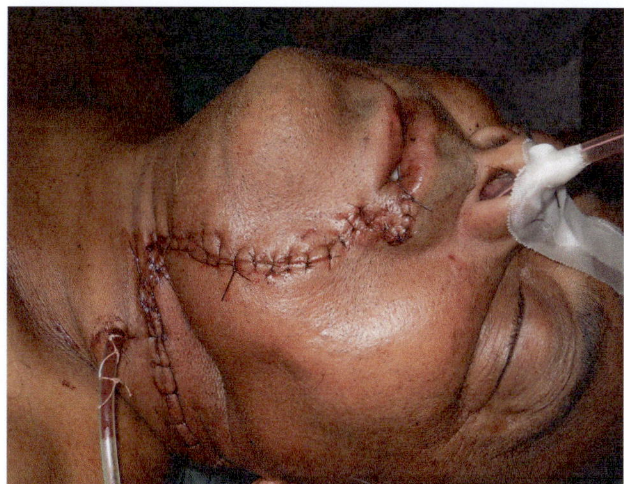

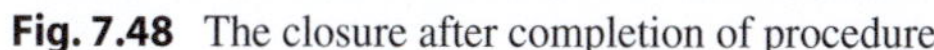

Fig. 7.48 The closure after completion of procedure

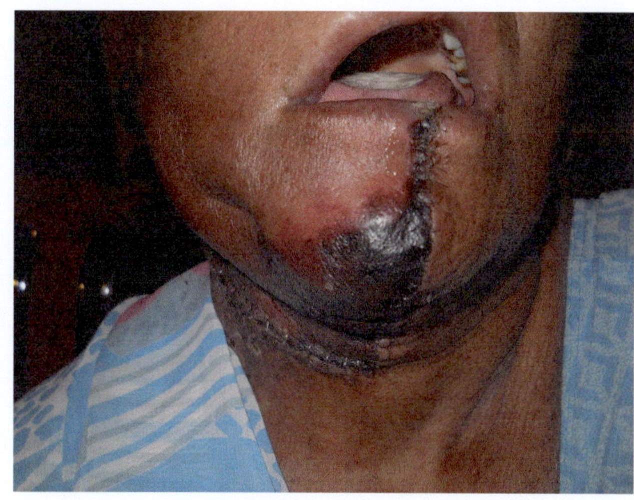

Fig. 7.49 Devascularized portion of skin leading to skin necrosis when erroneous planning of midline split was performed

T3-T4 Lesion

Approach: Composite resection involving soft tissue of buccal mucosa and mandible–maxilla depending upon their involvement

Marginal mandible resection can be performed for lesion abutting mandible but not grossly infiltrating mandible. Segmental mandibulectomy needs to be performed for gross cortical erosion or marrow involvement. Relative contraindications for marginal resection are edentulous mandible, post-radiotherapy case, or coexisting severe trismus.

Marginal Mandible Resection

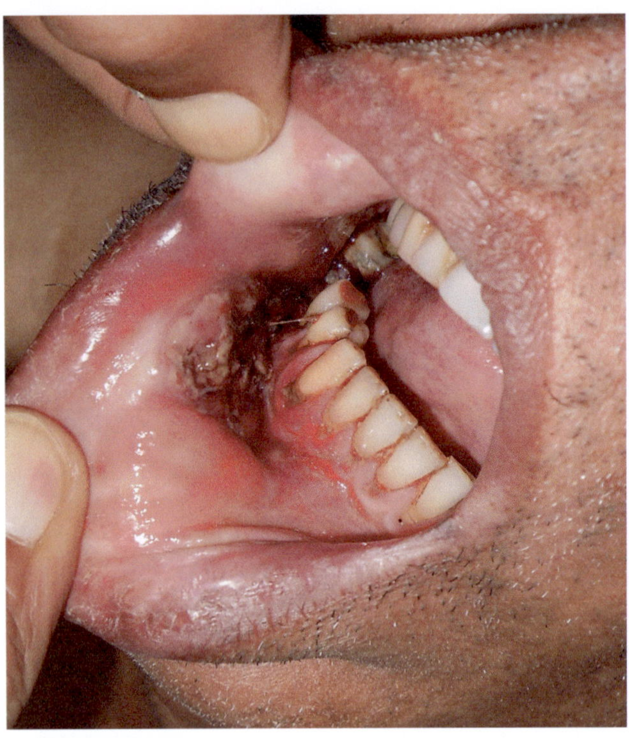

Fig. 7.50 Gingivo-buccal sulcus lesion abutting mandible. There is no gross involvement of mandible providing opportunity to perform marginal mandibulectomy. It is our philosophy that posteriorly located lesions with associated severe trismus (submucous fibrosis) are better suited for segmental mandibulectomy

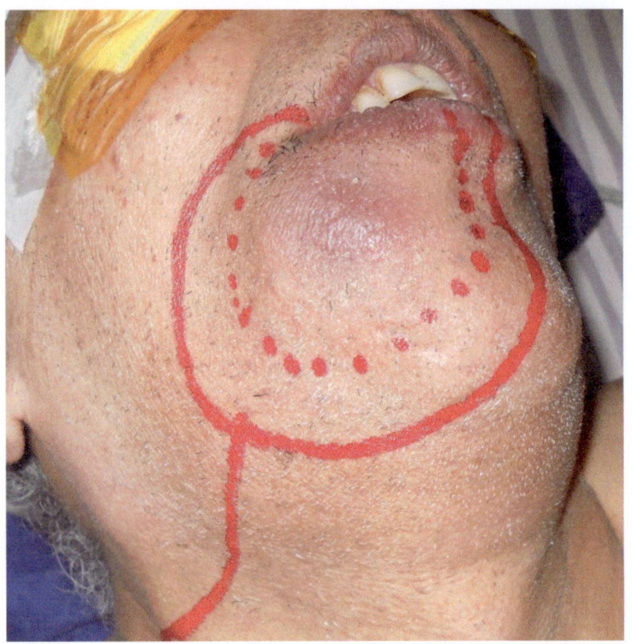

Fig. 7.51 Lesion showing skin induration and involvement. These factors are considered in planning the incision

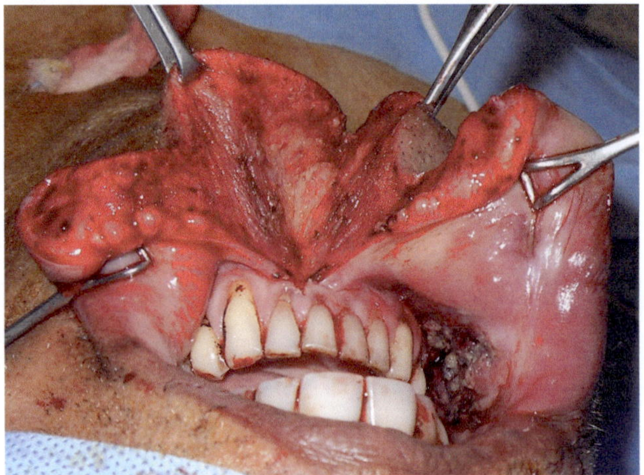

Fig. 7.52 Midline lip split with adequate margins

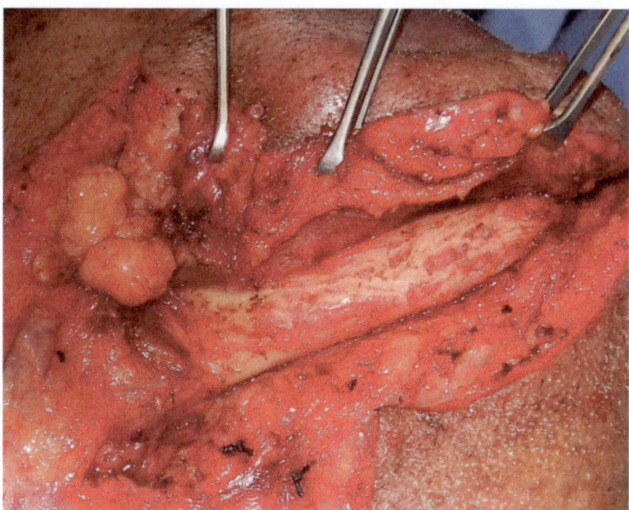

Fig. 7.53 Exposing lower border of mandible. It is essential to preserve at least 8 mm of lower mandible height after marginal resection. The bone is weakest at angle of mandible

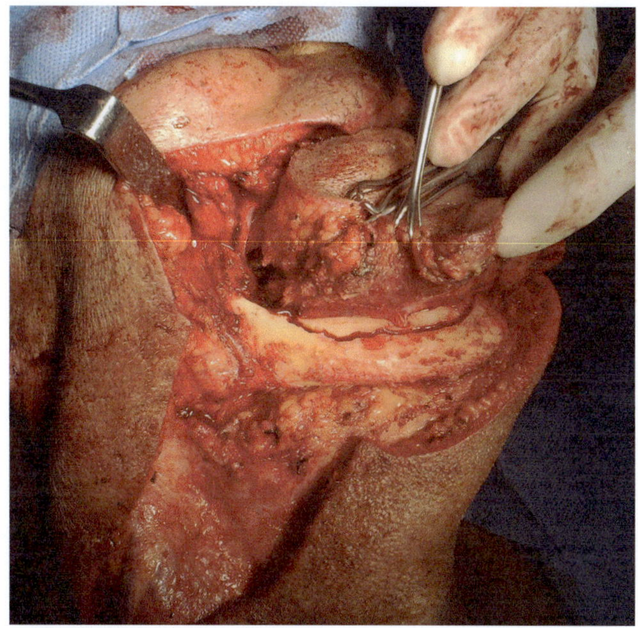

Fig. 7.54 Proposed bone cuts

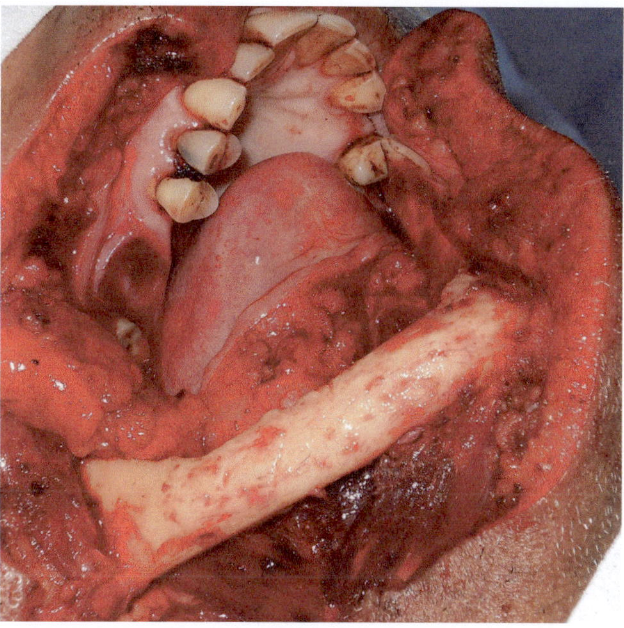

Fig. 7.55 Remaining portion of mandible after resection of lesion. All the sharp edges of mandible are smoothened. The bleeding from marrow is stopped with bone-wax application

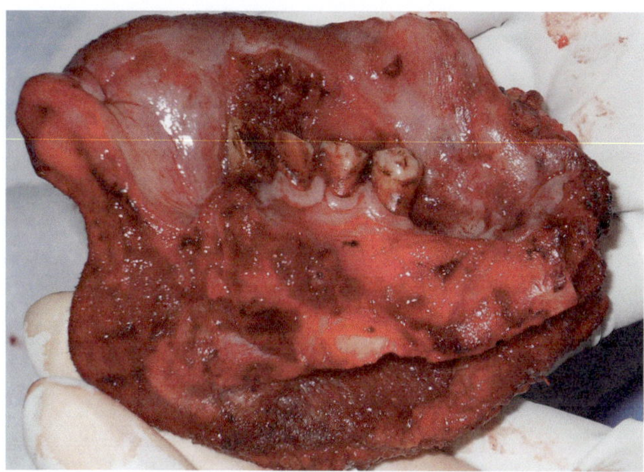

Fig. 7.56 Specimen showing resection of tumor with adequate margins in three dimensions

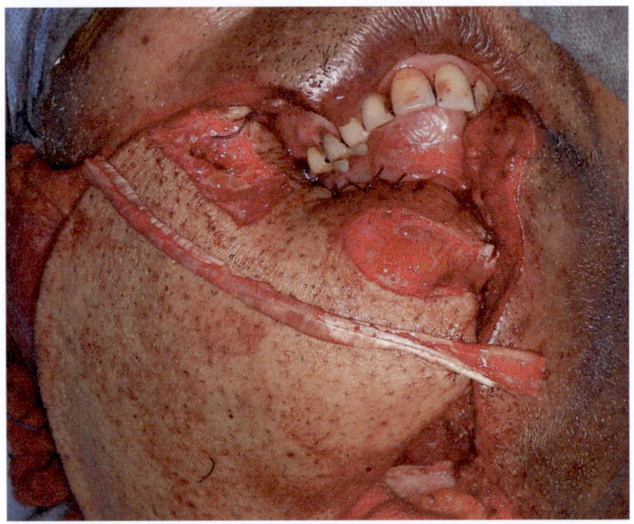

Fig. 7.57 Reconstruction of through and through cheek defect with bi-paddled anterolateral thigh free flap. The angle of mouth is reconstituted with fascia lata sling

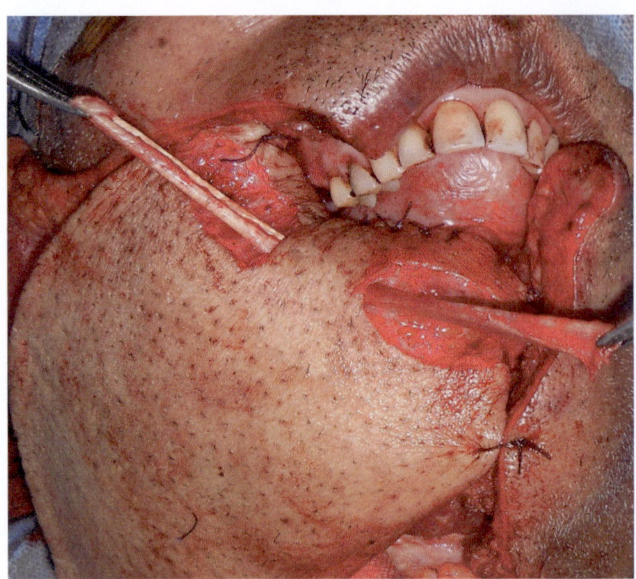

Fig. 7.59 Facial sling is ready to support new commissure

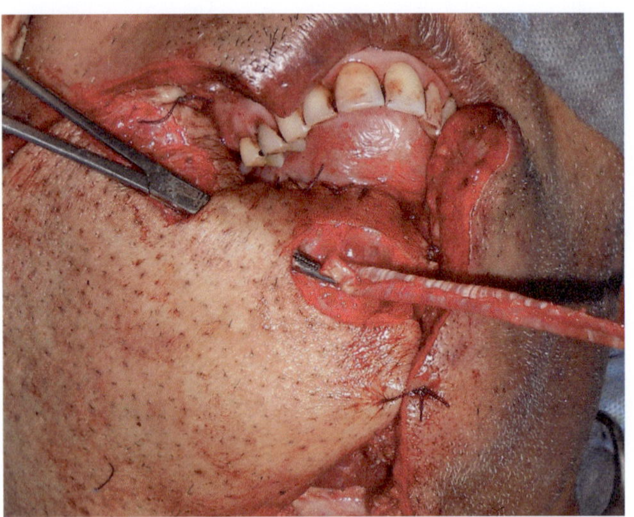

Fig. 7.58 Facial sling is tunneled through subdermal plane

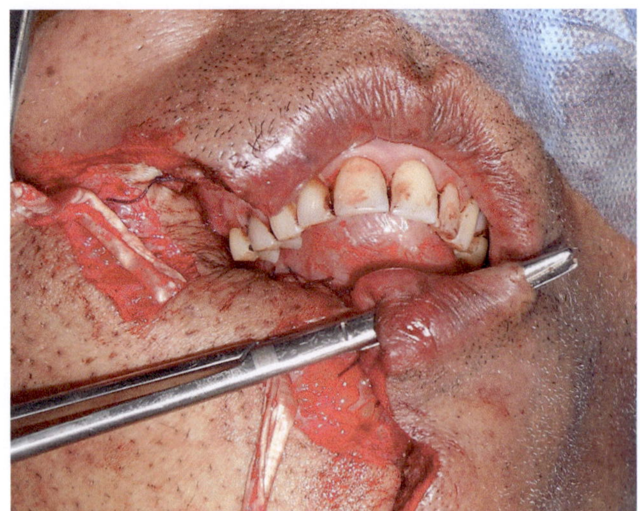

Fig. 7.60 Sling is tunneled into lower lip with help of artery forcep

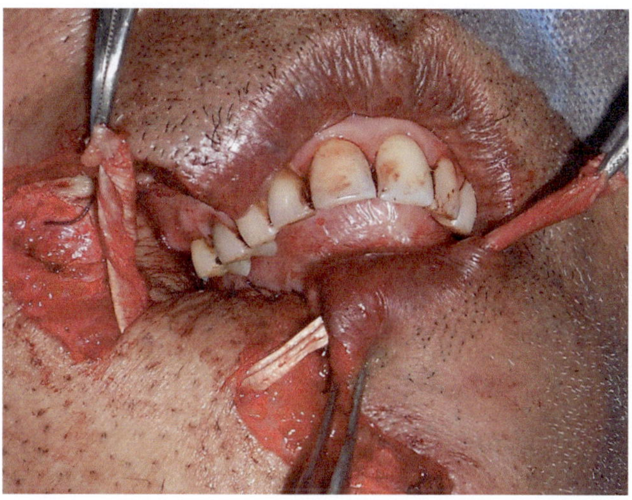

Fig. 7.61 Adjusting length of facial sling in lower lip

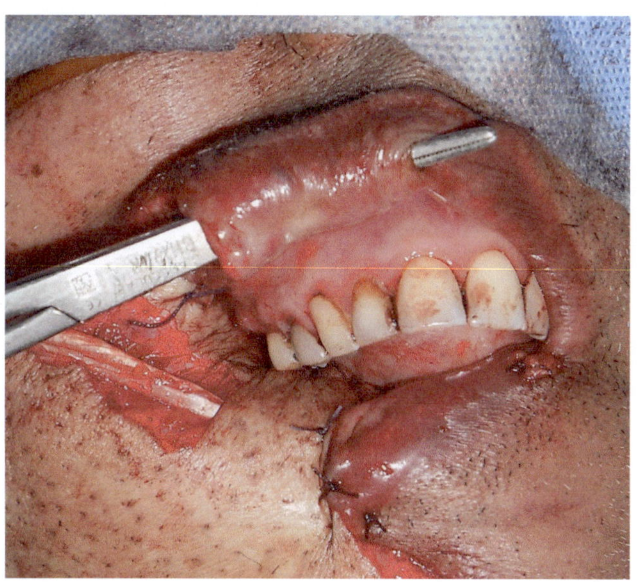

Fig. 7.62 Sling insertion in upper lip

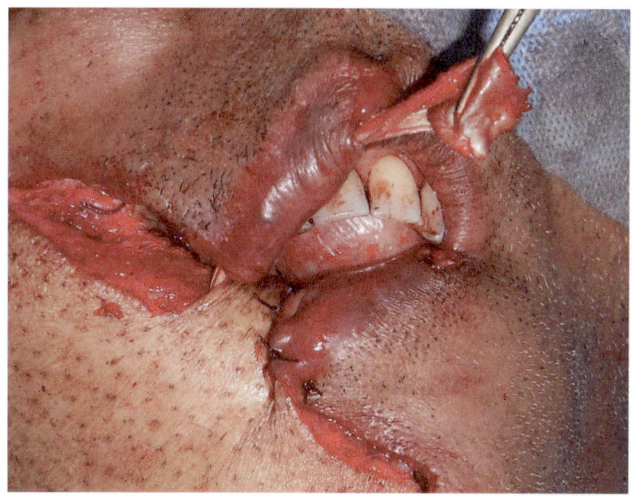

Fig. 7.63 Tightening of sling to provide optimum tension to commissure. It is important to have balance between adequate mouth opening and competent oral commissure

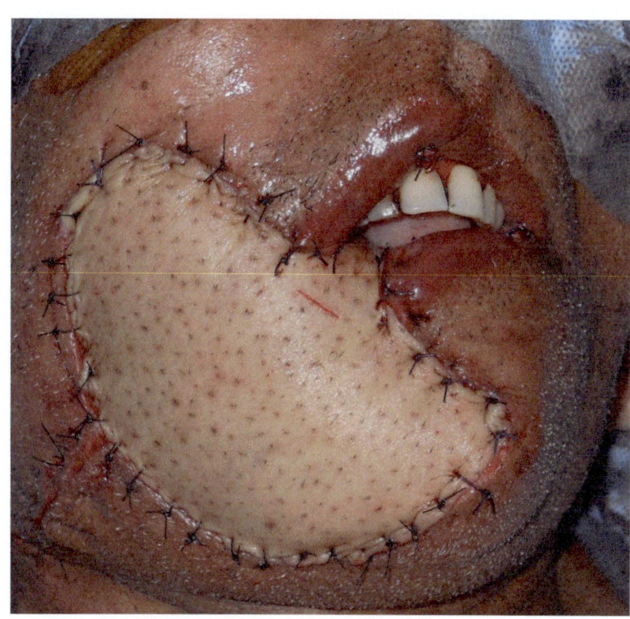

Fig. 7.64 Final outcome after flap suturing

Segmental Mandible Resection

Concept: The composite resection is performed for advanced tumors. The soft tissue clearance with adequate margins in third dimension forms the basis for improved local control rates. We prefer to perform compartment resection involving entire anatomical subunit containing tumor rather than removing tumor with one cm margins. The anterior lesions can be resected in conventional manner as shown in this section. The posterior located lesions that infiltrate into the masticator space can be resected by performing compartment infratemporal fossa (ITF) clearance. This procedure is described in a separate section.

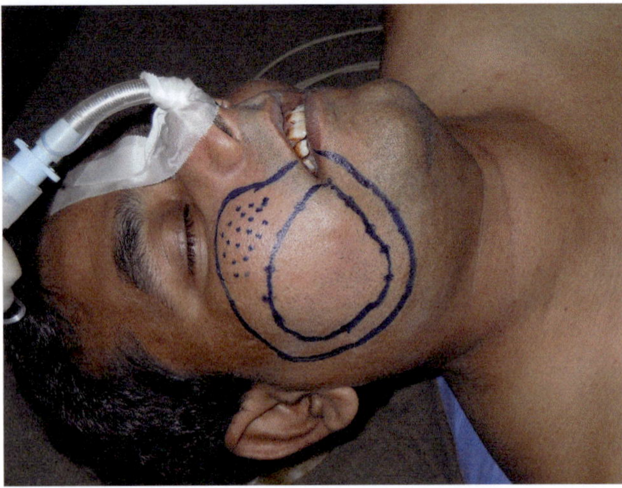

Fig. 7.65 Photo shows advanced buccal cancer with skin involvement. The entire skin with edema and induration is included in resection

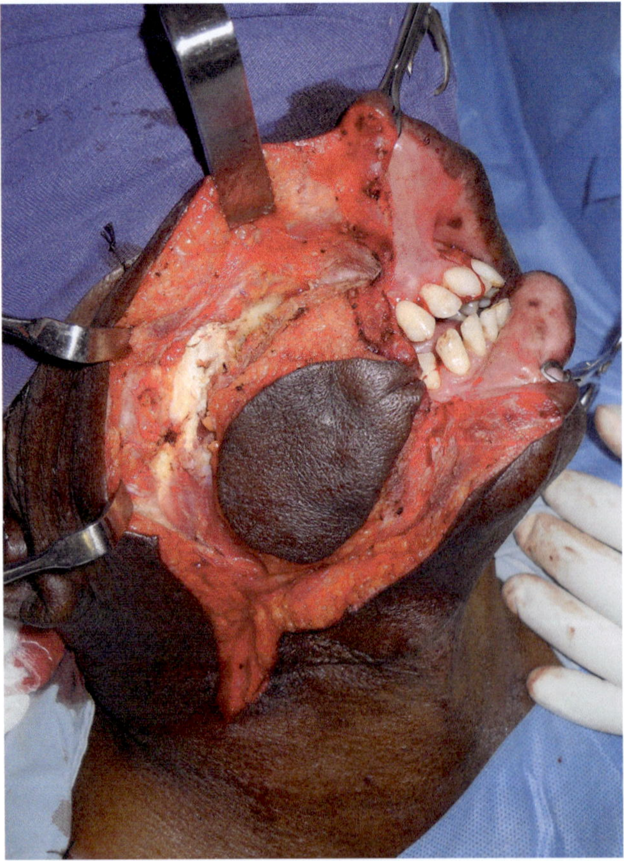

Fig. 7.66 Upper and lower flaps are raised. We perform composite resection as compartment resection removes entire soft tissue in involved compartment

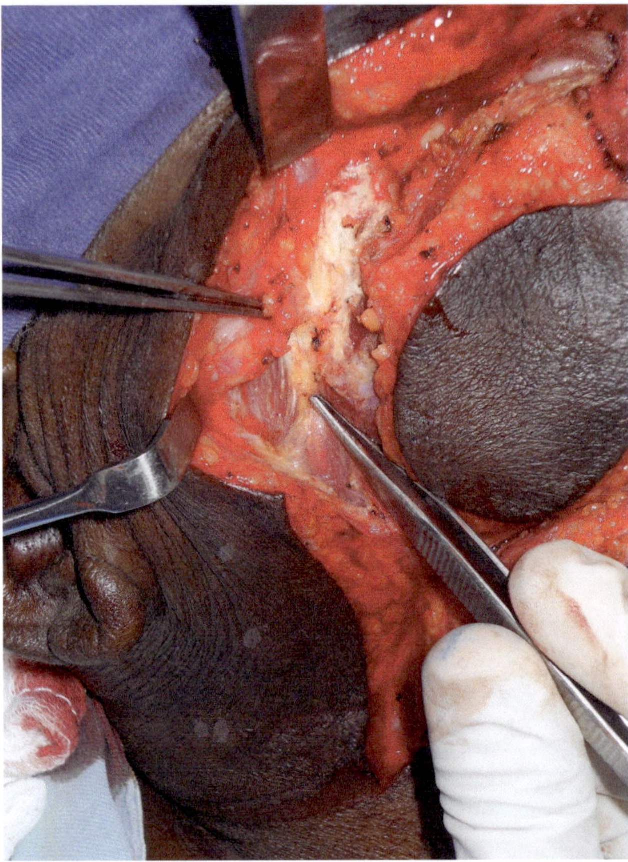

Fig. 7.67 The upper flap is raised to expose zygoma and posterolateral wall of maxilla. The photograph shows insertion of masseter on zygoma

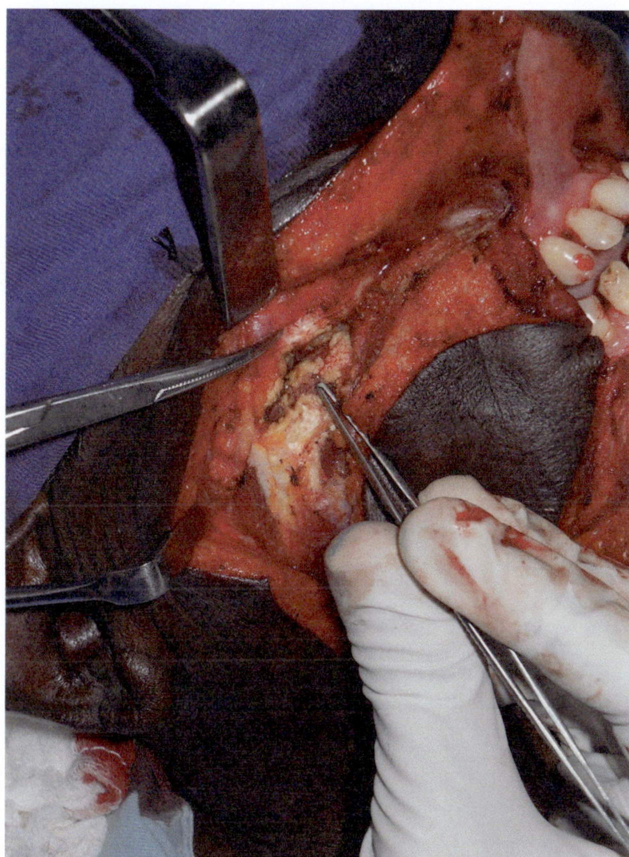
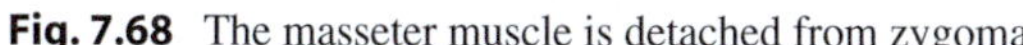

Fig. 7.68 The masseter muscle is detached from zygoma

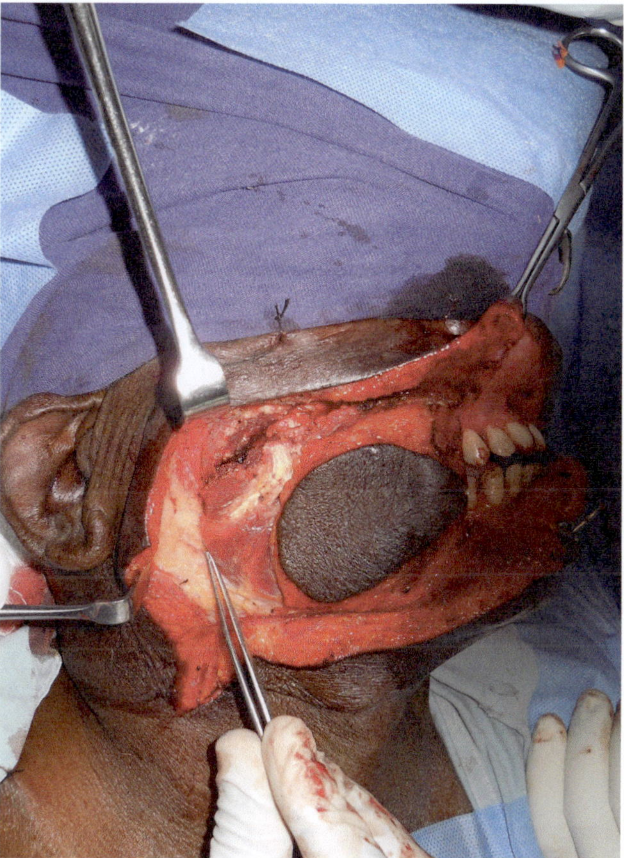

Fig. 7.69 The masseter muscle has been separated from parotid tissue. Buccal branch of the facial nerve is resected and eye branch is preserved. There are numerous small blood vessels in this plane, and care is taken to achieve a clean field

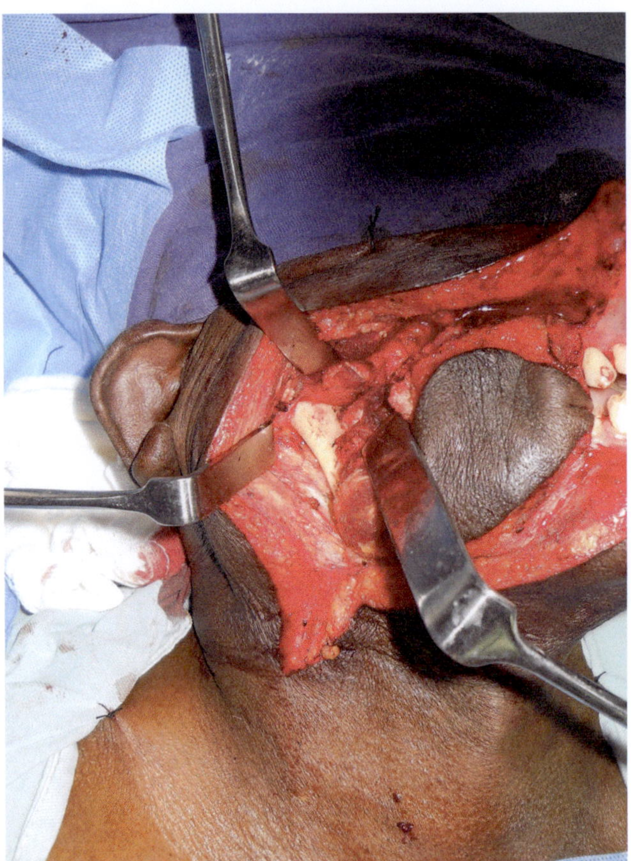

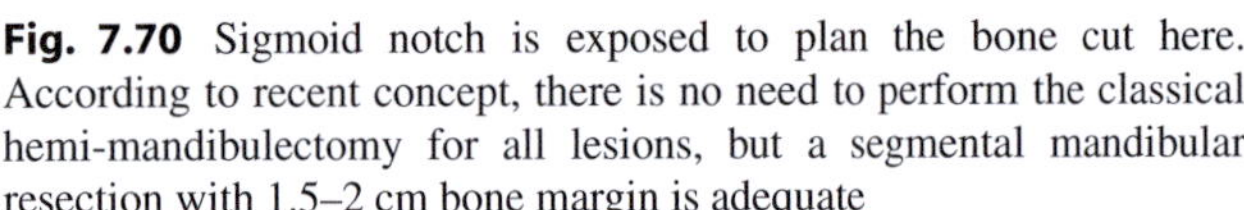

Fig. 7.70 Sigmoid notch is exposed to plan the bone cut here. According to recent concept, there is no need to perform the classical hemi-mandibulectomy for all lesions, but a segmental mandibular resection with 1.5–2 cm bone margin is adequate

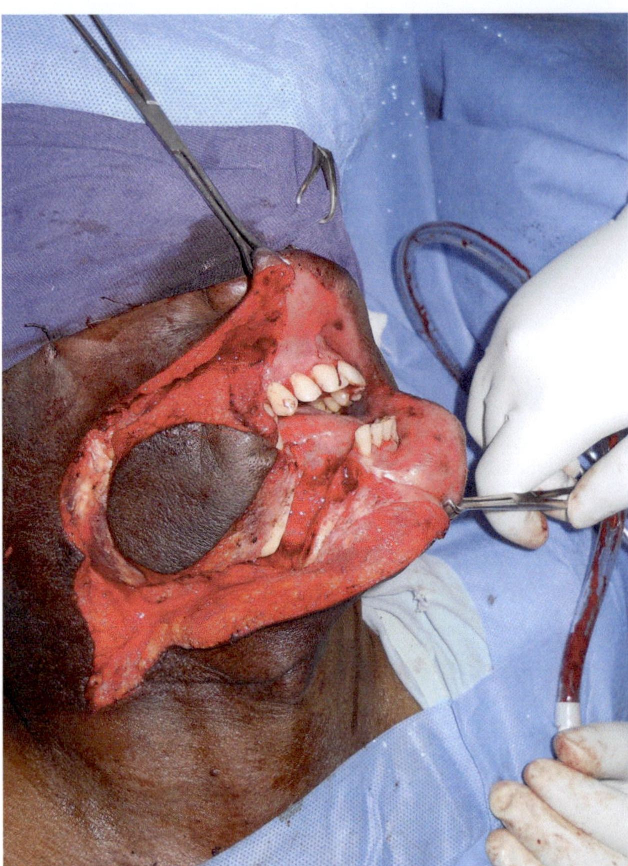

Fig. 7.71 Anterior mandible cut is planned with 2 cm of bone margin

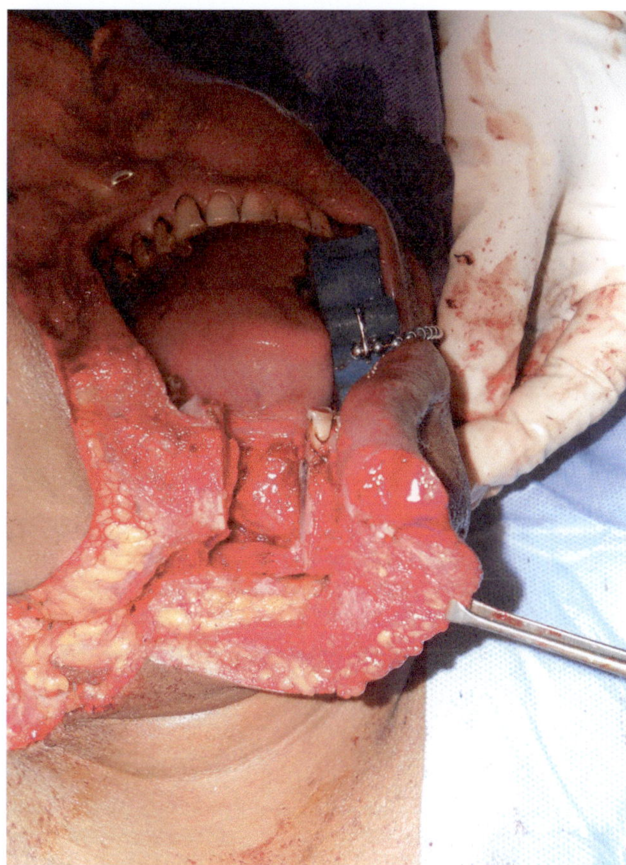

Fig. 7.72 The mandible is retracted to expose mylohyoid muscle and sublingual gland. Bone wax is useful in stopping bleeding from edges of cut mandibular

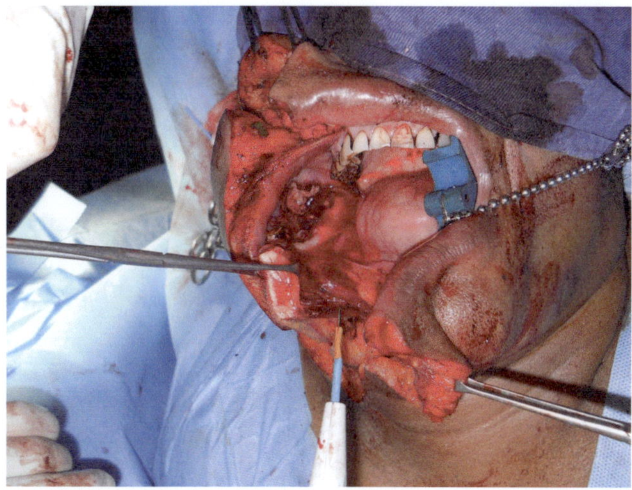

Fig. 7.73 Mylohyoid muscle is sectioned

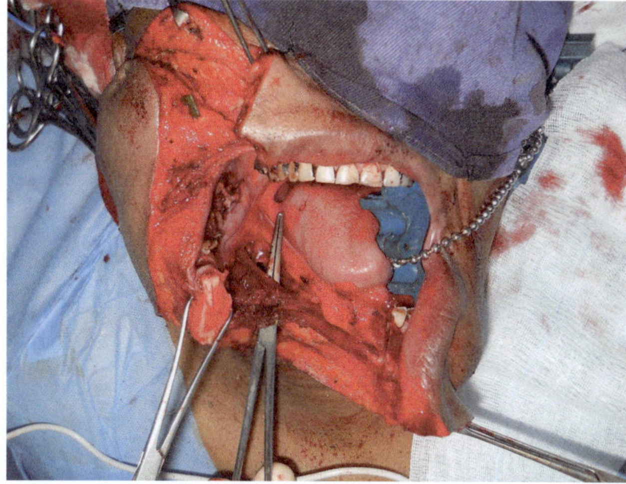

Fig. 7.74 The lingual nerve is identified and preserved while transecting mylohyoid and medial pterygoid muscle

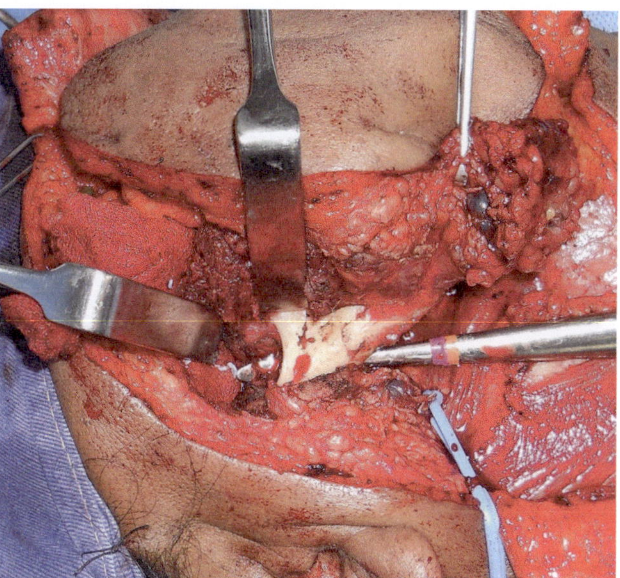

Fig. 7.75 Posterior mandible bone cut is made at level of sigmoid notch

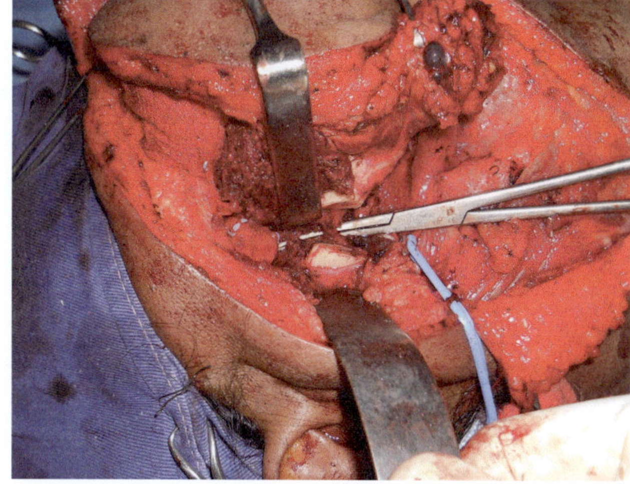

Fig. 7.76 Internal maxillary artery is ligated that reduces bleeding to a significant extent

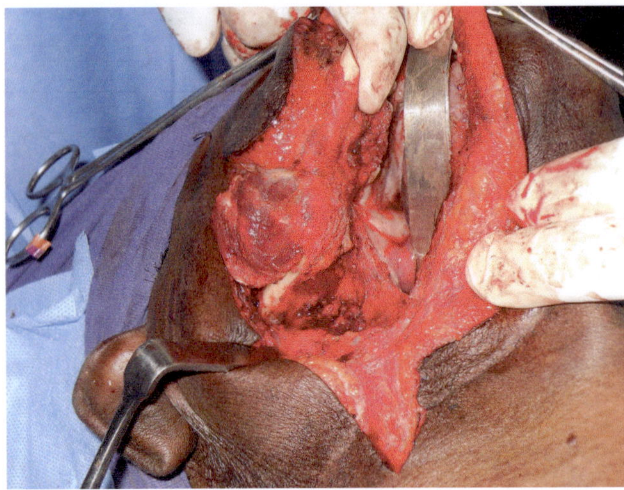

Fig. 7.77 The mandible is mobilized after releasing stylomandibular ligament

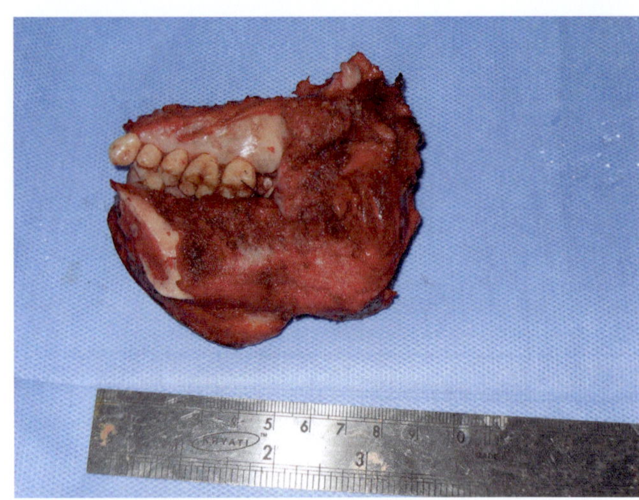

Fig. 7.79 The specimen. The photo shows all the soft tissue structures resected in anatomical planes with intact facial barriers

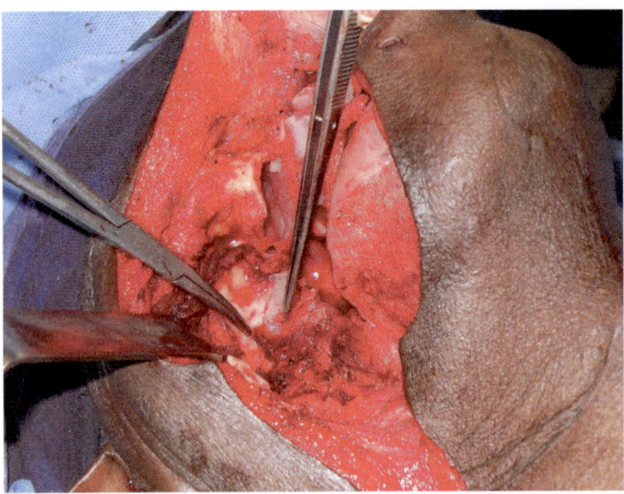

Fig. 7.78 The medial pterygoid muscle is resected from the pterygoid plate to remove the entire specimen with involved soft tissues (masseter and medial pterygoid muscle) en bloc. The photograph shows exposed skull base bone

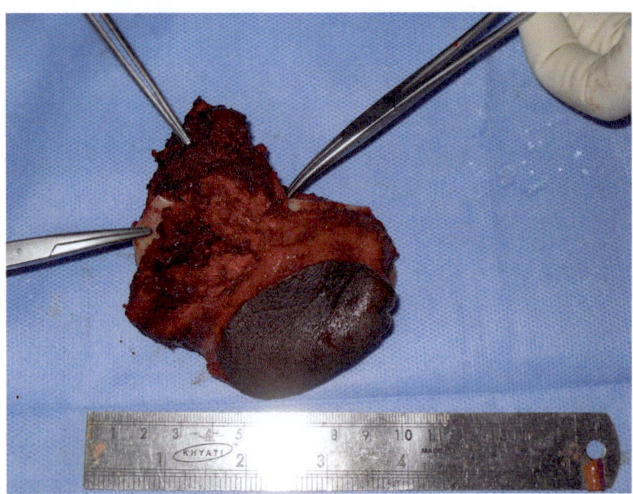

Fig. 7.80 Photo demonstrating soft tissue margin at depth

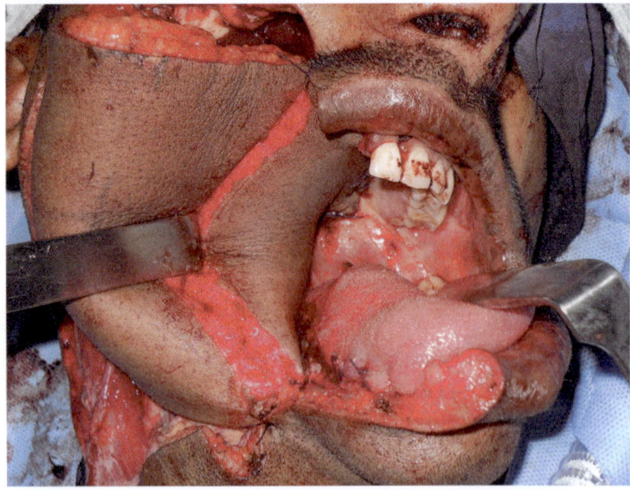

Fig. 7.81 The defect has been reconstructed with bi-paddle anterolateral thigh flap. The middle portion of the flap is de-epithelized

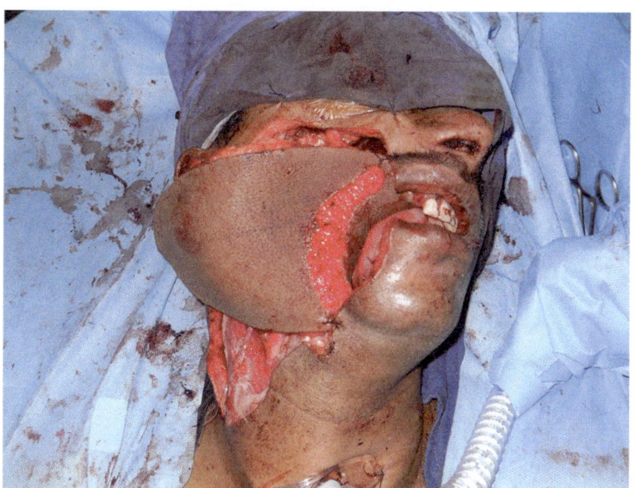

Fig. 7.82 Reconstruction of commissure

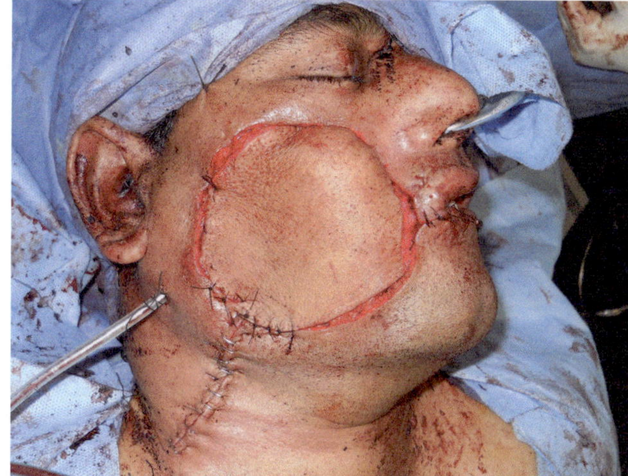

Fig. 7.83 Final outcome

Reconstruction Algorithm

Figure 7.84 demonstrates reconstructive algorithm for buccal–alveolus cancers. Small defects can be managed by local or free flaps. It is essential to advise aggressive postoperative physiotherapy to avoid trismus. The larger composite defects require complex reconstruction. The mainstay of lateral composite defect is the pectoralis flap. It is very easy and quick to raise, is reliable, and can be used to reconstruct a variety of defects ranging from lining the oral cavity to bi-paddled flap. The anterolateral thigh (ALT) flap serves as an alternative to the pectoralis flap. The ALT allows better range of movement and doesn't have drag of pectoralis flap. Large ALT flap can cover most of complex defects quite comprehensively, and it has become the mainstay of composite defects in our unit.

The central arch mandible defects and some lateral mandible defects require bone reconstruction. Pure lateral alveolar defects with little soft tissue component are ideal for bone reconstruction. There is no role for non-vascularized bone in current reconstructive algorithm, and vascularized bone reconstruction has become standard of care. Fibula flap with skin paddle remains the primary option for majority of bone defects.

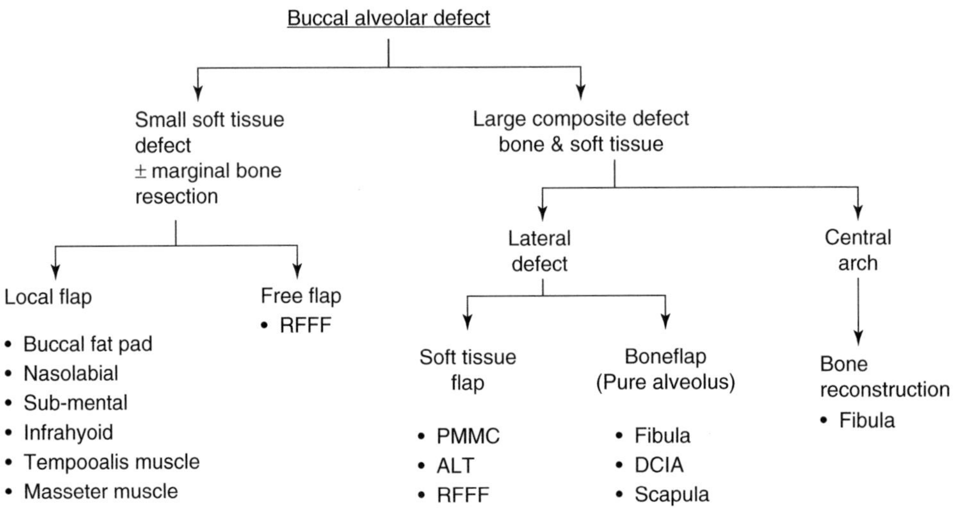

Fig. 7.84 Reconstruction algorithm

Reconstruction of Central Arch Mandible

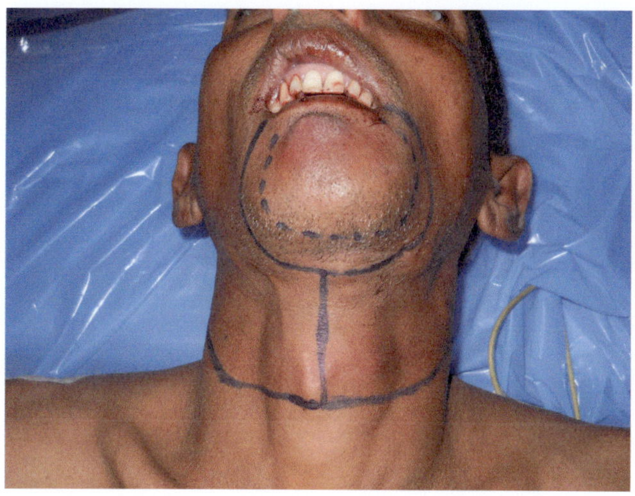

Fig. 7.85 Lower lip cancer with involvement of skin central arch of mandible

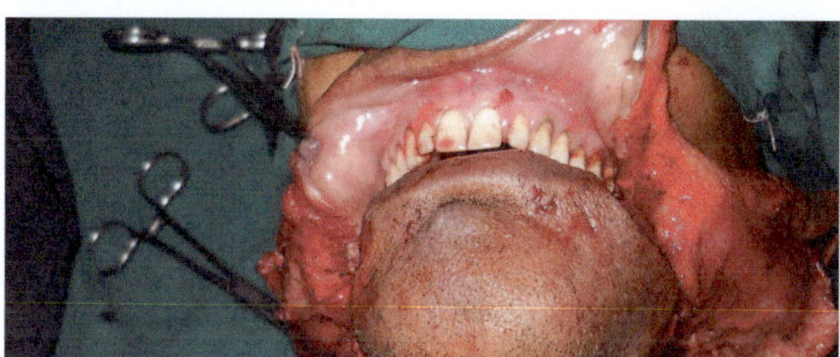

Fig. 7.86 Flap being raised

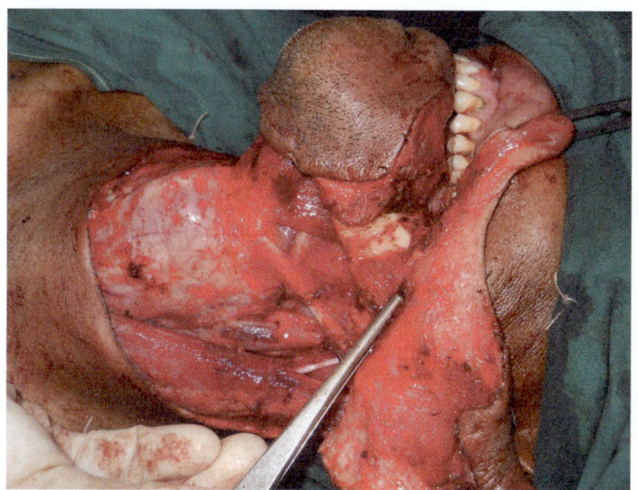

Fig. 7.87 Lateral mandible is exposed for plating. It is essential to put mandible in occlusion with interdental fixation before cutting it

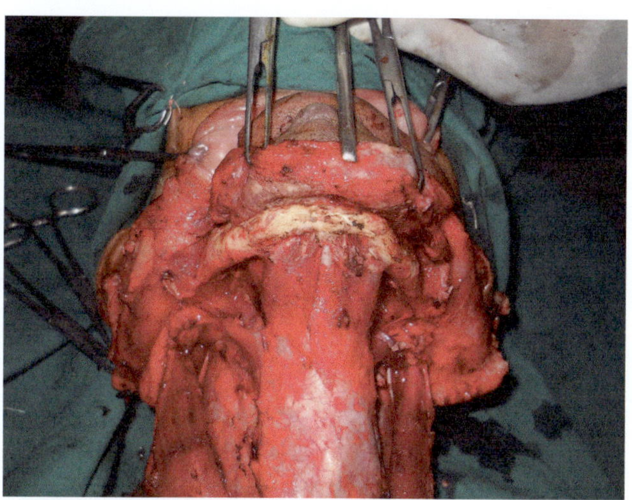

Fig. 7.88 Lower border of mandible is exposed for pre-plating

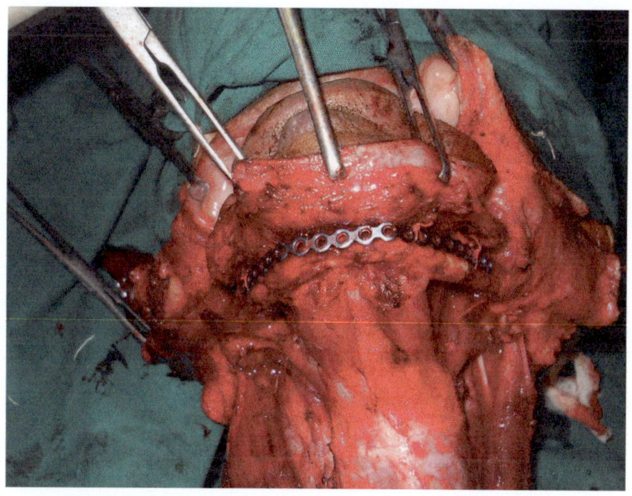

Fig. 7.89 Plate is adapted according to countering of bone

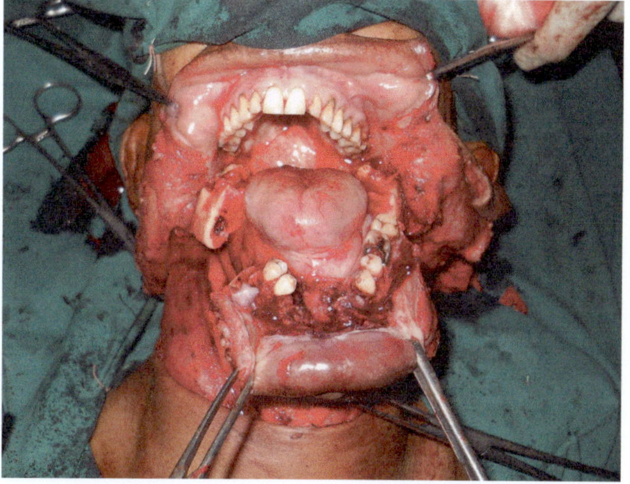

Fig. 7.90 The lesion is mobilized

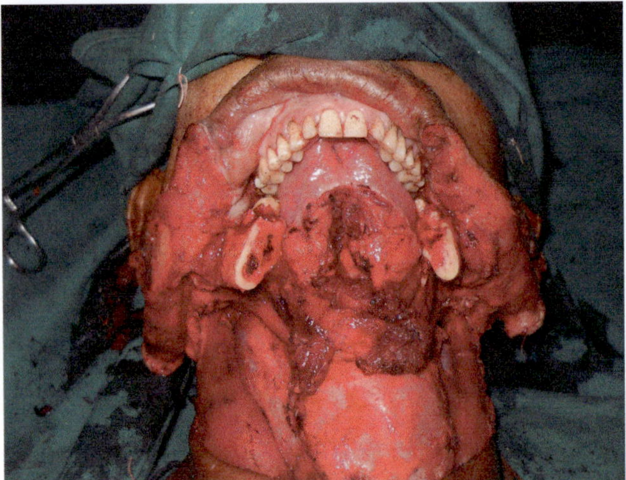

Fig. 7.91 Complete resection. The tongue muscle needs support so that patient can swallow

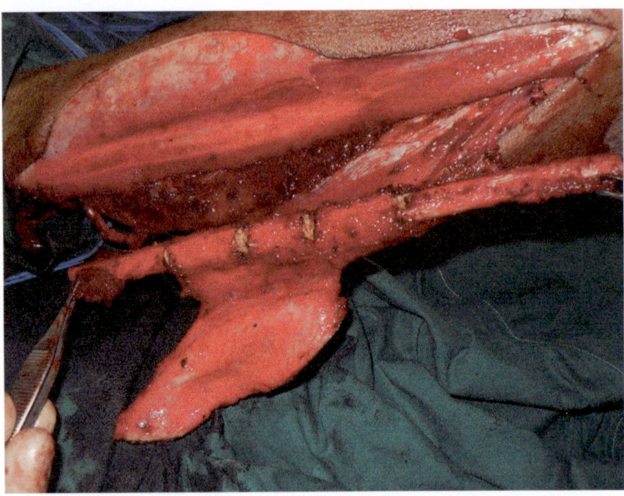

Fig. 7.92 Fibula flap being raised along with skin paddle. The markings are made for osteotomy based on pre-adopted plate

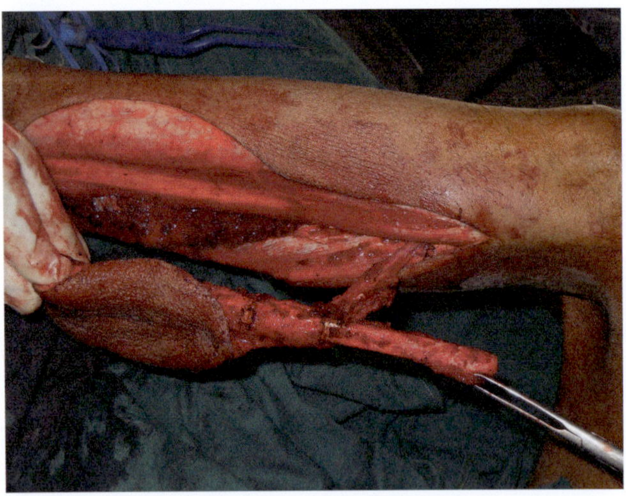

Fig. 7.93 Extra bone being separated and resected

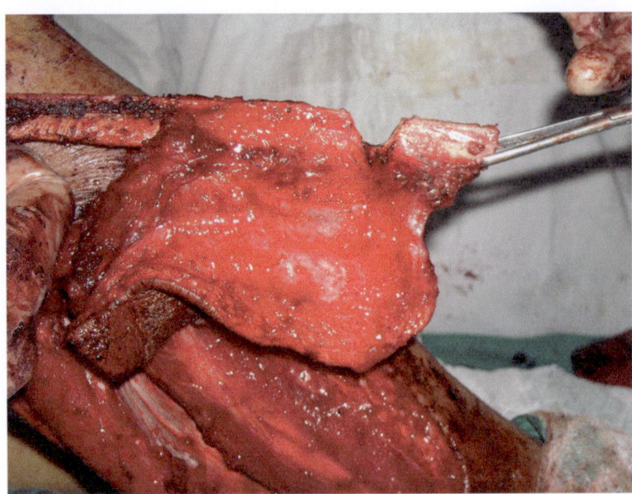

Fig. 7.94 The osteotomy being performed. It is essential to protect vascular pedicle while performing bone cuts

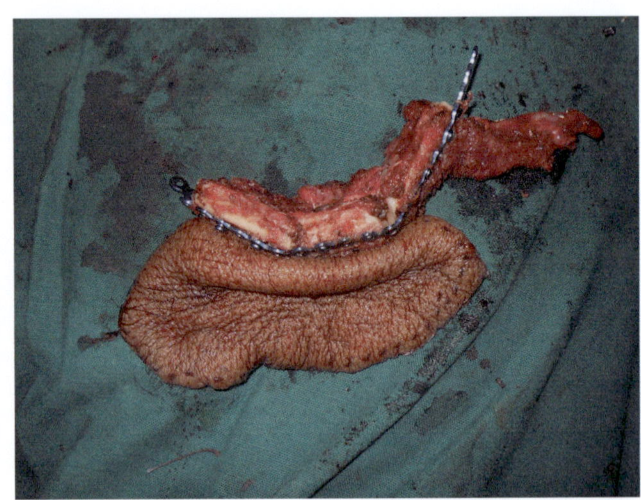

Fig. 7.95 The fibula is being fixed on prebended plate

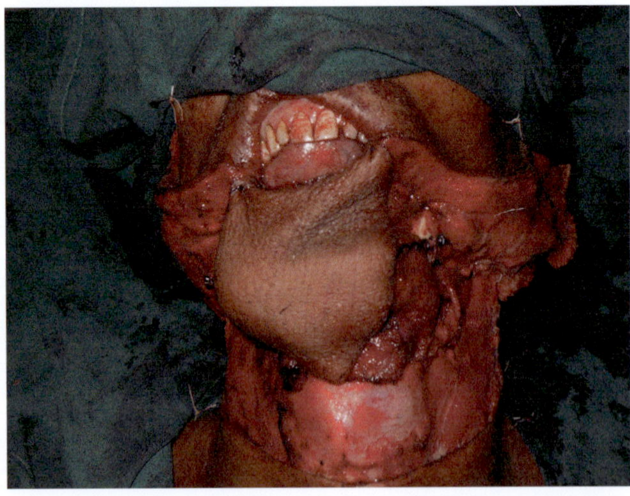

Fig. 7.96 The flap is inserted

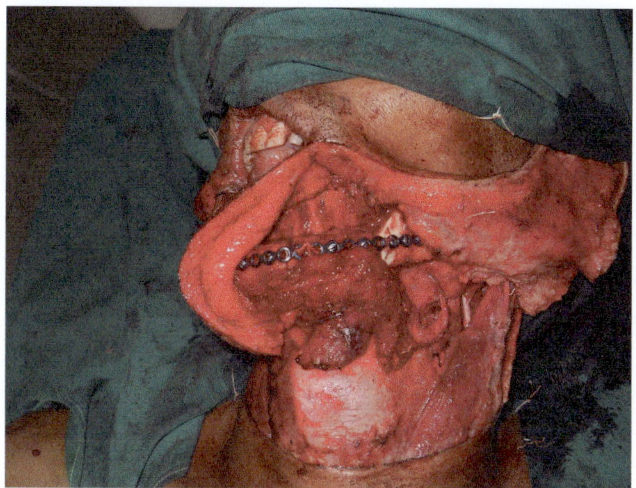

Fig. 7.97 Plate fixation

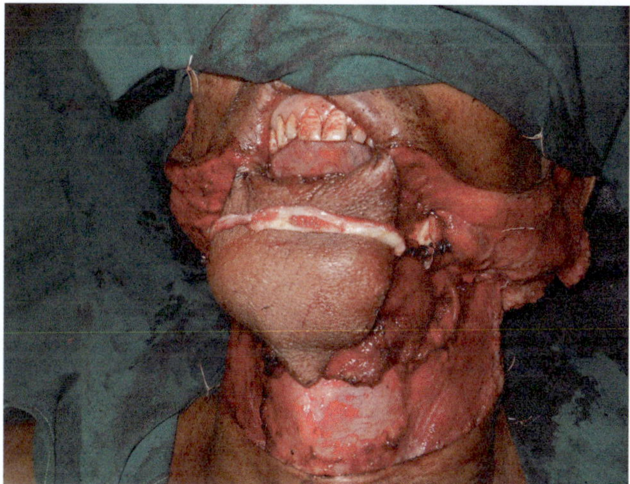

Fig. 7.98 Facial sling for lower lip continence

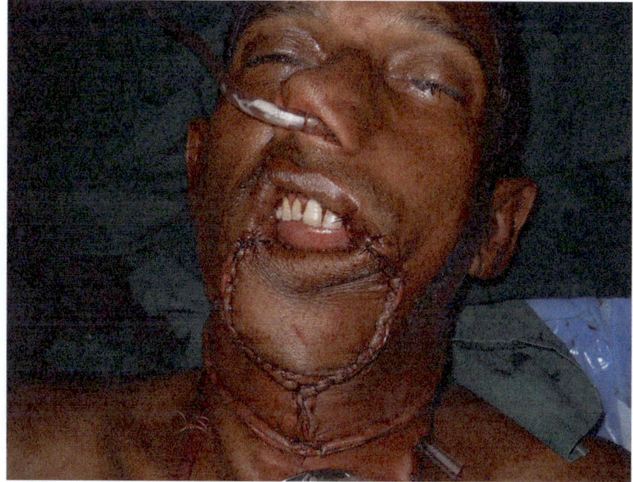

Fig. 7.99 The final closure

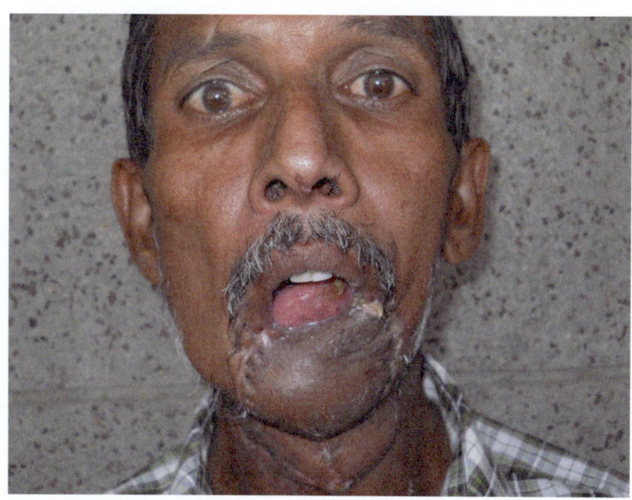

Fig. 7.100 Photograph after 10 days of procedure

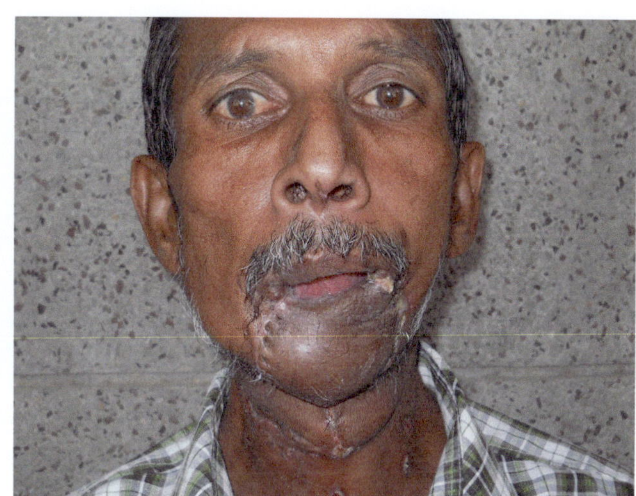

Fig. 7.101 Good mouth competence

8 Tumors of the Tongue and Floor of the Mouth

Surgical Anatomy

Carcinoma of the tongue and floor of the mouth are one of the more aggressive oral cancers. The tumors have a tendency to spread locally as well to the lymph nodes and to the distant parts of the body. These characteristics make treatment of this tumor tricky. The tongue has a unique anatomy with muscle fibers crisscrossing allowing it to move in all directions. These muscles are broadly divided into intrinsic and extrinsic groups of muscles. This area is also rich in its vascular supply and lymphatic network and tumor has tendency to spread beyond local area at relatively earlier stages. The part near the midline has bilateral lymphatic drainage.

The tongue is broadly divided into the anterior tongue and base of the tongue which is rather considered as part of the oropharynx. The anterior 2/3rd is divided into two halves by median raphe. Lateral tongue mucosa continues beyond to floor of the mouth and to the alveolus (Fig. 8.1a). The mylohyoid muscle forms the infero-lateral diaphragm separating the sublingual gland from the submandibular gland. The genioglossus muscle attaches the tongue to the anterior mandible, while the hyoglossus muscle curves anteriorly to the hyoid (Fig. 8.1b). The entire unit is supplied by two lingual arteries entering through the hyoglossus muscle. The hypoglossal nerve provides the motor supply to the tongue running deep to the mylohyoid muscle entering the hyoglossus muscle.

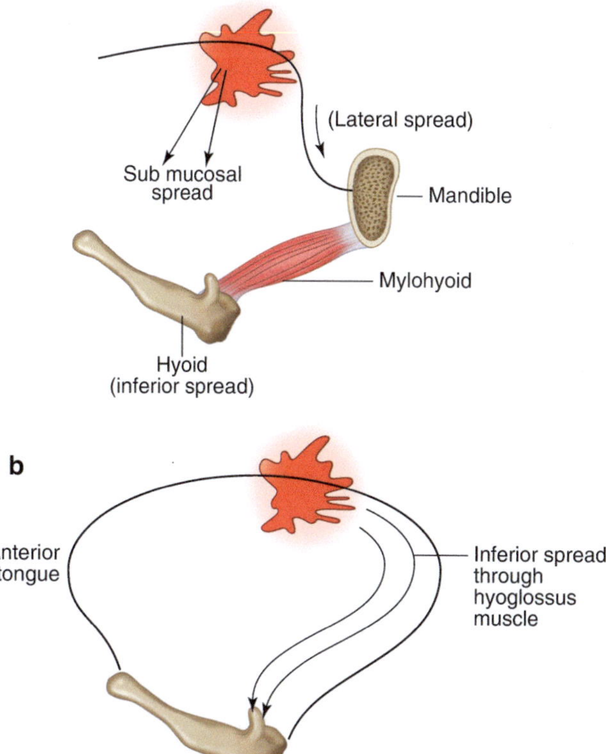

Fig. 8.1 Surgical anatomy and pattern of spread

N. Trivedi, *Atlas of Head and Neck Cancer Surgery: The Compartment Surgery for Resection in 3-D*, DOI 10.1007/978-81-322-2050-3_8, © Springer India 2015

Pattern of Spread

Tongue cancers are known for its aggressive and infiltrative nature and its submucosal spread. It is essential to palpate the induration around tumor before marking resection margin and a good habit is to continuously palpate the tumor while resecting. The lateral border of the tongue is mostly the first site to be involved, and then the tumor spreads laterally to the floor of the mouth and alveolar ridge (Fig. 8.1a). Mylohyoid insertion on the mandible usually limits its spread below and forms the basis for performing oblique marginal mandible resection. The deeply infiltrative tumor has the tendency to spread along hyoglossus muscle inferiorly, and this is the most common site for failure while performing intraoral tumor ablation (Figs. 8.1b and 8.2a).

The aggressive tumors also have tendency to spread across the midline though majority of lesions spread vertically. The inferior spread through the hyoglossus muscle is the most difficult area to address by conventional surgical approach. This forms the third dimension for infiltrative tongue or floor of mouth (FOM) tumors. Figure 8.2a, b proposes a concept for compartment tongue resection for deeply infiltrative lesions. The hyoglossus muscle is transected from its base, and thus the entire anatomical unit can be resected en bloc. This resection is also known as vertical resection compared to conventional horizontal resection. The chance of positive inferior margin is very rare.

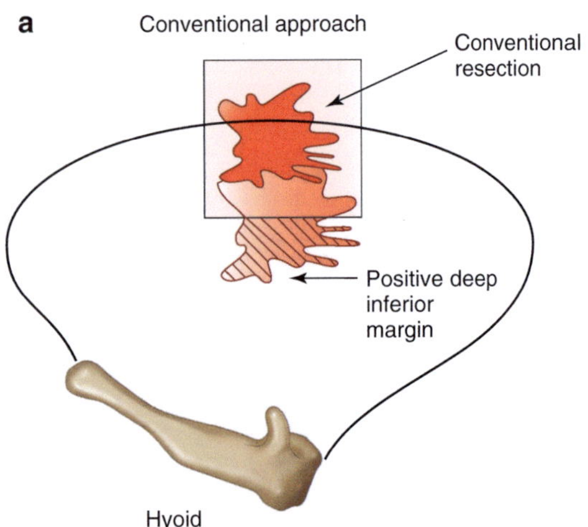

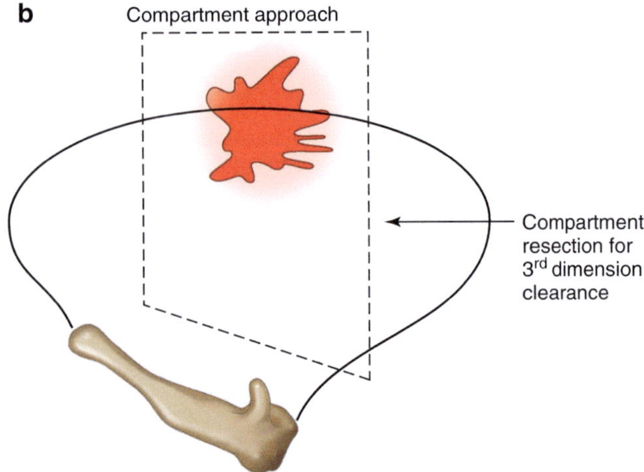

Fig. 8.2 Comparison between conventional and compartment (3D) surgical approach

Surgical Concepts

Figure 8.3 shows the algorithm for management of tongue cancers. Early T1 lesions can be managed by wide excision. The T2 lesion needs to be managed more aggressively with consideration for clearing deep margins. The larger T3 and T4 lesions need total glossectomy (TG) or near total glossectomy (NTG) preserving one side of the base of the tongue. More complex lesions can be managed by extended glossectomy along with mandible or larynx resection.

- Consider submucosal spread while planning resection margins.
- Palpate the tumor all the time during surgery.
- Infiltrative tumor has the tendency for inferior spread through hyoglossus, and removal of this muscle from hyoid is essential in achieving negative margins.
- Ligation of lingual artery before primary resection significantly reduces bleeding during surgery.
- Be aggressive on lymph node removal and consider bilateral removal for lesions crossing midline.

Algorithm				
	T1	T2	T3,T4	Complex
Resection	Wide excision	WLE $\bar{c}$ Compartment Clearance ± marginal mandible	Total glossectomy or Near total glossectomy	total glossectomy ± mandible ± larynx
Reconstruction	1° closure	• RFF • Regional flap • SCM • Infrahyoid • PMMC	• PMMC • ALT	• PMMC • ALT • Fibula + PMMC/ALT

Fig. 8.3 Treatment algorithm for tongue and FOM cancer

T1 Lesion

This section demonstrates surgical procedure for tongue and FOM cancers.

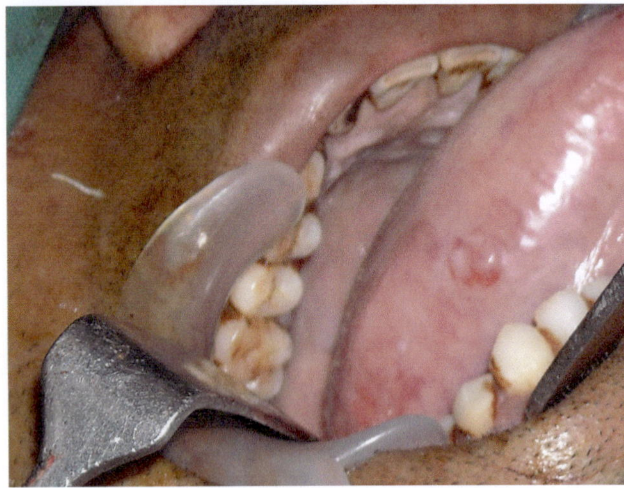

Fig. 8.4 Small primary lesion on lateral border of tongue

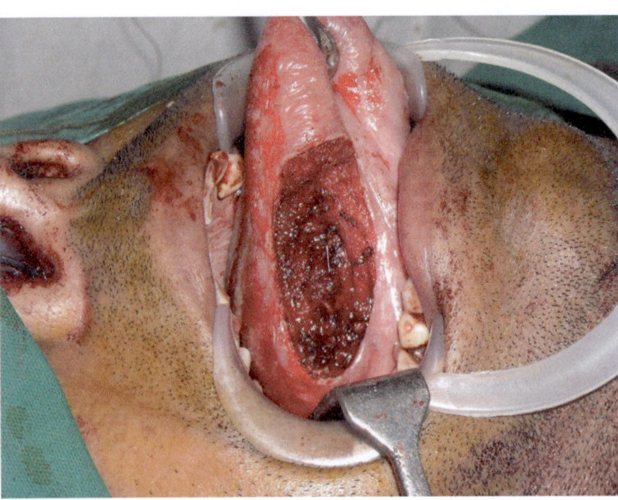

Fig. 8.5 Wide excision demonstrating 1.5 cm margin in all direction

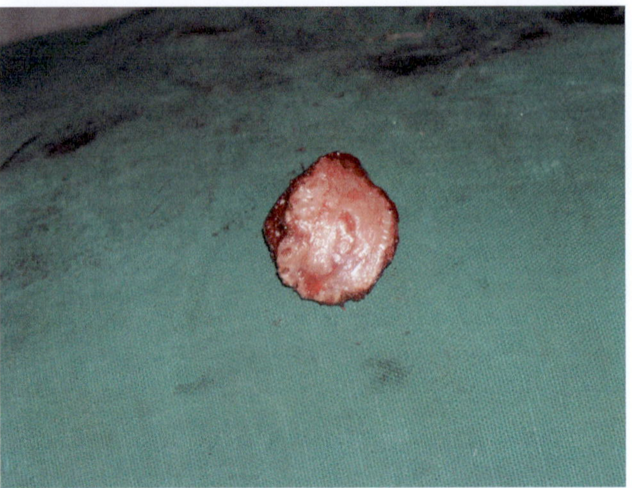

Fig. 8.6 Photograph showing specimen

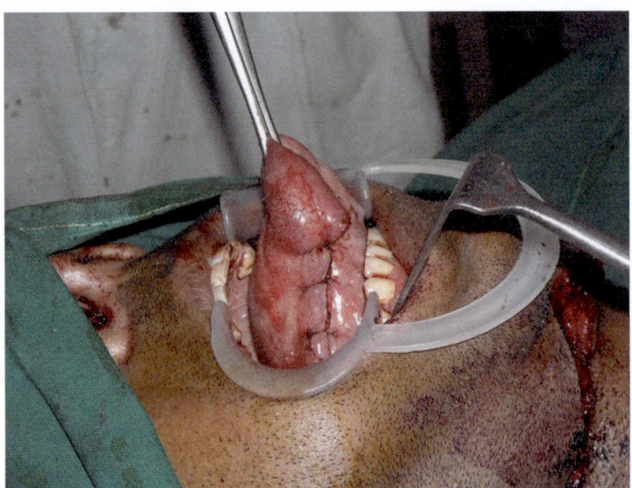

Fig. 8.7 Primary closure of lesion. There is a great chance that these stitches will give way in postoperative phase. Alternatively one can leave this area raw to heal with secondary intention

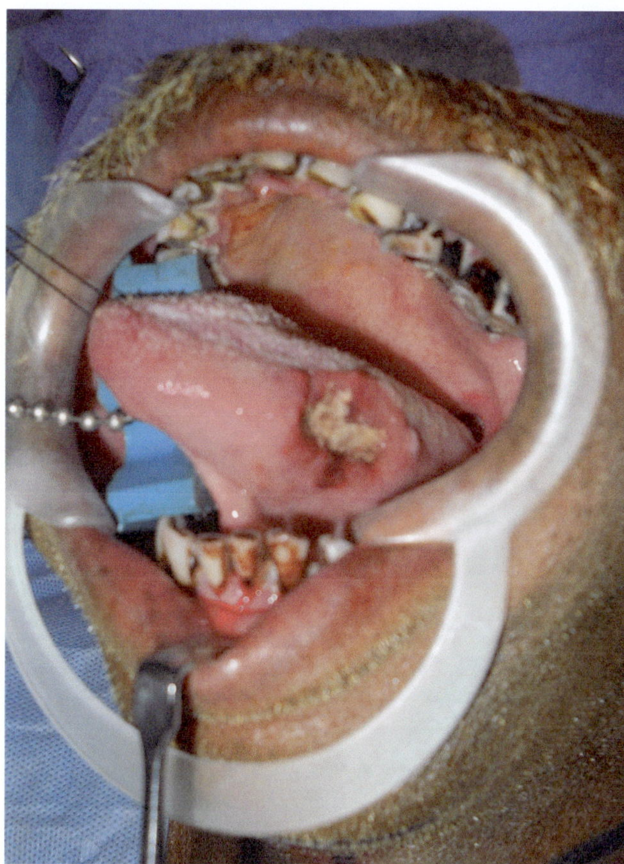

Fig. 8.8 Photograph showing another lesion on lateral border of the tongue. This is an infiltrative lesion

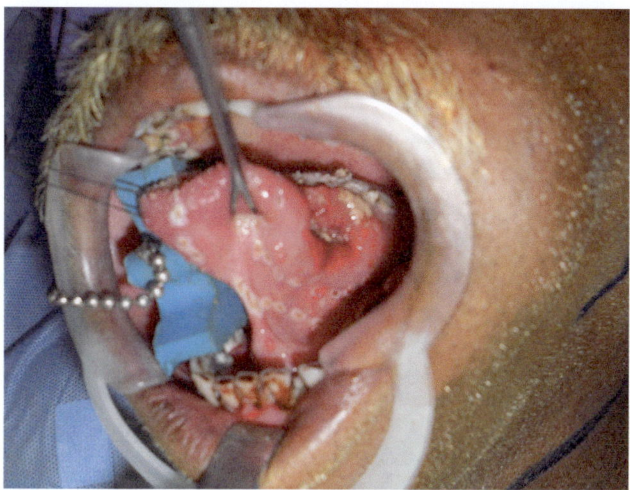

Fig. 8.9 The inner marking is for induration. It is very important to palpate the induration and mark it. The 1–1.5 cm wide margin is removed from this marking and not from the visible ulcer margin

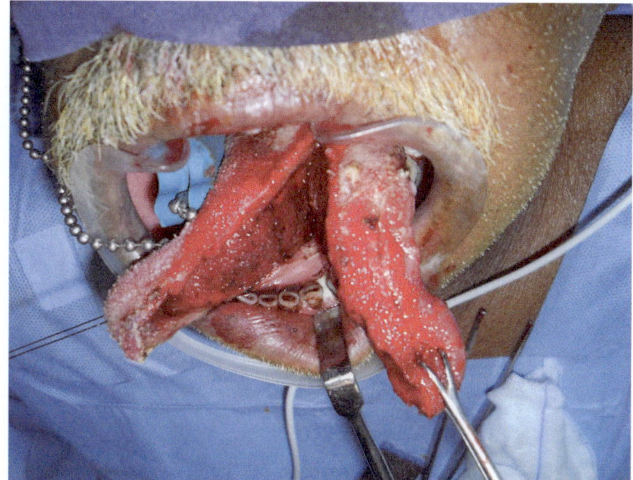

Fig. 8.10 Wide excision is performed

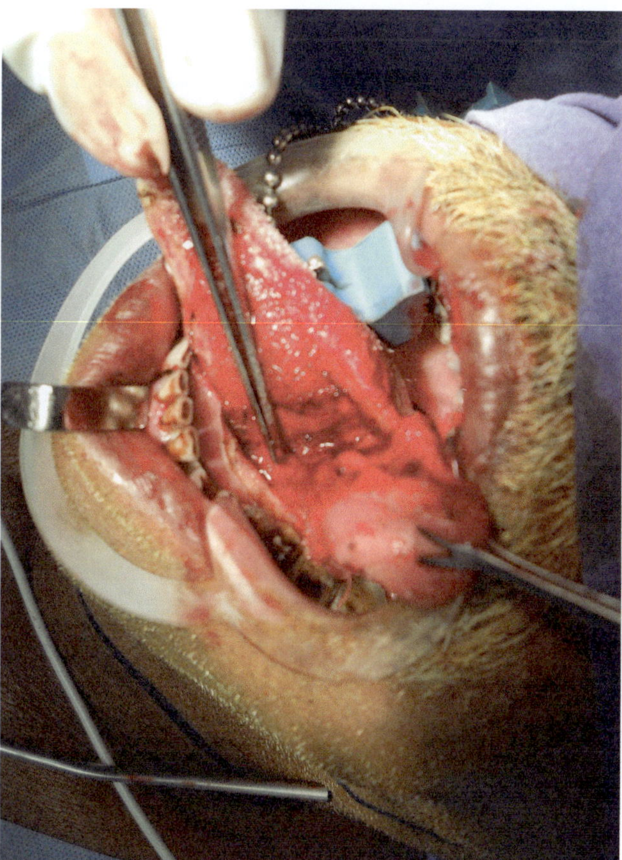

Fig. 8.11 The lingual artery is identified and ligated in depth

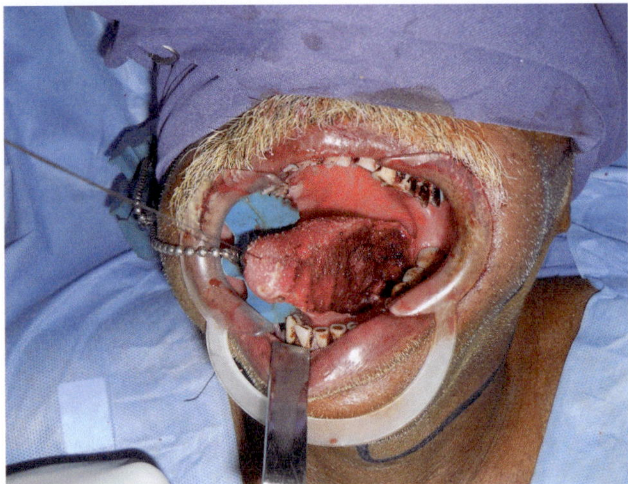

Fig. 8.12 Photograph shows complete resection superficially eroding mandible cortex with adequate hemostasis

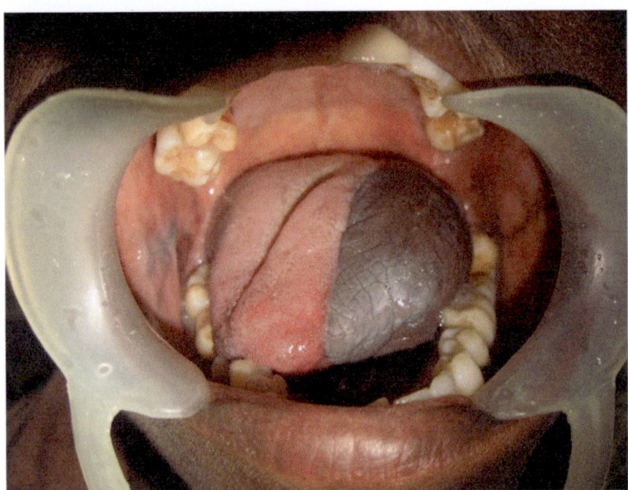

Fig. 8.13 Reconstruction of the defect with lateral arm flap. This flap is ideal for such defect. Alternatively, one can use infrahyoid flap as local–regional flap for such defects

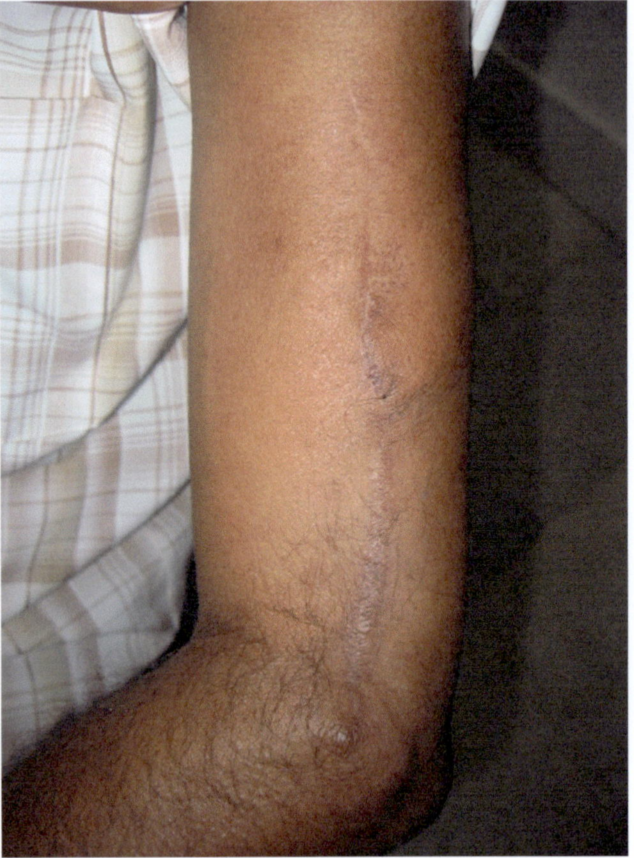

Fig. 8.14 The healed scar for lateral arm flap

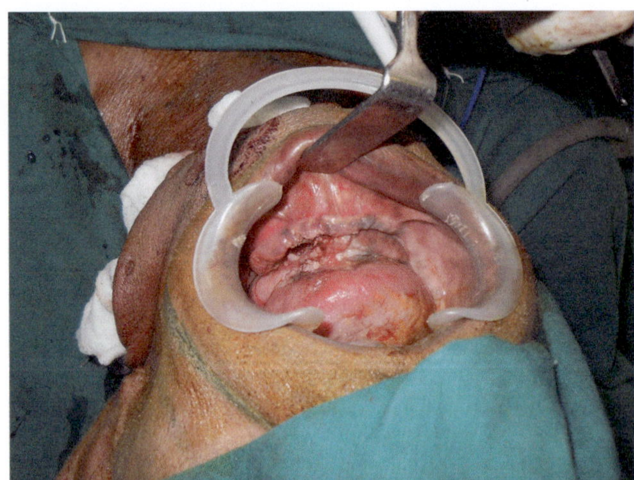

Fig. 8.15 The anterior FOM lesion superficially eroding mandible cortex

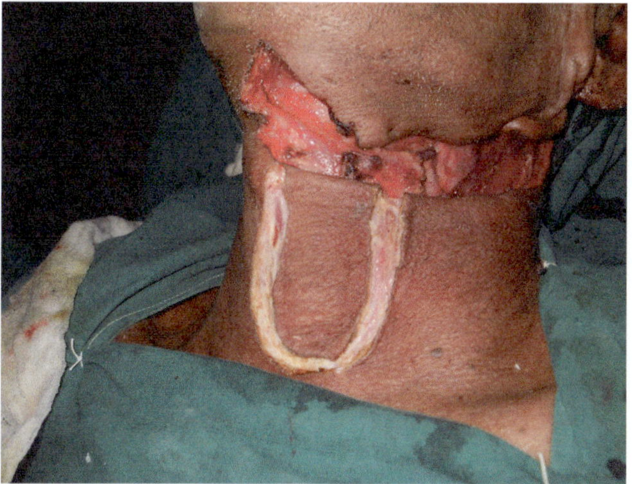

Fig. 8.16 Proposed infrahyoid flap

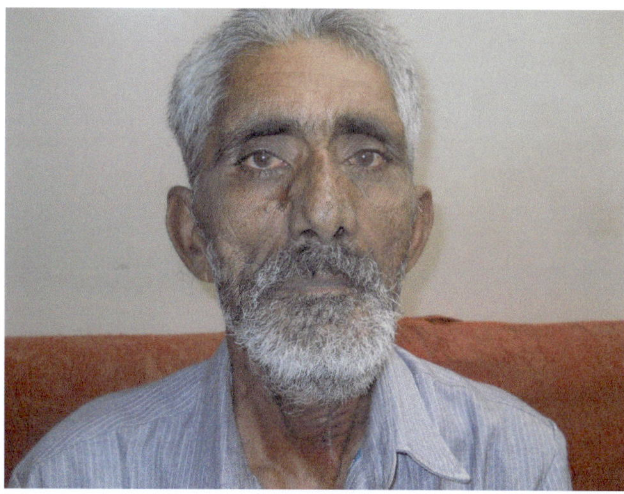

Fig. 8.19 The final outcome of this patient

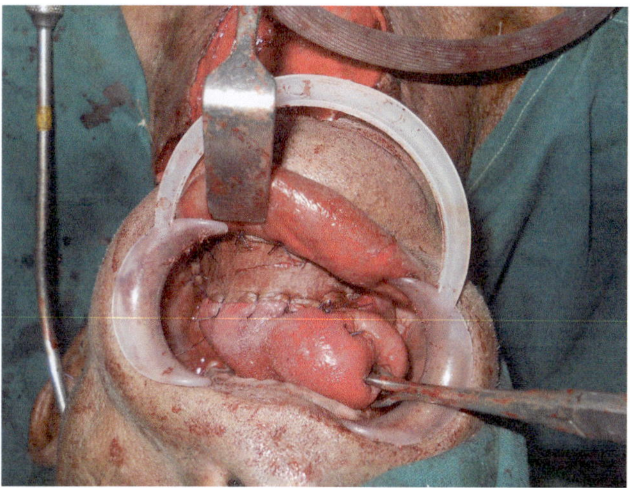

Fig. 8.17 Flap insertion to reconstruct defect

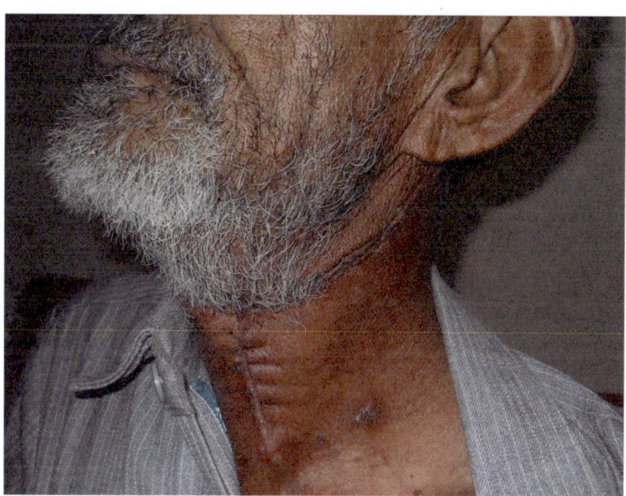

Fig. 8.20 Healed scar for donor site. This flap is preferred over submental flap as donor site doesn't involve any lymph node area

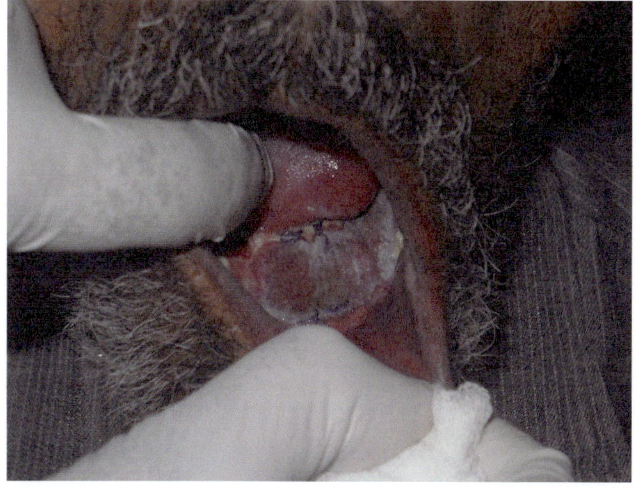

Fig. 8.18 Healed flap

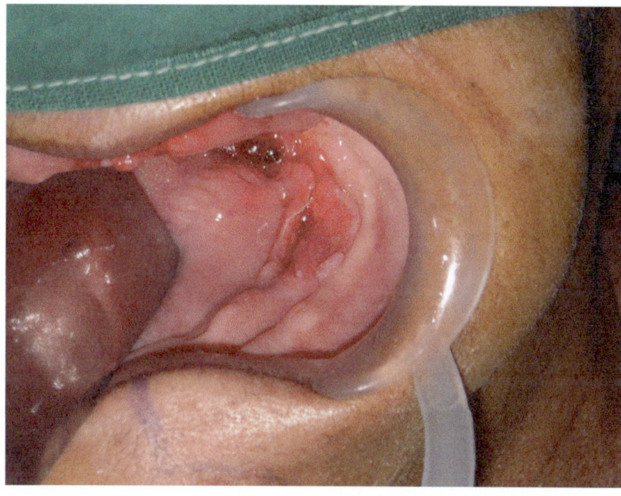

Fig. 8.21 Posterior FOM lesion abutting mandible

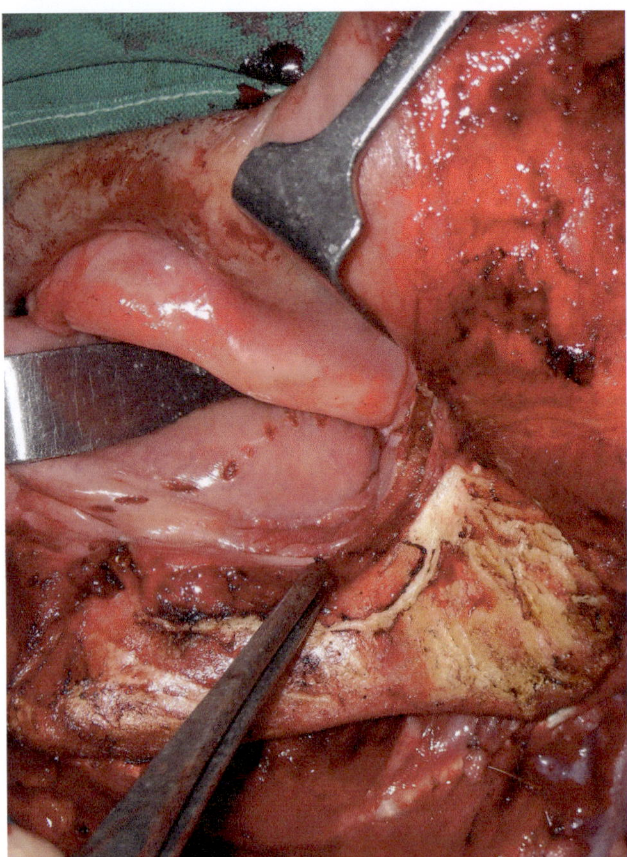

Fig. 8.22 Cheek flap is raised to have adequate exposure

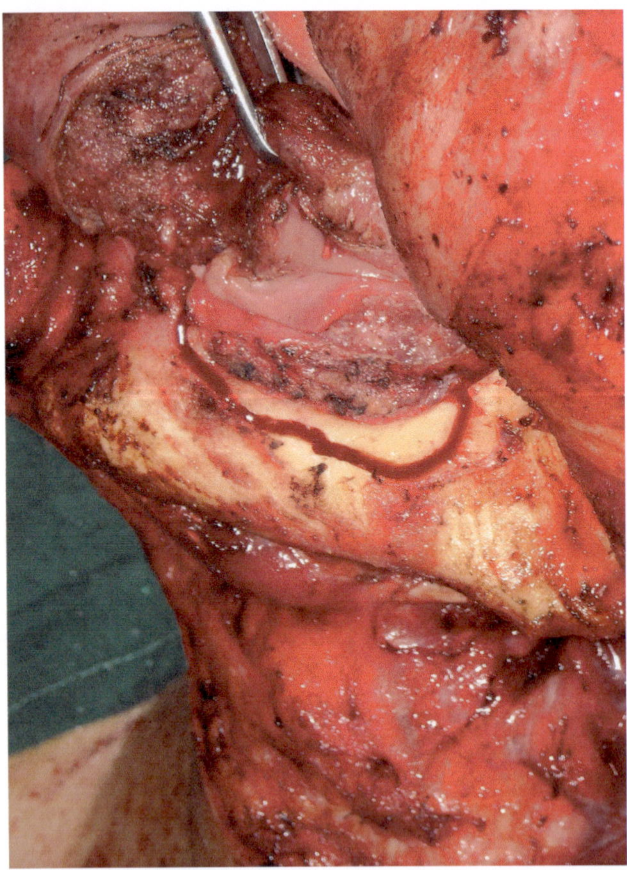

Fig. 8.23 Marginal mandibular resection

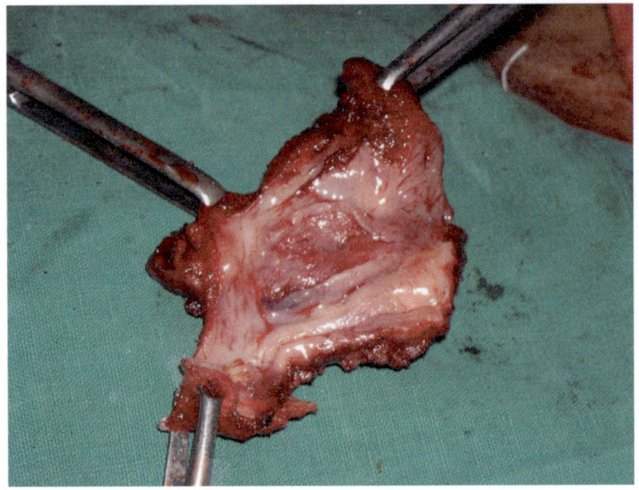

Fig. 8.24 Resected specimen with adequate tumor free margins

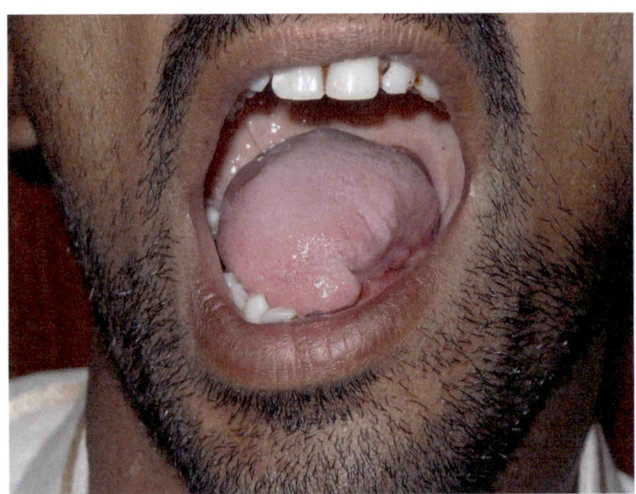

Fig. 8.25 The final outcome

T2 Lesion

This section demonstrates surgical procedure for T2 lesion. The procedure is performed with concept of compartment resection for 3-D resection.

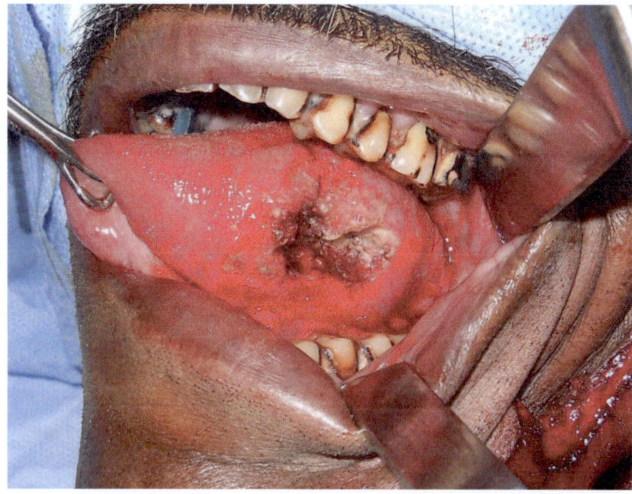

Fig. 8.26 Large infiltrative lesion involving lateral half of the tongue

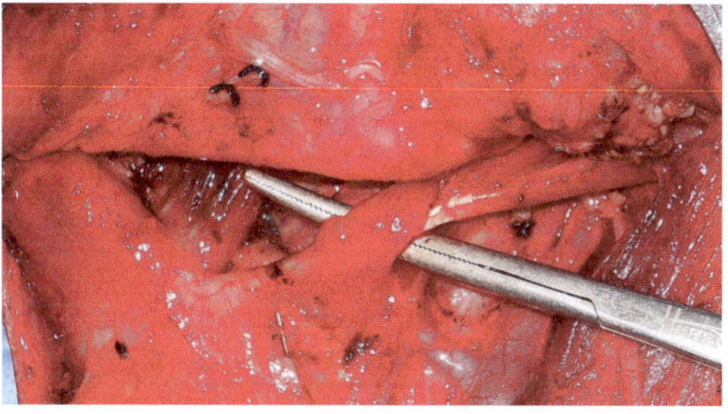

Fig. 8.27 After performing SND (level I to IV), resection for primary tumor starts in retrograde manner (deep margin first). The digastric muscle is divided

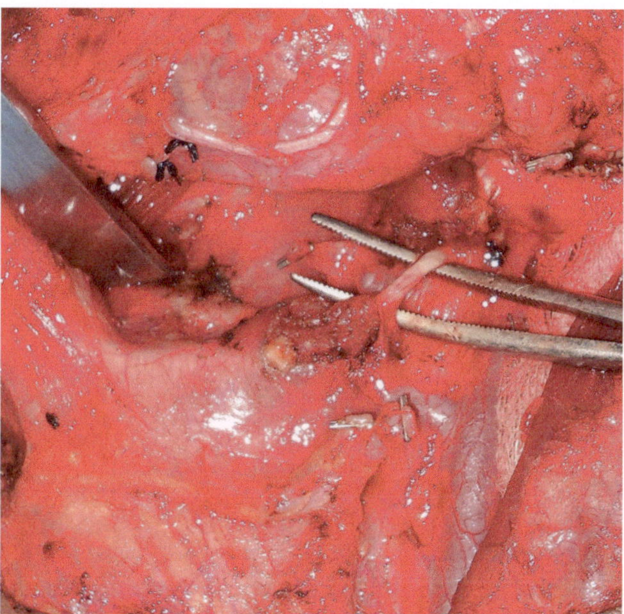

Fig. 8.28 Hypoglossal nerve is identified and transected

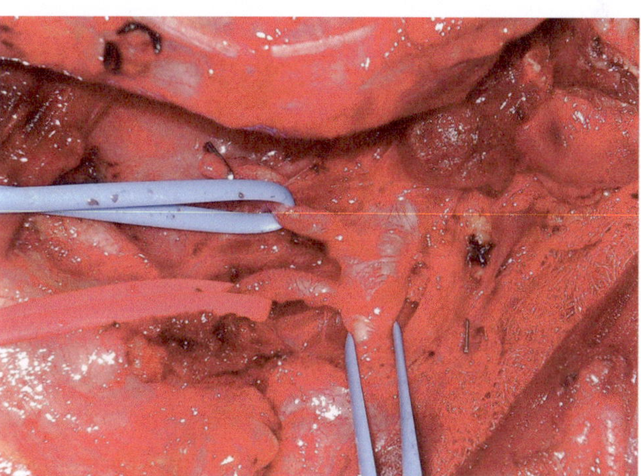

Fig. 8.29 Identification of external carotid artery and ligation of lingual and facial artery. This helps in reducing bleeding while resecting the tongue. This manoeuver also helps in opening up the parapharyngeal space to allow resection of hyoglossus muscle from hyoid bone

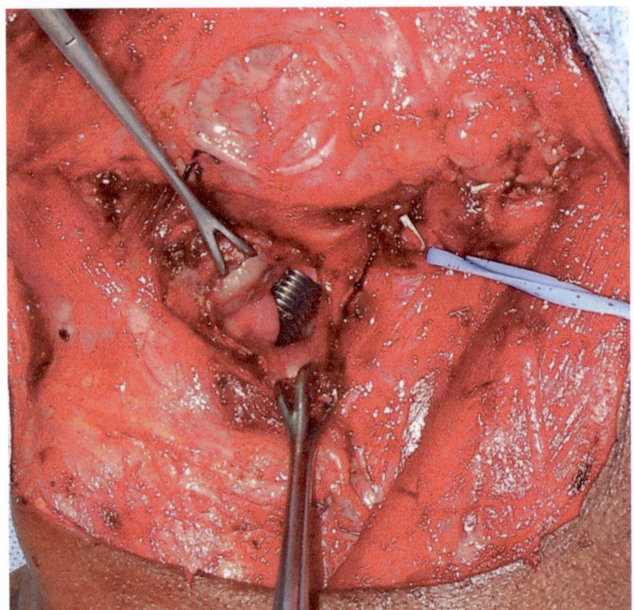

Fig. 8.30 The hyoglossus muscle is completely detached from hyoid bone

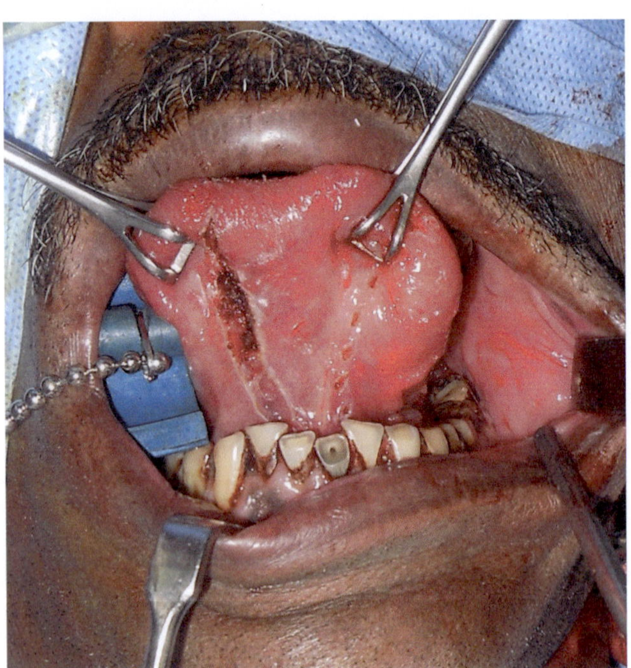

Fig. 8.31 Proposed resection margin 1.5 cm away from marked induration

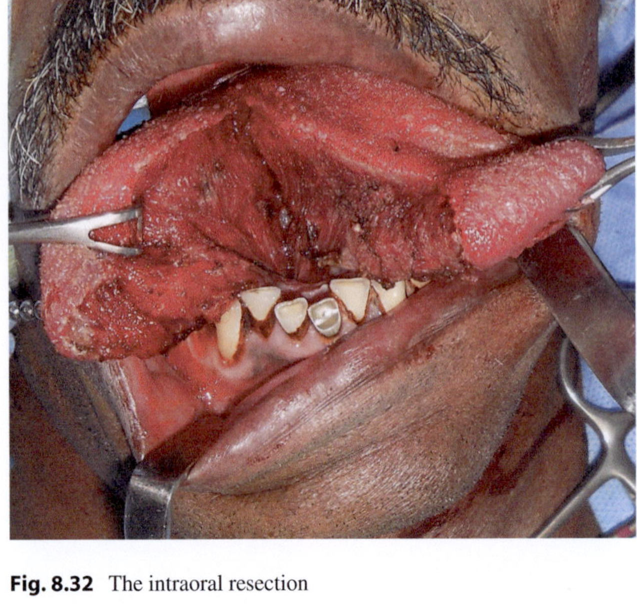

Fig. 8.32 The intraoral resection

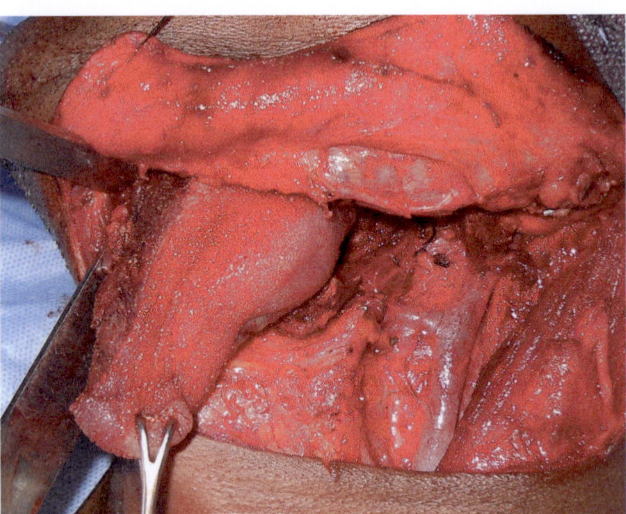

Fig. 8.33 The tongue is mobilized through neck

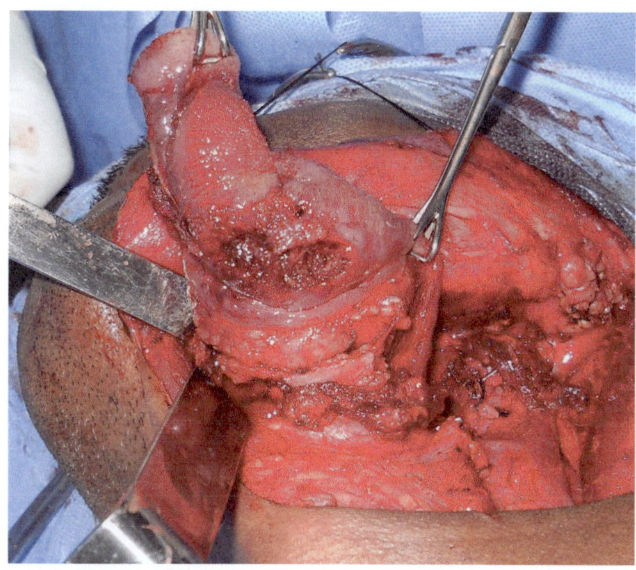

Fig. 8.34 The entire compartment is showing tumor clearance in all three dimensions. It is difficult to achieve this type of clearance by any other approach. This also enables us to remove lymphatics in the sublingual region in en-bloc manner and may help in better local control

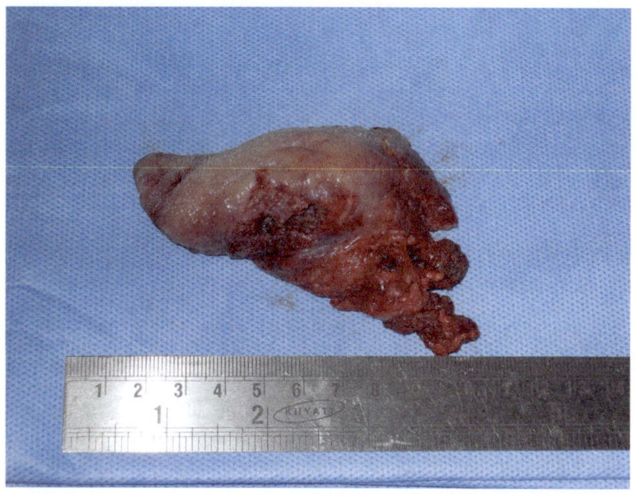

Fig. 8.35 Photograph showing entire hyoglossus muscle in its anatomic position. This demonstrates that the inferior margin can rarely be positive with this approach

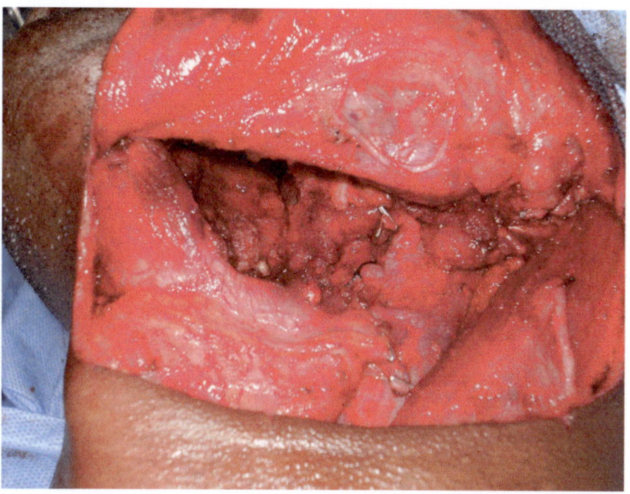

Fig. 8.36 Through and through defect from below. This needs reconstruction with flap

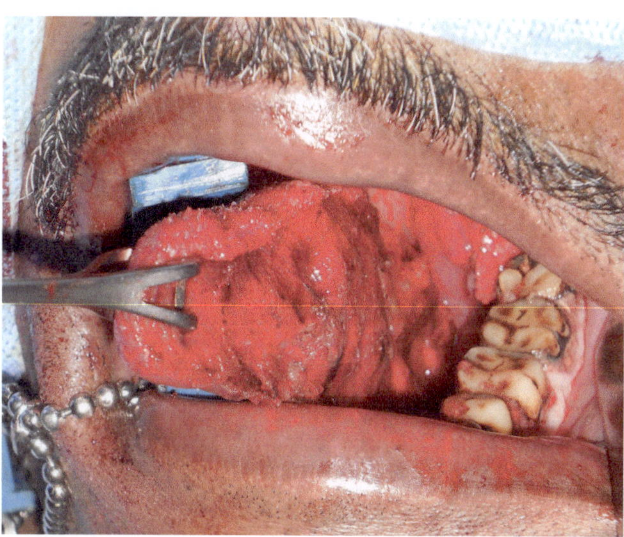

Fig. 8.37 Extent of intraoral resection. The entire vertical compartment is removed

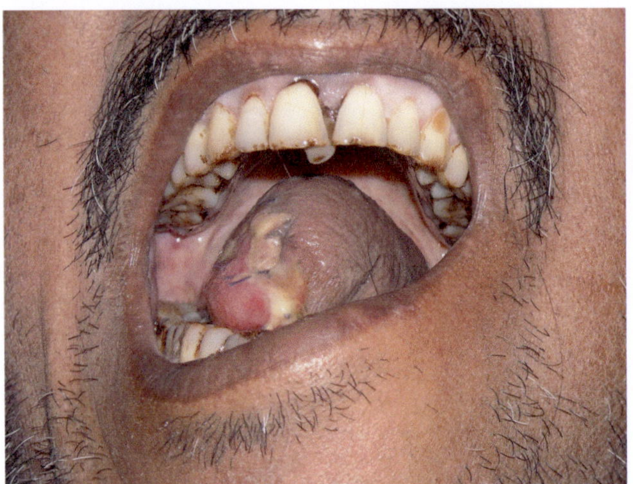

Fig. 8.38 Reconstruction with radial forearm flap. This defect can also be reconstructed with PMMC flap if facility for free flap is not available. The extent of resection should not be compromised in fear of difficult reconstruction

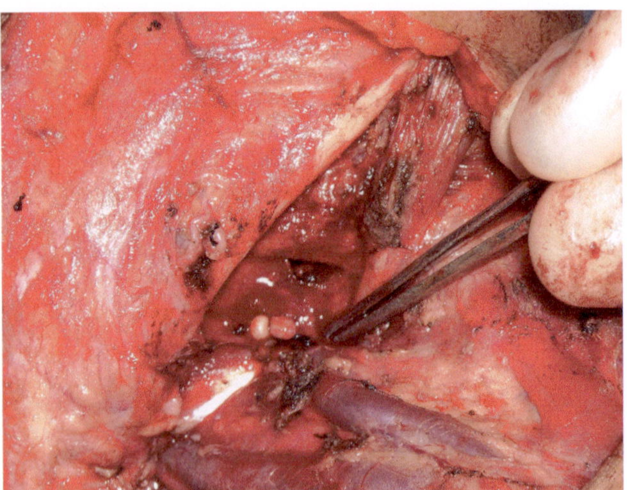

Fig. 8.39 In less infiltrative lesions, the mylohyoid muscle can be preserved and the resulting defect is much less severe

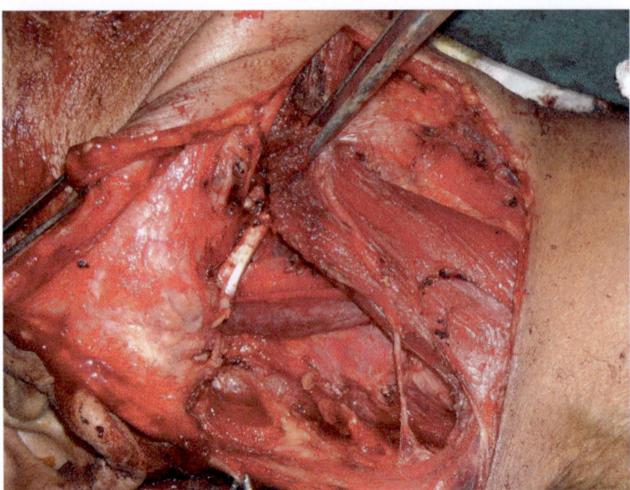

Fig. 8.40 This defect can be reconstructed by using the upper end of the SCM muscle. The muscle is separated from the mastoid and rotated to fill the FOM defect. The spinal accessory nerve is preserved in entire length

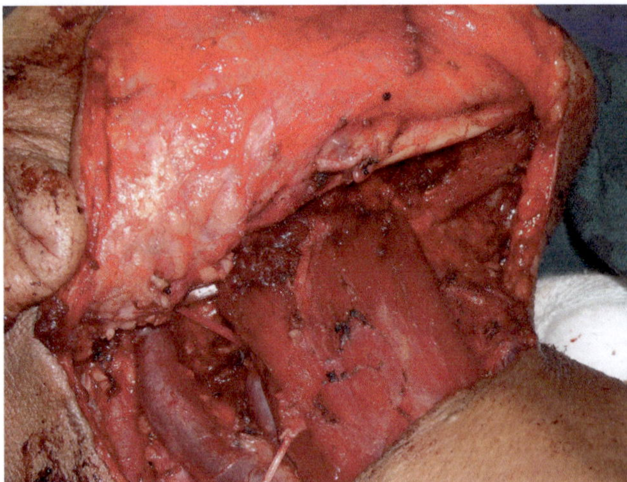

Fig. 8.41 The muscle is sutured to mylohyoid muscle and medial pterygoid muscle laterally. This seals the FOM defect and intraoral tongue is left to heal by secondary intention. This mode of reconstruction is particularly useful in high volume centers and in resource constrained environment. This allows us to be more aggressive with 3-D resection and allows easy reconstruction

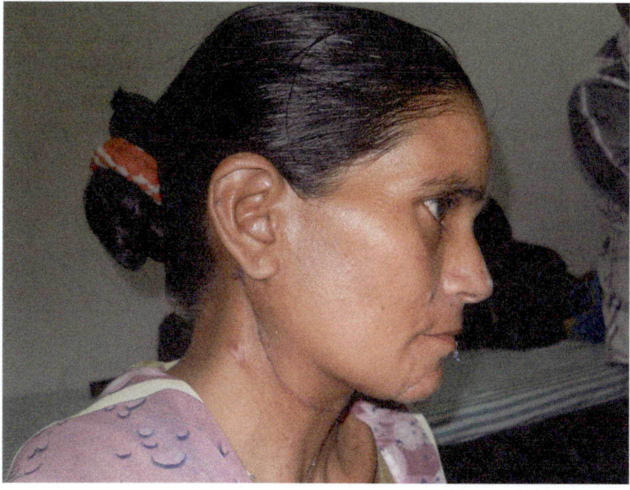

Fig. 8.42 The long-term outcome

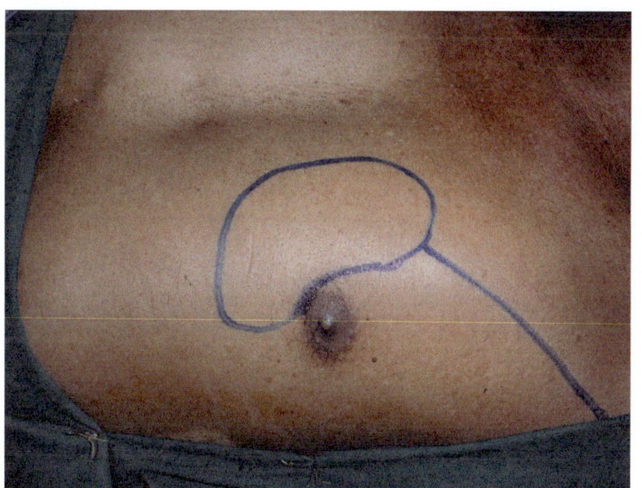

Fig. 8.43 Proposed PMMC flap for similar defect

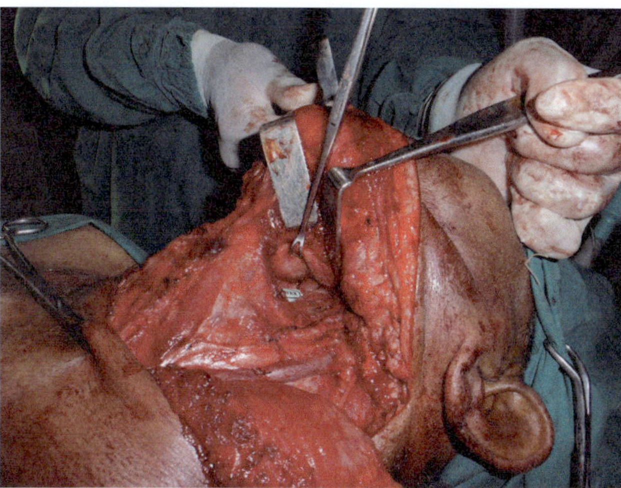

Fig. 8.44 Defect extending to the base of the tongue

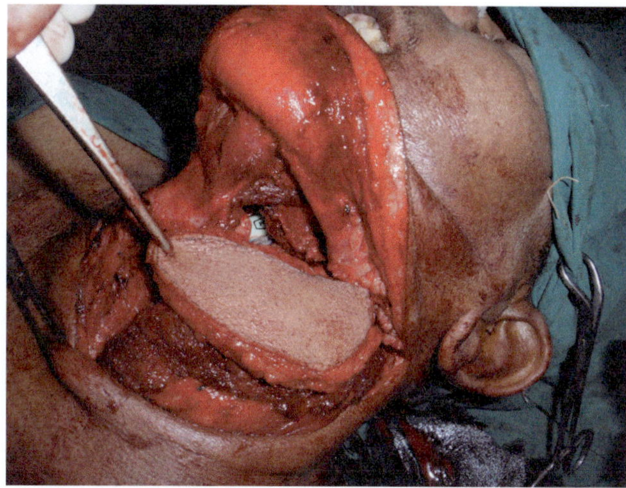

Fig. 8.45 The PMMC flap

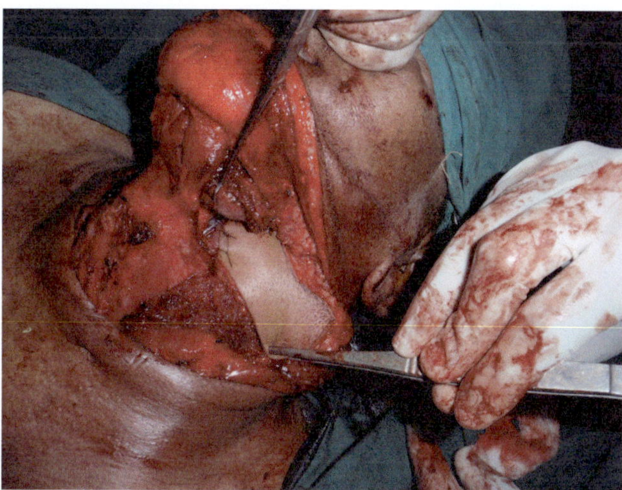

Fig. 8.46 Flap suturing. This is challenging as part of suturing is achieved from the neck while the other half is sutured through the intraoral approach

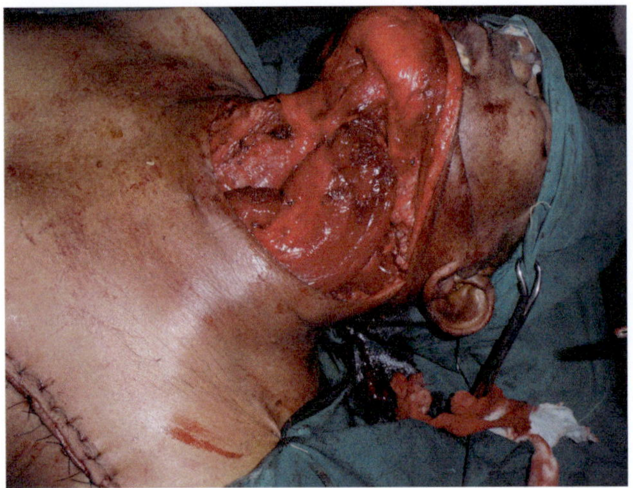

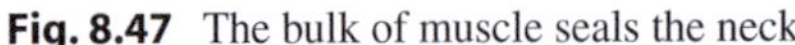

Fig. 8.47 The bulk of muscle seals the neck

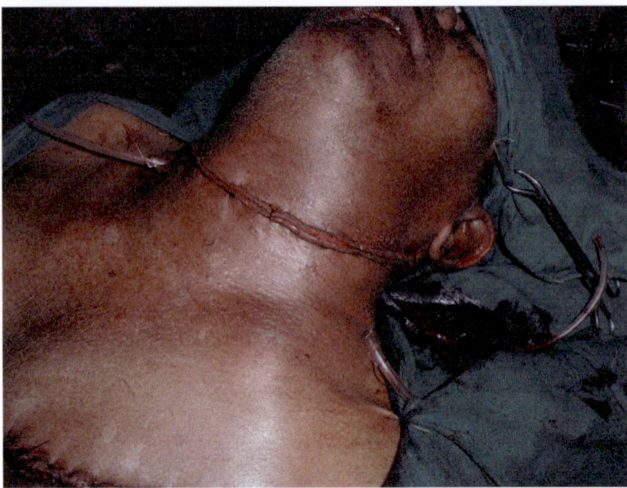

Fig. 8.48 The final closure

T3 and T4 Lesion

This section demonstrates resection of large tongue tumors needing total glossectomy. The concept is similar to 3-D resection with entire tongue, FOM with bilateral submandibular and sublingual glands removed en bloc.

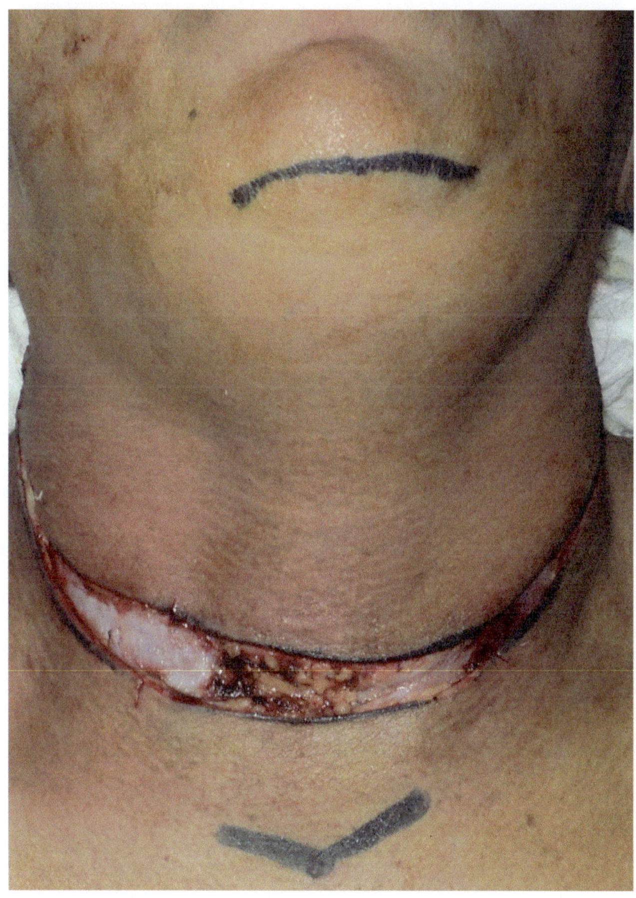

Fig. 8.49 Transverse cervical incision in neck

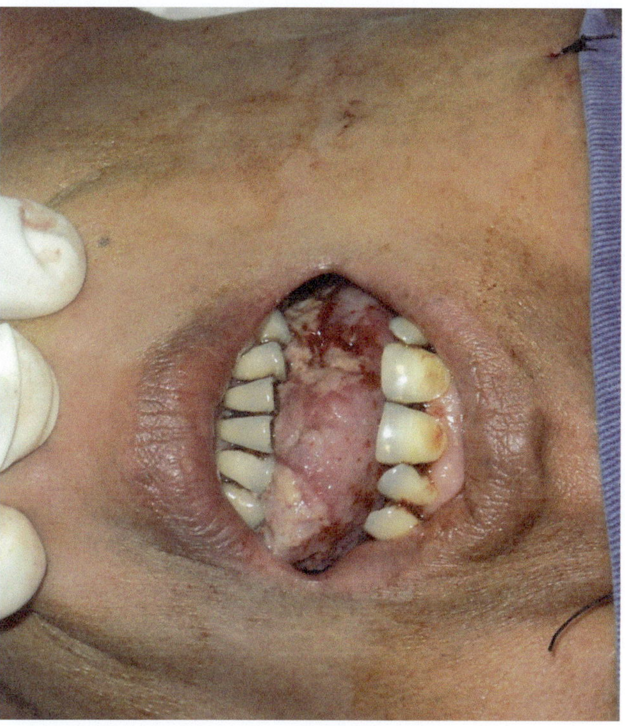

Fig. 8.50 The entire tongue is infiltrated by tumor

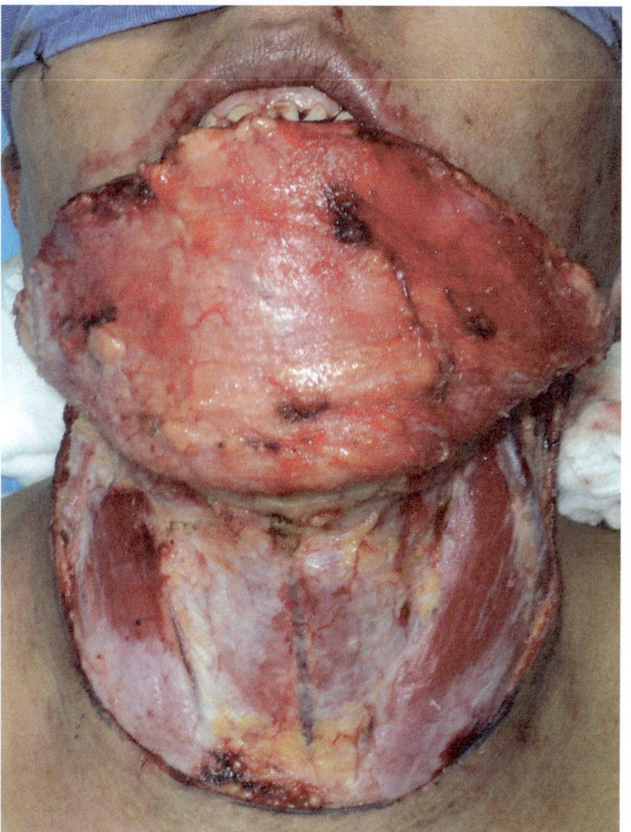

Fig. 8.51 The neck flap is raised. Care should be taken not to expose the buccal surface of the mandible. The blood supply to the mandible is maintained through its buccal attachments after the entire tongue is removed

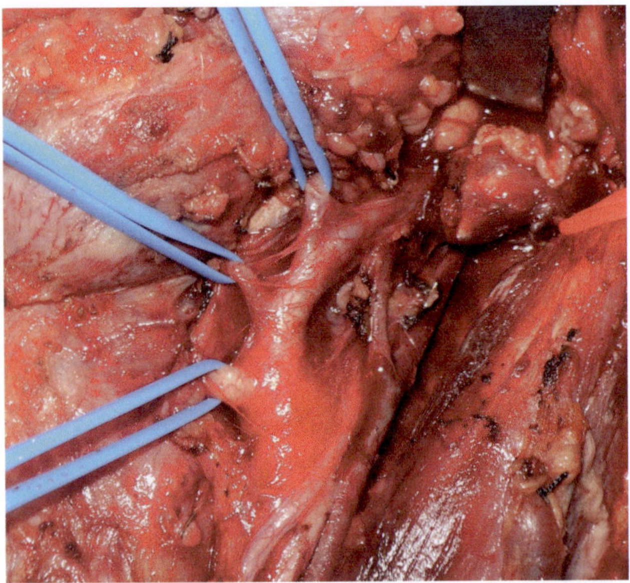

Fig. 8.52 Identification of the external carotid artery and ligation of lingual and facial artery

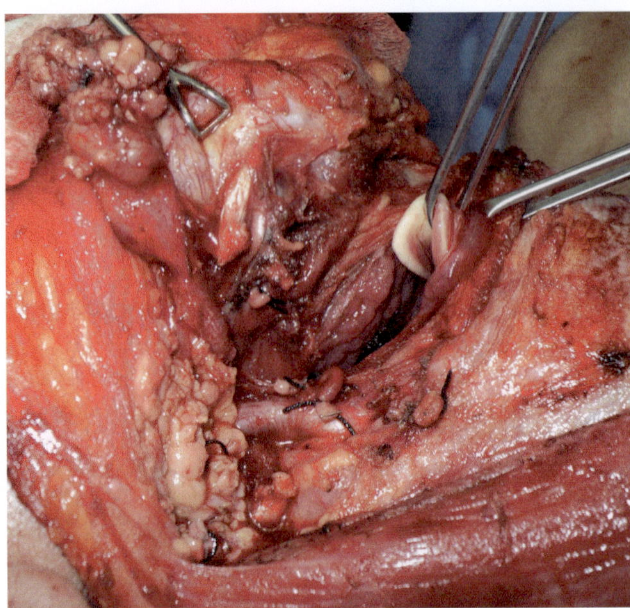

Fig. 8.54 The tongue base is freed from hyoid bone

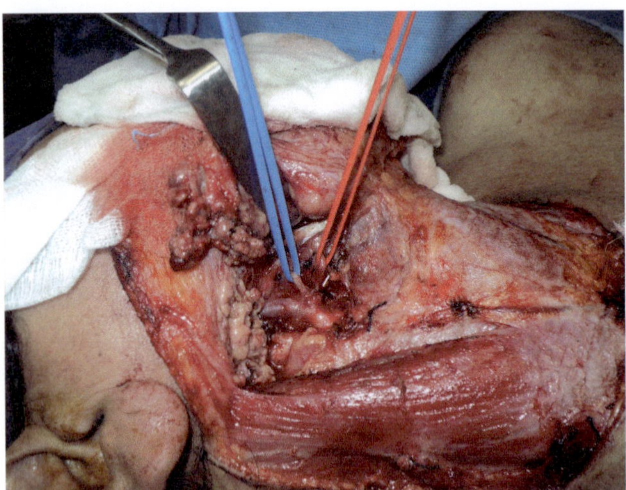

Fig. 8.53 This is done on either side of the neck. This helps in mobilizing the tongue from below and also makes the tongue avascular. This reduces bleeding while removing the tongue

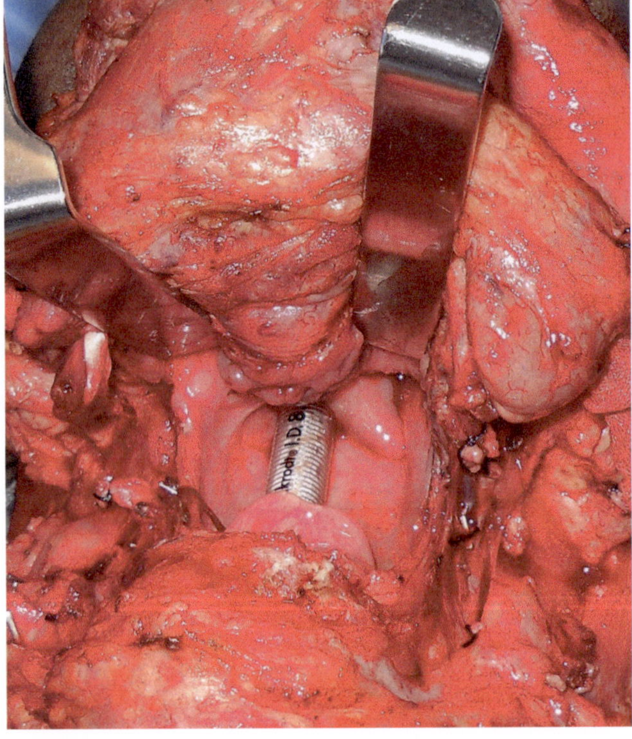

Fig. 8.55 The entire compartment of the tongue is separated from its base

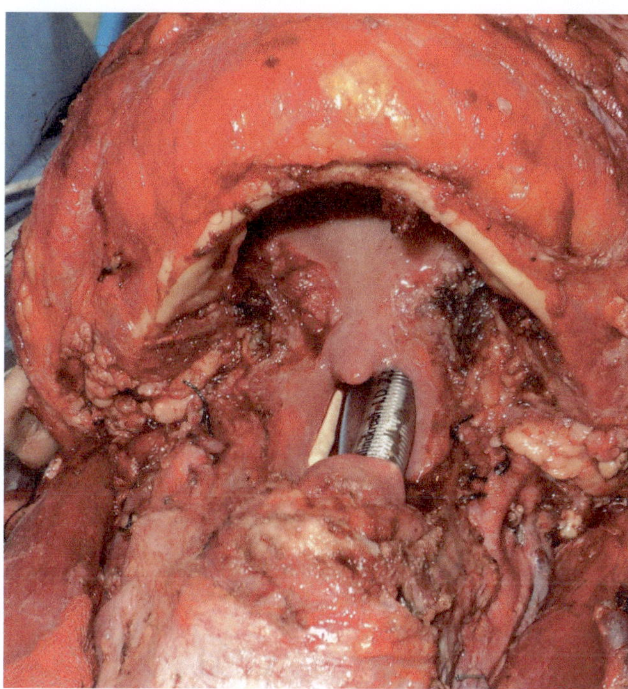

Fig. 8.56 The entire compartment is resected from one lateral pharyngeal wall to another lateral pharyngeal wall and from mandible to hyoid. This ensures negative margins in all directions

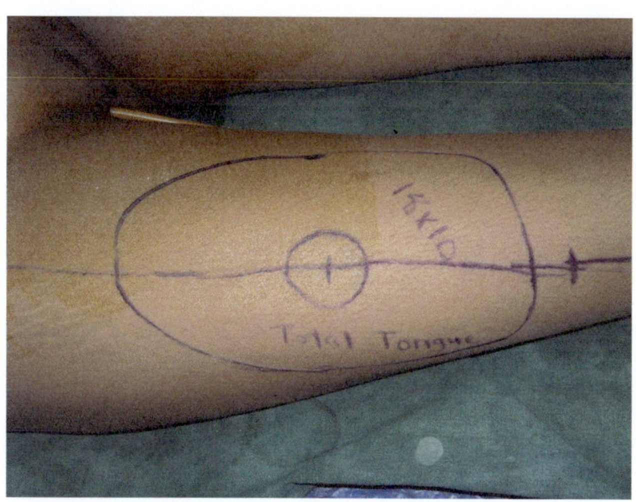

Fig. 8.57 The ALT flap is raised and ready for insertion

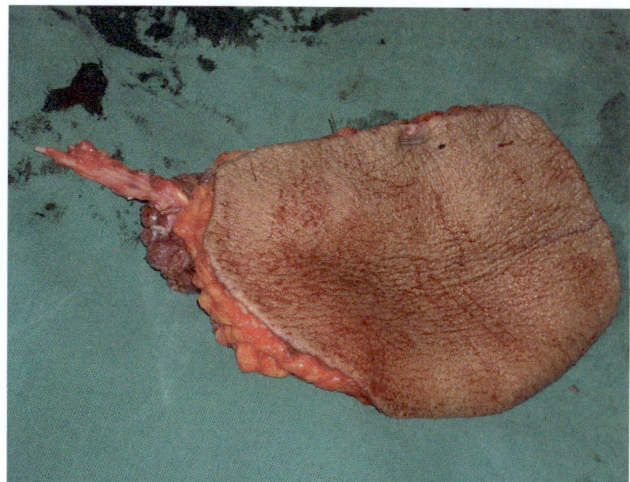

Fig. 8.58 The ALT flap with its vascular pedicle

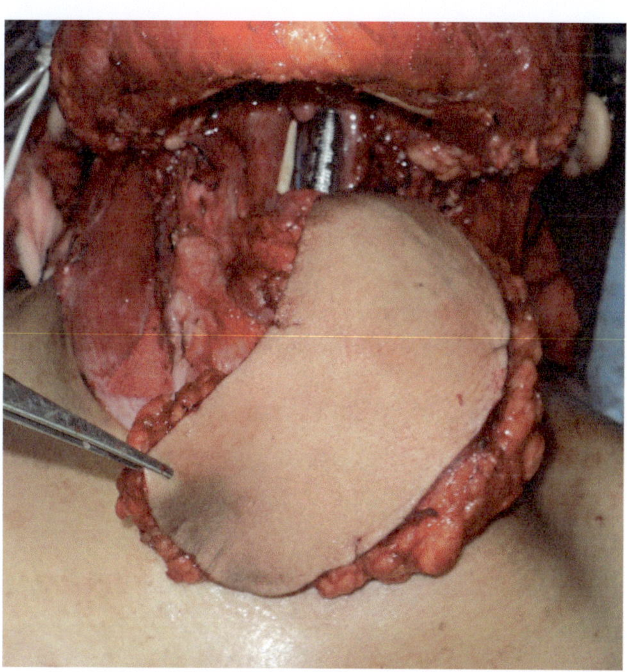

Fig. 8.59 The flap is ready for insertion

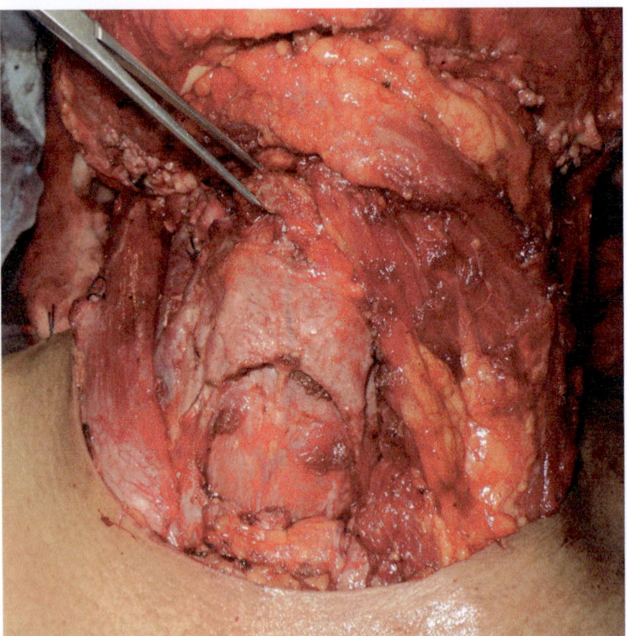

Fig. 8.60 The larynx pull-up procedure. The infrahyoid strap muscles are released to free the larynx and hyoid. The hyoid is pulled up to push the larynx anteriorly, and this manoeuver helps in reducing postoperative aspiration. This is the single most important factor in improving swallowing function of total glossectomy patient

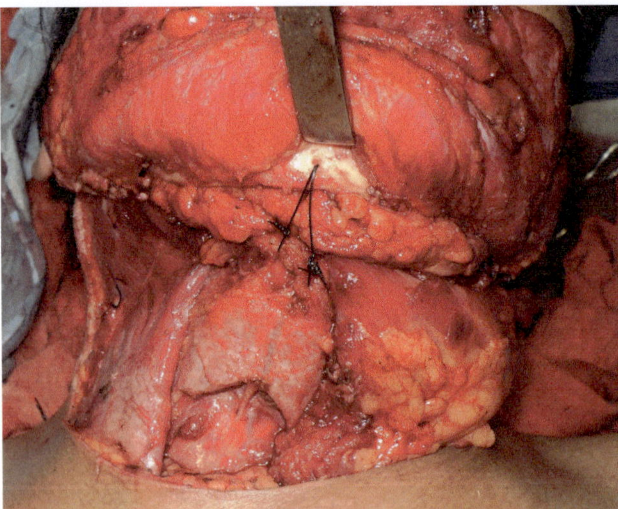

Fig. 8.61 Holes are made in the mandible by drill. Now hyoid bone is suspended by passing thick ethilon sutures through these holes and tied

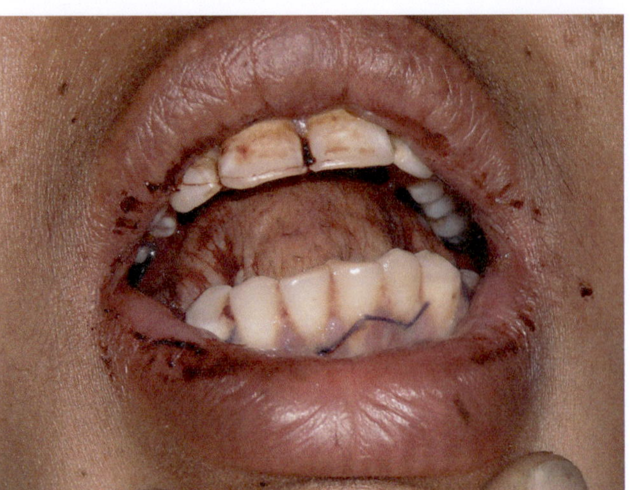

Fig. 8.62 The final outcome. It is advisable to have bulky flap in oral cavity as flap volume reduces with time. Swallowing is better with large and bulky flap

Complex Tongue Tumors

This section demonstrates surgical approach for large, complex lesions involving surrounding structure.

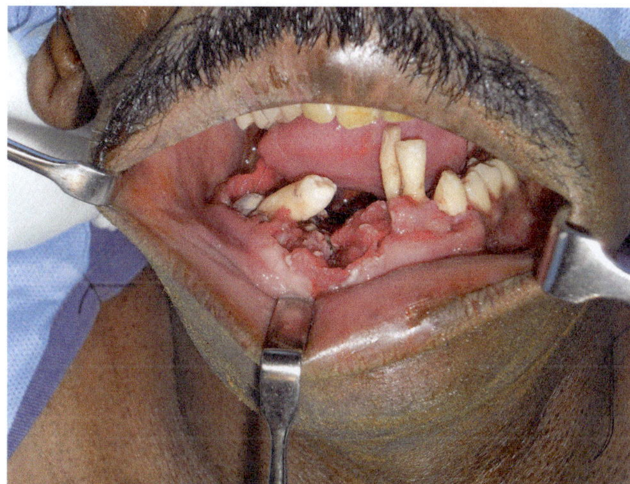

Fig. 8.63 Tumor involving tongue and eroding mandible causing pathological fracture

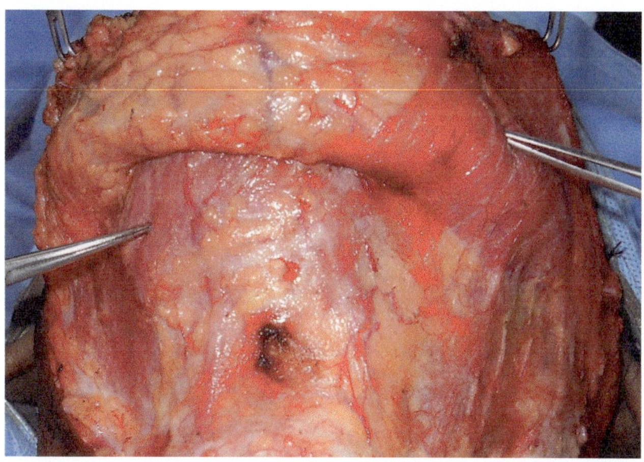

Fig. 8.64 Neck flap being raised. One can notice that flap is raised in the subcutaneous plane leaving platysma on large mass underneath

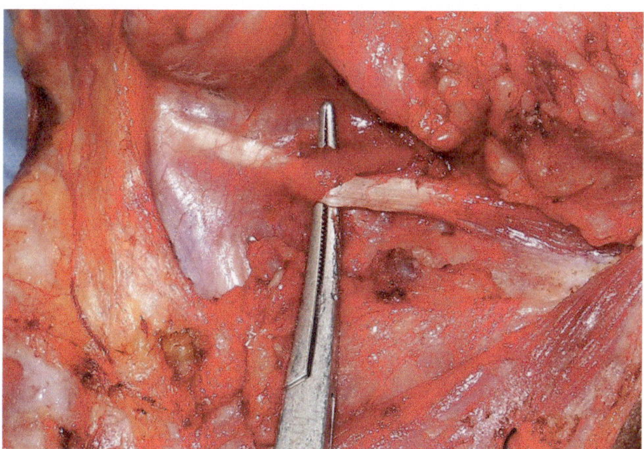

Fig. 8.65 The digastric is divided

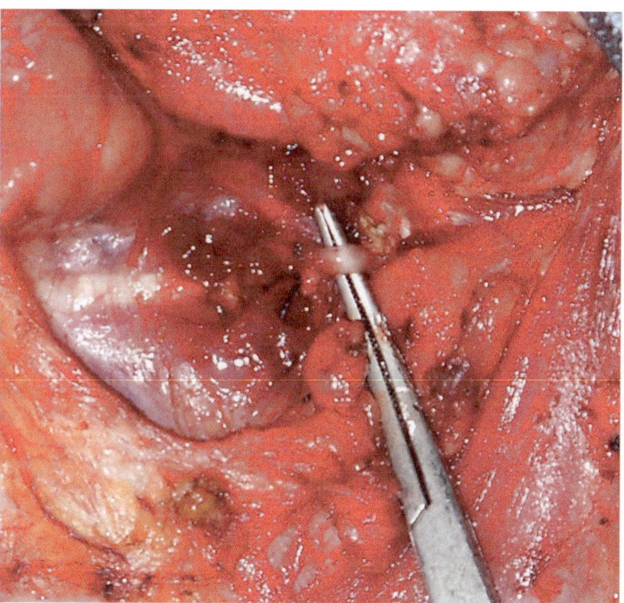

Fig. 8.66 Hypoglossal nerve is transected and lingual and facial vessels are ligated

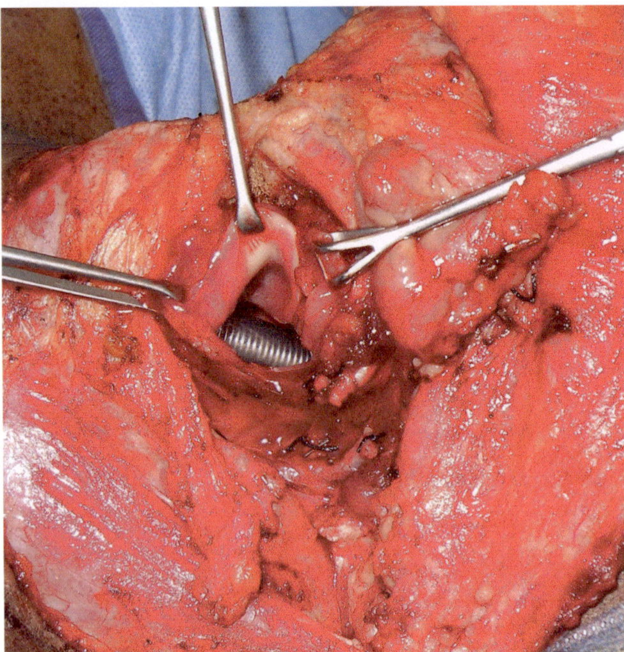

Fig. 8.67 The tongue base is mobilized as described earlier

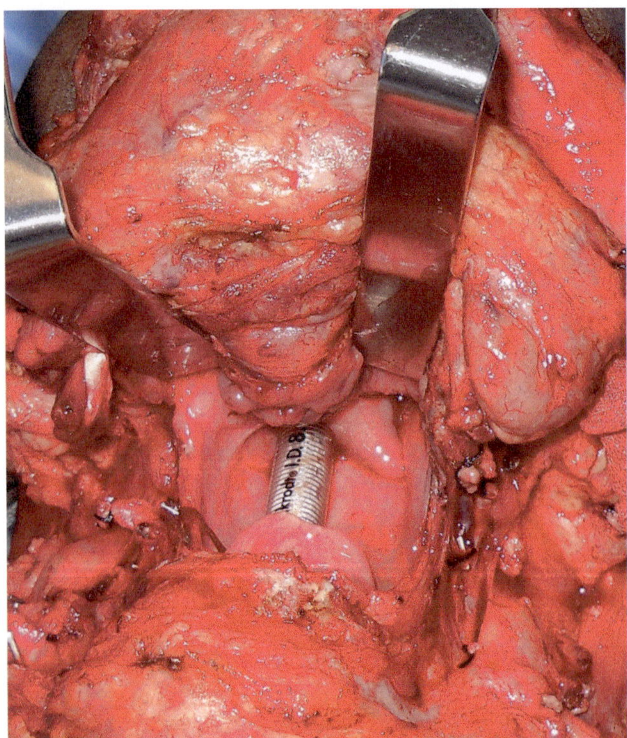

Fig. 8.68 The entire tongue lifted from hyoid

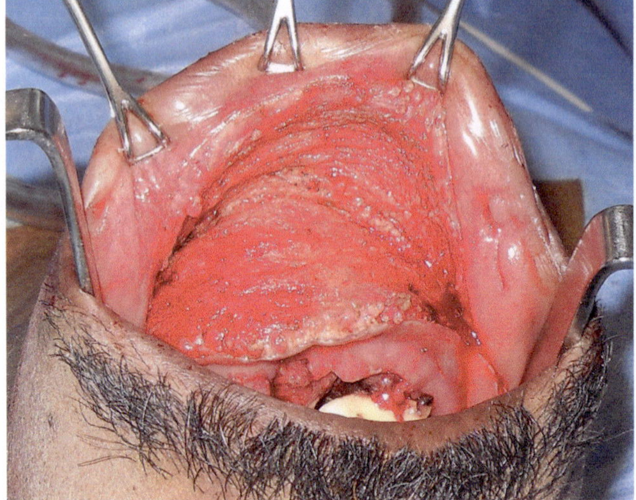

Fig. 8.69 Intraoral flap is raised

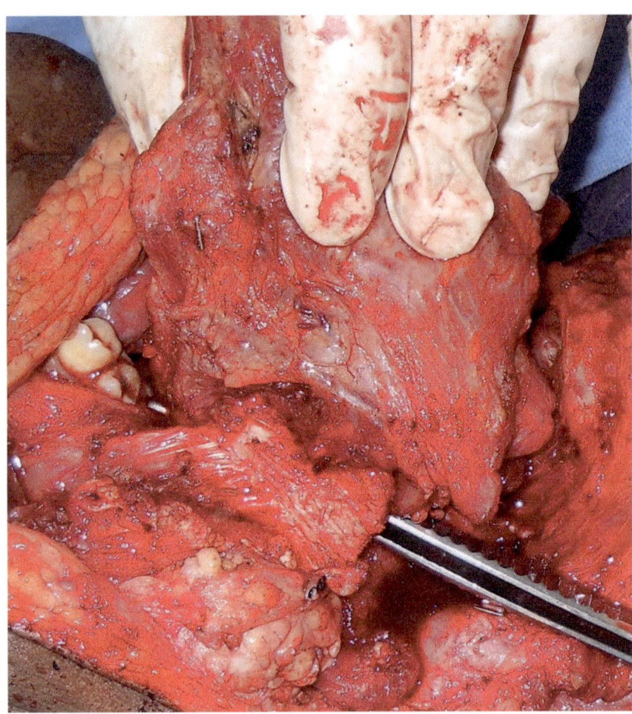

Fig. 8.70 Segmental mandibulectomy is being performed

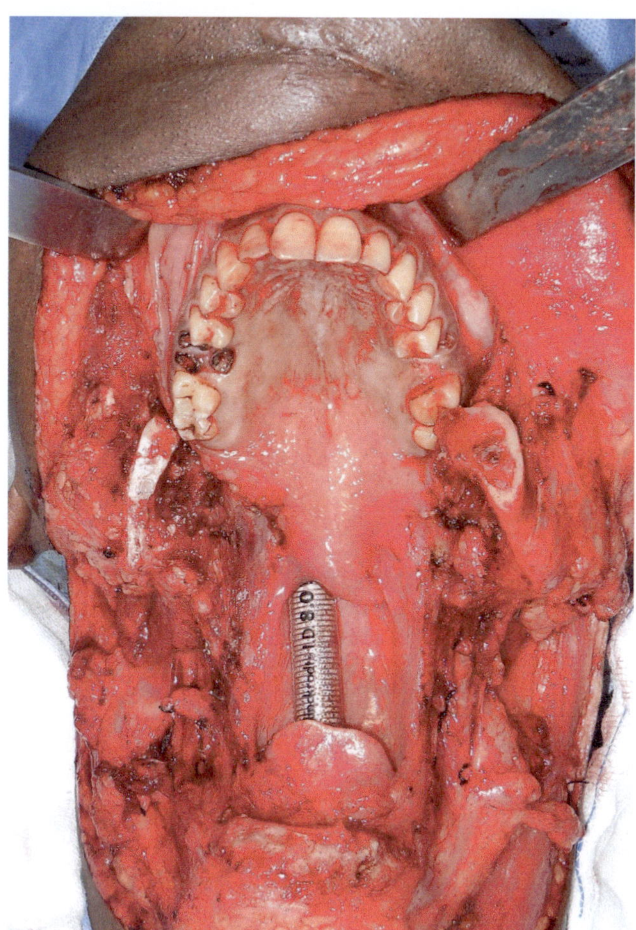

Fig. 8.71 The entire lower mandible and tongue are resected. The resulting defect needs reconstruction with two flaps. Bone flap is needed to provide support and soft tissue flap to provide tongue bulk

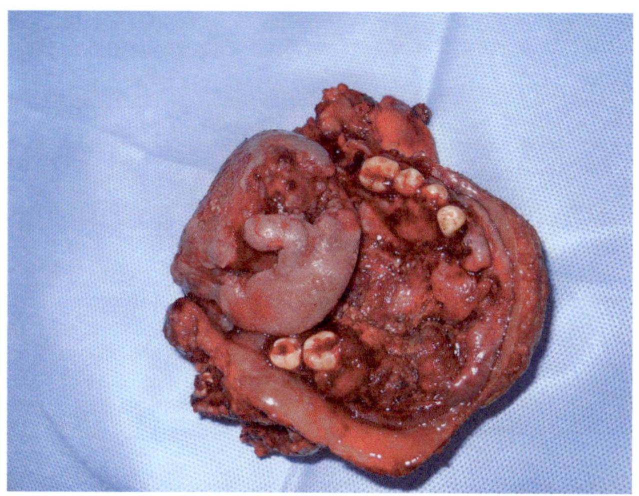

Fig. 8.72 Photograph showing specimen

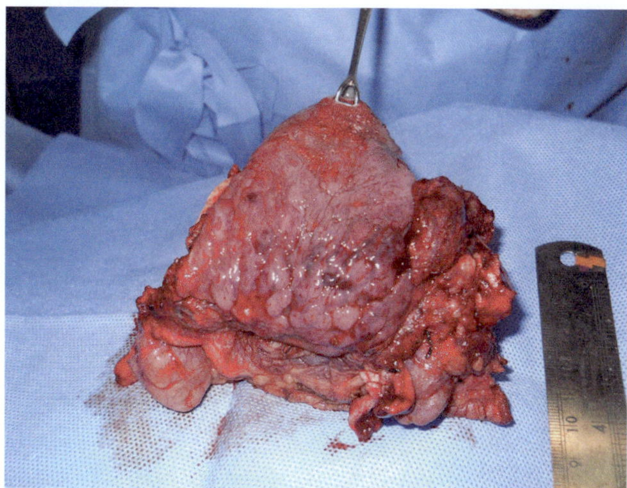

Fig. 8.73 The base of tumor

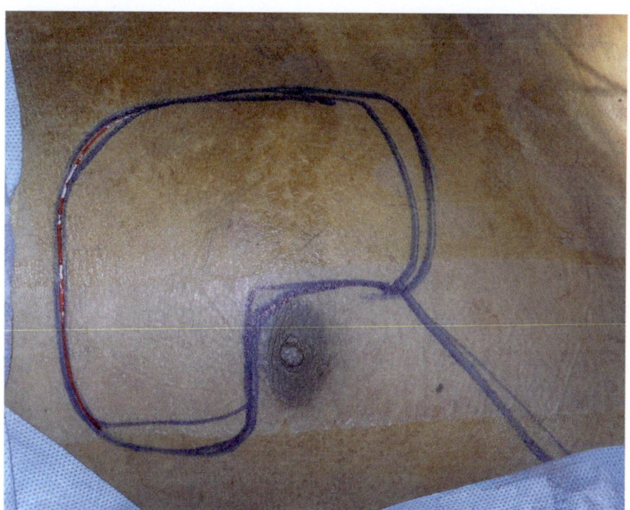

Fig. 8.74 The PMMC flap design

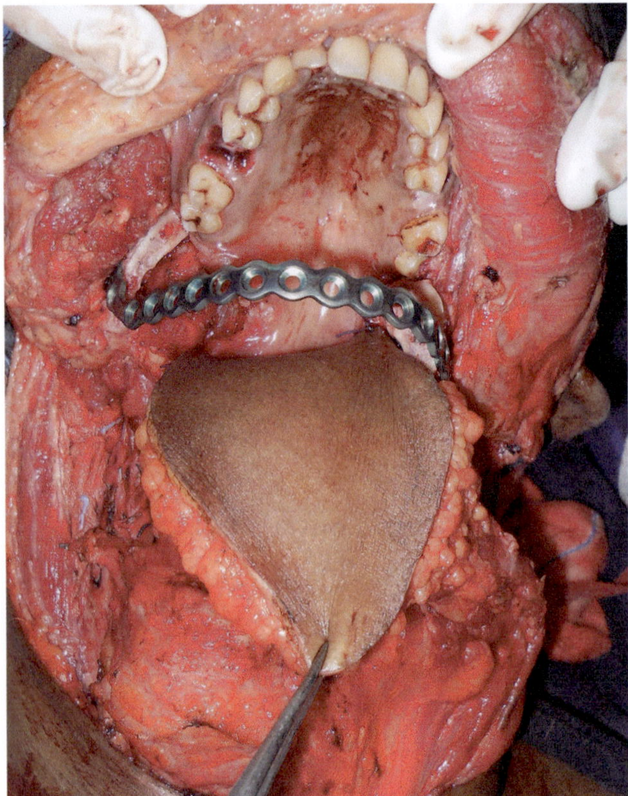

Fig. 8.75 The PMMC flap is inserted in the neck and plate is placed to fix fibula

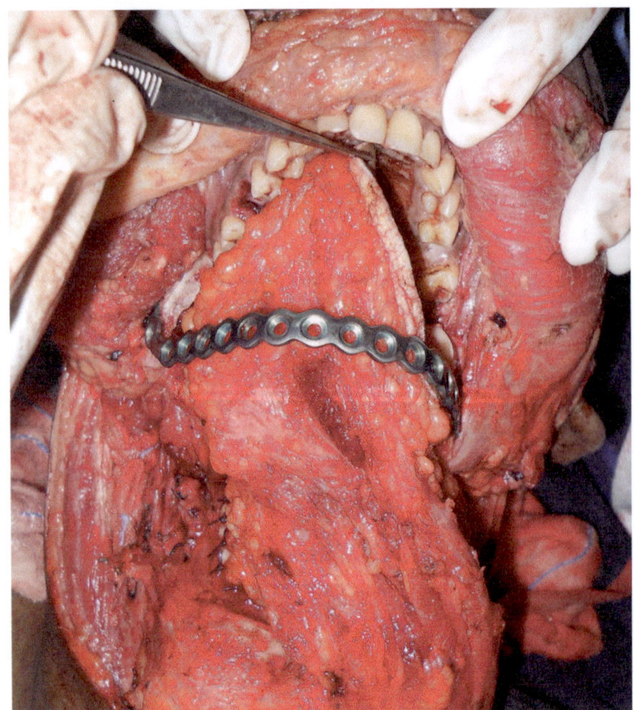

Fig. 8.76 Photograph showing pharynx suture line

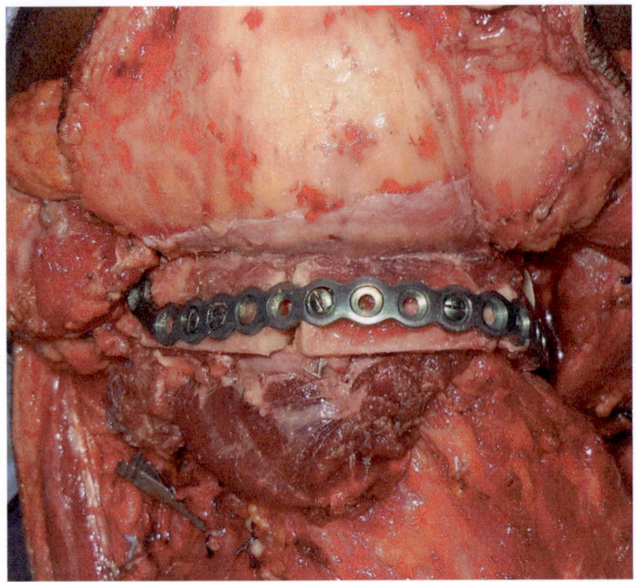

Fig. 8.77 The fibula flap is inserted and ready for anastomosis

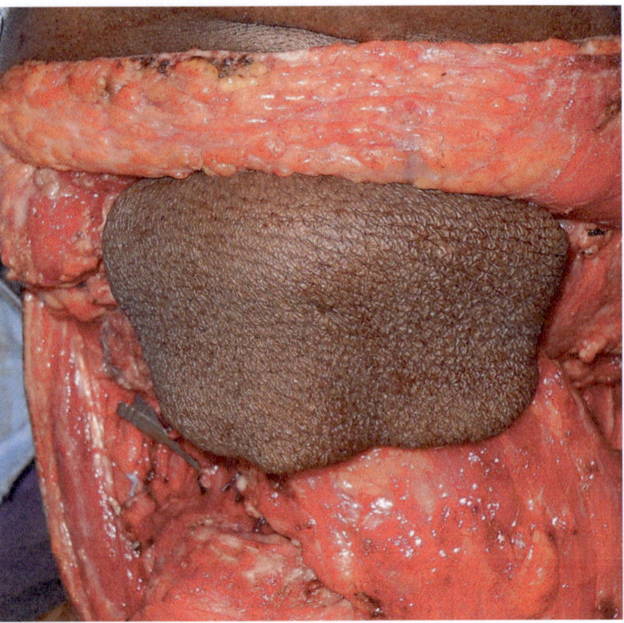

Fig. 8.78 Skin paddle of fibula flap will provide anterior floor of the mouth

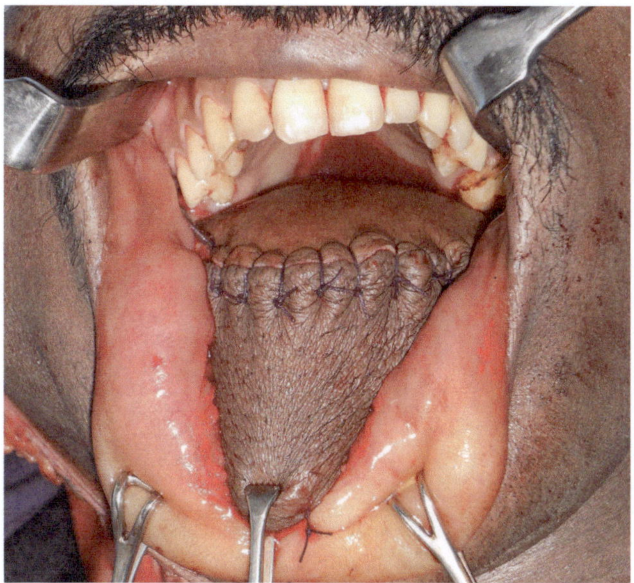

Fig. 8.79 Both flaps are sutured together

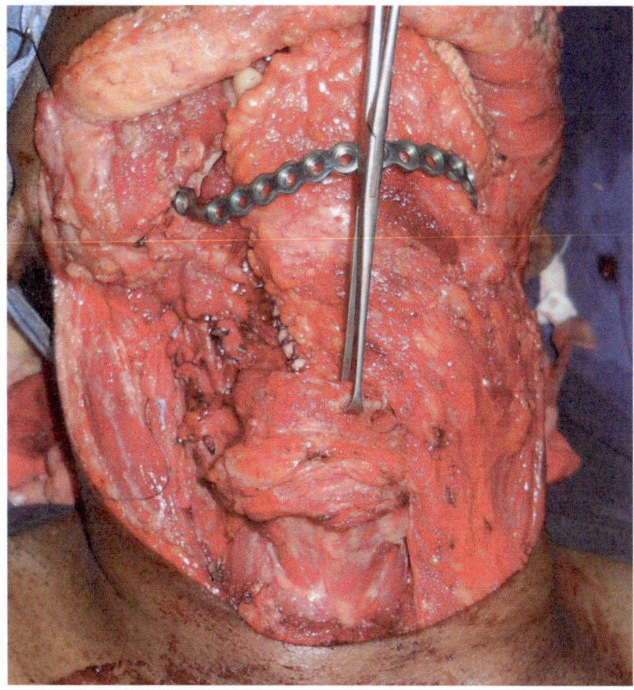

Fig. 8.80 The larynx suspension is prepared

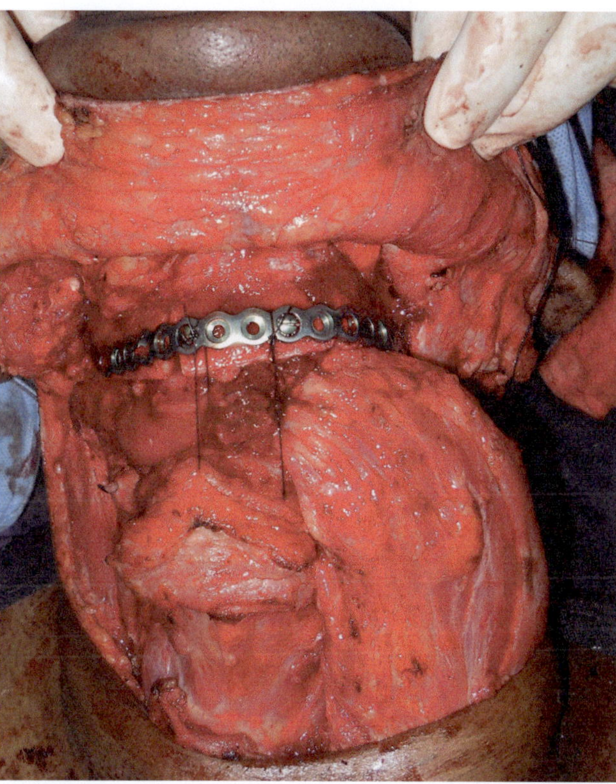

Fig. 8.81 The final suspension of hyoid to reconstructed mandible

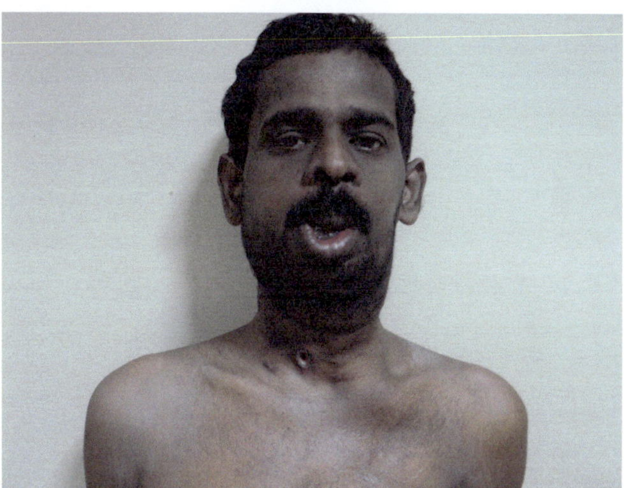

Fig. 8.82 Patient photograph after 1 month of procedure

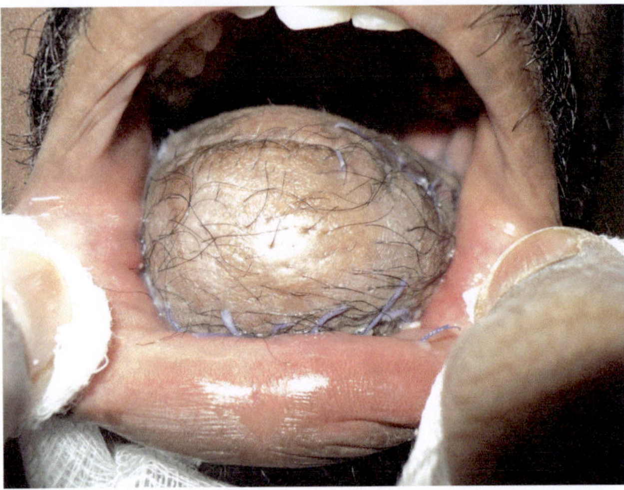

Fig. 8.83 Both flaps have healed well. This patient is rehabilitated to swallow semisolids and can communicate adequately. He has completed 2 years of follow-up and is doing fine

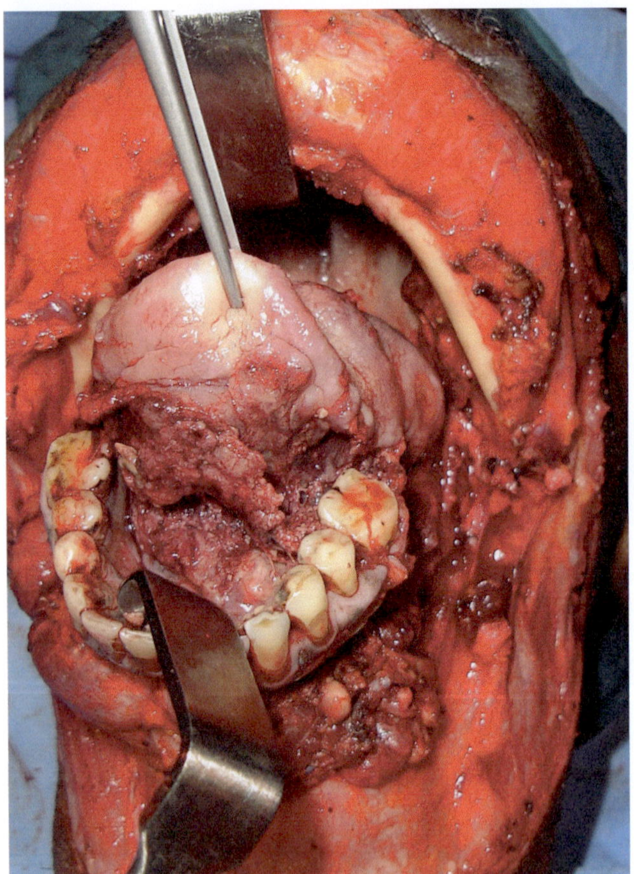

Fig. 8.84 This is another large tumor of the FOM abutting the mandible but not eroding it. Angle to angle marginal mandibular resection with total glossectomy is performed. This makes reconstruction significantly easy and recovery speedy

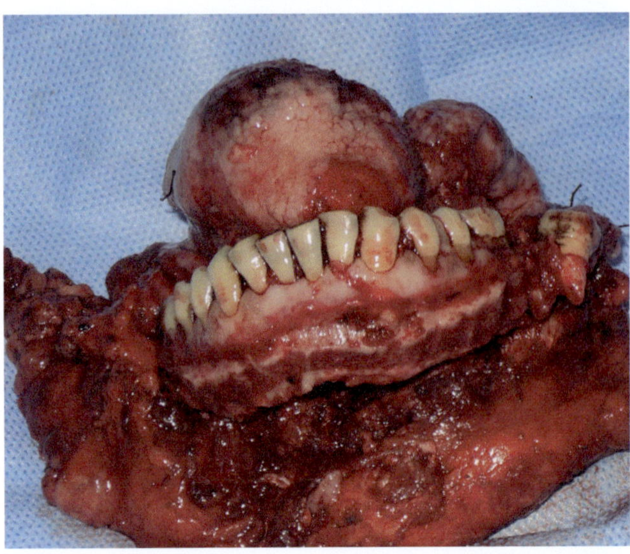

Fig. 8.85 The resected specimen showing entire lingual cortex being included in marginal resection

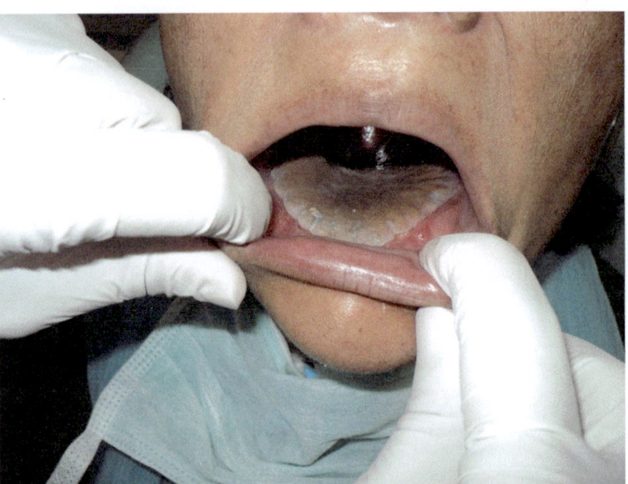

Fig. 8.86 The long-term outcome after complete healing

Reconstruction Algorithm

The tongue is a very important organ for speech and swallowing. The reconstruction of defect after tongue removal is very important for good quality of life. There are no set guidelines for reconstruction, and very few studies have compared functional outcomes after different reconstructive methods. Figure 8.87 demonstrates the algorithm that we follow at our institute.

Two major factors are to be considered while planning for reconstruction – tongue movement and tongue volume. Tongue movement is more important in the anterior portion as it affects speech. The tongue volume is more important in the posterior aspect as it affects swallowing function. The entire algorithm is developed keeping these factors in mind. The options include a variety of local flaps, regional flaps, and free flaps, and one should use them according to their training and resources available. The functional and cosmetic outcome remains acceptable as far as principles of tongue reconstruction are maintained.

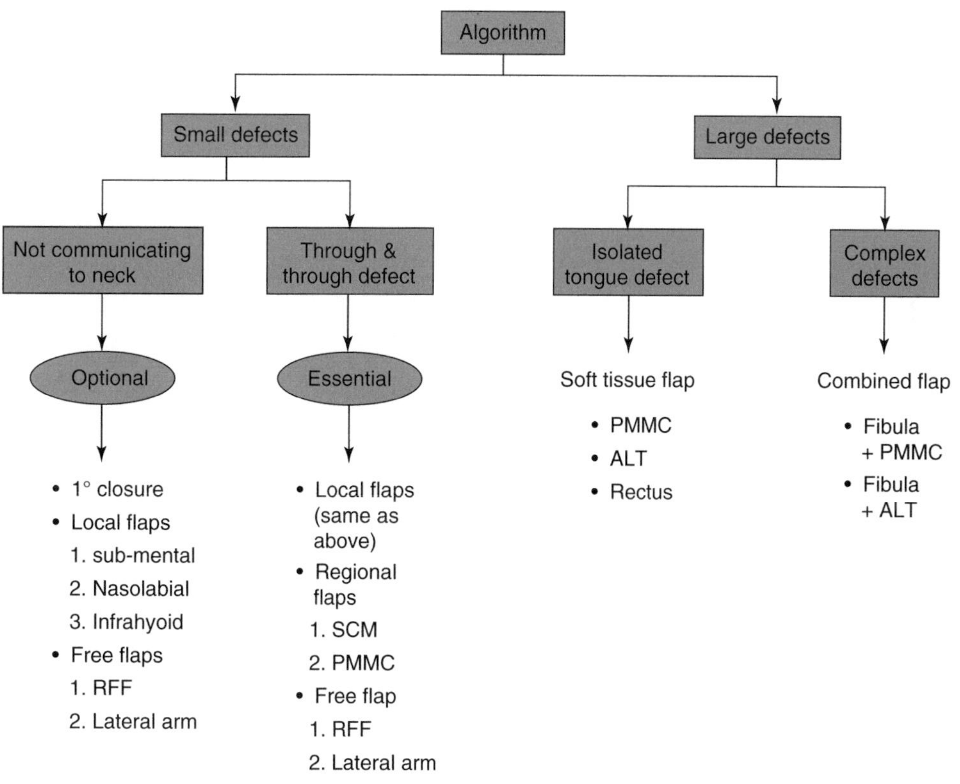

Fig. 8.87 Reconstruction algorithm for tongue/FOM defects

9 Tumors of the Oropharynx

Surgical Anatomy

The oropharynx is one of the most complex anatomical sites in the head and neck region. It consists of various subsites – base of the tongue (BOT), tonsil, soft palate, and pharyngeal wall (Fig. 9.1). Tumor in each of these subsites has different biology but is grouped as one in majority of the head and neck studies. The oropharynx forms circular envelop in posterior aspect of oral cavity working as an inlet for pharynx. The base of the tongue is the most inferior structure and is in close relation to the hyoid bone inferomedially and lateral pharyngeal wall and tonsil laterally. The tonsil occupies lateral position and is connected inferiorly to BOT and superiorly to the soft palate. It is separated by the medial pterygoid muscle by a fascia, and this plane can be exposed to resect early oropharyngeal lesions. The soft palate hangs on top of the pharynx inlet and is important in speech and swallowing.

The oropharynx is supplied by branches of the external carotid artery which traveres the parapharyngeal space. This space can be exposed to clear the lateral margin that is the deep margin for oropharynx tumors.

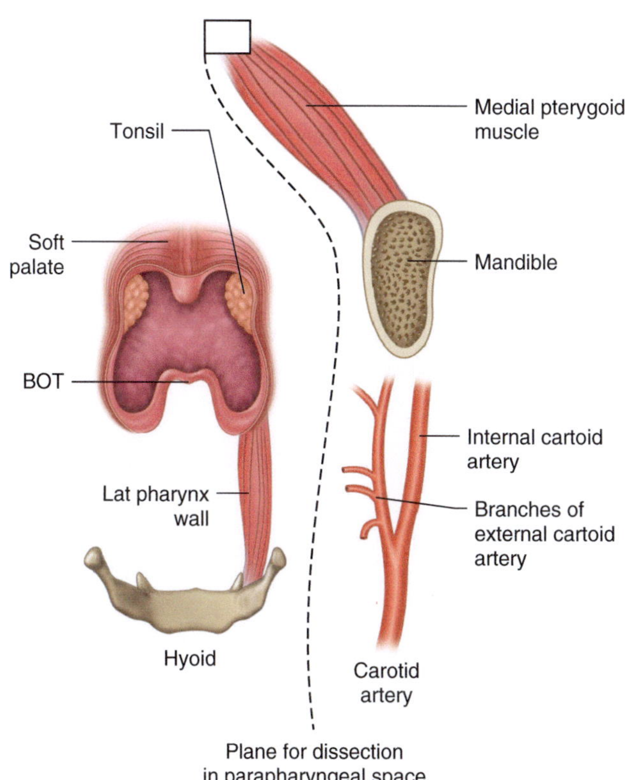

Fig. 9.1 Surgical anatomy of the oropharynx

N. Trivedi, *Atlas of Head and Neck Cancer Surgery: The Compartment Surgery for Resection in 3-D*, DOI 10.1007/978-81-322-2050-3_9, © Springer India 2015

Surgical Pathology

The early lesions of oropharynx are generally confined to the pharyngeal wall and spread laterally to neighboring subsite. Their lateral spread is limited by the parapharyngeal space. These early lesions can be resected by entering the parapharyngeal space and mobilizing the lesion from deep to superficial. This also helps in controlling bleeding as branches of the external carotid artery are already ligated.

The advanced lesions of the oropharynx pose a difficult surgical challenge. The anatomy is multidimensional and tumor spread involves critical areas. The spread can be in two directions (Fig. 9.2). The superior and lateral spread is towards the ITF. The medial pterygoid muscle is the first one to be involved, and the tumor can spread further to high ITF. The second ie inferior spread is directed medially towards hyoid bone. The surgical resection can be planned depending upon the compartment involved. The resection includes the base of the tongue when spread is inferior and ITF when spread is superior. Both compartments need to be resected for very advanced tumors.

Figure 9.3 demonstrates the treatment algorithm for management of oropharynx tumors. The oropharynx is essentially managed by a nonsurgical approach in current era of human papilloma virus (HPV), and surgery is generally reserved for recurrent cases. However, surgery can still be considered as one of the options in primary treatment. The newer surgical techniques in the form of robotic surgery and endoscopic laser surgery have again shifted the focus towards surgical approach. This chapter essentially focuses on the conventional open surgical approach for treatment of these tumors. The advanced tumors generally respond well to nonsurgical treatment compared to other subsites, though certain infiltrative and very advanced lesions do much better with upfront surgery.

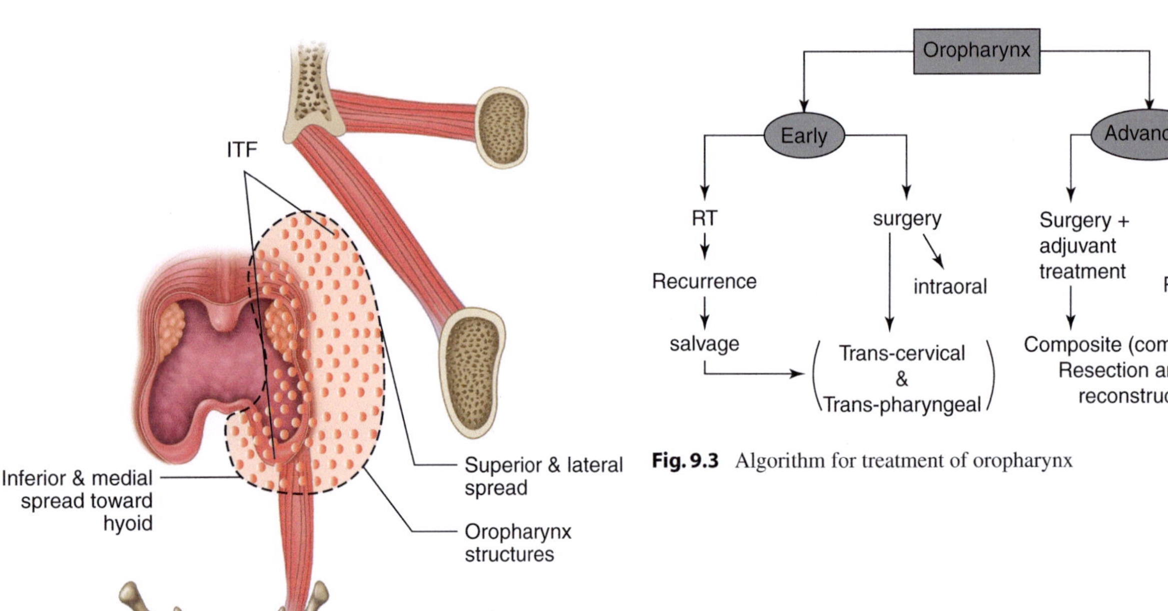

Fig. 9.2 Pattern of disease spread outside the oropharynx

Fig. 9.3 Algorithm for treatment of oropharynx

Surgical Concepts

- The lateral pharyngeal wall forms the deep margin for oropharynx tumor. This space can be exposed and cleared to achieve negative margins.
- The advanced tumors have two potential ways for spread. The superior and lateral spread is towards the ITF, and this can be cleared with compartment clearance. The inferior spread is towards the hyoid bone and can be addressed by resecting the base of the tongue area.
- The mandibulotomy approach has been traditionally used to address large oropharynx tumors. This is becoming less popular and these tumors can be addressed by combination of transpharyngeal and transoral approaches.
- The anatomy of the parapharyngeal space is of paramount importance, and mobilization begins with clearing this area. Once the base is mobilized, the involved compartments can be addressed.
- The SND is performed on the same side for lateralized lesions, while bilateral neck dissection is done for more centralized lesions.

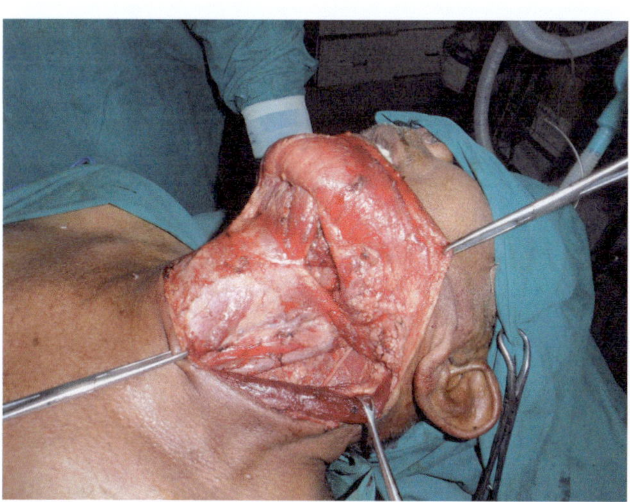

Fig. 9.4 SND level I to IV is complete

Early Lesion

This procedure demonstrates resection of early oropharynx tumor with transcervical–transpharyngeal approach. These tumors can be addressed by open intraoral approach or by robotic assisted surgery. We come across many patients in clinical practice who come with trismus due to sub-mucus fibrosis, and these can be best addressed by the transpharyngeal approach.

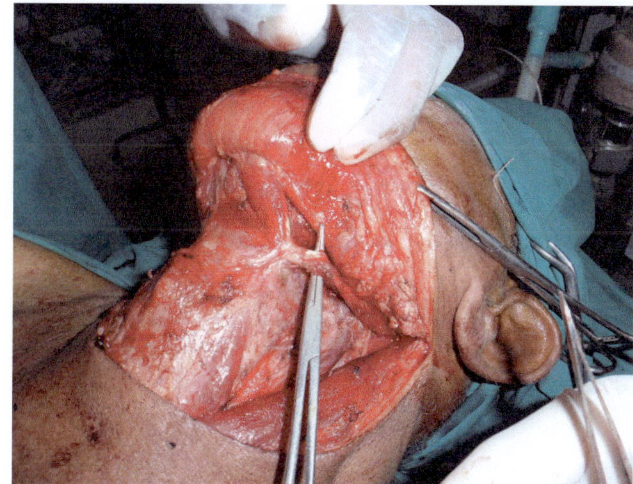

Fig. 9.5 The digastric muscle is cut

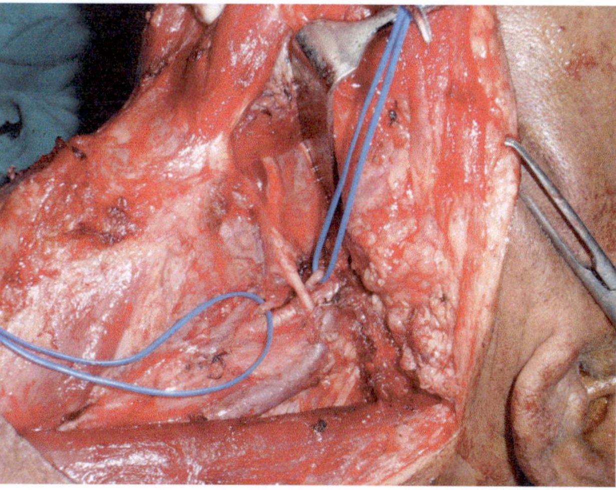

Fig. 9.6 The branches of the external carotid artery are identified and ligated. There are parapharyngeal veins coming from the IJV that needs to be secured as well

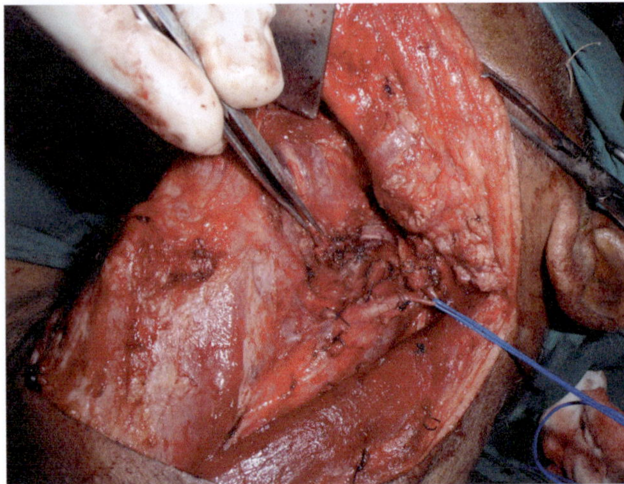

Fig. 9.7 The ligated branches of ECA are retracted laterally to expose the parapharyngeal space. The dissection can run upwards to separate the medial pterygoid muscle from tonsil and lateral pharyngeal wall. This provides complete exposure of oropharynx subsites and achieves clearance in depth

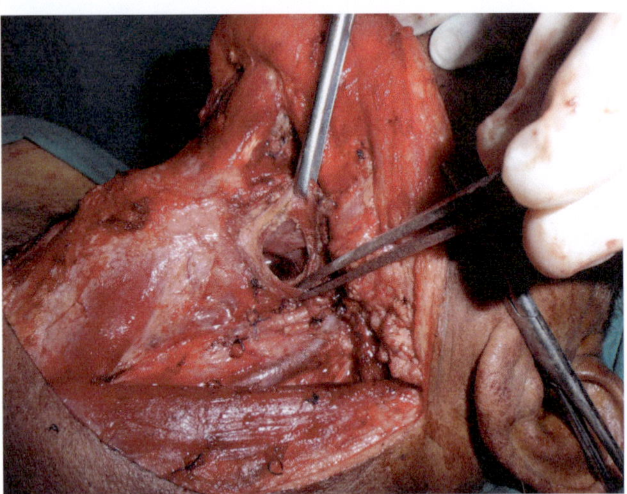

Fig. 9.8 The pharynx is opened from BOT area

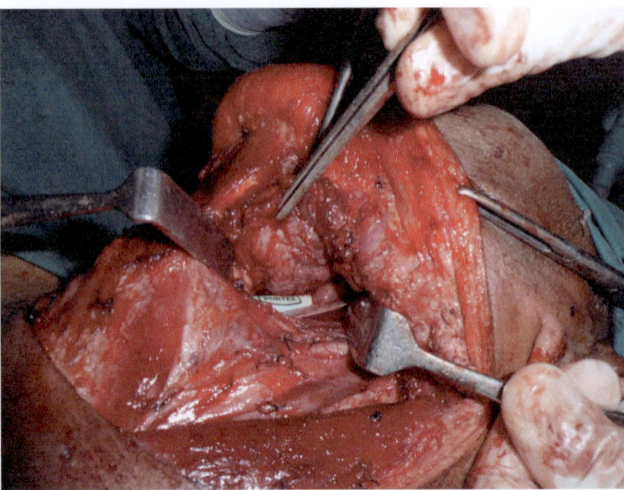

Fig. 9.9 The tumor involving the BOT can be seen in this photograph. The tumor can be palpated all around, and wide excision can be performed under control. The resection for superficial lesions need not involve removal of the entire BOT muscle but selective excision of the involved area. This helps in preserving the function

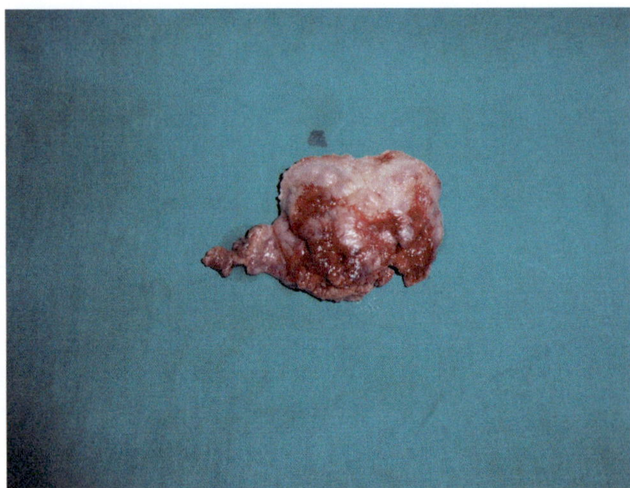

Fig. 9.10 The photograph showing negative mucosal margins

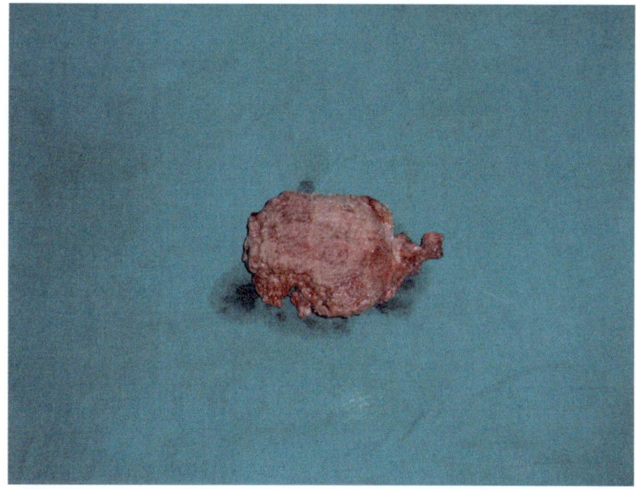

Fig. 9.11 The deep muscle margin seems clear

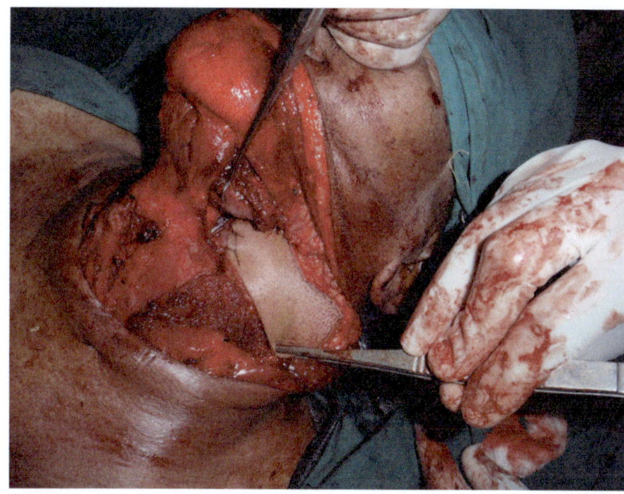

Fig. 9.14 The flap suturing

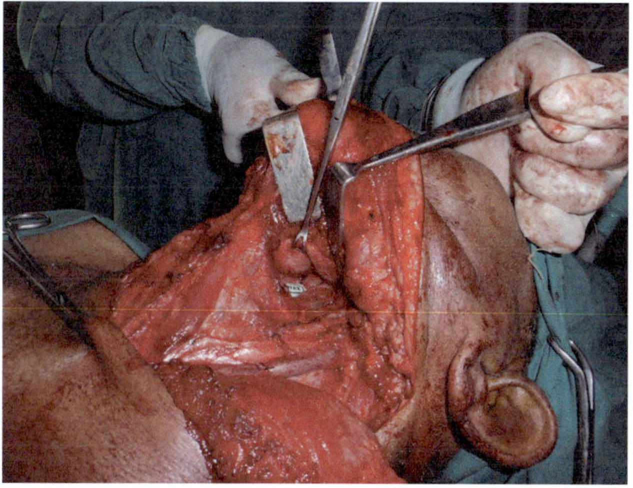

Fig. 9.12 The resulting defect needs flap reconstruction

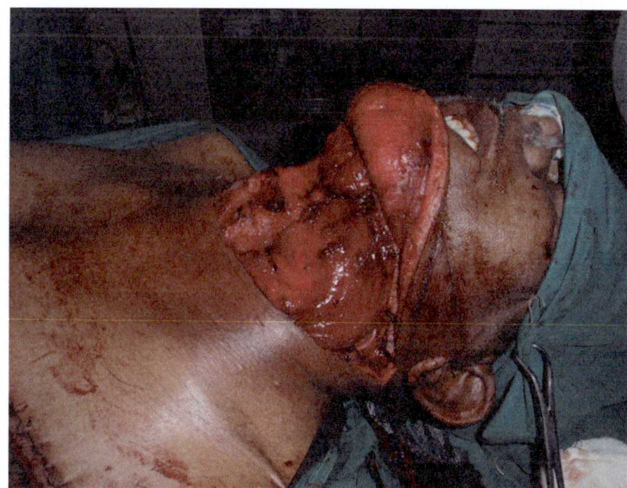

Fig. 9.15 Flap insertion covers the entire defect

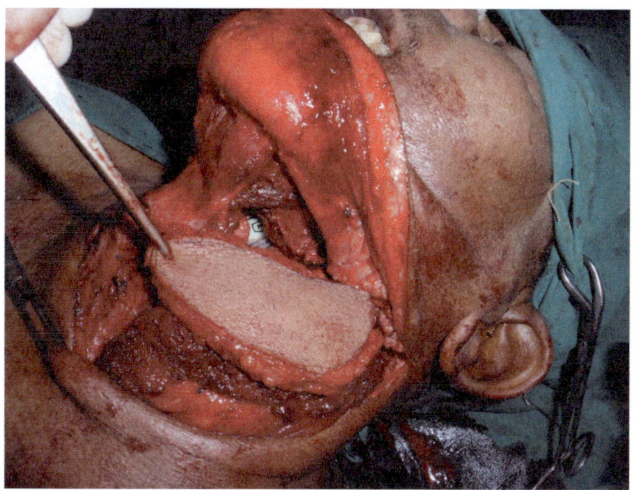

Fig. 9.13 The PMMC flap is raised

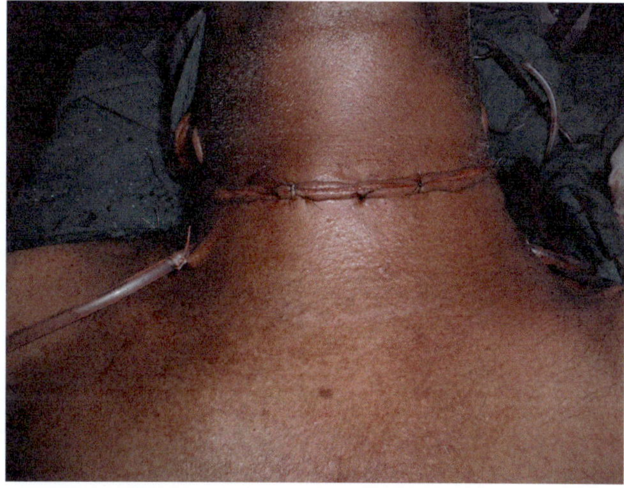

Fig. 9.16 Completed bilateral SND and closure

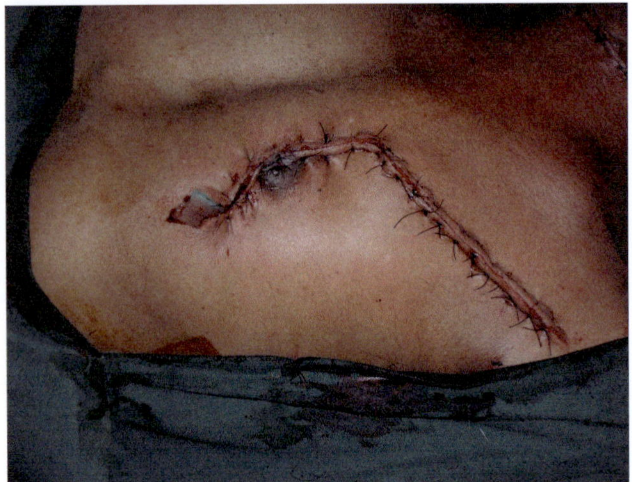

Fig. 9.17 Donor site defect is closed primarily

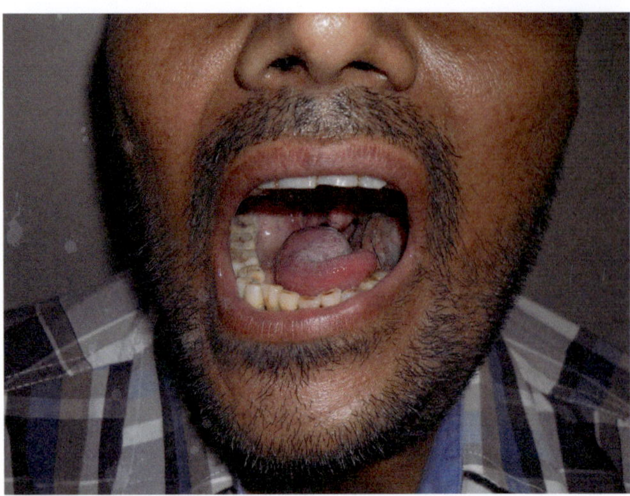

Fig. 9.18 The final long-term outcome. This patient can eat full diet and has good quality of speech. There are a few infiltrating, deep BOT lesions (non-HPV) that don't respond well to radiotherapy, and this approach serves good for this group in our experience

Salvage Surgery for Recurrent Early Oropharynx

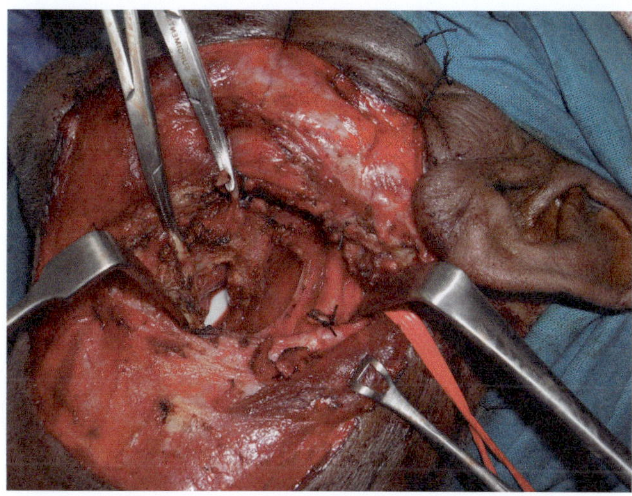

Fig. 9.19 This photograph shows exposed parapharyngeal space for a recurrent oropharynx cancer

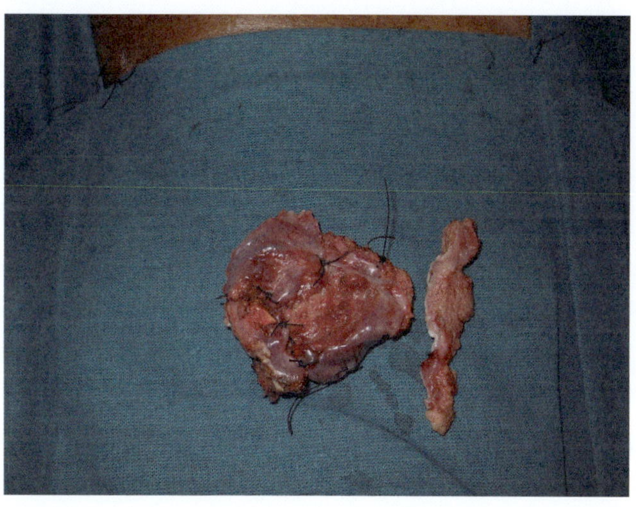

Fig. 9.20 The completed resection of BOT and lateral pharyngeal lesion with adequate margins

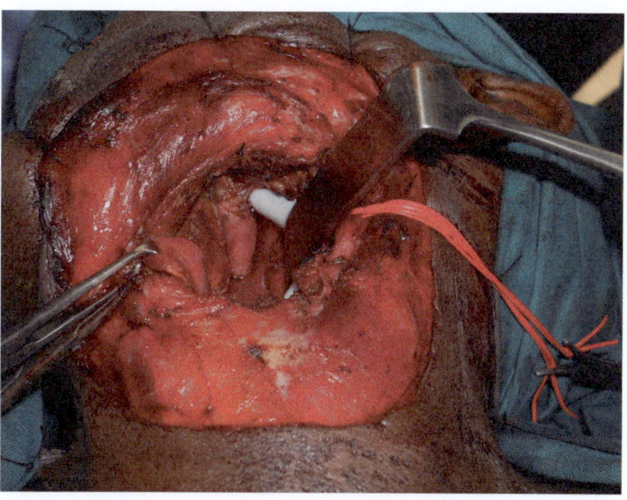

Fig. 9.21 The photograph shows resected area which inlcudes resection of entire lateral pharyngeal wall, tonsil and part of soft palate

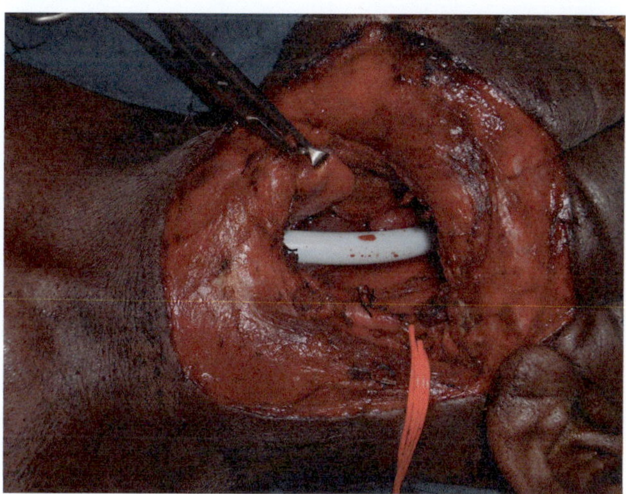

Fig. 9.22 Photograph showing resected portion of BOT

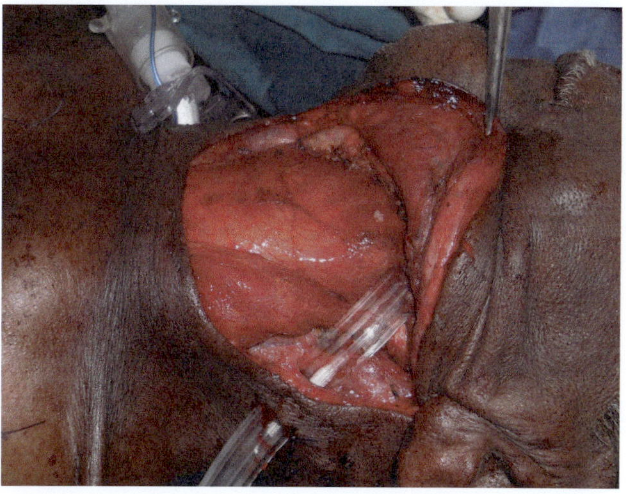

Fig. 9.23 The PMMC flap reconstruction. The PMMC is preferred over RFFF for salvage cases as muscle provides additional vascularity for healing

Complex Oropharynx

This section demonstrates compartment resection of advanced oropharynx tumors to achieve negative margins for soft tissues all around.

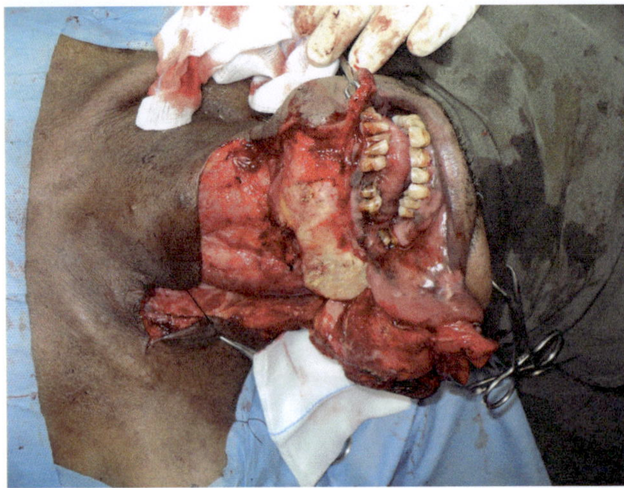

Fig. 9.24 The cheek flap is raised

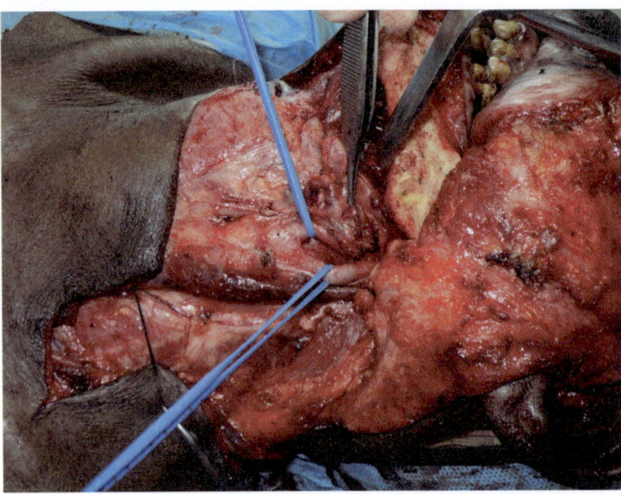

Fig. 9.25 The external and internal carotid artery is identified

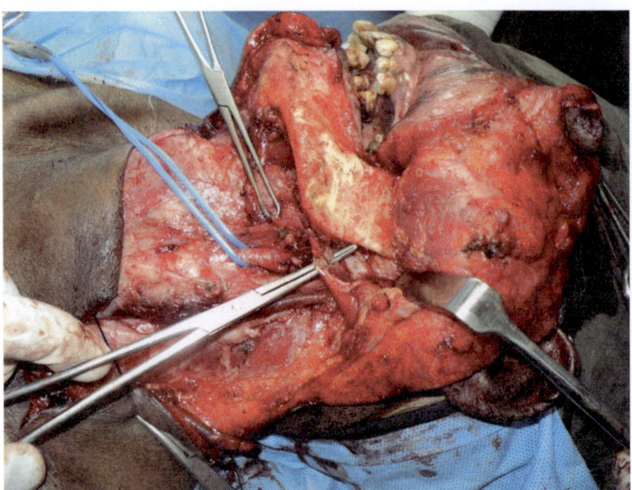

Fig. 9.26 The digastric muscle is divided

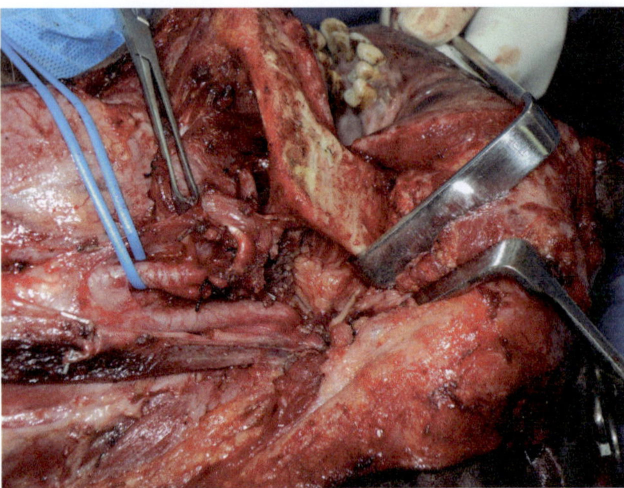

Fig. 9.27 The branches of the external carotid artery are ligated and shifted laterally to expose the parapharyngeal fat

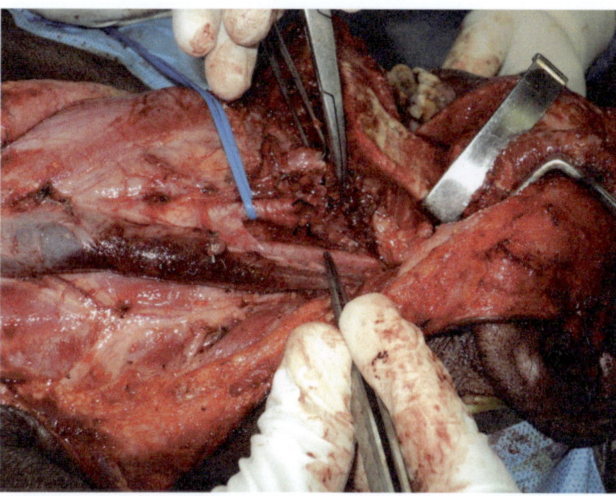

Fig. 9.28 The photograph shows internal carotid artery in the parapharyngeal space. The muscle attached to the styloid is transected, and deep fascia over the internal carotid is exposed to dissect it in entire length till the skull base. This helps in mobilizing the lateral pharyngeal wall in its entire length till the eustachian tube and nasopharynx. The base is prepared for pharyngeal resection this way safeguarding carotid artery

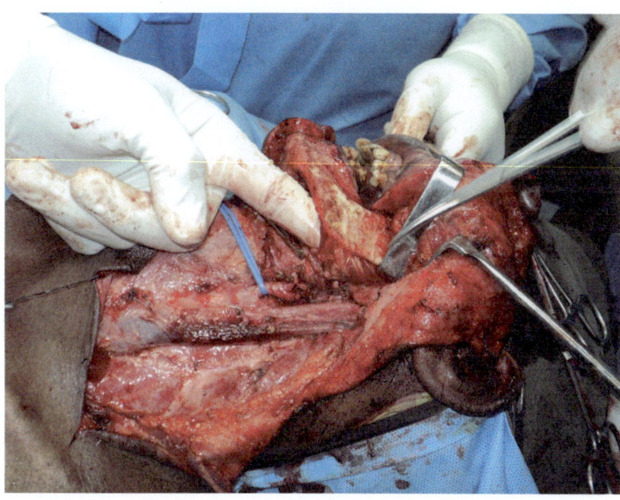

Fig. 9.29 The medial pterygoid muscle is lifted from the pharyngeal space to be included in resection. The finger is in the parapharyngeal space and pterygoid plate can be palpated at the skull base

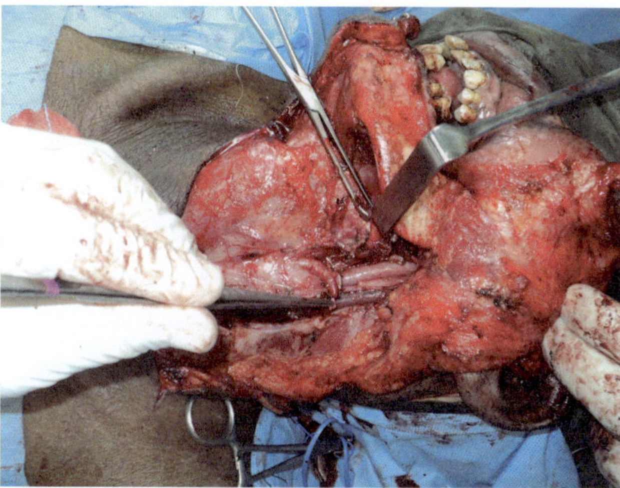

Fig. 9.30 The internal carotid artery being exposed

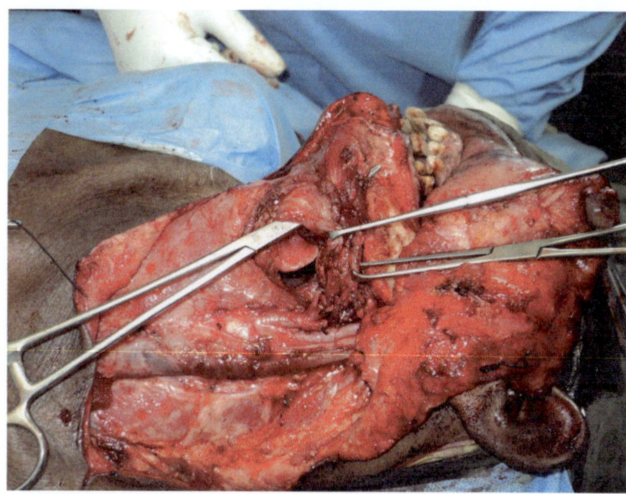

Fig. 9.31 This tumor is primarily involving the inferomedial compartment. The BOT compartment is resected from the hyoid bone. The advantage of performing this out-to-in resection is that your deep margin is always secure. The soft tissue is resected from its base and chances of positive margin are negligible. One can notice that we haven't performed any intraoral cuts, and base of resection is prepared first

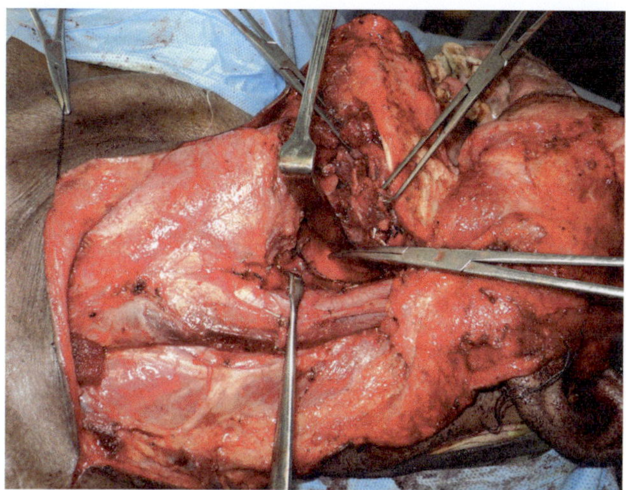

Fig. 9.32 The base is free

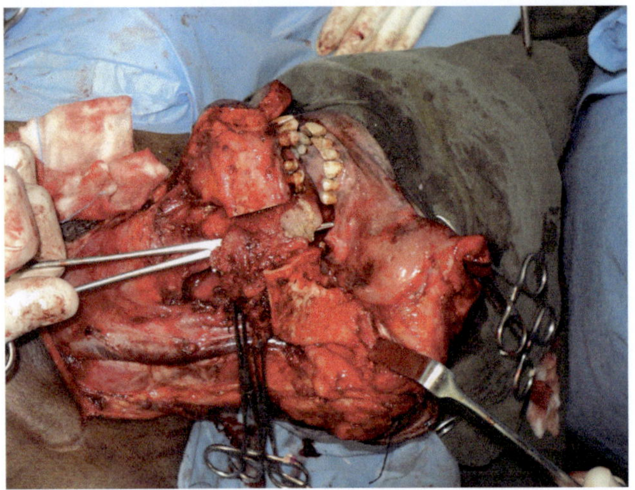

Fig. 9.33 The resection of the intraoral part of the tongue. The tumor is under constant palpation to have adequate margins

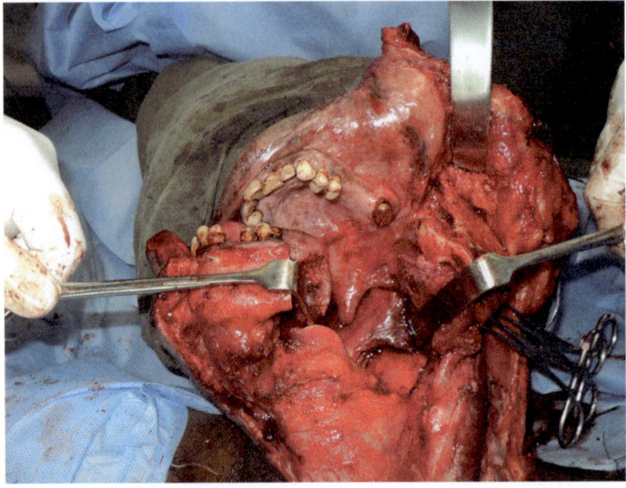

Fig. 9.34 The mandible cut is made to expose the entire oropharynx. The lateral margin is already dissected in the parapharyngeal space and inferior margin from hyoid bone. The tumor free mucosal margins can be achieved by appropriate cuts under vision

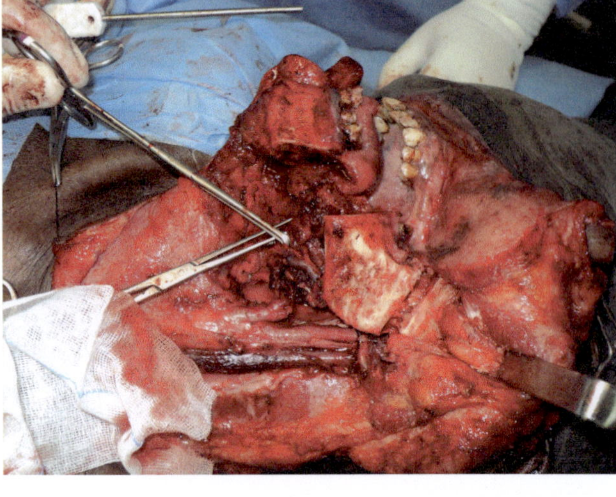

Fig. 9.35 The lesion has involved the medial pterygoid muscle and abutted the mandible, and hence part of the mandible was sacrificed. If the medial pterygoid muscle was free, there is no need to have mandibular cuts. Mandibulotomy can be avoided by combining transpharyngeal and trans oral resection

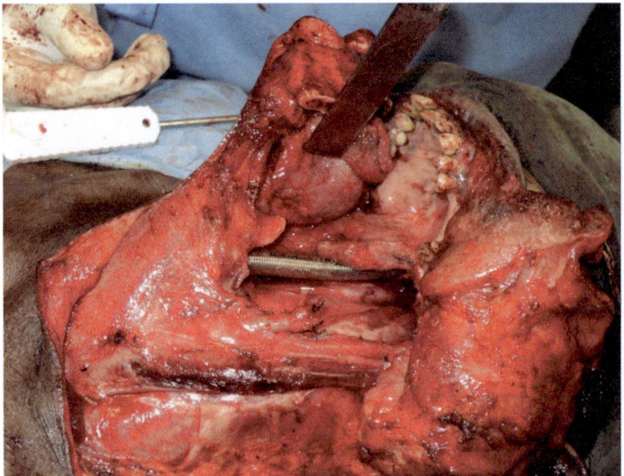

Fig. 9.36 The resection is complete. The entire oropharynx with involved compartment is resected en bloc

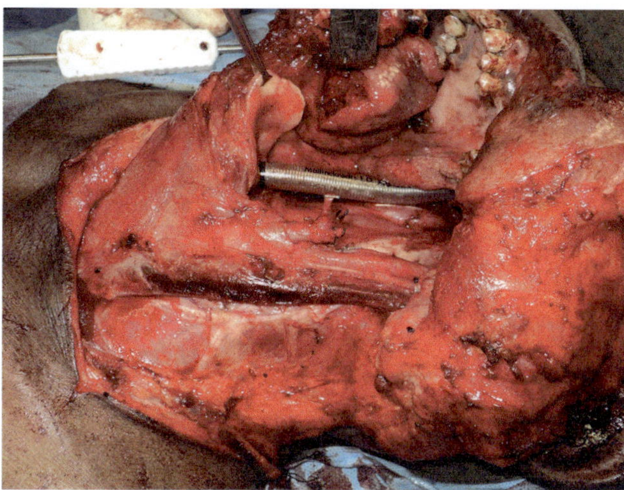

Fig. 9.37 The photograph shows resection from hyoid to soft palate and lateral pharyngeal wall upto nasopharynx. The internal carotid forms the lateral boundary for this resection

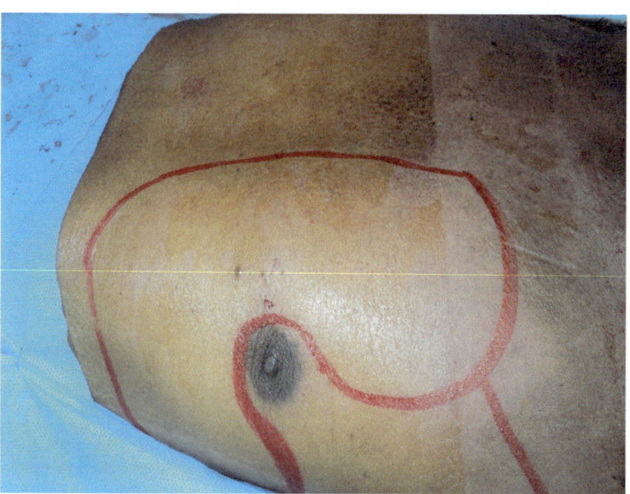

Fig. 9.38 Proposed PMMC flap

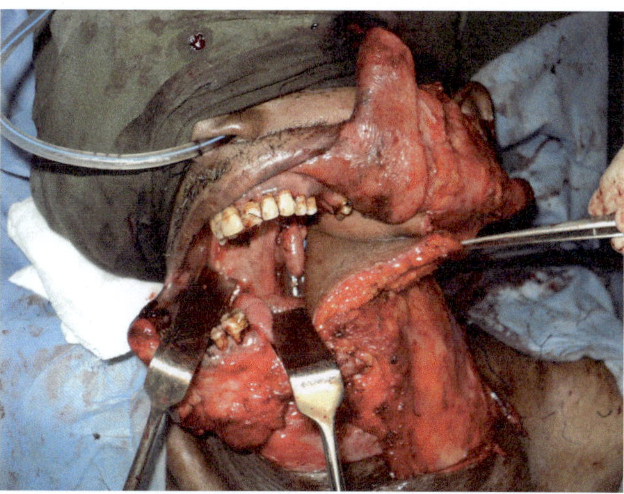

Fig. 9.39 The flap is sutured to pharyngeal wall

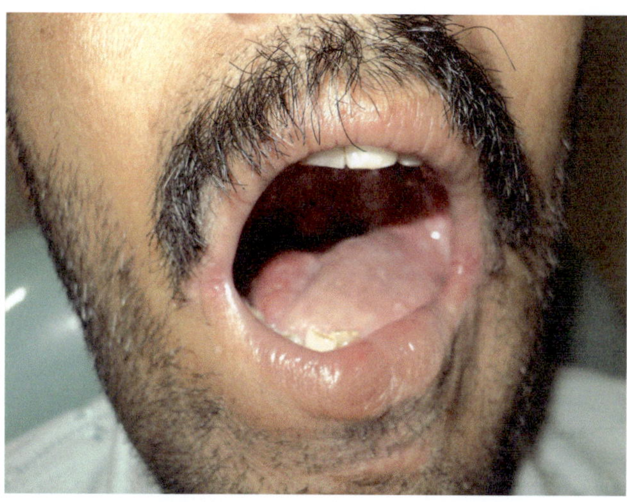

Fig. 9.40 The long-term outcome. These patients have a risk of aspiration in the postoperative phase and need percutaneous endoscopic gastrostomy (PEG) tube for feeding. But with appropriate rehabilitation they can eat semisolid food with relative ease and have reasonable quality of life

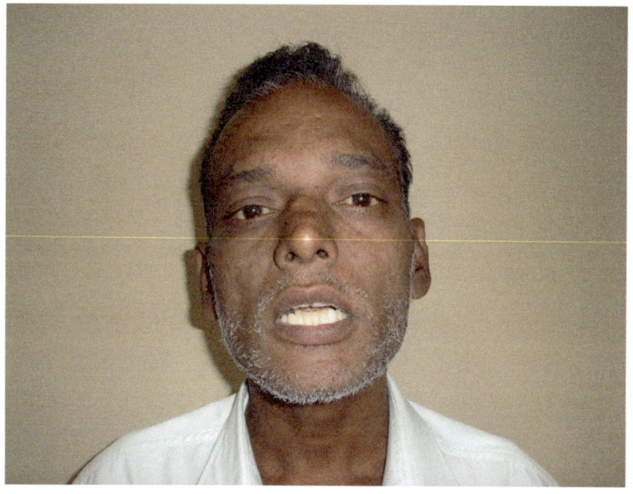

Fig. 9.41 The patient with severe trismus due to involvement of the superolateral ITF from spread of oropharynx tumor. The disease also had involved the inferior compartment and resection needed to involve both compartments. These large, infiltrative tumors (non-HPV) cannot be treated with nonsurgical organ preservation treatment and need surgical resection upfront

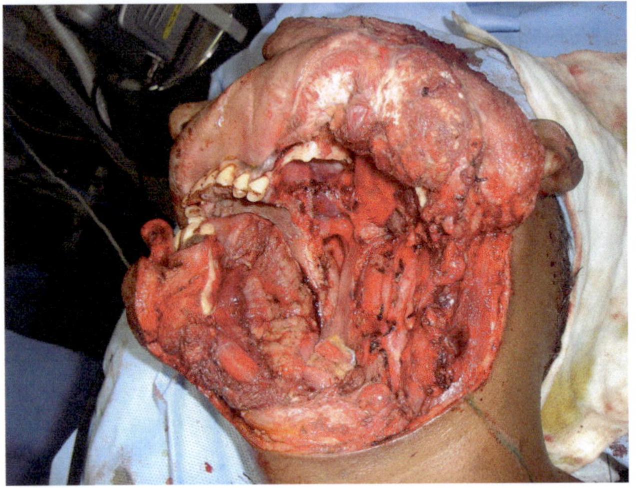

Fig. 9.42 The entire oropharynx showing both compartments are resected. The resection is from hyoid to the skull base

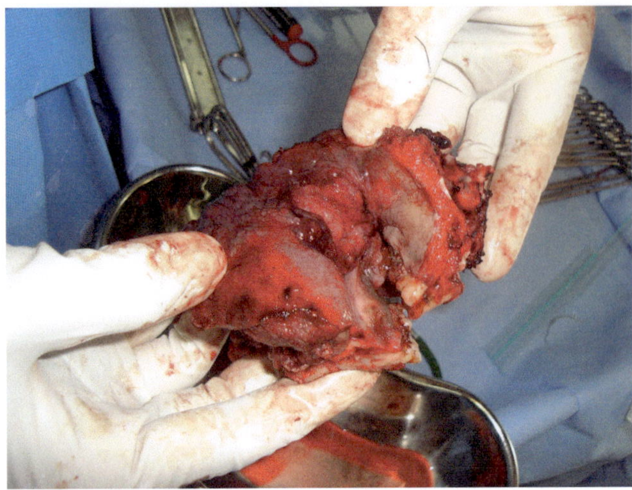

Fig. 9.44 The resected specimen showing very good resection margin in all direction. The compartment surgical approach is the most effective approach for clearing such extensive tumors

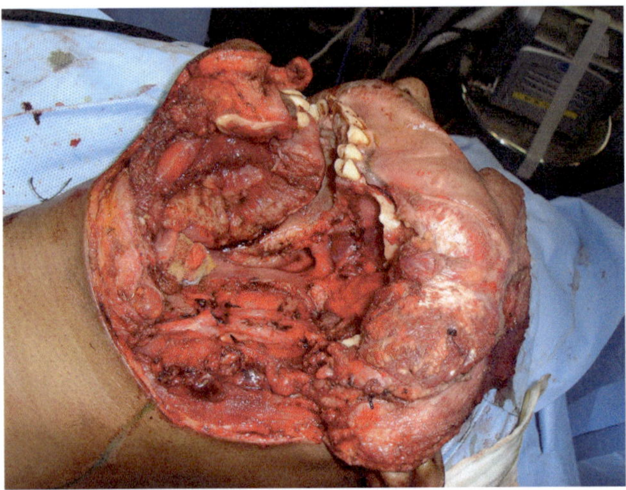

Fig. 9.43 The photograph shows exposed internal carotid artery in its entire length. The surgical procedure to clear ITF is described in a separate chapter in this book

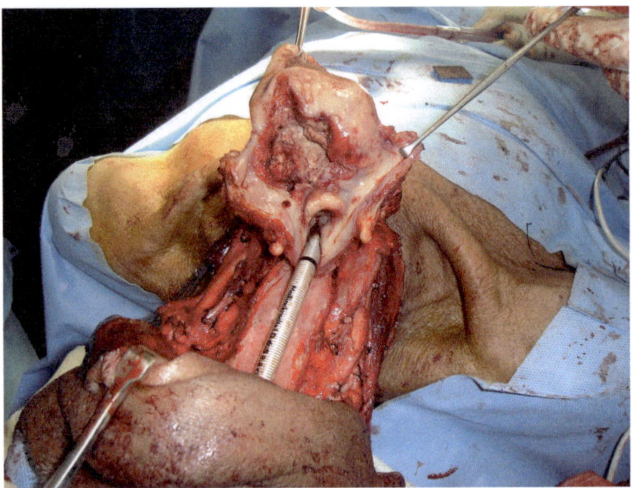

Fig. 9.45 The BOT tumor involving the supraglottis. These are also called junctional tumors and need total glossectomy with total laryngectomy

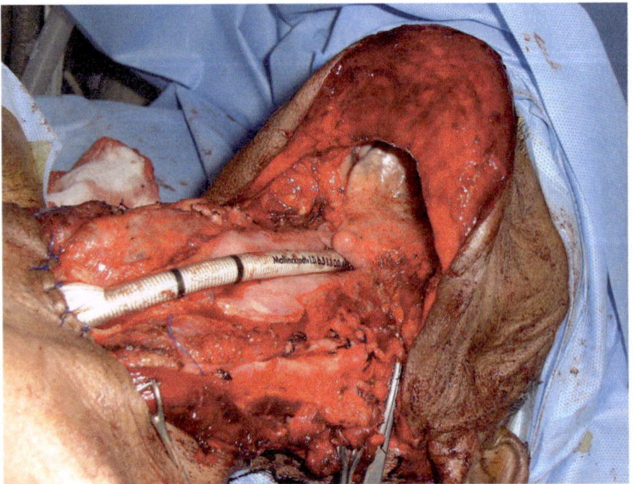

Fig. 9.46 The photograph shows post resection status

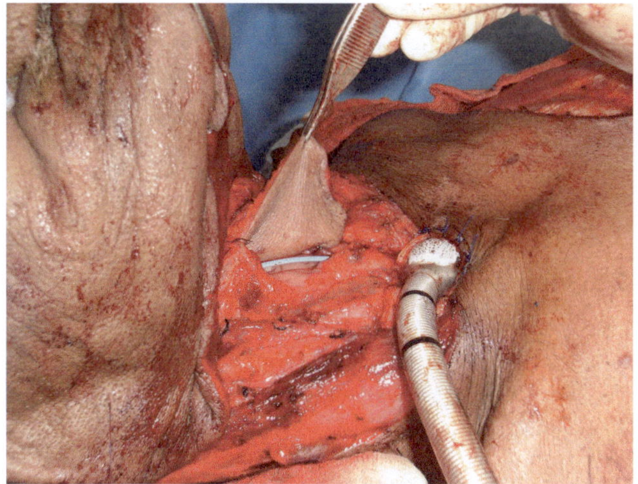

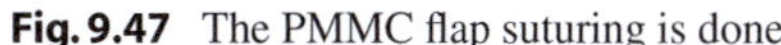

Fig. 9.47 The PMMC flap suturing is done

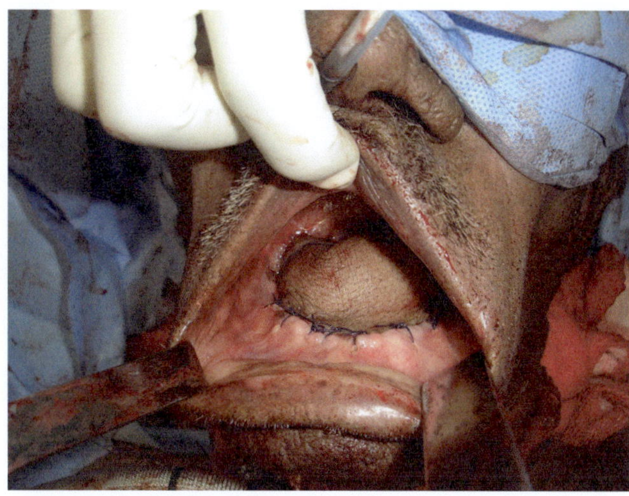

Fig. 9.48 Photograph showing final closure

Tumors of the Larynx and Hypopharynx

10

Surgical Anatomy and Pathology

The larynx is one of most critical organ in the human body responsible for voice production. The larynx is subdivided into supraglottis, glottis, and subglottis. The tumor from each subsite has different biological behavior and has different pattern of spread. The supraglottic tumor has higher tendency to have lymphatic spread compared to glottic tumor. Treatment algorithm for laryngeal cancer has changed significantly with majority of tumors being treated by nonsurgical organ preservation approach. Early laryngeal lesions are managed either by radiotherapy or by endoscopic laser surgery. The minimally invasive surgery is beyond the scope of this book. The moderately advanced tumors are managed by concurrent chemoradiotherapy in majority of cases. The conventional total laryngectomy (TL) can be offered to this group in select cases. The very advanced tumors require TL and voice rehabilitation with tracheoesophageal prosthesis (TEP). Open conservative laryngeal procedures have become almost obsolete with the advent of endoscopic laser procedures and concurrent chemoradiotherapy regimens. Near total laryngectomy (NTL) is almost like total laryngectomy but voice quality is inferior to TEP and majority of clinicians prefer TL with TEP over NTL.

The management of hypopharynx tumor is almost similar to laryngeal tumor with majority of lesions treated with chemoradiotherapy. The hypopharynx tumors have poor biology with the tendency for distant metastasis. These tumors are known for their submucosal spread and skip lesions in adjacent areas. These factors should be kept in mind while performing the surgery. Total laryngectomy with partial pharyngectomy is the standard operation for the majority of pyriform fossa tumors. The advanced post-cricoid tumors require total laryngopharyngectomy with or without esophagectomy depending upon the lower extent of tumor spread.

There are many issues to discuss in the treatment of the larynx and hypopharynx cancer, but the focus of this book is on surgical approach, and the following procedures will be discussed in this chapter:

1. Total laryngectomy
2. Total laryngopharyngectomy
3. Repair of pharyngeal fistula

N. Trivedi, *Atlas of Head and Neck Cancer Surgery: The Compartment Surgery for Resection in 3-D*,
DOI 10.1007/978-81-322-2050-3_10, © Springer India 2015

Total Laryngectomy

This section deals with TL procedure for a case of advanced cancer of the larynx.

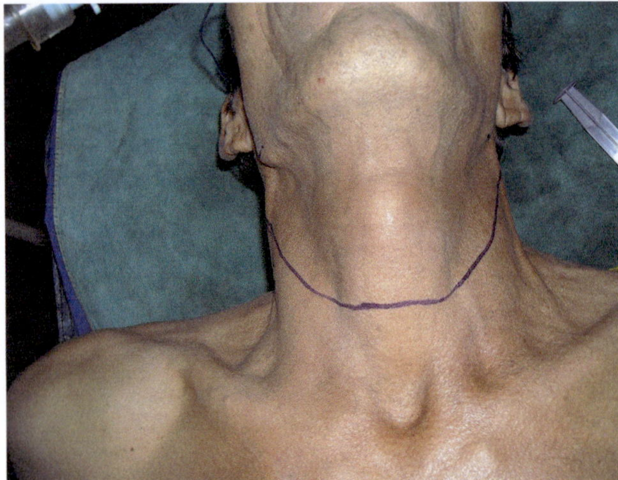

Fig. 10.1 The U-shape incision for TL. Alternatively one can use transverse incision

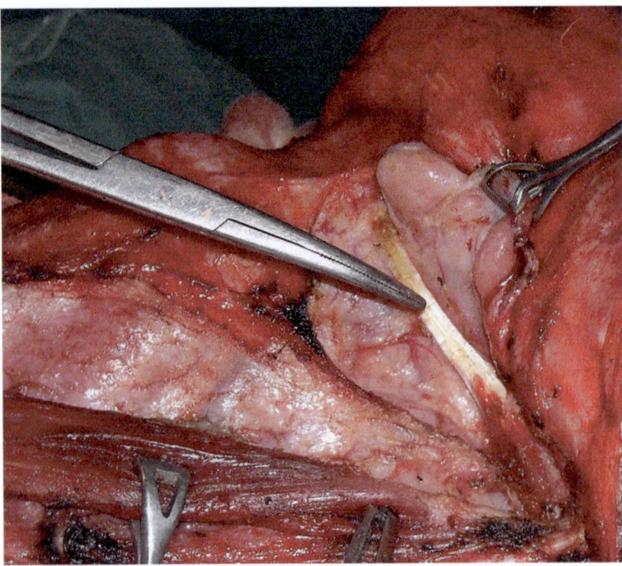

Fig. 10.2 The flap is raised till the digastric muscle is exposed in its entire length

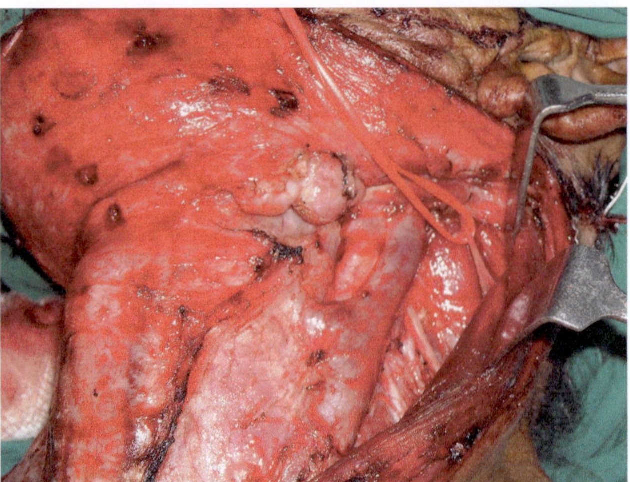

Fig. 10.3 The SND level II to IV is performed

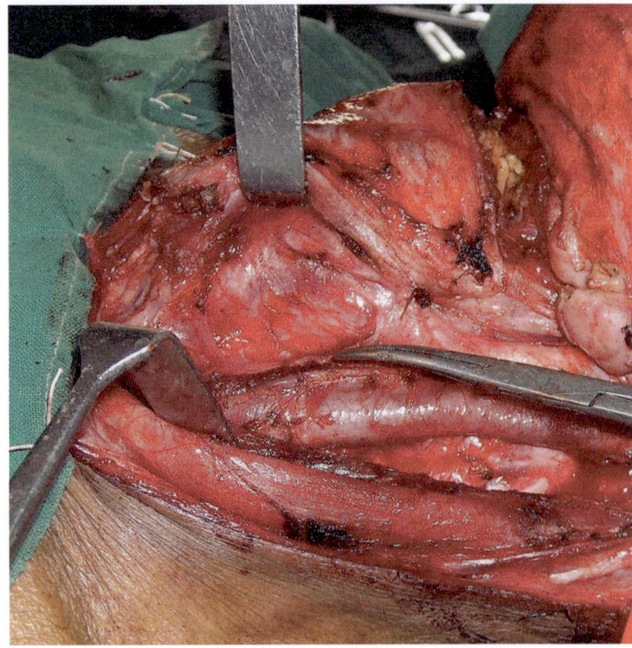

Fig. 10.4 The carotid artery is separated from the thyroid gland and cartilage

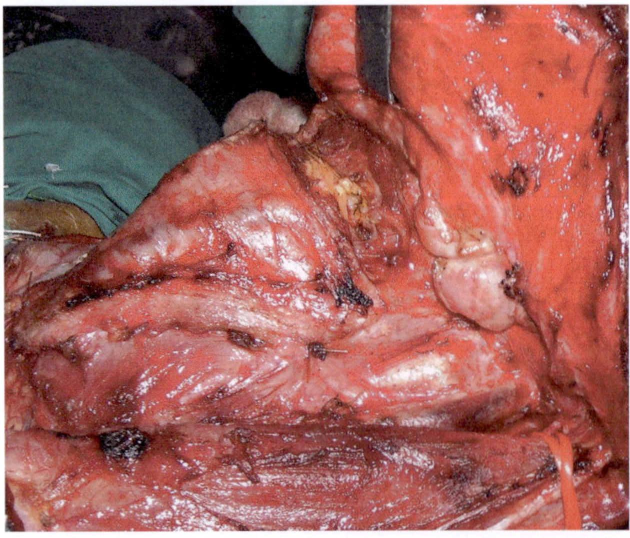

Fig. 10.5 The hyoid bone is exposed

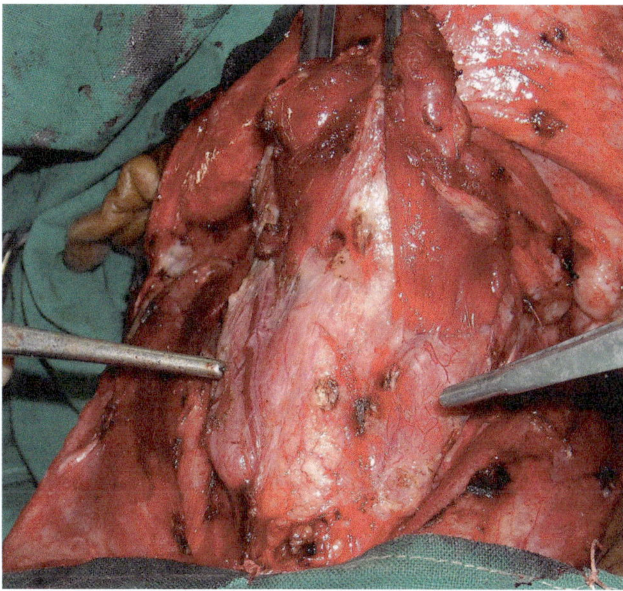

Fig. 10.6 The strap muscle is divided above the trachea and the thyroid gland is exposed. It is a standard practice to save the thyroid gland on the contralateral side. When both lobes of the gland are involved in the tumor, efforts are made to save the parathyroid glands on either side

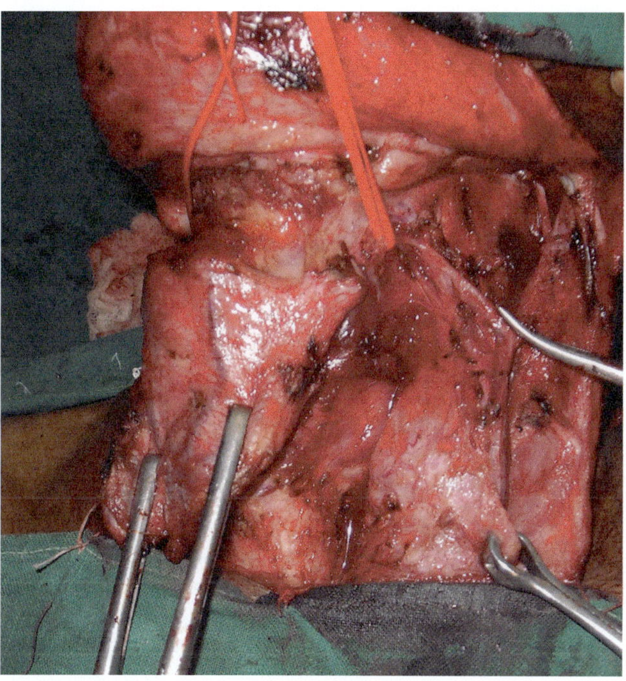

Fig. 10.8 The gland is lateralized away from thyroid cartilage with intact vascular pedicle

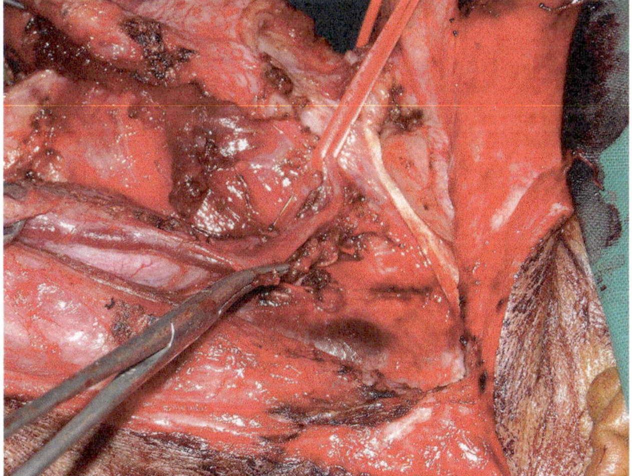

Fig. 10.7 Pedicle of the superior thyroid is dissected. Branch supplying strap muscle is clipped

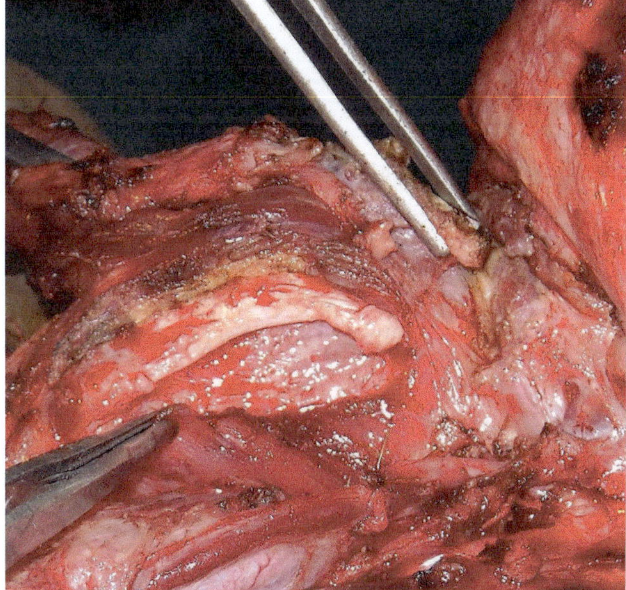

Fig. 10.9 The lateral border of thyroid cartilage is dissected and pyriform fossa mucosa is exposed. This maneuver is done on the side where the disease is not there we can preserve pharyngeal mucosa on non-disease side this way. The pharynx cavity is entered from normal side

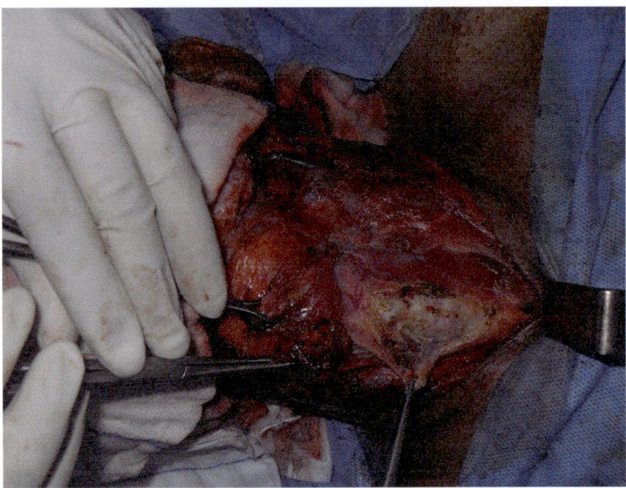

Fig. 10.10 The lower end of trachea is exposed to perform end tracheostomy

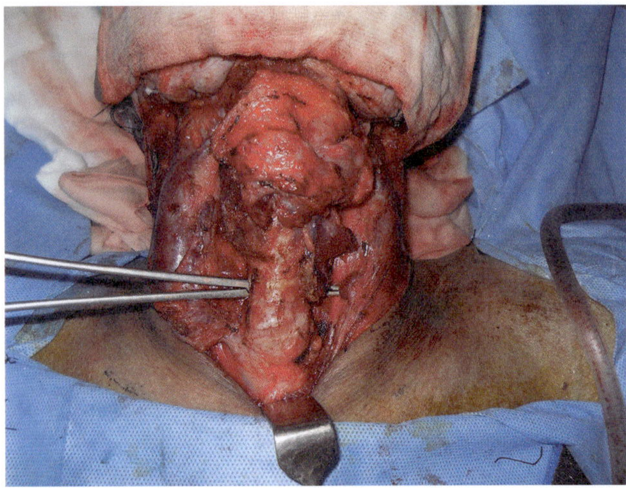

Fig. 10.11 Proposed site for tracheostomy. In cases where subglottis has significant disease extension, this site can be much lower and care should be taken to have a secure lower end of the trachea

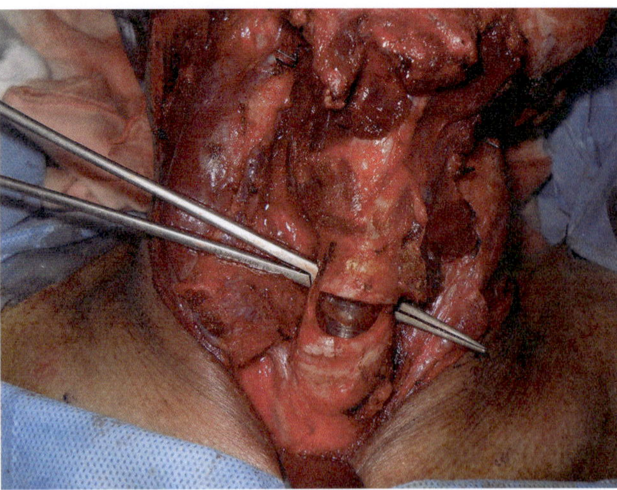

Fig. 10.12 The anesthetic tube should be de-cuffed and withdrawn before cutting the trachea. Try and have cut curving upwards in the posterior wall for easy suturing of stoma

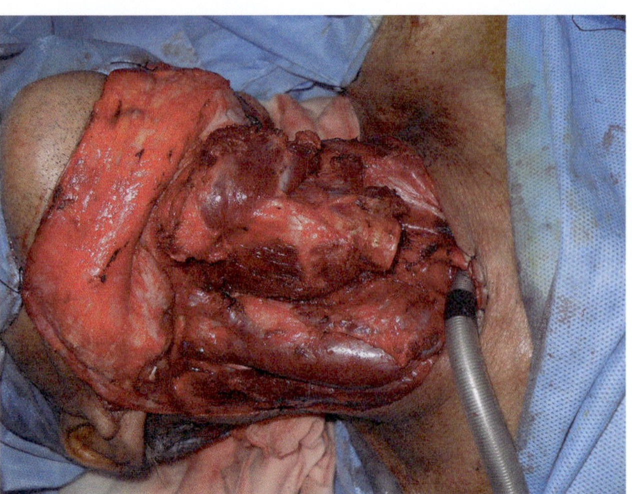

Fig. 10.13 The lower end of the trachea is sutured to the chest wall, and an endotracheal tube is shifted to this end. The sterile endotracheal tube should be ready before transecting the trachea

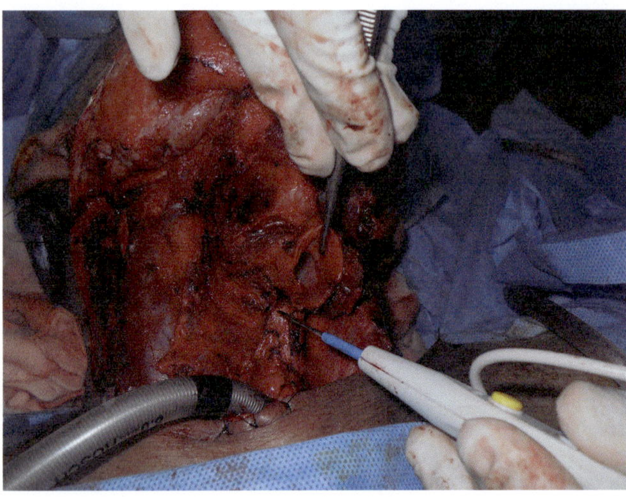

Fig. 10.14 The larynx and trachea being separated from the esophageal wall

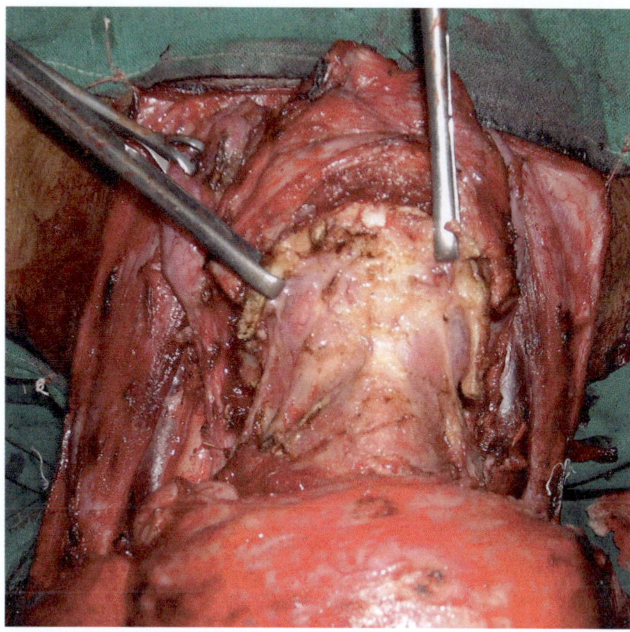

Fig. 10.15 The hyoid bone is separated and vallecula is exposed

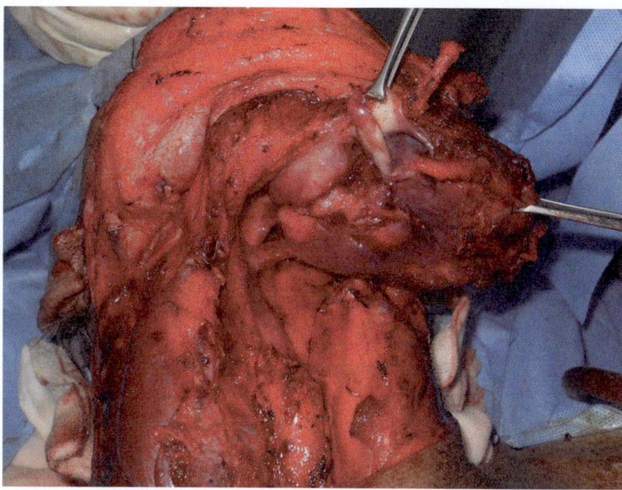

Fig. 10.17 The specimen being removed. This tumor was involving a part of the base tongue, and entry into the larynx was from pyriform sinus instead from vallecula. It is important to plan the resection in such a way that entry into the cavity is from the tumor-free part and the part containing bulk of tumor is addressed in a proper way. For this particular tumor where part of BOT was involved, it is important to preserve at least one side of the lingual artery which runs very close to hyoid bone

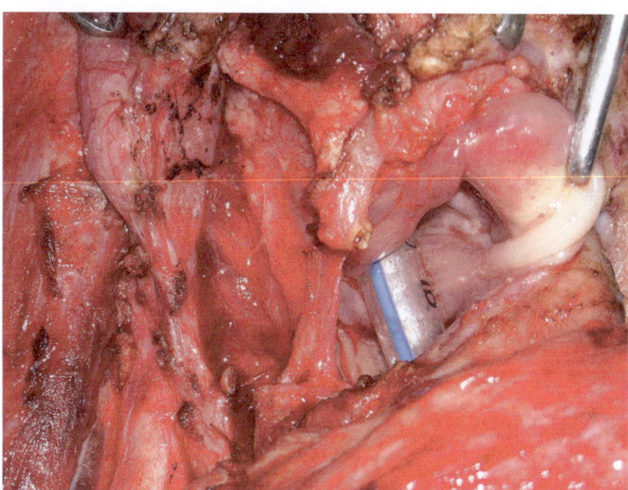

Fig. 10.16 The pharynx is opened and dissection is completed to remove the larynx. It is advisable to preserve as much pharyngeal mucosa as possible to facilitate primary closure

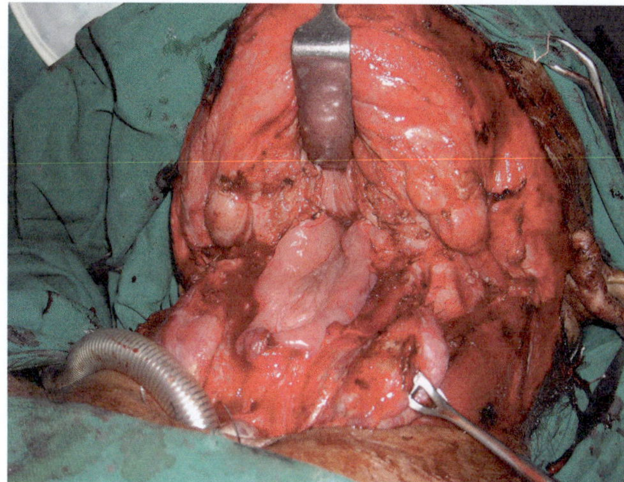

Fig. 10.18 Resection is complete and one can see the remaining pharyngeal mucosa. The feeding tube needs to be inserted at this stage. The pharynx mucosa can be closed primarily if not under tension (roughly 3 cm of unstretched mucosa)

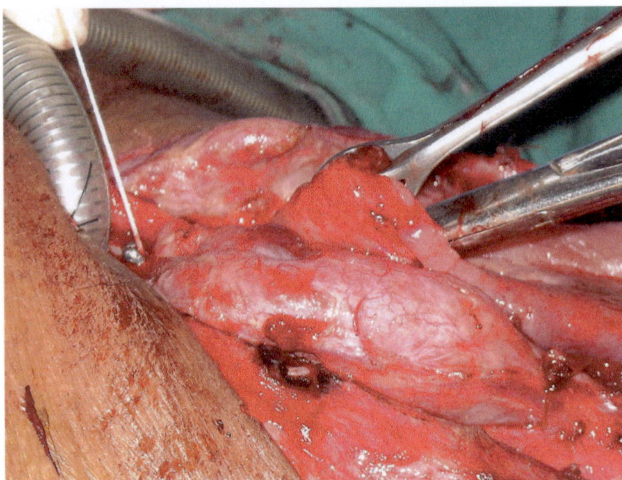

Fig. 10.19 Procedure to create primary tracheoesophageal puncture. The right angled forceps is inserted through the esophagus into the posterior wall of the trachea. A silk thread is pushed into the esophagus

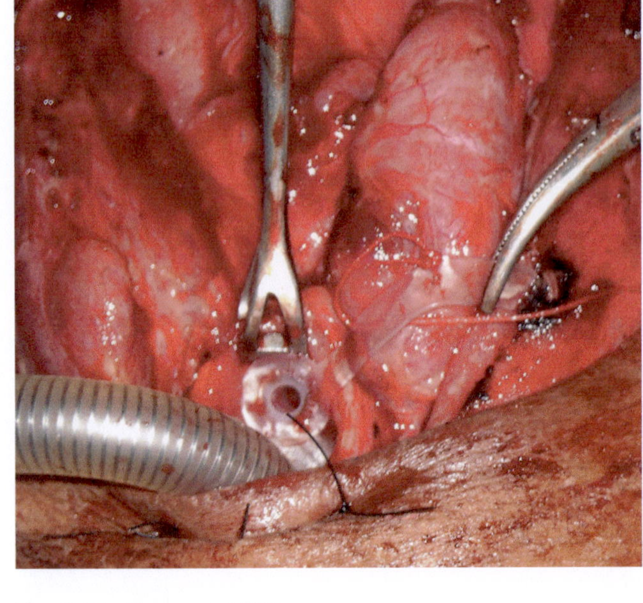

Fig. 10.21 The inserted TEP

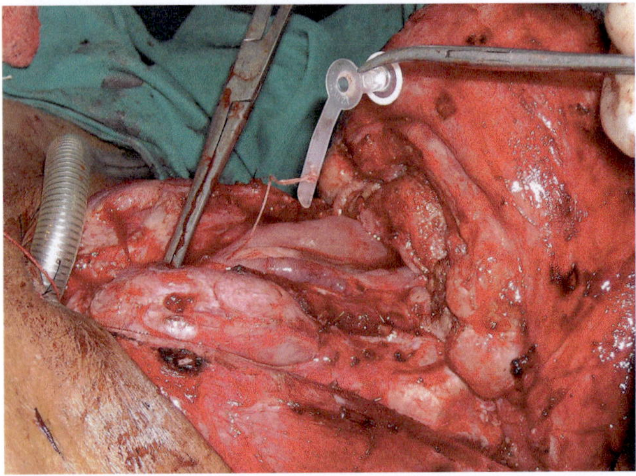

Fig. 10.20 The TEP is pulled through the posterior wall of the trachea. This is a gentle manouever, and care should be taken not to tear the posterior tracheal wall

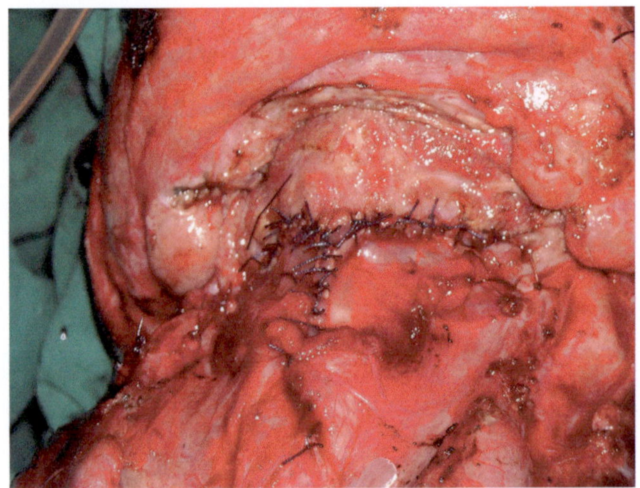

Fig. 10.22 The pharynx was closed in T shape in two layers. Tension-free repair and vascular mucosa are key factors in preventing leak. One should never hesitate in using PMMC flap to patch the pharyngeal defect when in doubt. Pharyngeal fistula is a notorious problem and takes long time to settle and causes great problem to patients in postoperative period. All care and efforts should be taken to avoid it. We have a policy to use PMMC flap for all salvage cases and the majority of advanced pyriform fossa cases

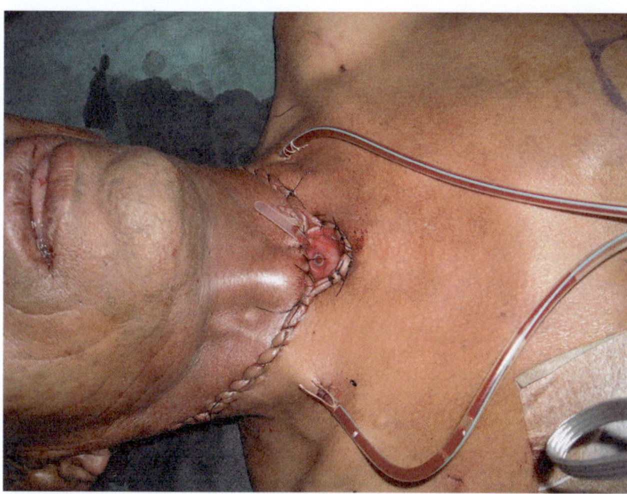

Fig. 10.23 The final outcome after closure

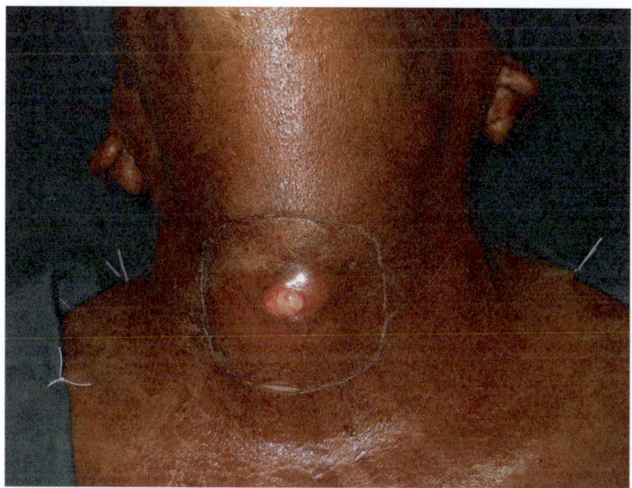

Fig. 10.24 A patient with advanced laryngeal cancer with skin involvement

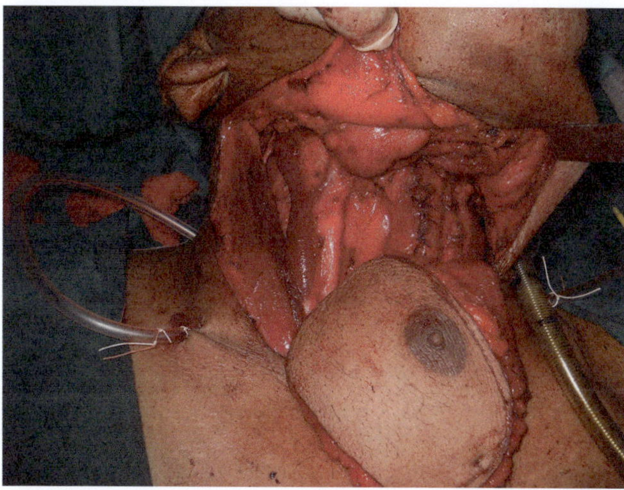

Fig. 10.25 The PMMC flap is used for external cover. One can see completed primary pharyngeal closure

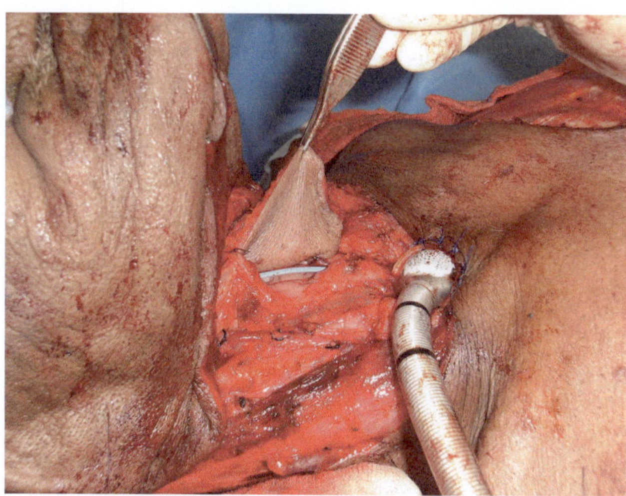

Fig. 10.26 Alternatively the skin can be used for inside lining, and STG can be used over the muscle for external cover

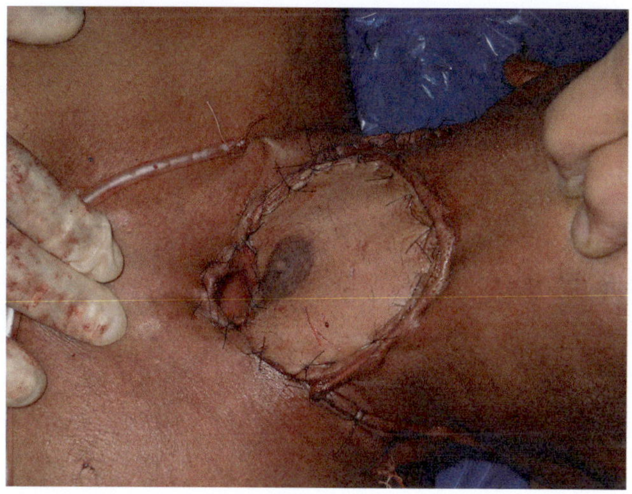

Fig. 10.27 The final outcome

Total Laryngopharyngectomy (TLP)

The procedure demonstrates important steps in performing TLP for post-cricoid cancer.

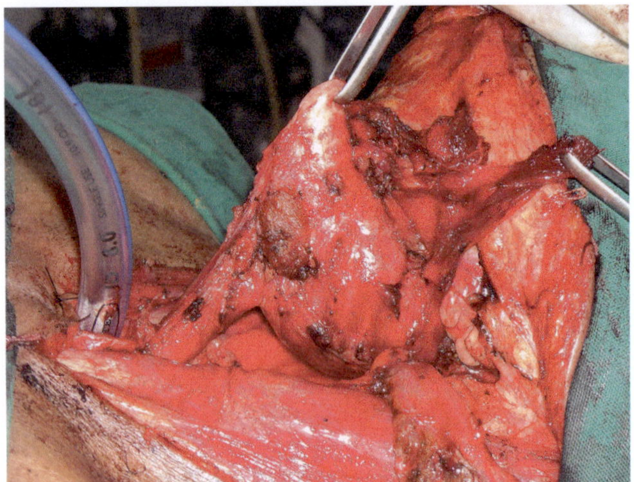

Fig. 10.28 The procedure is similar to TL. This photograph shows that the larynx is mobilized and the upper end of esophagus is exposed. The lesion is located in the post-cricoid region. The lower extent of the tumor decides if total esophagectomy is required. One needs to have 4 cm clear margin in the esophagus to take into account for the submucosal spread. Total esophagectomy is not required if tension free anastomysis can be performed in the neck

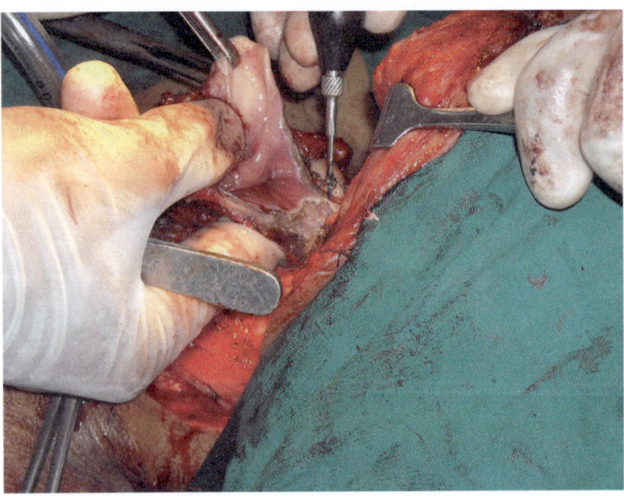

Fig. 10.29 The upper end has been divided in full circumference in contrast to TL where posterior pharyngeal wall is left intact

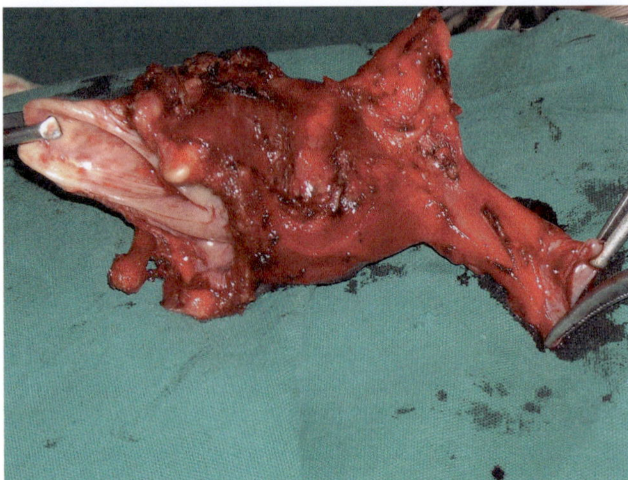

Fig. 10.30 The resected specimen

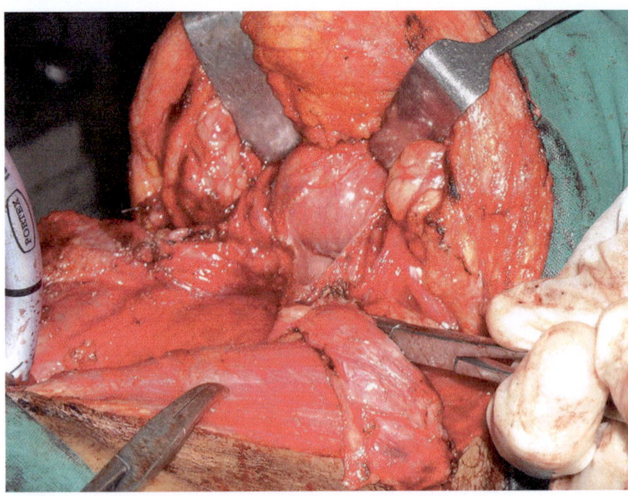

Fig. 10.31 The resulting defect needs tube reconstruction. The options are free jejunum, free ALT/RFFF, and tube PMMC flap. The tube ALT and free jejunum are the most suitable options. The ALT has become the flap of choice as donor site morbidity is less and swallowing outcomes are better. Free jejunum flap is reserved for fatty patients where ALT flap cannot be tubed due to excessive thickness. TLP with esophagectomy defects is reconstructed with stomach pulled up flap

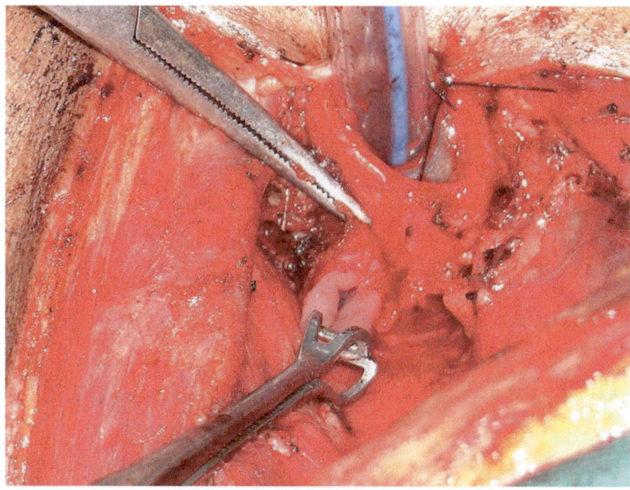

Fig. 10.32 The lower end of the esophagus prepared for anastomosis

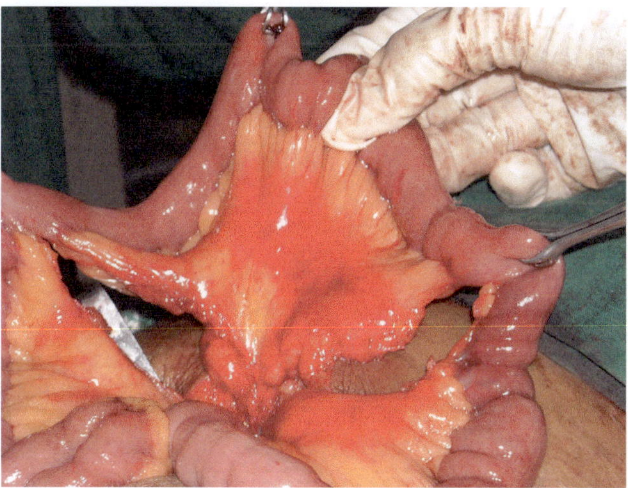

Fig. 10.33 The photograph is showing harverst of jejunal free flap

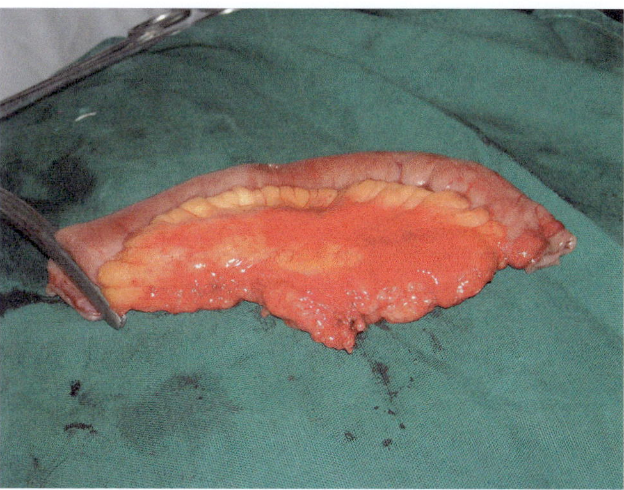

Fig. 10.34 The flap is ready for insertion. It is important to have a sentinel loop for the monitoring of vascularity of flap

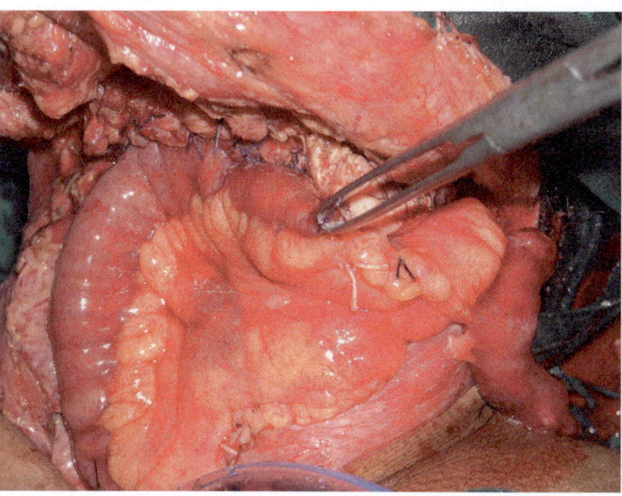

Fig. 10.35 Completed flap suturing. The upper end is anastomosed in the end to side manner while the lower end is sutured in the end to end manner

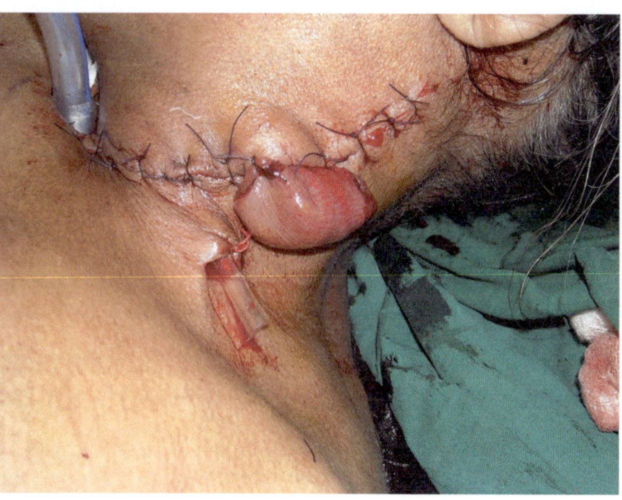

Fig. 10.36 The sentinel loop for monitoring of flap

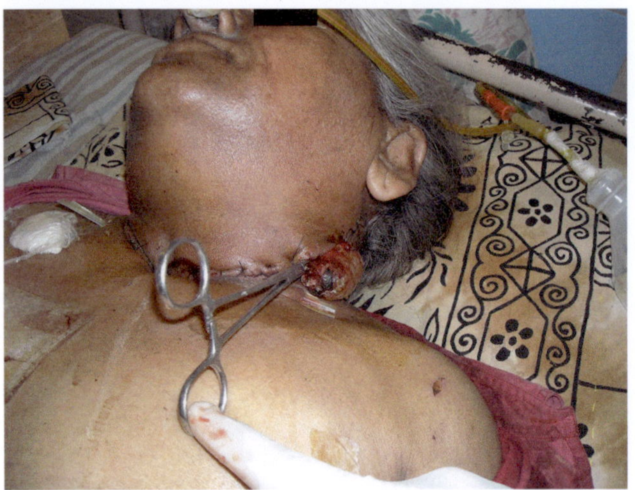

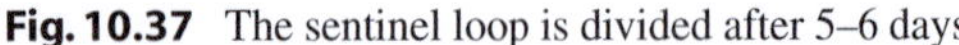

Fig. 10.37 The sentinel loop is divided after 5–6 days

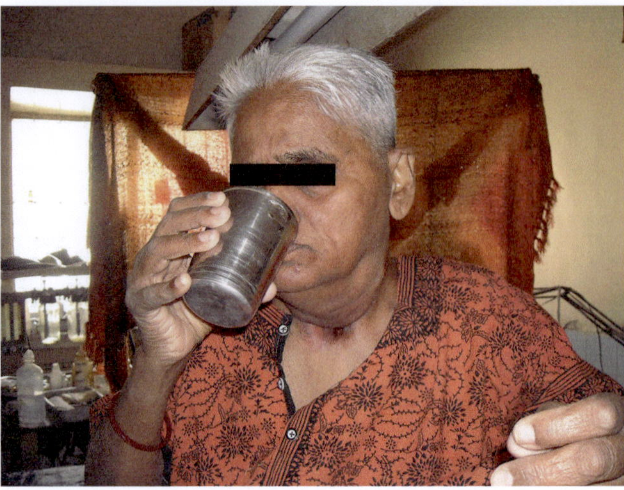

Fig. 10.38 The long-term outcome

Pharyngeal Fistula

The pharyngeal fistula leading to salivary leak is one of the most common and challenging problems of laryngeal surgery. All the efforts should be made to avoid the leak, and this includes prompt use of patch PMMC flap whenever in doubt. The fistula can be classified into two categories. One is major fistula that occurs in immediate postoperative period and threatens to cause carotid blowout. These are relatively rare, happen due to gross surgical error, and need immediate surgical exploration and PMMC flap reconstruction. The second is minor leak occurring on the 7th to 10th postoperative day. This can happen on the 14th to 20th day in post-radiotherapy surgery. Their management requires lots of patience and common sense. It is important to lateralize the leak to avoid aspiration. Subsequent management is conservative for 8–10 weeks. Many of these fistulas heal by themselves with time. We use tight bandage around the neck to hold the tissue together, and this helps in speedy recovery.

Few fistulas don't heal and need surgical intervention. The intervention should be done only when a track is formed and all inflammation is gone. The preference is to use local tissue but PMMC flap may be needed in some cases.

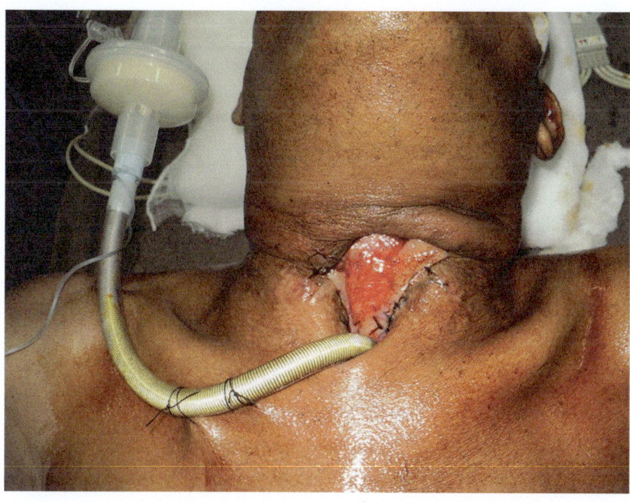

Fig. 10.39 A case of chronic fistula not responding to conservative treatment

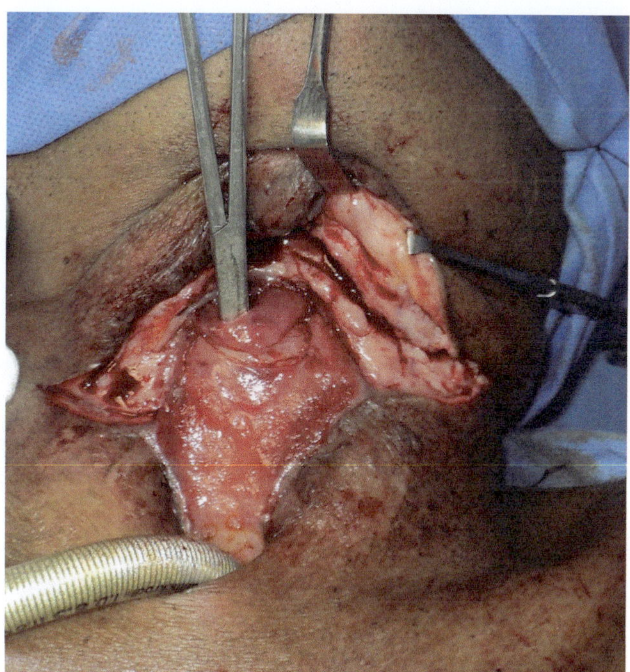

Fig. 10.40 The everted mucosa can be seen with pharyngeal tube underneath

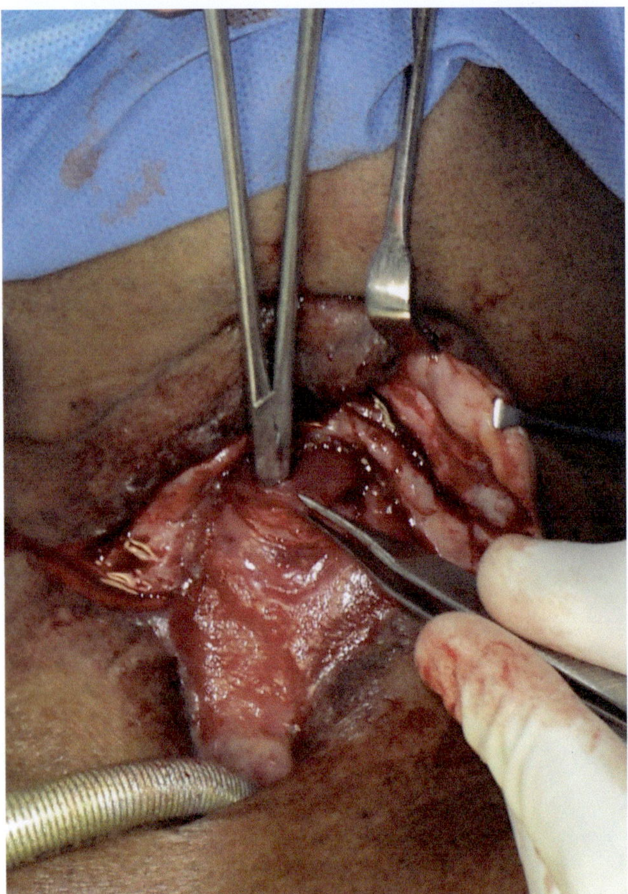

Fig. 10.41 The mucosa has been lifted with knife dissection preserving its base for adequate blood supply

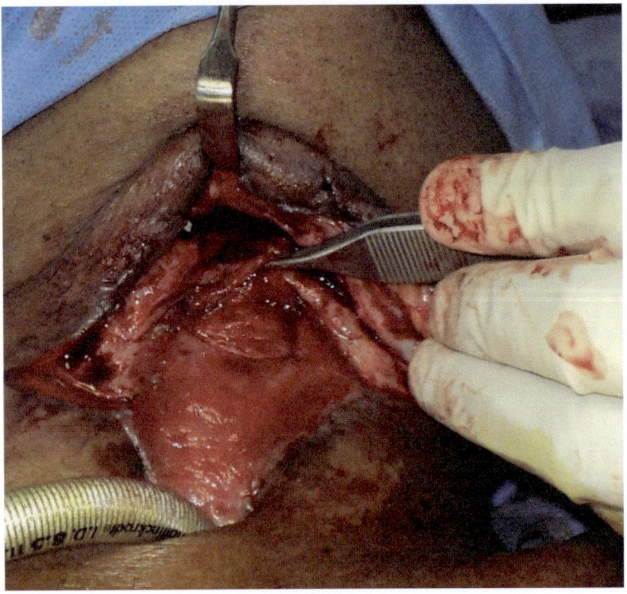

Fig. 10.42 The mucosa is ready for suturing

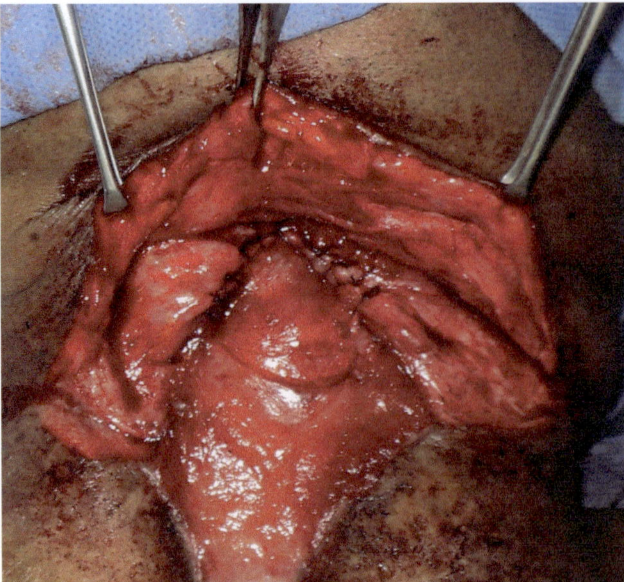

Fig. 10.43 The fistula track is closed by mucosal flap. It is always advisable to provide a second layer of closure. The overlying skin can be sutured to the soft tissues of the neck to provide this layer

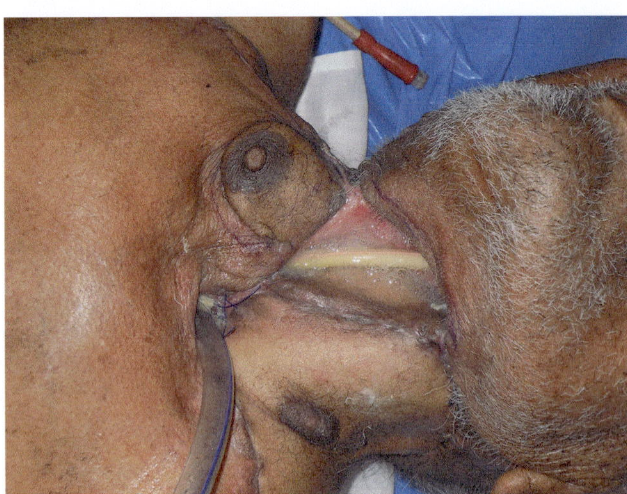

Fig. 10.44 A case of major fistula. Both the PMMC flaps were used in the first surgery to reconstruct extensive defect. Both flaps fell apart in the postoperative phase and resulted in open pharyngeal tube

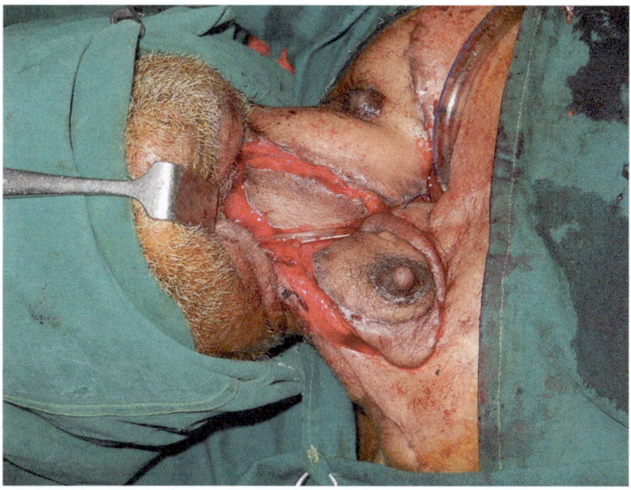

Fig. 10.45 The posterior skin of PMMC flap is refreshed to prepare for suturing. The skin of one side of PMMC flap has been used as a rotation flap. Care should be taken to keep the base of the flap attached in a way to provide adequate blood supply

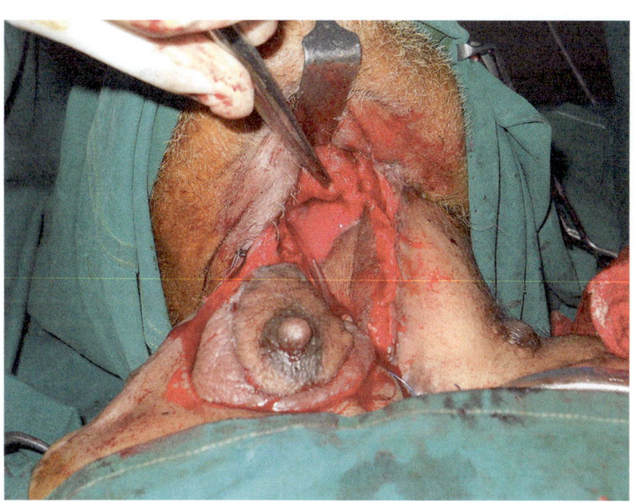

Fig. 10.46 The bed is refreshed for suturing

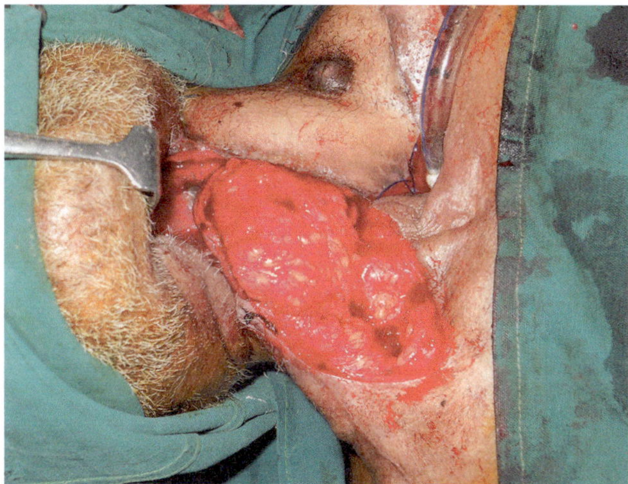

Fig. 10.47 The flap is sutured and the skin graft is placed over it to cover the soft tissue

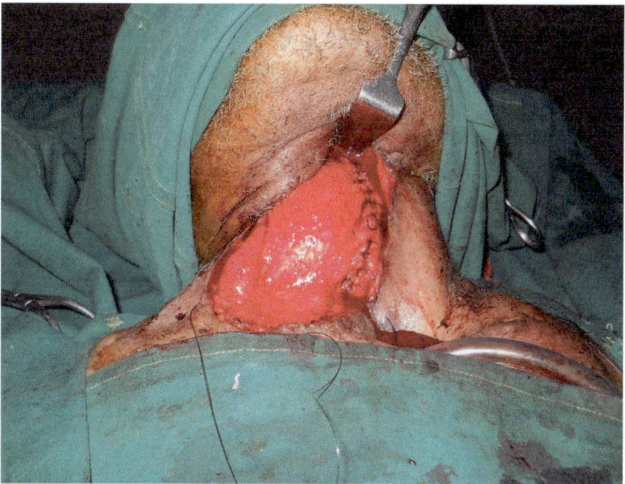

Fig. 10.48 The complete closure of pharyngeal defect

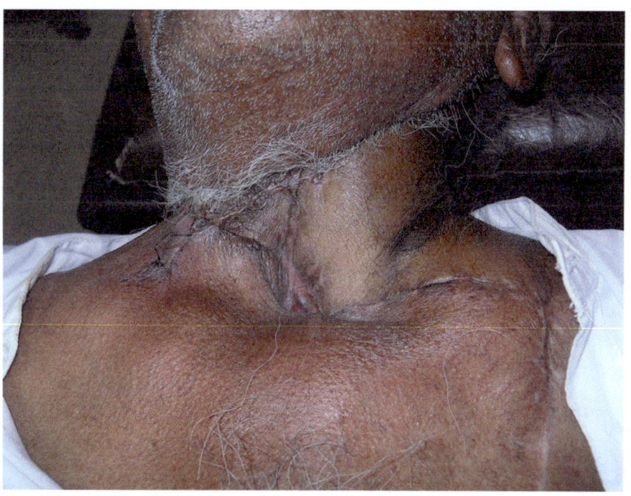

Fig. 10.49 A photograph showing complete healing and closure of the fistula

11 Tumors of the Nose and Paranasal Sinus

Surgical Anatomy

The nose and paranasal (PNS) sinus have complex anatomy. It is related to various important structures that serve vital functions. It is essential to have clear understanding of the anatomy of this region to adequately address these tumors. The paranasal sinus is a common term used for group of sinuses that drains into the nasal cavities. The maxillary sinus is the largest and the most common to be involved in the pathology. The frontal, ethmoid, and sphenoid sinuses do get involved by pathology occasionally, and this mostly happens due to the extension of tumor from the nasal cavity. Primary tumor can occur in these sinuses but is relatively less common, and discussion in this chapter will focus on maxillary sinus and its pathology.

Figure 11.1 demonstrates the schematic anatomy of the nose and PNS and their relation to surrounding structures. The inferior part is formed by the palate and alveolus. The superior part is related to the ethmoid sinus, to the skull base and frontal sinus medially, and to the orbital floor and eye laterally. The posterior compartment is formed by the muscle of mastication in ITF.

N. Trivedi, *Atlas of Head and Neck Cancer Surgery: The Compartment Surgery for Resection in 3-D*,
DOI 10.1007/978-81-322-2050-3_11, © Springer India 2015

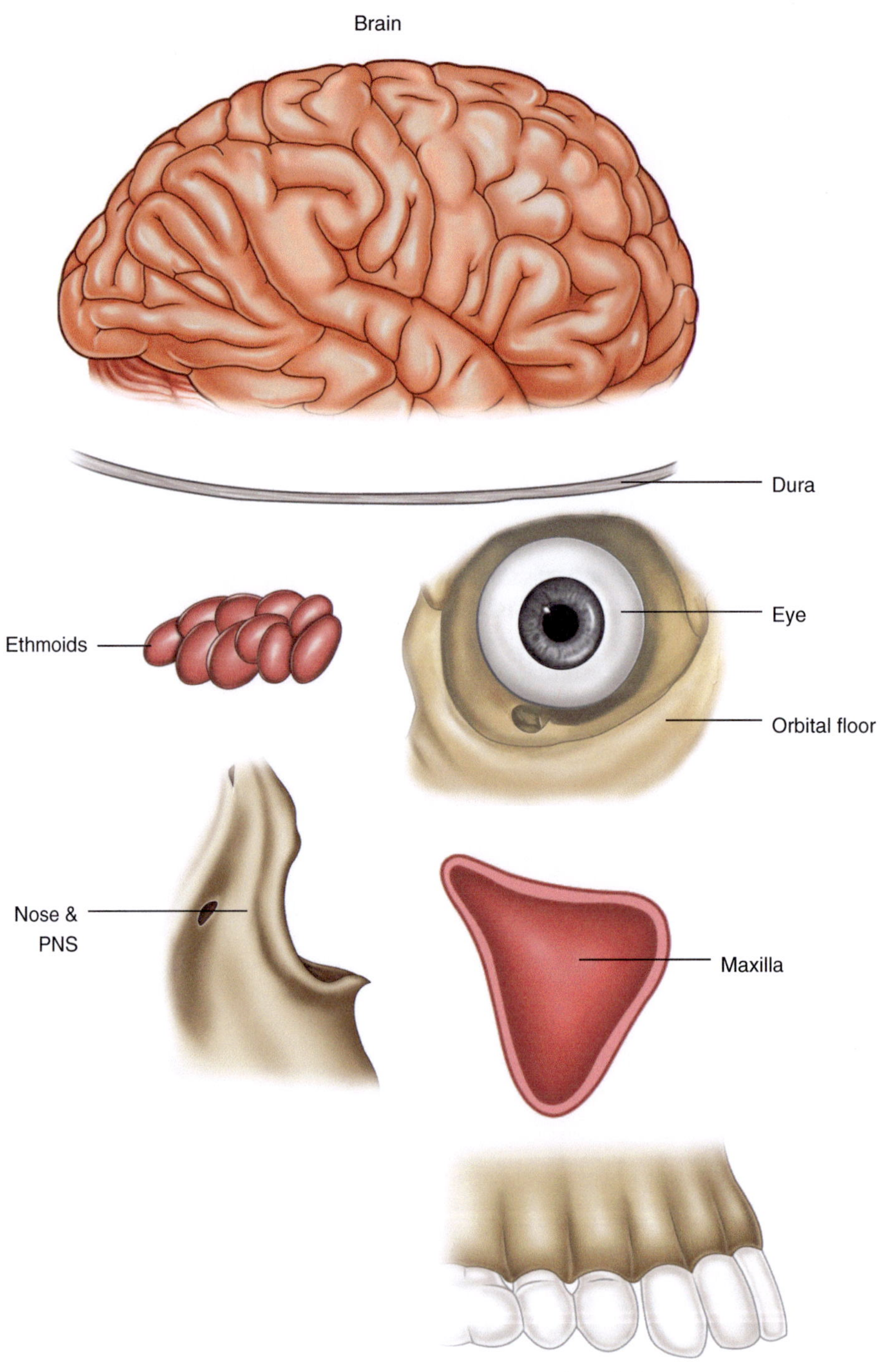

Fig. 11.1 Schematic representation of paranasal sinus

Surgical Pathology

This is one of the most challenging areas to deal with surgically, and understanding the pattern of spread of the tumor is critical in achieving clear margins. Figure 11.2 shows the path of spread of the tumor in a schematic manner. It is mandatory to have imaging studies in the form of CT scan and MRI to evaluate the extent of disease spread. Many times both CT scan and MRI are needed for detailed evaluation. CT scan is always the first imaging modality that outlines the extent of spread. MRI is done to see soft tissue involvement in relation to the orbit and optic nerve, dura, and brain involvement and assess perineural spread. There is possibility of variety of tumor pathology. It is essential to know exact tumor pathology, and one should not hesitate to ask for immunohistochemistry studies to confirm the histopathology result. This is important to plan treatment protocol and overall prognosis depends upon the tumor biology.

The surgical planning is in accordance with the extent of disease spread. Figure 11.3 demonstrates various surgical approaches to address these tumors. Tumor spreading inferiorly is addressed by infrastructure maxillectomy, while tumor spreading upwards needs maxillectomy with orbital exenteration. If the skull base is involved, anterior skull base resection is required. The tumor limited to anterior ethmoid can be cleared by trans-facial resection, while combined approaches are required for posterior and superior ethmoid involvement of the lesion. The posterior spread into ITF is the most challenging and requires posterior to anterior approach (compartment approach) to address the 3rd margin. This procedure is described in the chapter addressing ITF resection.

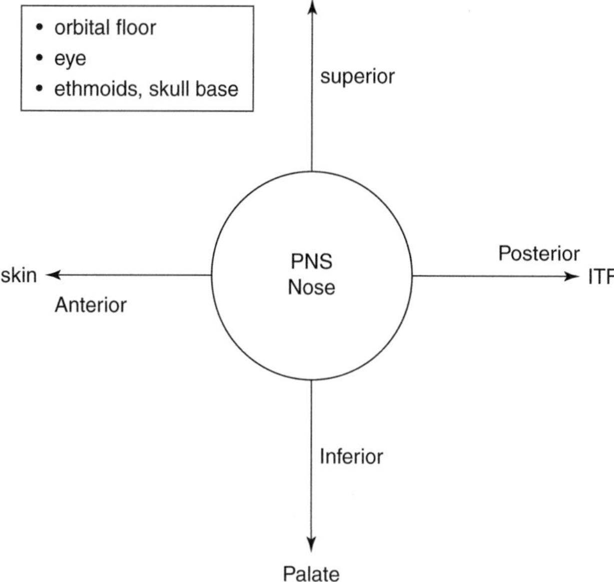

Fig. 11.2 Pattern of spread of paranasal sinus tumors

Treatment algorithm for PNS tumors.

	I	II	III
Category	Confined to Nose & maxilla cavity	Inferior spread (palate + olveolus)	Superior to orbital floor & eye
Resection	WLE c̄ medial maxillotomy	Infrastructure Maxillectomy	Suprastructure maxillectorny
Reconstruction	Primary closure	• RFF • Temporalis • Obturator	• Temporalis • RFF

	IV	V	VI
Category	Posterior spread to ITF	Total maxilla (palate + orbital floor)	Skull base
Resection	Maxillectomy c̄ ITF clearance (Transmandibular) approach	Total maxillectomy	Anterior skull base resection
Reconstruction	• ALT • Rectus • Fibula • PMMC/ Forehead	• Rectus • ALT • Fibula • Scapula • Forehead • Obturator	

Fig. 11.3 Treatment algorithm for PNS tumors

Surgical Concepts

- Imaging studies with CT scan and MRI are essential before planning the surgery.
- It is advisable to accurately map the tumor and outline various structures involved by the tumor. This helps in planning the surgical approach and reconstruction.
- Surgery remains the primary treatment approach, but long-term outcome depends upon tumor biology.
- Removal of the eye is a sensitive issue and every chance should be given to conserve it. The eye needs to be resected if the tumor involves the rectus muscle, ocular fat, and optic nerve. Involvement of periorbita is not an indication for orbital exenteration.
- The majority of tumors are addressed by lateral rhinotomy incision. One can have vertical extension (lynch extension) or lateral extension (Weber–Ferguson extension) depending upon the structures to be removed.
- It may be difficult to achieve wide margins for tumor in this area. It is essential to dissect in a clear tissue plane between the tumor and vital structure. The decision to sacrifice structure is taken when clear plane is not available.
- The tumor with posterior spread needs transmandibular approach.
- Combined craniofacial resection is reserved for lesions involving the cribriform plate, dura, and brain.
- Trans-nasal endoscopic approach has become popular in recent time. One needs to be very careful in applying this approach to malignant neoplasm, and surgical clearance should not be compromised at any cost. It is essential to have the capacity to perform extensive endoscopic sinus surgery and open anterior skull base surgery before attempting endoscopic removal of malignant lesion. It is best reserved for early, low-grade malignancy in experienced hand.
- The reconstruction poses a difficult challenge and one has to plan carefully to have a good functional outcome.

Wide Excision

This section demonstrates a surgical procedure for early nose and paranasal sinus tumor.

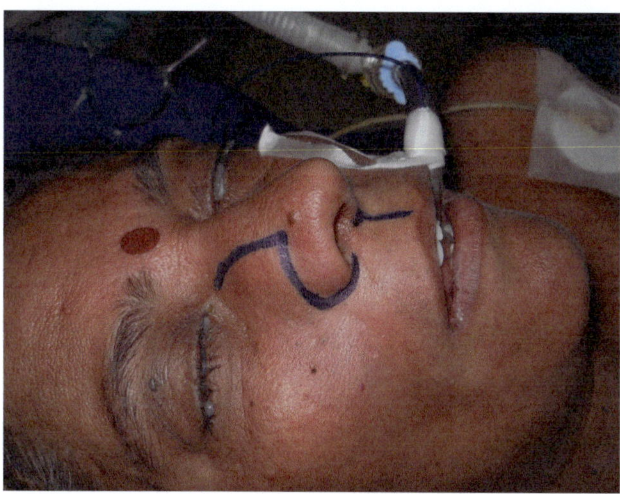

Fig. 11.4 This is a lateral rhinotomy incision with lip split extension. The lip split is not essential in all cases but does provide good excess to perform bone cuts

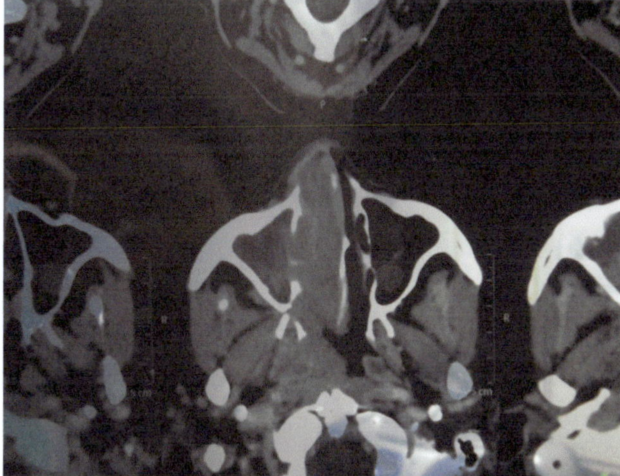

Fig. 11.5 Tumor extension on a CT scan plate showing involvement of the lateral nasal wall in the entire length. This lesion can be addressed endoscopically provided the surgeon has adequate experience of doing endoscopic surgeries and performing open cancer surgeries

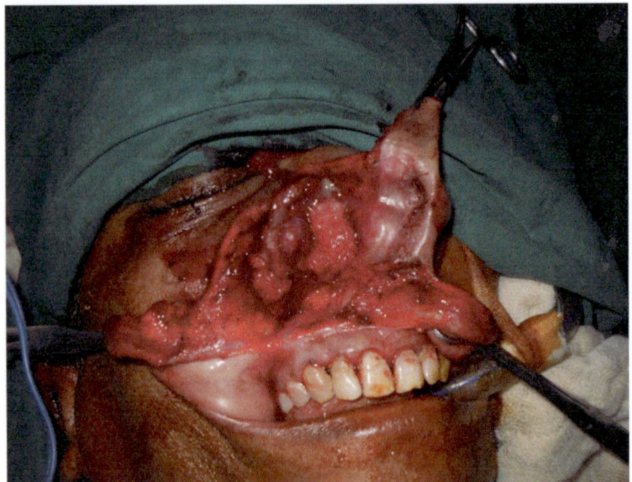

Fig. 11.6 The flaps are raised to expose the lesion and anterior maxilla

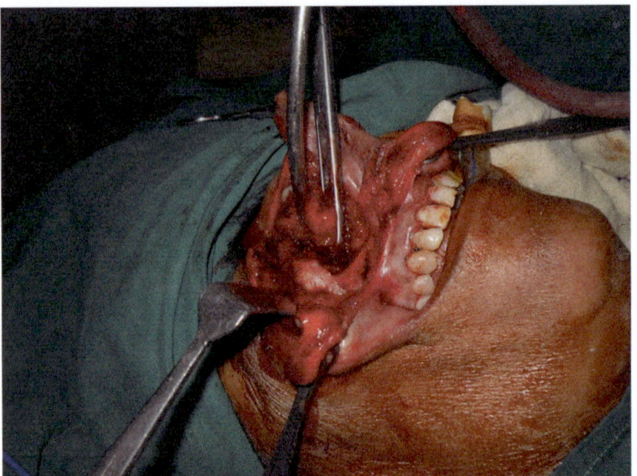

Fig. 11.7 The medial wall of the maxilla is exposed for bone cuts

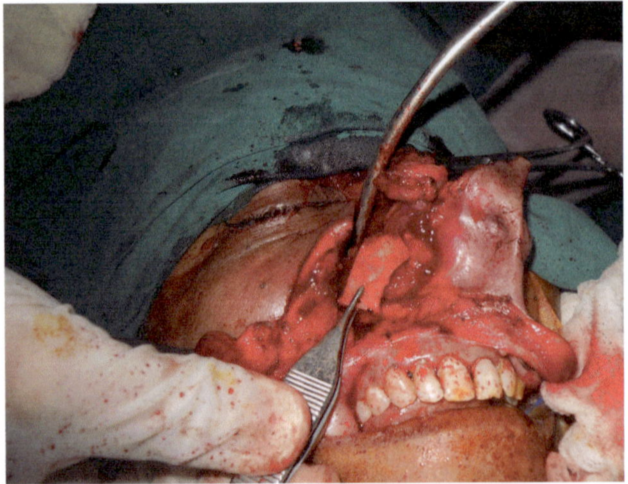

Fig. 11.8 Cuts are made to perform medial maxillotomy. The removal of the anterior wall of the maxilla in medial part allows easy access to the lateral nasal wall in the entire length

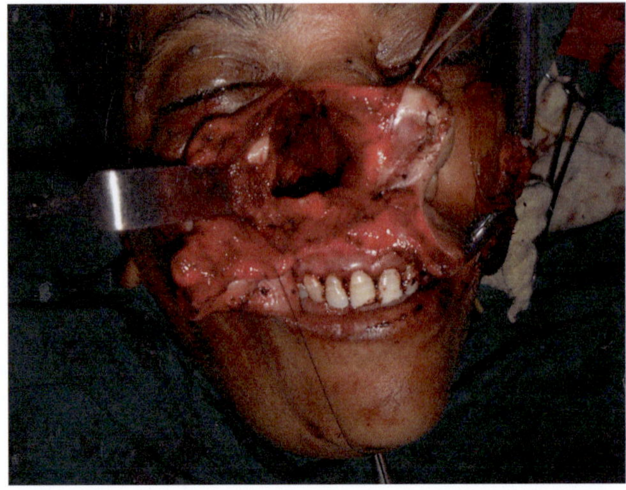

Fig. 11.9 The resection is complete. This surgery results in bleeding and one has to learn to work with bleeding. The systolic blood pressure can be kept low to reduce the bleeding. It stops once the lesion is completely out

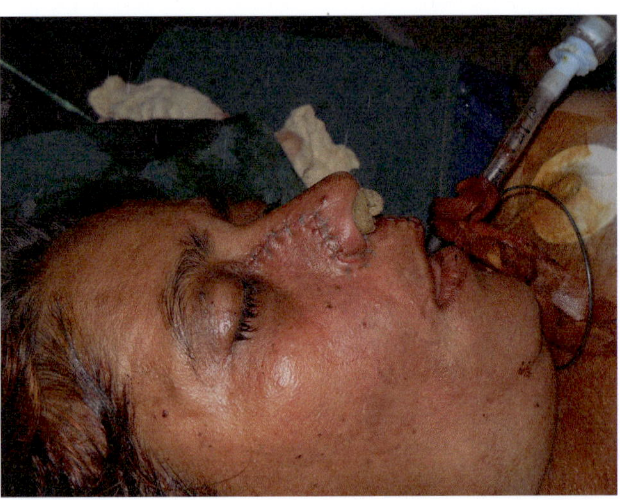

Fig. 11.10 The closure of the wound. The nasal cavity is packed for 2–3 days, and the patient is advised to clean the cavity with salt water in postoperative period to avoid crusting

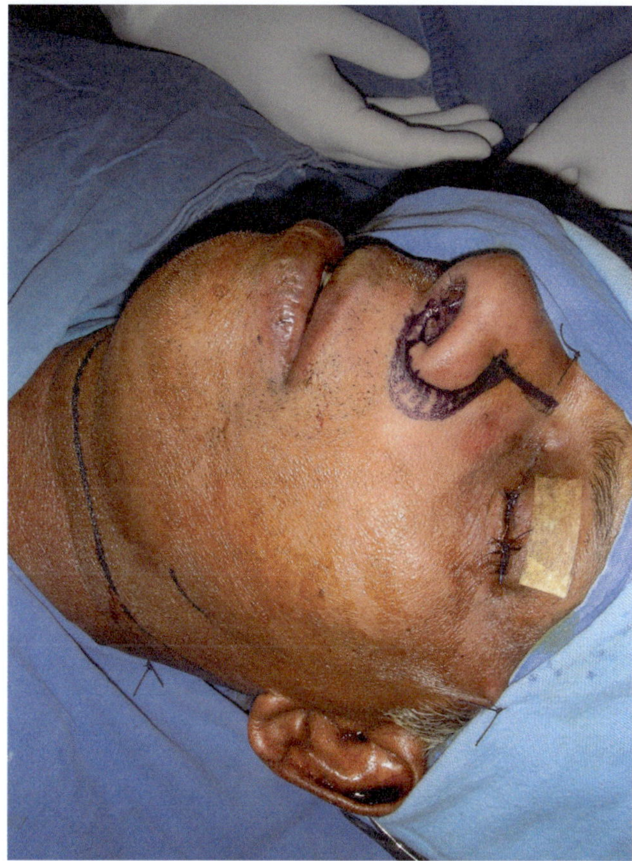

Fig. 11.11 Patient with nasal tumor involving part of the skin

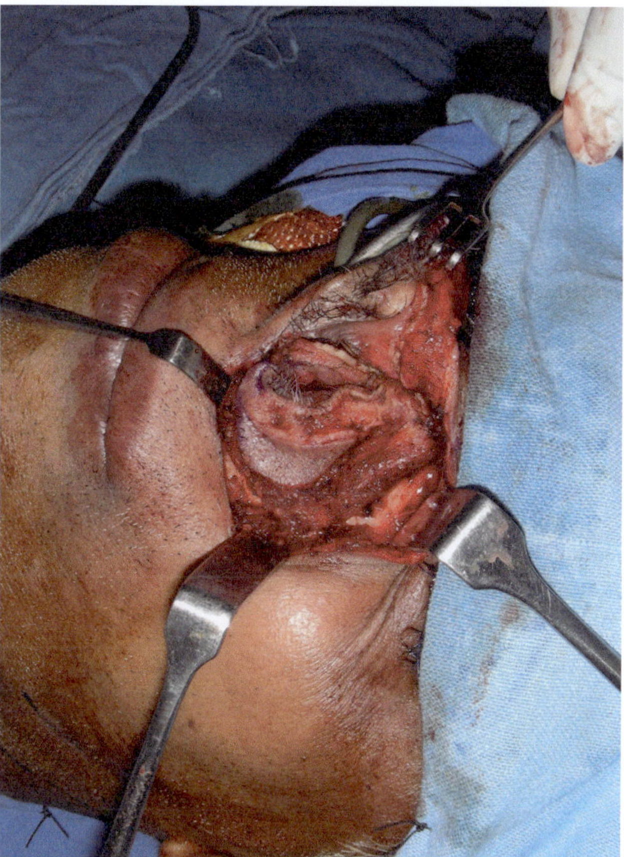

Fig. 11.12 Similar approach to the first case to perform wide excision of lesion including the skin

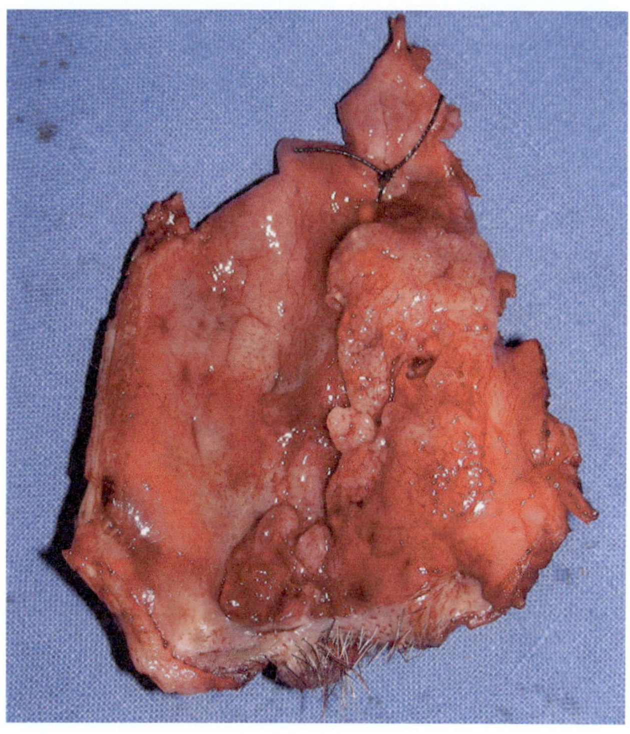

Fig. 11.13 Photograph showing specimen

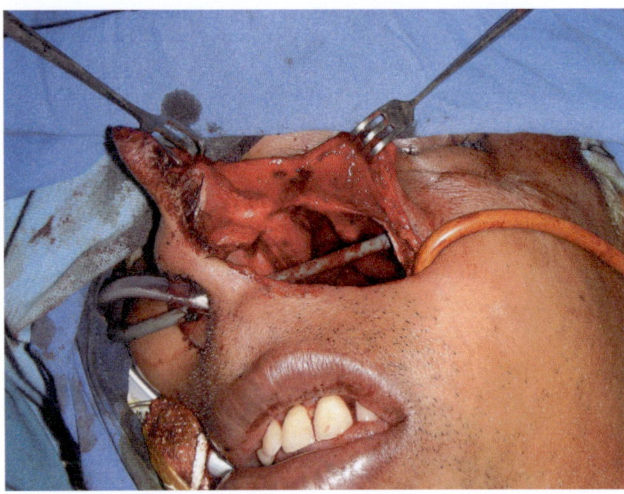

Fig. 11.14 The reconstruction was planned with radial forearm free flap

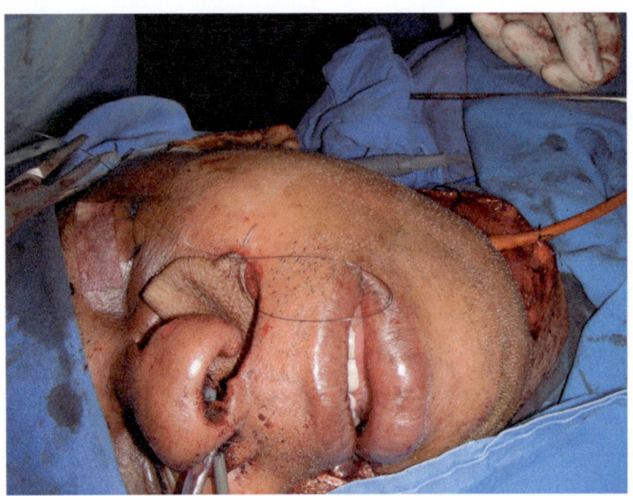

Fig. 11.15 The flap is inserted to cover the skin defect

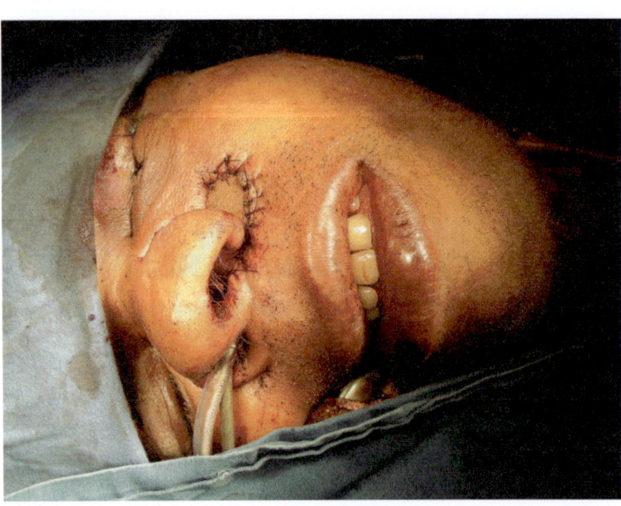

Fig. 11.16 The closure is complete. This defect could have been closed primarily with an advancement flap

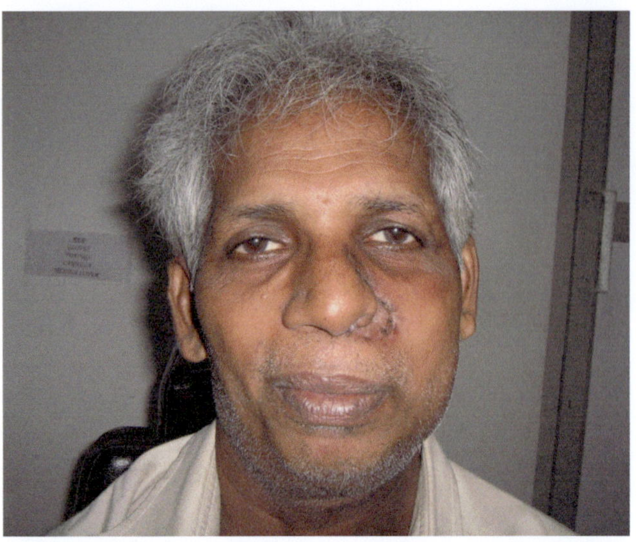

Fig. 11.17 Long-term outcome

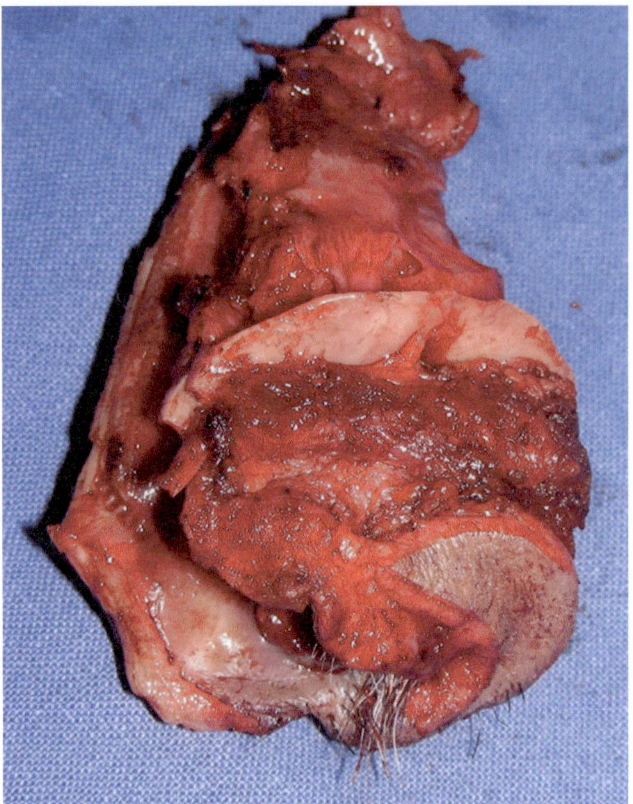

Fig. 11.18 Patient with lesion in the hard palate. The biopsy result suggested malignant neoplasm, and CT scan showed palatal bone was not involved. It is important to remember that one needs to take extra layer of tissue in depth to have a clear margin. Removal of the palatal bone for all malignant neoplasm is mandatory

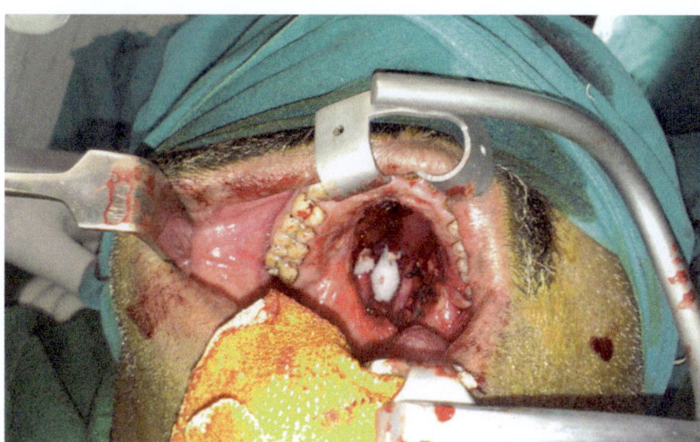

Fig. 11.19 Wide excision with palatal bone is complete and hemostasis is achieved

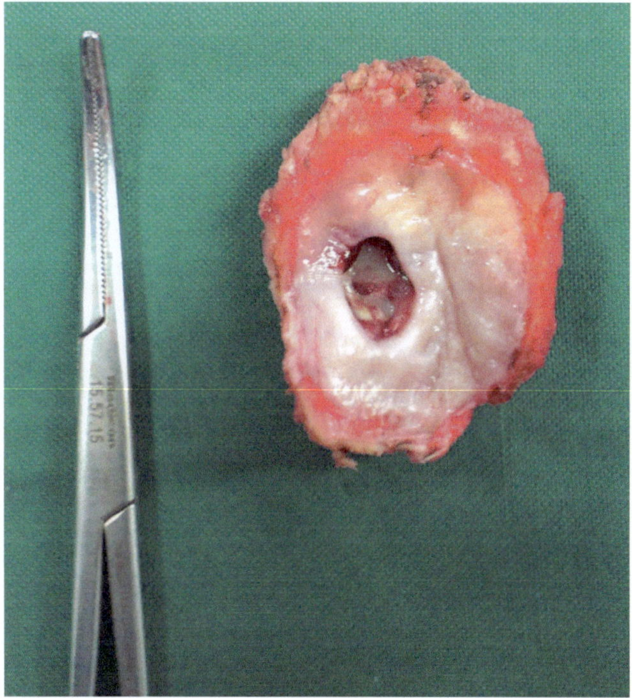

Fig. 11.20 Specimen showing clear margins

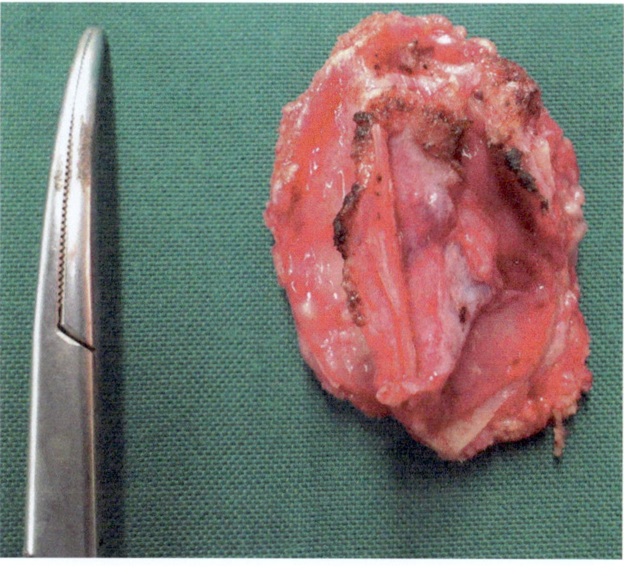

Fig. 11.21 The septum side showing normal anatomy confirming clear margins

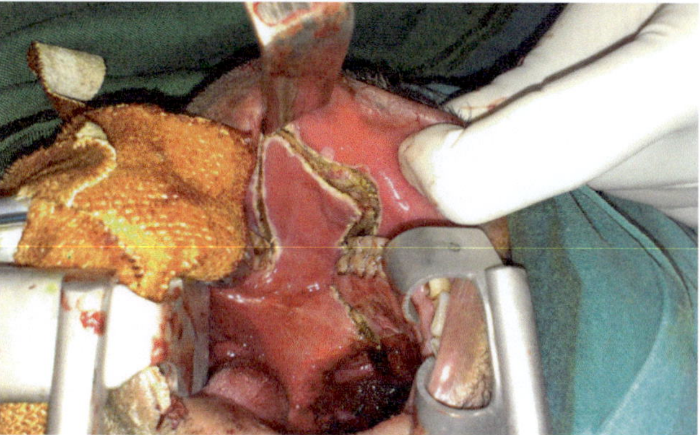

Fig. 11.22 The reconstruction was planned with a combination of buccal rotation flap and palatal rotation flap. Smaller defects can be addressed with palatal rotation alone or facial artery myomucosal flap (FAMM)

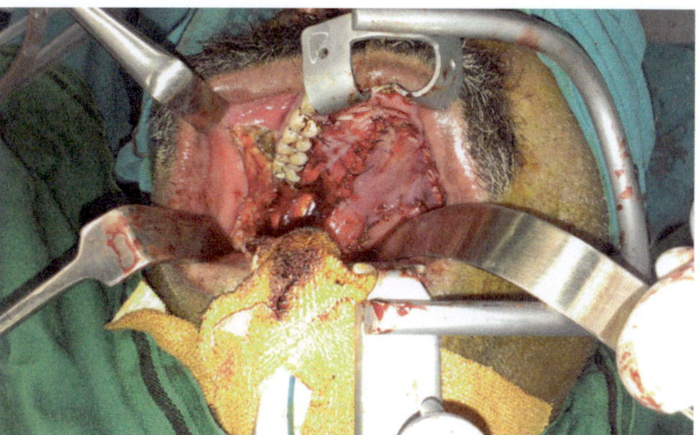

Fig. 11.23 Both the flaps are sutured together to have complete seal for palatal defect

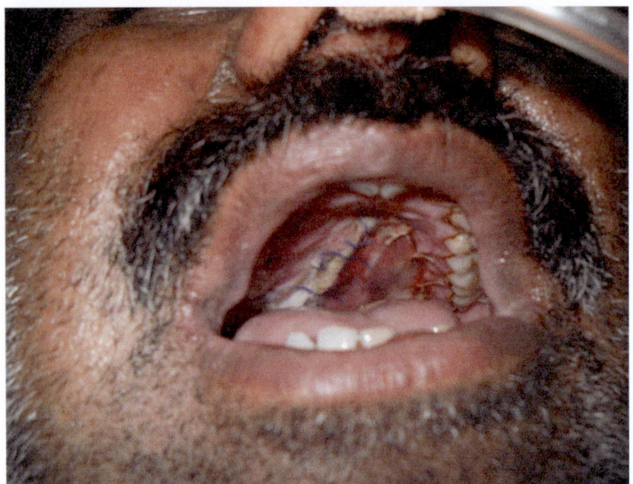

Fig. 11.24 Photograph showing completed procedure

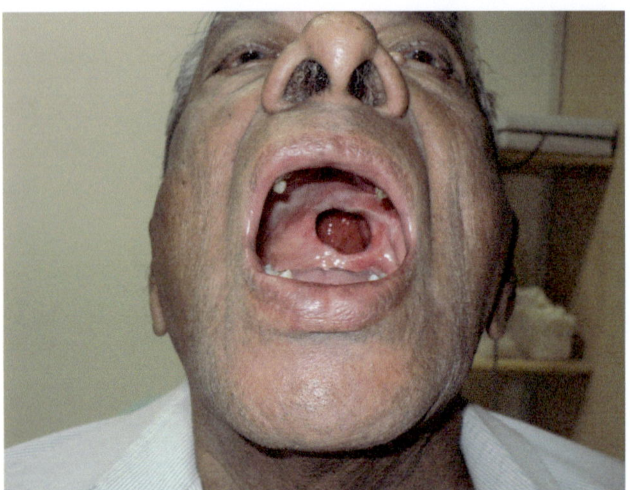

Fig. 11.25 Patient with palatal defect

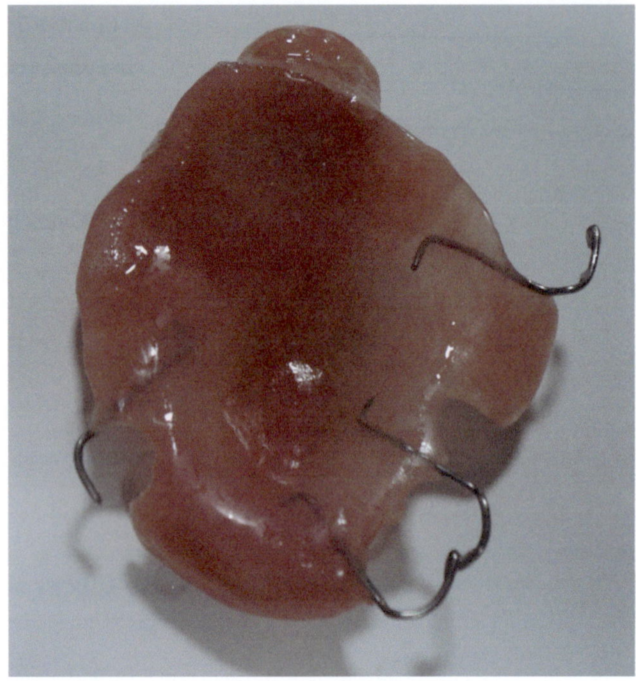

Fig. 11.26 The reconstruction was performed with obturator

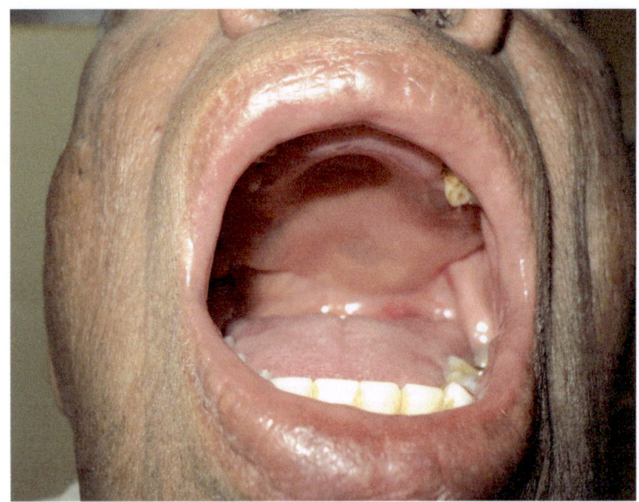

Fig. 11.27 The final outcome. The obturator is a simple method to rehabilitate these patients and gives very good outcome in the majority of cases

Infrastructure Maxillectomy

This section shows surgical procedure to remove PNS tumor that spreads inferiorly and involves the palate and alveolus.

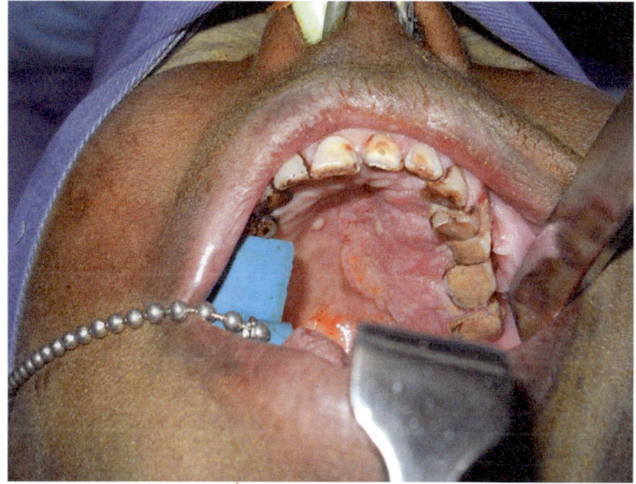

Fig. 11.28 Photograph showing lesion involving the hard palate reaching the alveolus. It is essential to get CT scan in this case to evaluate the upper extent of the lesion

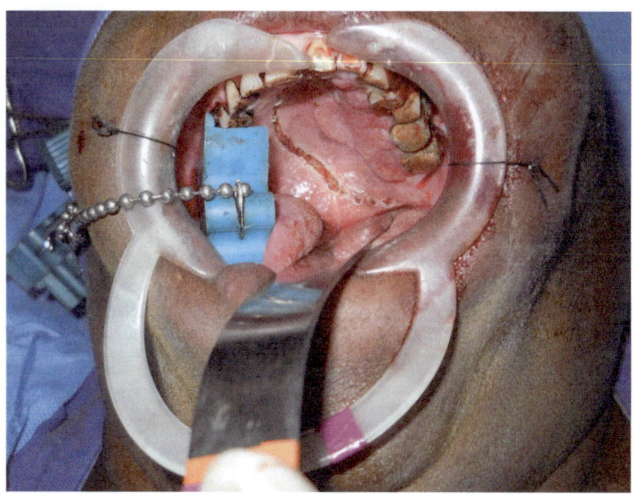

Fig. 11.29 Proposed mucosal and bone cuts with 1 cm margin

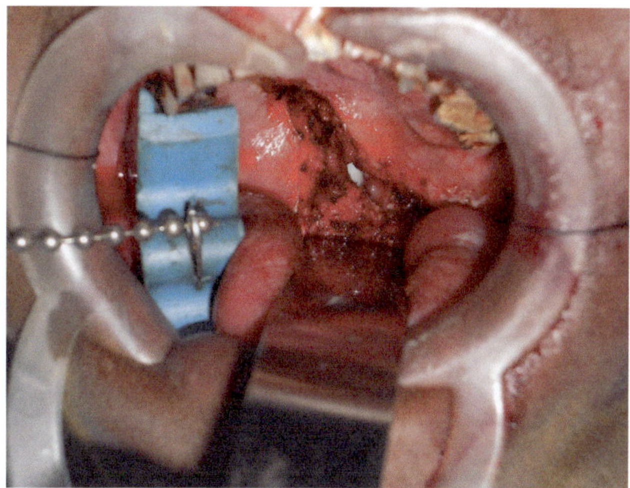

Fig. 11.30 The soft palate has been separated and one can see the endotracheal tube. It is convenient to have endotracheal tube from the opposite nostrils instead having it through the oral cavity. One needs to be careful of not injuring it while performing palatal bone cuts

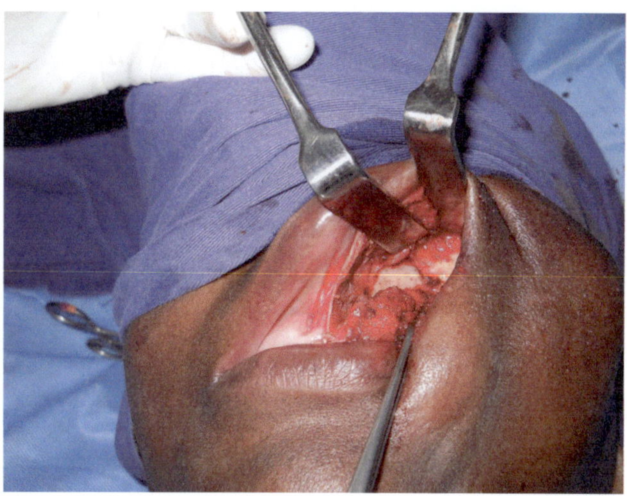

Fig. 11.31 Anterior sublabial flap is raised. One can also perform lateral rhinotomy incision to have better exposure. The exposure should be adequate to perform appropriate bone cuts and control bleeding

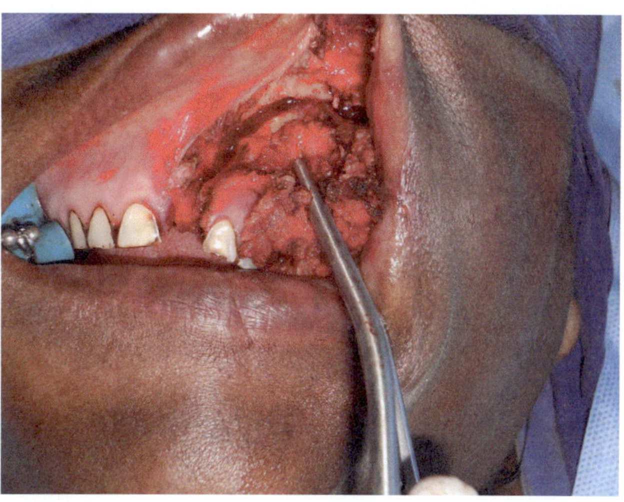

Fig. 11.32 The anterior bone cut extending posteriorly and laterally

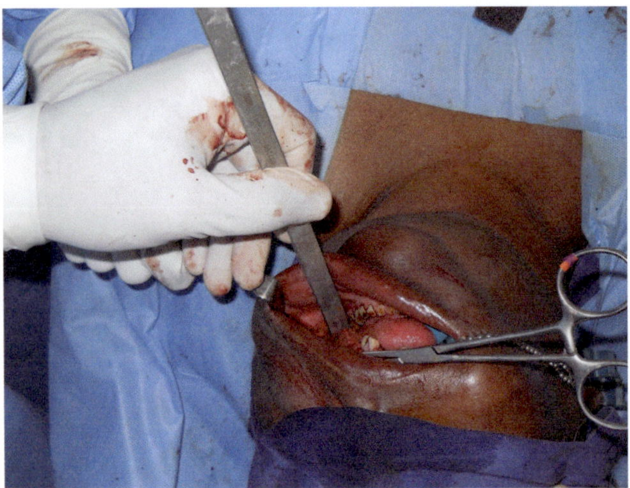

Fig. 11.33 The posterior cut is placed at pterygomaxillary junction. This can be achieved by curved pterygoid chisel. One needs to be careful not to break pterygoid plate too high or else it can lead to cerebrospinal fluid (CSF) leak

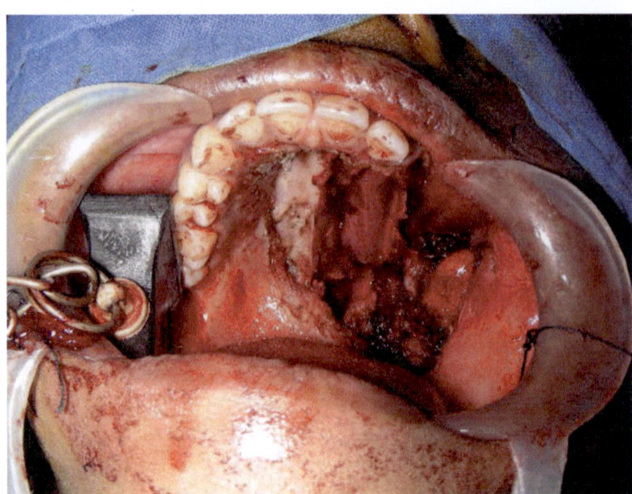

Fig. 11.35 Photograph showing a defect for reconstruction. The patient has good remaining dentition and can do with an obturator

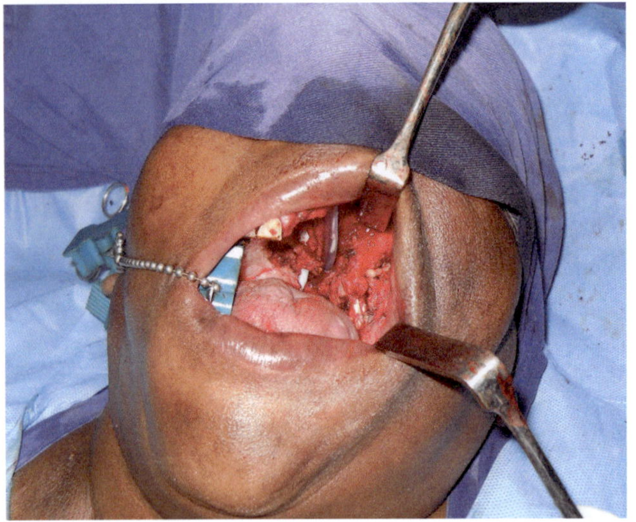

Fig. 11.34 The procedure is complete and feeding tube is in place. The bleeding happens from the nasal wall and greater palatine artery, and appropriate measures should be taken to control it

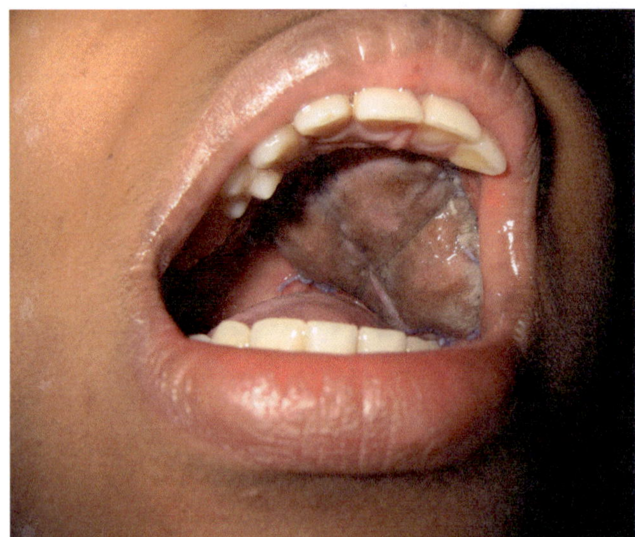

Fig. 11.36 This patient received radial forearm free flap. One can also use temporalis rotation flap for such defects

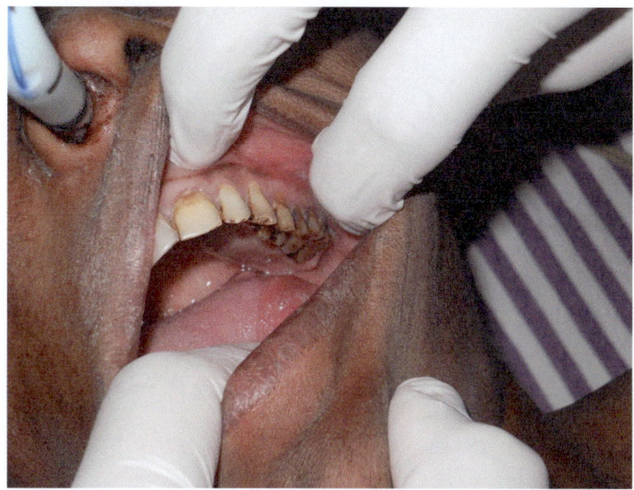

Fig. 11.37 Patient with minor salivary malignant neoplasm in the palate

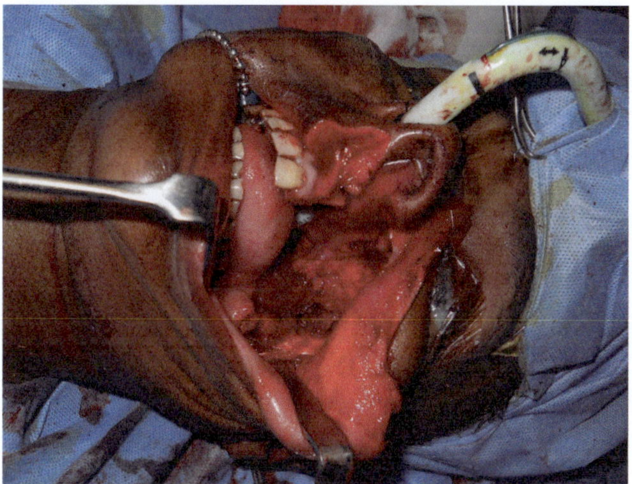

Fig. 11.38 The patient had severe submucous fibrosis and intraoral resection was difficult. Lateral rhinotomy incision was used to achieve adequate exposure. The resection was completed as described earlier

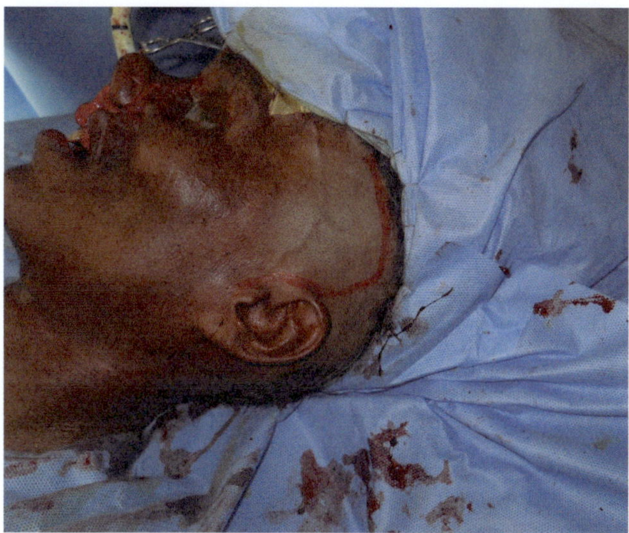

Fig. 11.39 Proposed incision for temporalis muscle flap

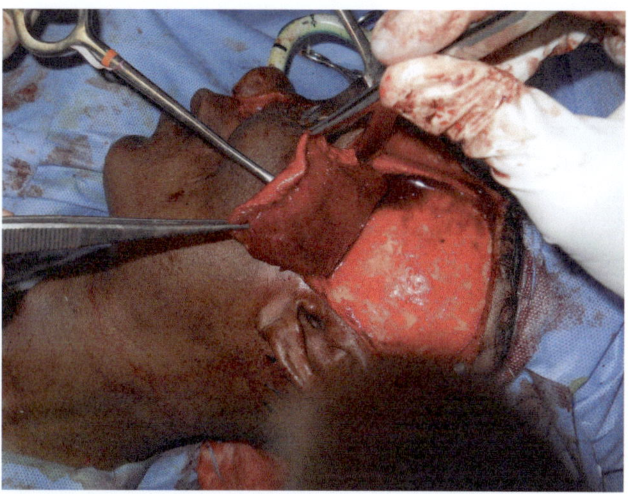

Fig. 11.40 The flap is being raised from the skull bone. One has to take the entire muscle in the posterior extent to increase its reach in the palate. The deep surface is preferably separated from the bone with periosteal elevator instead of cautery

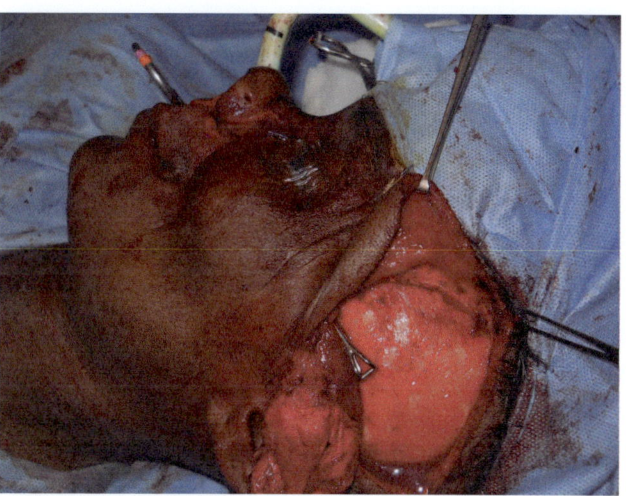

Fig. 11.41 The tunnel is made to rotate the muscle. Removal of maxillary tubercle area creates adequate space for muscle rotation. One must take appropriate precaution to protect blood supply deep to muscle in the coronoid process area

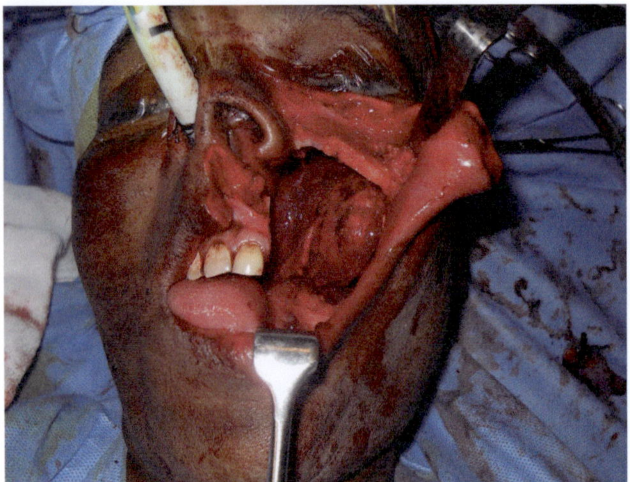

Fig. 11.42 The muscle is rotated in the cavity

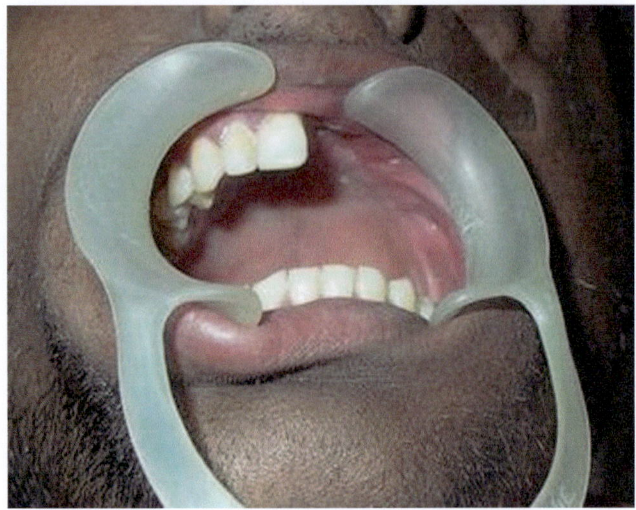

Fig. 11.44 Long-term outcome. One should notice the trismus that can happen in some cases, and aggressive mouth opening exercises are essential to prevent it

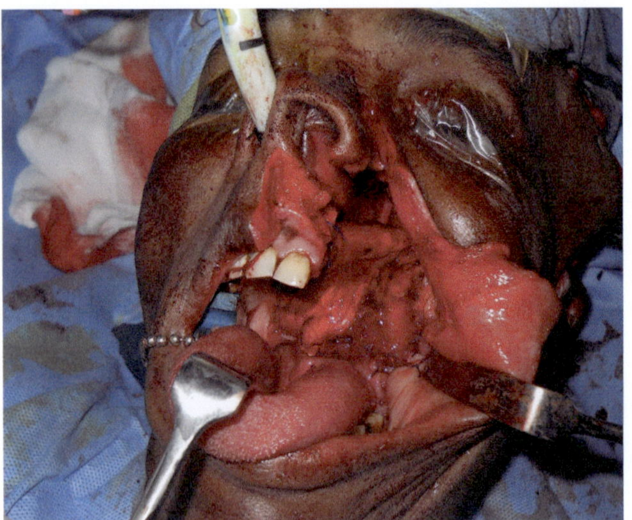

Fig. 11.43 The flap is sutured to the defect. It is a good practice to close the palate defect with secure sutures and avoid stitching the buccal defect. This avoids tension in the flap and helps in keeping flap in position

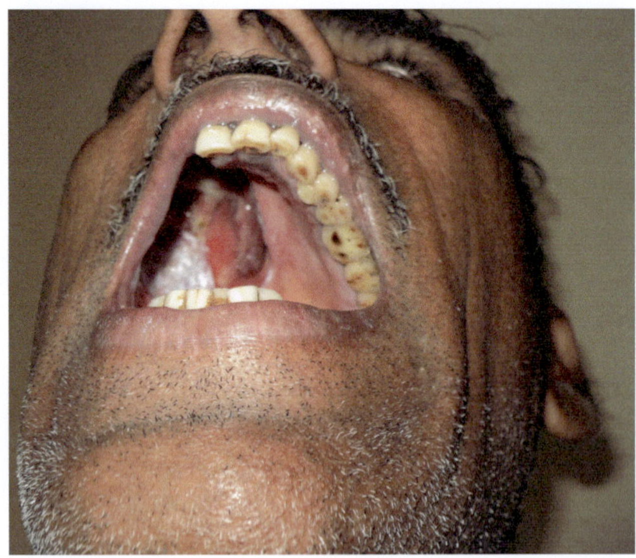

Fig. 11.45 A patient with healed infrastructure defect. It is advisable to use split thick skin graft to line the cavity if reconstruction is planned with obturator

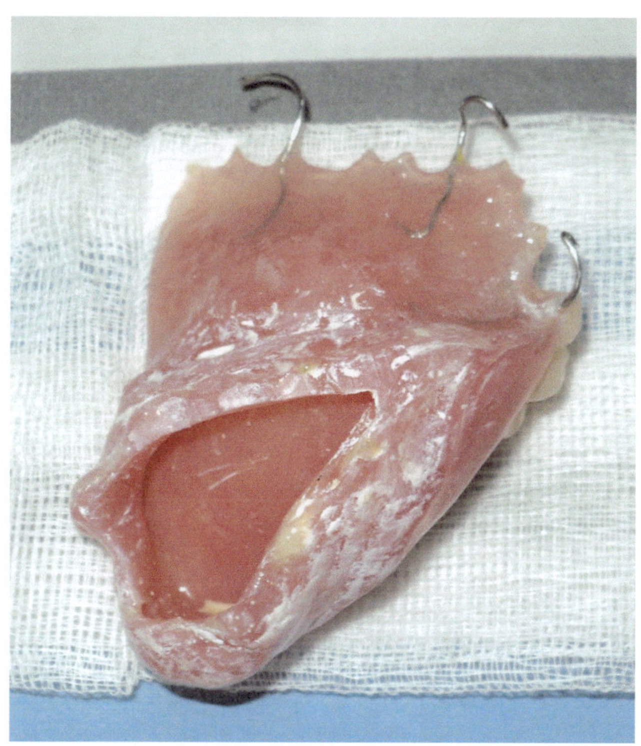

Fig. 11.46 The obturator is made. The patient can have interim obturator immediately after surgery if preoperative impression is taken

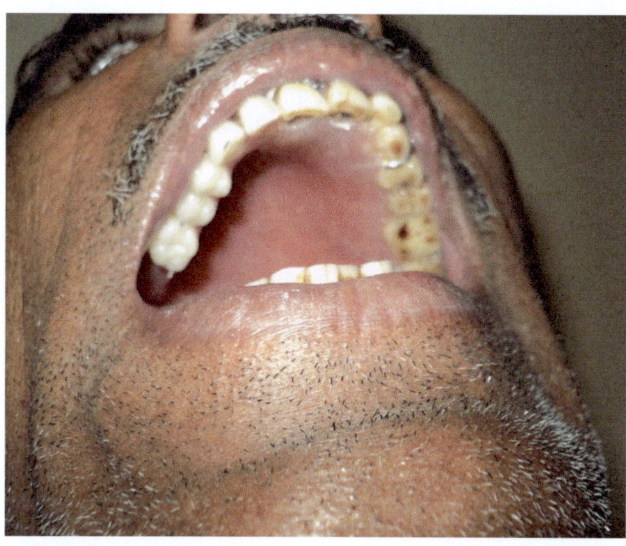

Fig. 11.47 The final outcome with obturator in place. This provides dentition that cannot be provided by flap but one needs to manage obturator for the rest of his or her life

Suprastructure Maxillectomy

This section demonstrates the procedure to address maxillary tumor spreading to the orbital floor and eye.

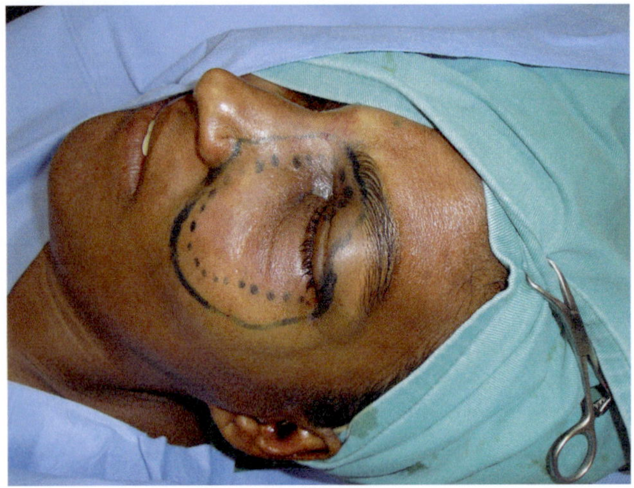

Fig. 11.48 A tumor involving the skin, orbital floor, and eye

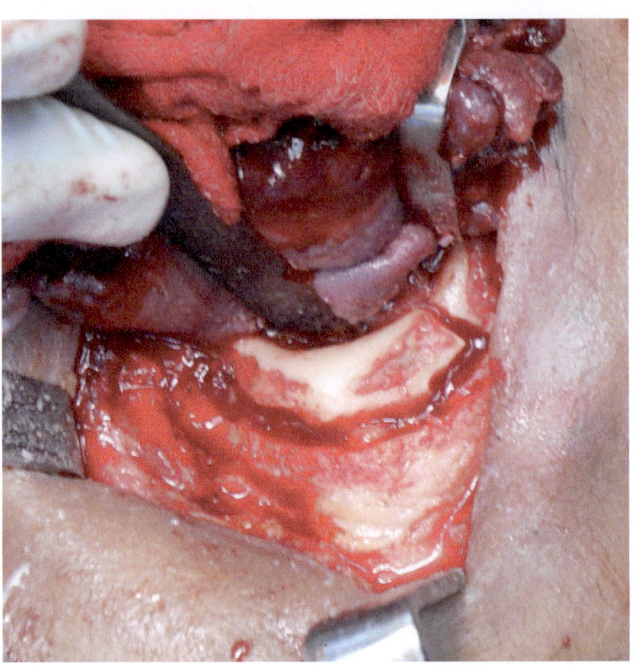

Fig. 11.50 The bone cuts are made to remove entire orbital floor. This also provides access to apex of orbit and clamping becomes easy

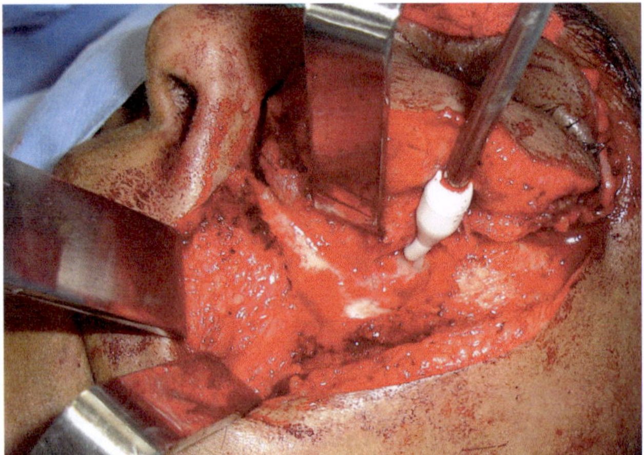

Fig. 11.49 The anterior wall of maxilla is exposed to perform suprastructure maxillectomy

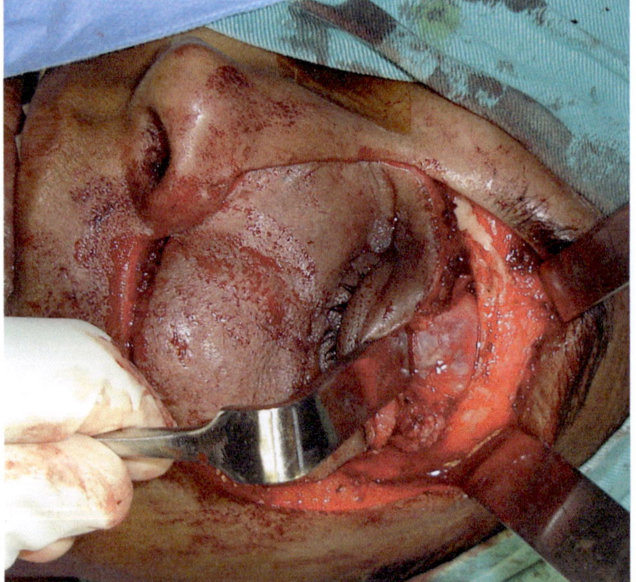

Fig. 11.51 The eye is mobilized from superior aspect

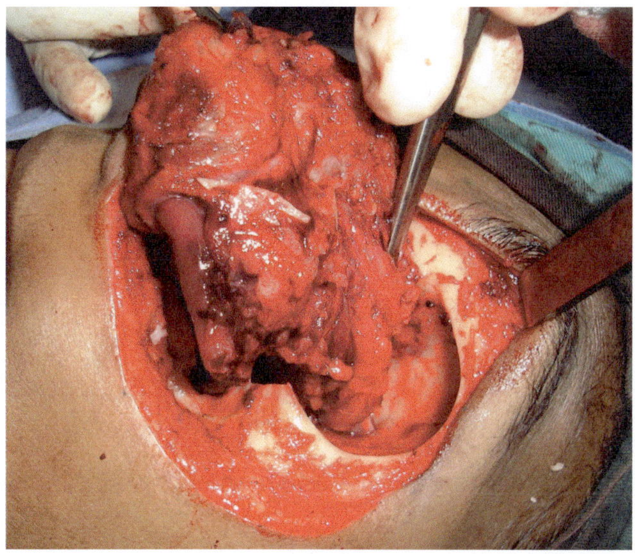

Fig. 11.52 The anterior and posterior ethmoid vessels are secured. The orbital apex is exposed. Right angled forceps is clamped to secure ophthalmic artery. The stump is trans-fixed with absorbable sutures

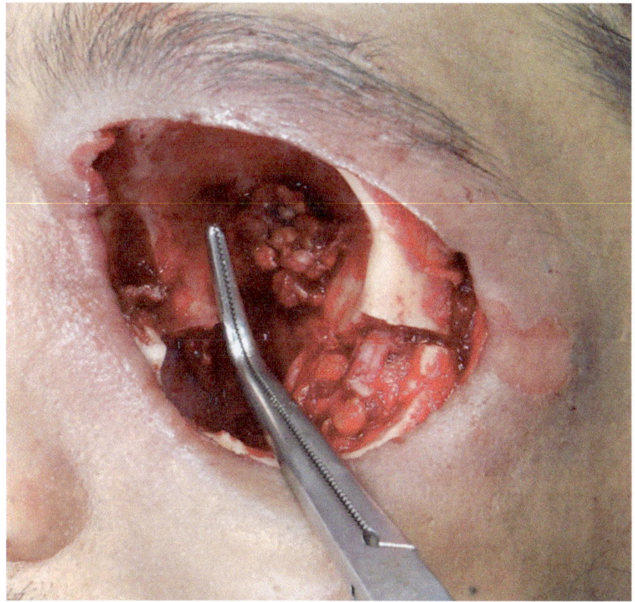

Fig. 11.53 The specimen is removed. The photograph is showing the advantage of performing suprastructure maxillectomy to have more space to apply forceps at apex

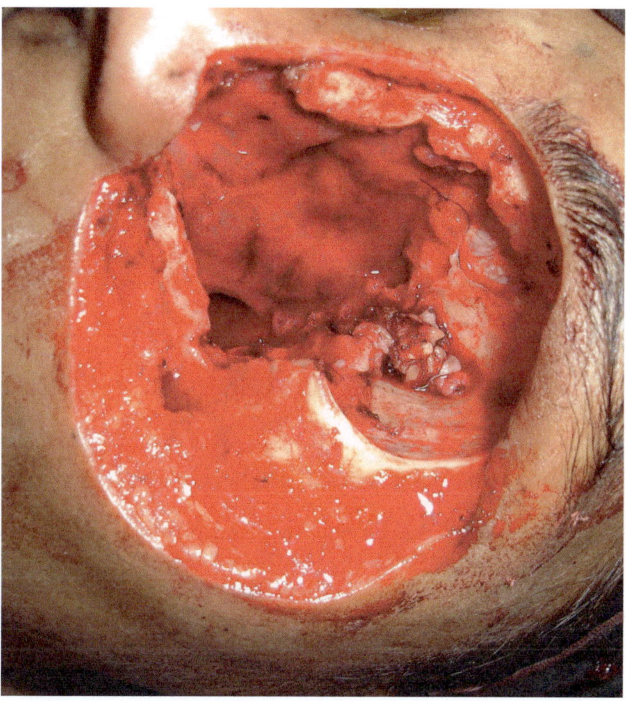

Fig. 11.54 Photograph is showing completed procedure

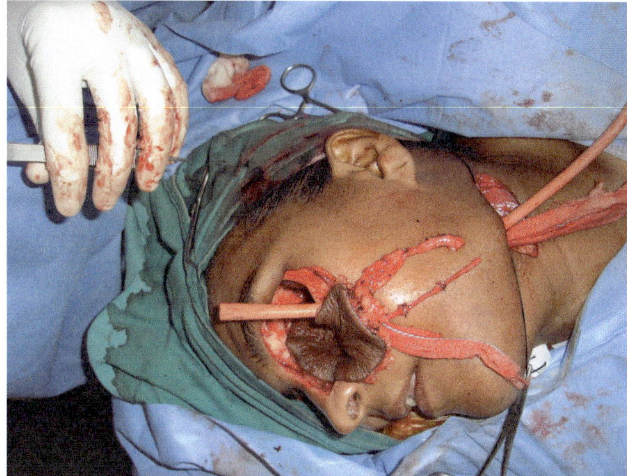

Fig. 11.55 Reconstruction was planned with RFFF

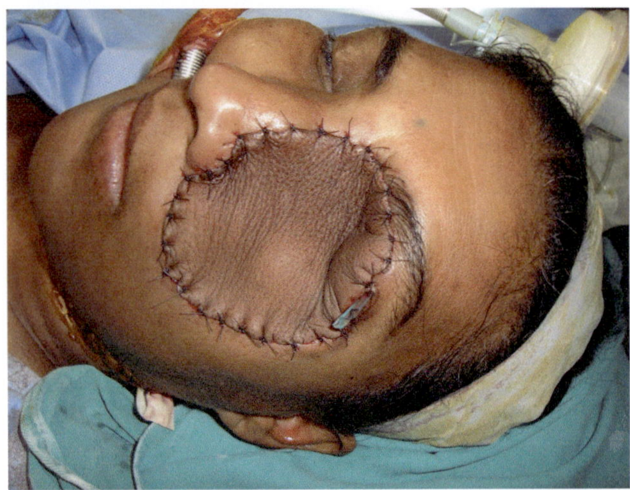

Fig. 11.56 Procedure is complete. The placement of eye prosthesis is reserved for the second stage and will require flap adjustment

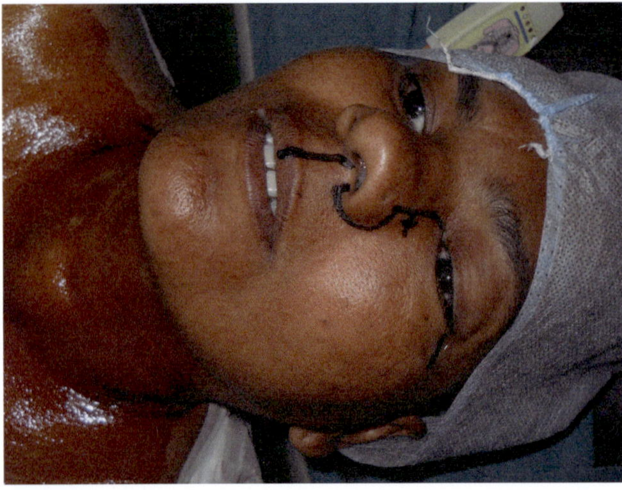

Fig. 11.57 Patient with Weber–Ferguson incision with trans-conjunctival extension

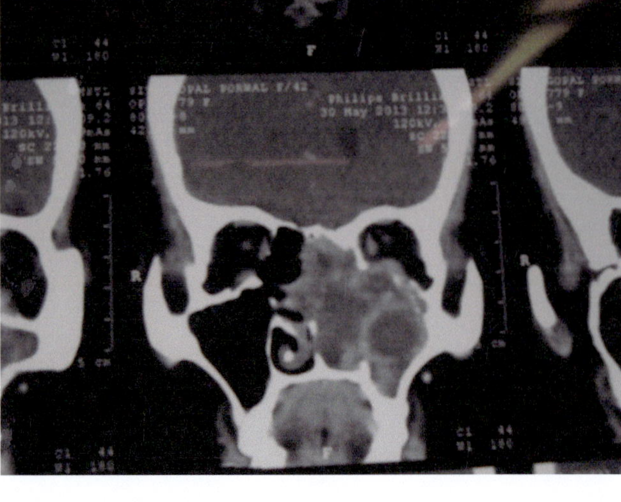

Fig. 11.58 The tumor involving the entire maxillary cavity, lateral nasal wall, and orbital floor. The hard palate seems free and can be preserved. The lesion does not involve the rectus muscle and orbital fat (MRI image), and hence exenteration is not required. It is advisable to leave the final decision on removal of eye for intraoperative period

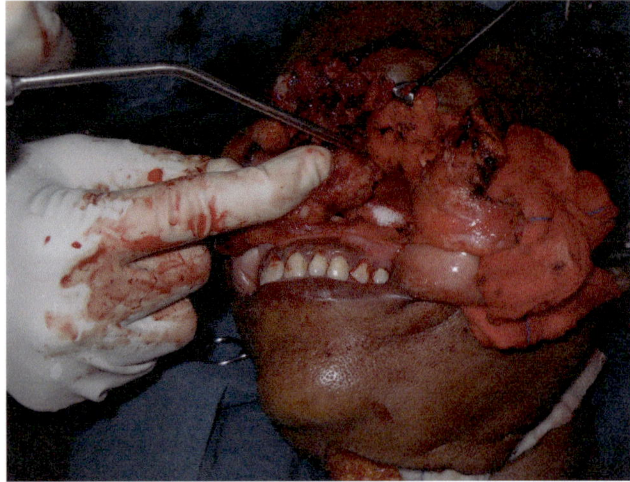

Fig. 11.59 The flap is raised. The anterior wall of the maxilla and orbital floor is removed to expose the maxillary cavity and lateral nasal wall which is filled with tumor. The tumor can be gently teased out from the cavity. The continuous bleeding can be controlled by packing as shown in the photograph

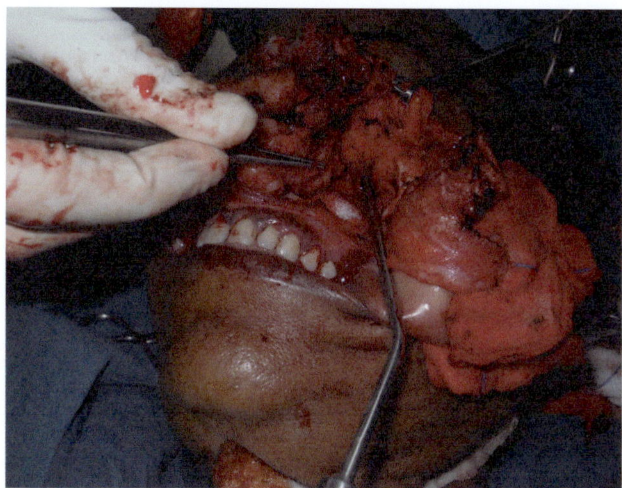

Fig. 11.60 One can see the tumor being separated from the eyeball. The periorbita was involved but the muscle and fats were free and there was a clear plane in between

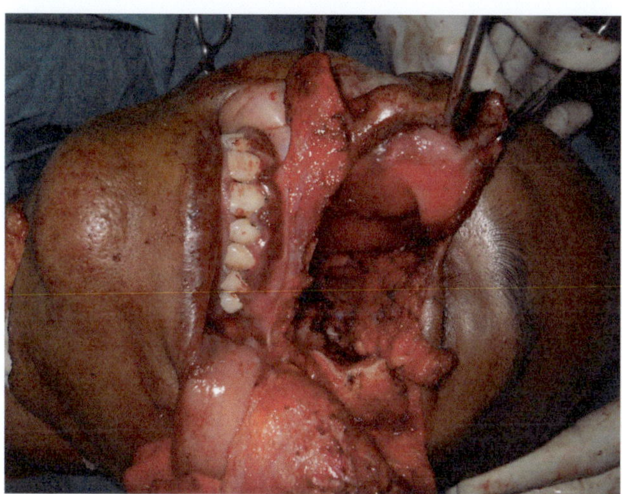

Fig. 11.61 Resection is complete with good clearance till the posterior wall of maxilla

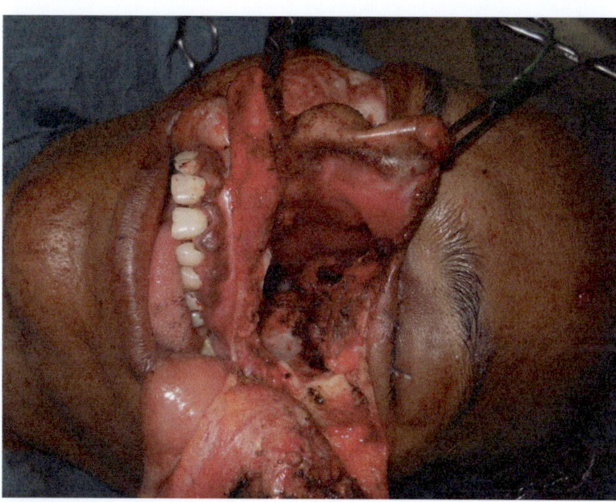

Fig. 11.62 Photograph showing the posterior wall of the maxilla and nasopharynx area

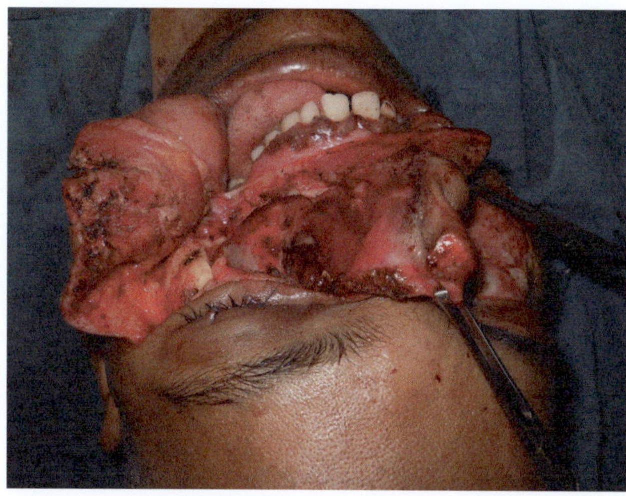

Fig. 11.63 Photograph showing floor of maxilla and nasal cavity completely cleared of tumor

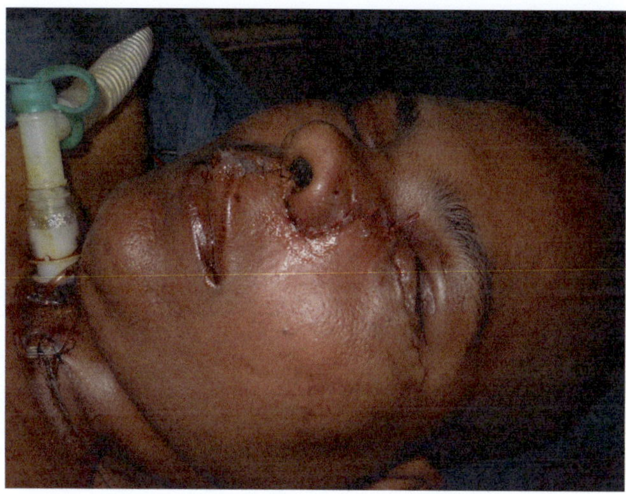

Fig. 11.64 Reconstruction of the orbital floor is done with fascia lata and titanium plate completely. The cavity is left open to heal on its own. The lateral part of the orbital floor is preserved, and only partial support for the eye is sufficient to prevent sinking of the orbit

Total Maxillectomy

This section demonstrates total maxillectomy procedure to remove more advanced lesions involving upper and lower wall of the maxilla.

The extended maxillectomy for PNS tumors involving adjoining structures is not described in this chapter. The operative procedure to clear anterior skull base tumors is described in skull base chapter. The transmandibular approach to address maxillary tumor with posterior spread and involving ITF is described in ITF chapter.

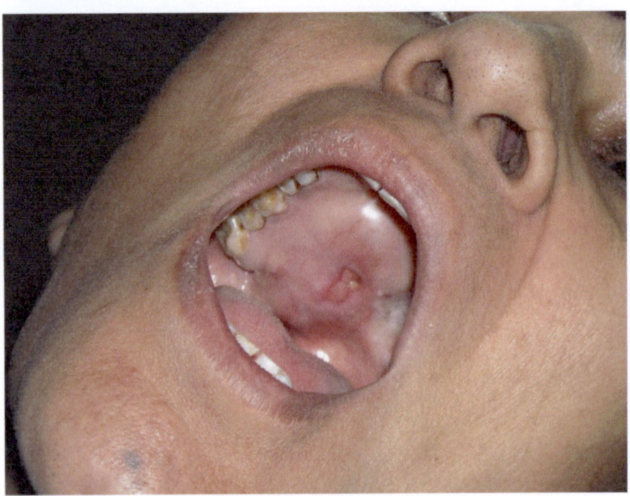

Fig. 11.65 Patient with advanced maxillary tumor

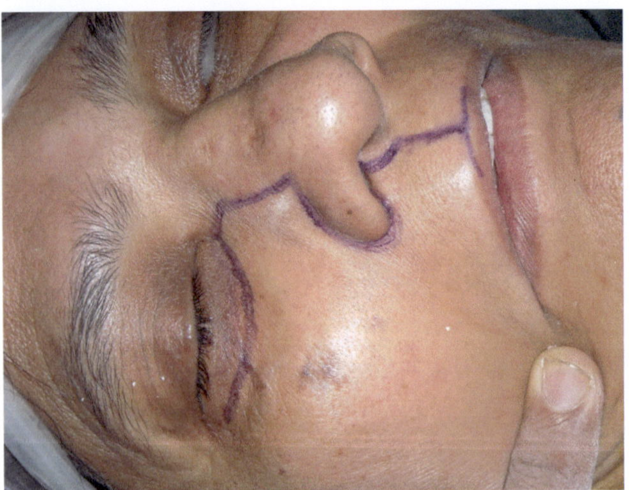

Fig. 11.66 Weber–Ferguson incision with sub-ciliary extension

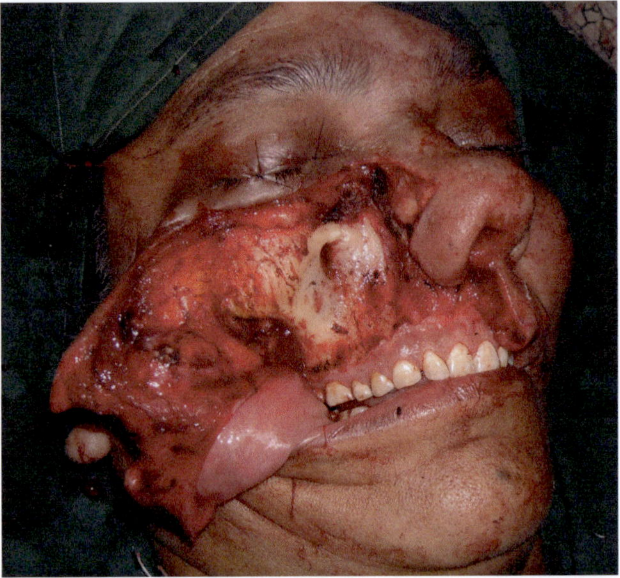

Fig. 11.67 The flap is raised. Infraorbital muscles need to be carefully divided

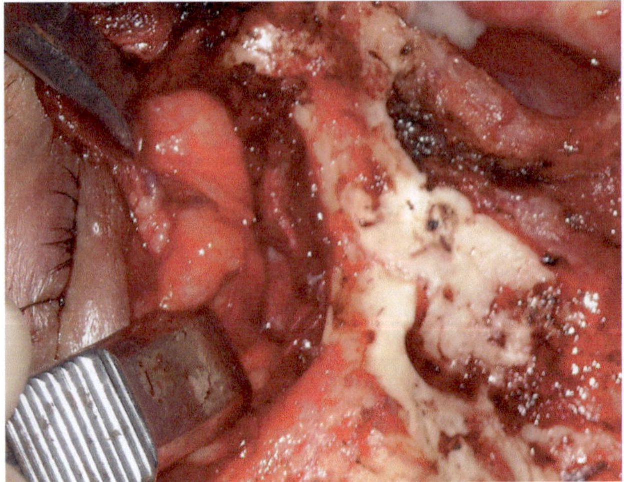

Fig. 11.68 Photograph showing the relation of the periorbita and orbital fat. The lesion is limited to the bone of orbital floor and periorbita and eye can be safely preserved

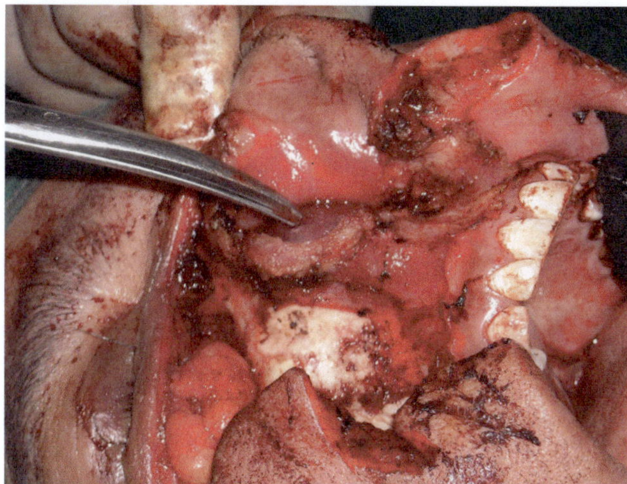

Fig. 11.69 The tumor involving lateral nasal wall

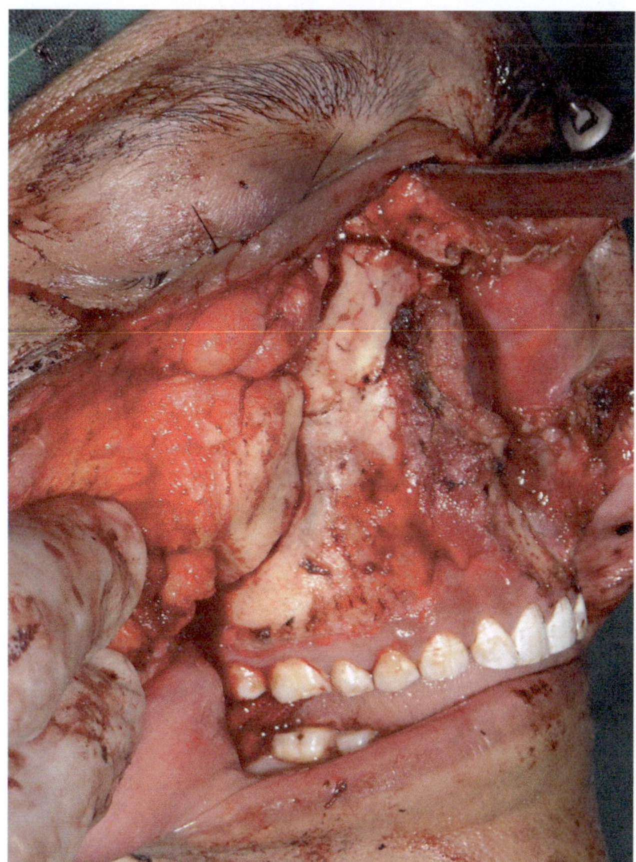

Fig. 11.70 Photograph shows bone cuts of maxilla. The nasal cut is placed first. The lateral cut is placed preserving the zygomatic buttress in this case. This improves the cosmetic outcome and helps in supporting the eyeball. If the tumor involves the lateral aspect of the maxilla, zygomatic buttress needs to be sacrificed

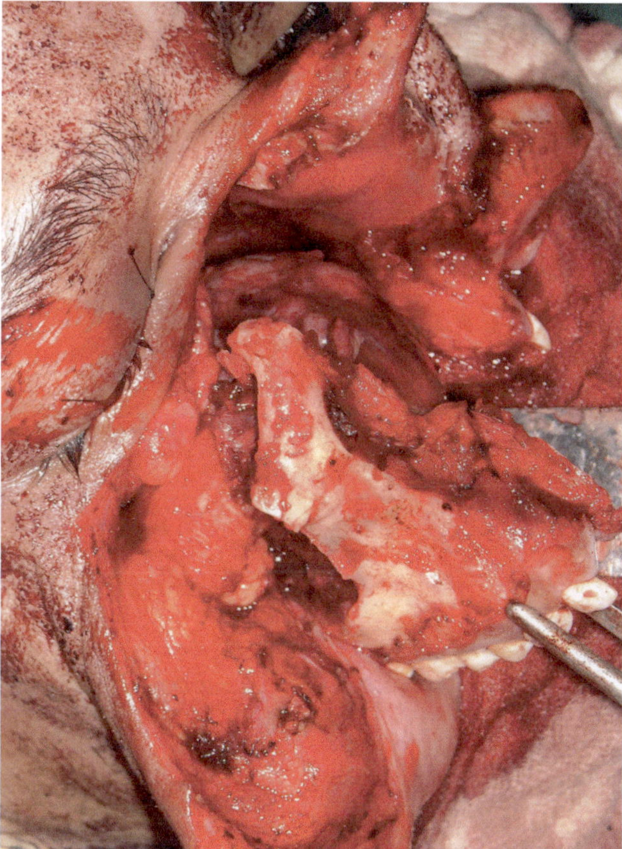

Fig. 11.71 Fractured maxilla is pulled down once palatal cuts are made. Constant gentle pressure in downward direction will help in this and posterior wall of maxilla is exposed. The pterygomaxillary disjunction is done to complete the procedure

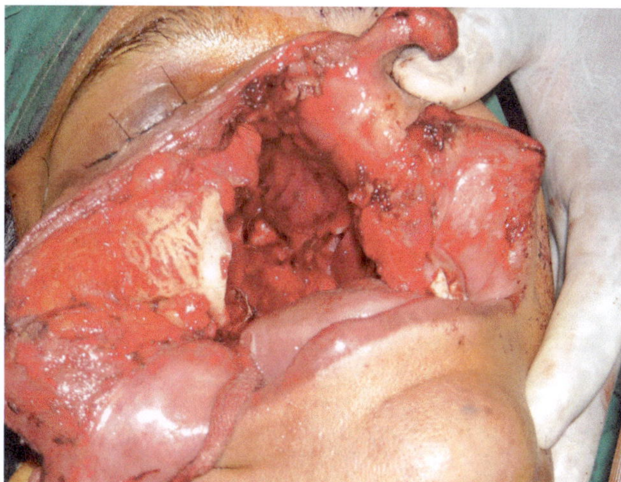

Fig. 11.72 Photograph showing completed procedure with good hemostasis. The bleeding stops automatically in the majority of cases with good pressure packing for some time

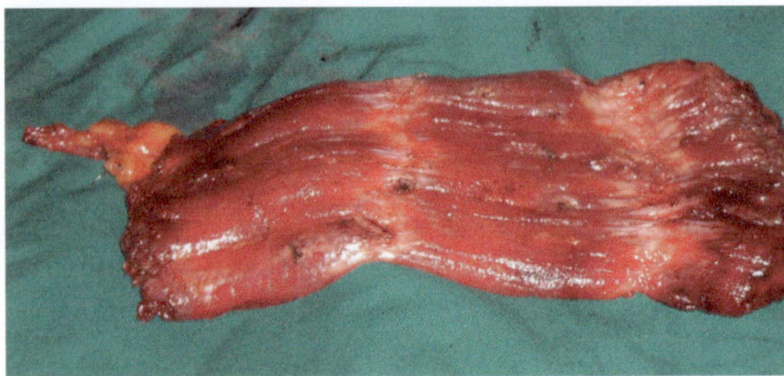

Fig. 11.73 The rectus muscle is harvested with vascular pedicle

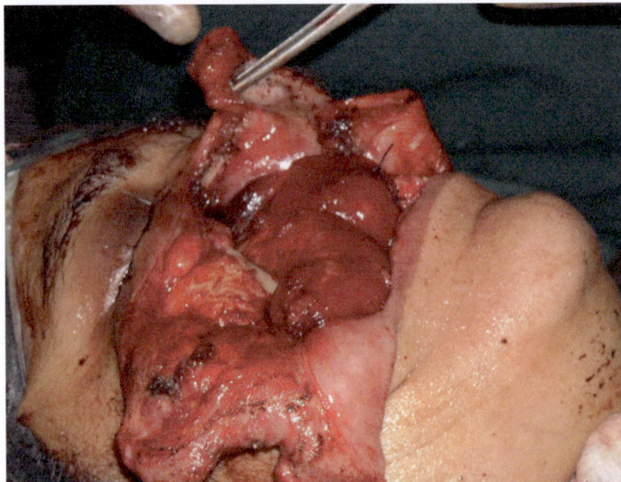

Fig. 11.74 The muscle is placed in the cavity. The orbital floor is reconstructed using fascia lata

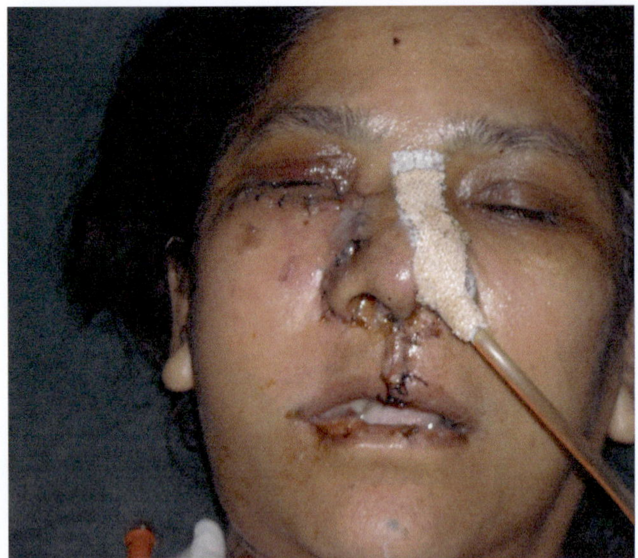

Fig. 11.75 Photograph showing completed procedure

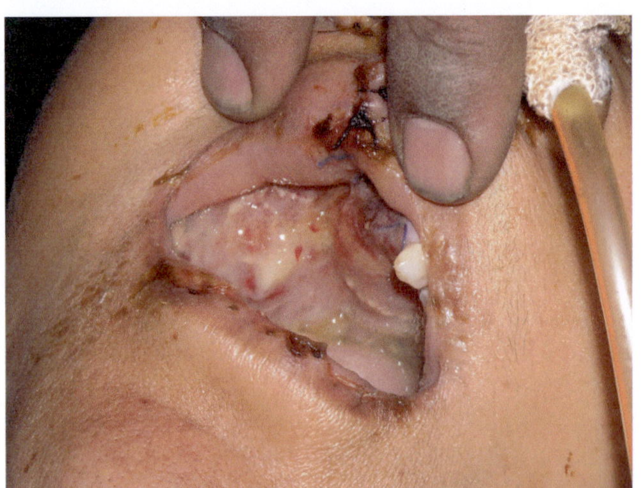

Fig. 11.76 The muscle is viable on the 3rd postoperative day

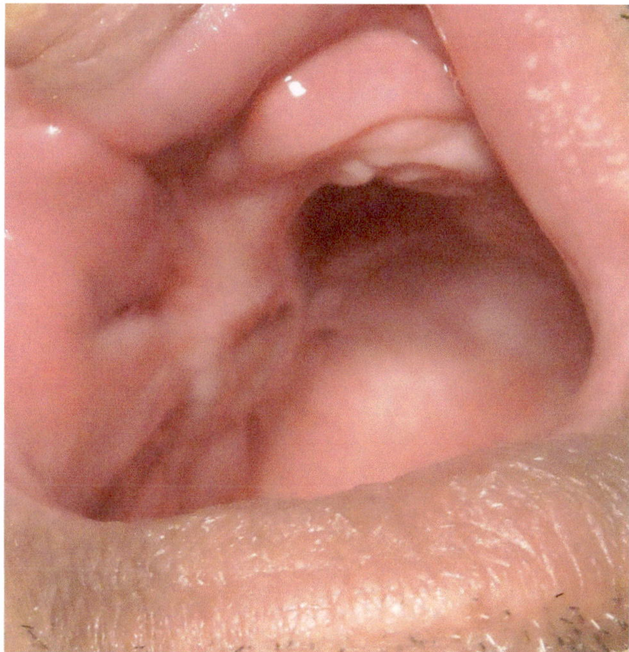

Fig. 11.77 Postoperative picture showing completely healed wounds. The mucosa cover is almost normal, and patient can have normal life with this reconstruction

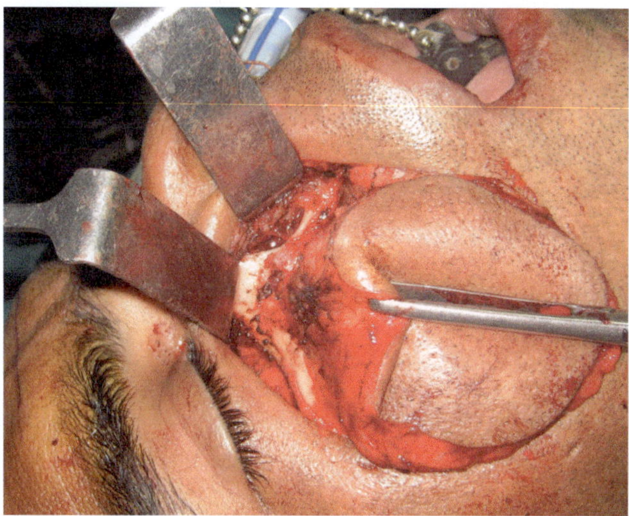

Fig. 11.78 Photograph showing exposed nasal bone and orbital floor for another lesion of the maxilla

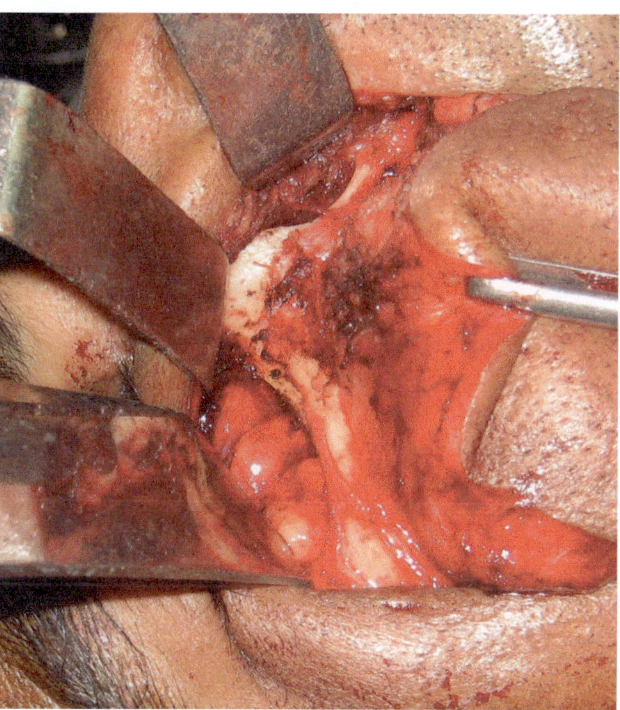

Fig. 11.79 The eyeball is free and can be separated from the floor

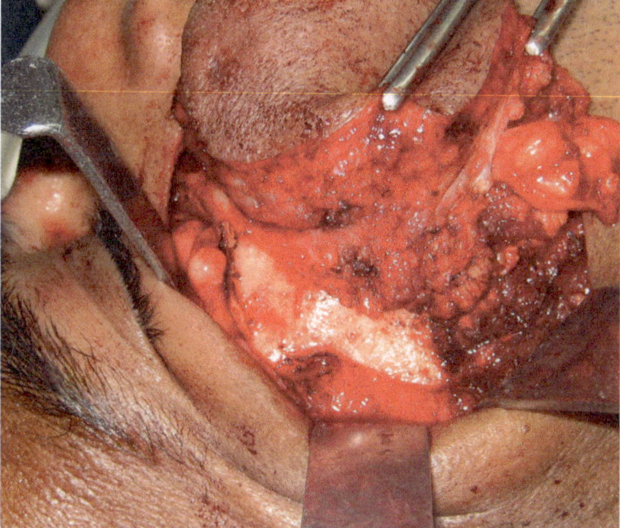

Fig. 11.80 The exposed zygomatic and frontal bone for planned cuts. This is done when the tumor involves entire orbital floor and lateral wall. These cuts can ensure complete clearance in this area

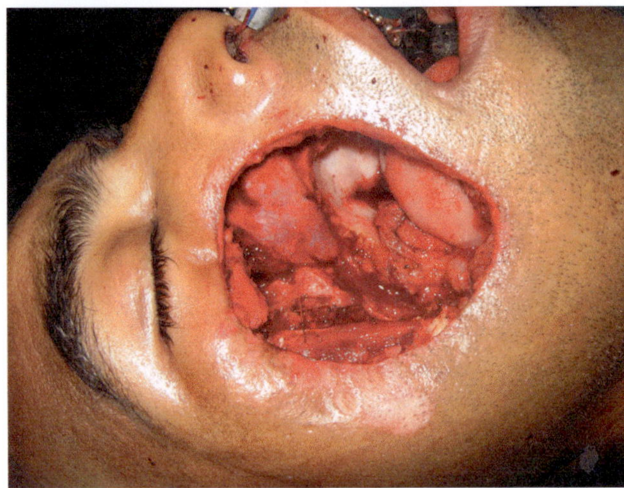

Fig. 11.81 The procedure is complete and reconstruction was achieved by rectus free flap

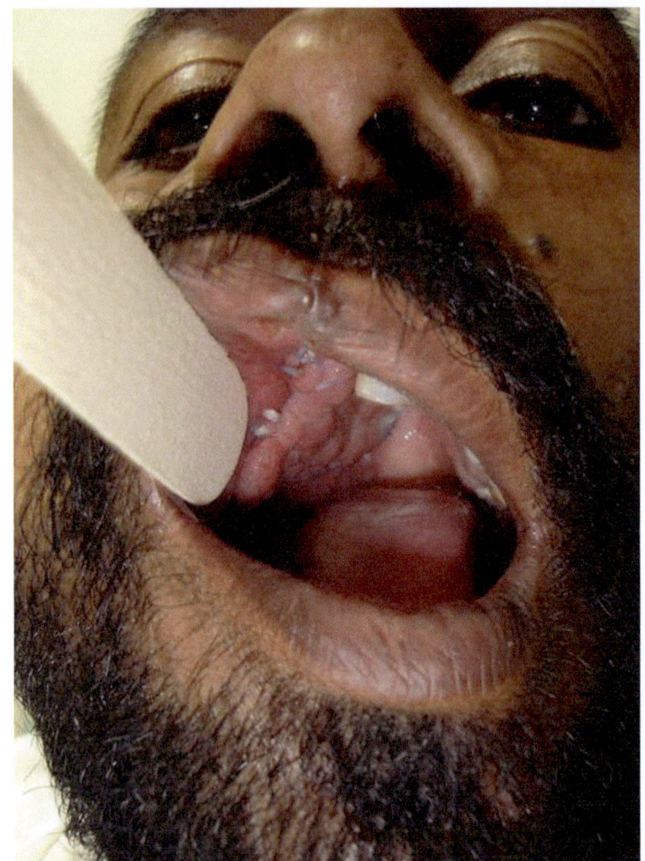

Fig. 11.82 The completed procedure showing final outcome

Orbital Exenteration

This section shows orbital exenteration procedure for very advanced cancers of the eye.

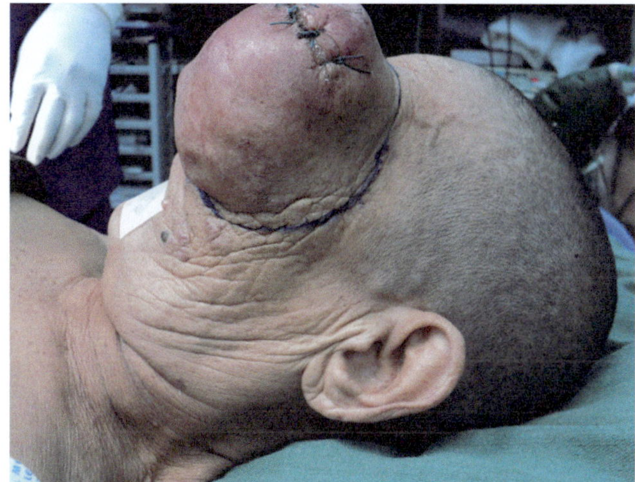

Fig. 11.83 Very advanced vascular tumor involving the eye. It is important to go around this tumor to minimize bleeding. Hypotensive anesthesia can help a great deal. The procedure needs to be completed as fast as possible. The entire content is mobilized from orbital cavity after removing the orbital floor. This can provide space to reach to orbital apex and apply clamp

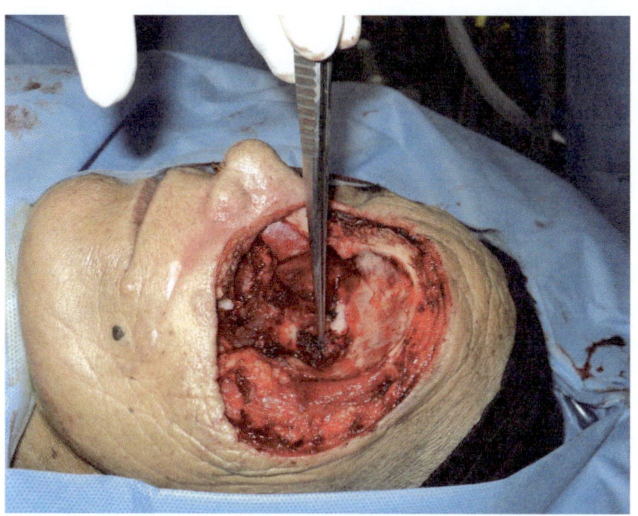

Fig. 11.84 The procedure is complete showing ligated orbital apex. In very rare cases, ligature of ophthalmic artery gets slipped off into the intracranial compartment and this can lead to troublesome bleeding. One can use the help of interventional radiologist to arrest bleeding with embolization. If this is not feasible and bleeding persists, one may have to perform craniotomy to achieve hemostasis

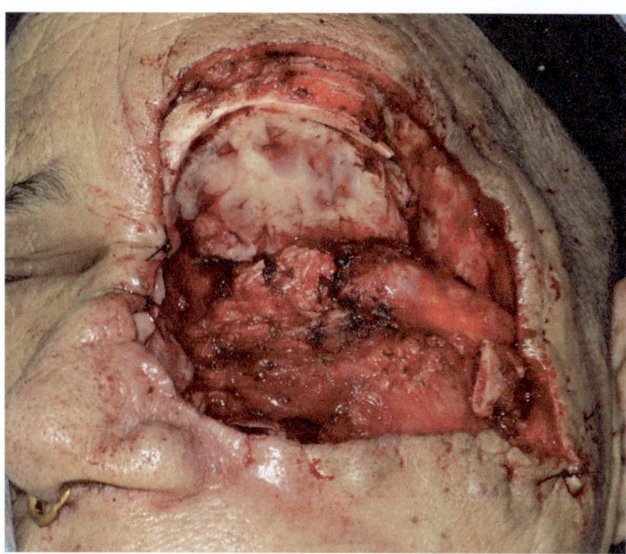

Fig. 11.85 Reconstruction was achieved with temporalis flap to fill the maxillary antrum

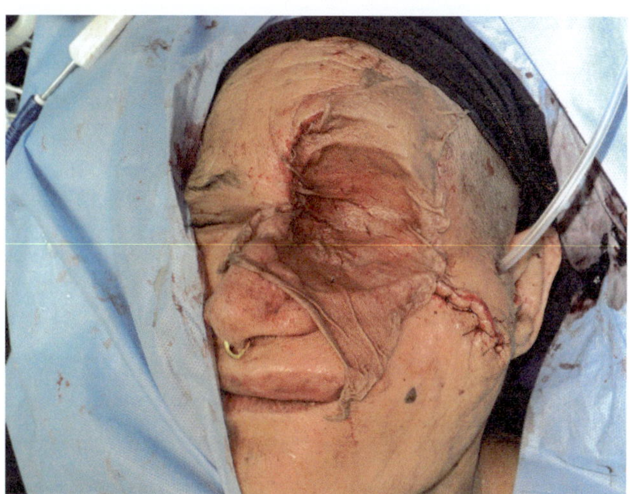

Fig. 11.86 The cavity was covered with split-thickness skin graft

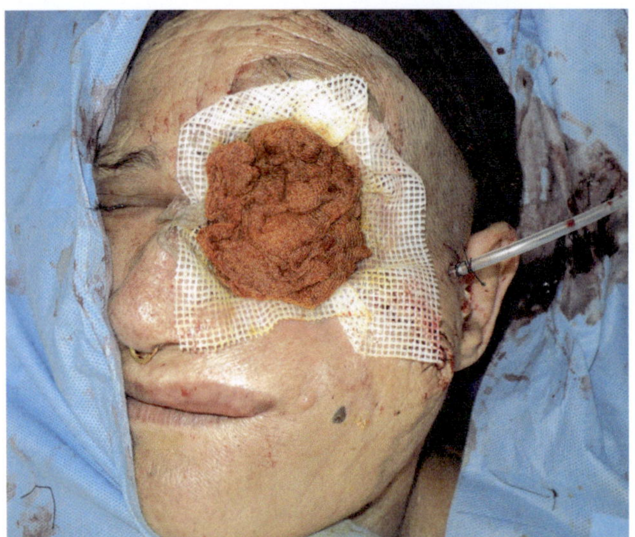

Fig. 11.87 Photograph showing dressing of the orbital cavity

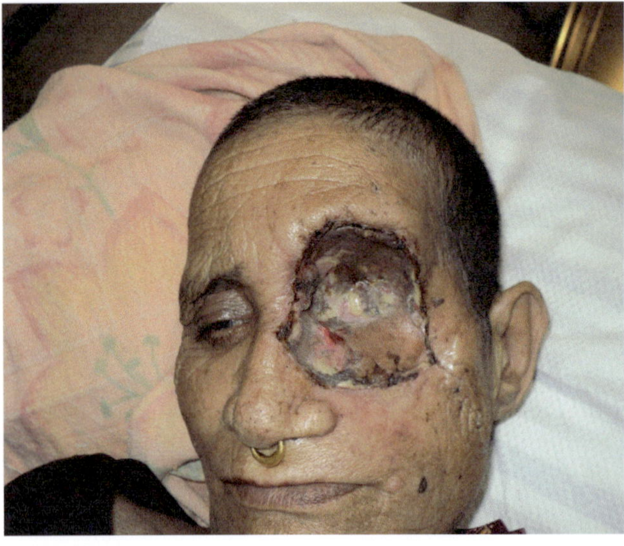

Fig. 11.88 Postoperative photograph after 1 week

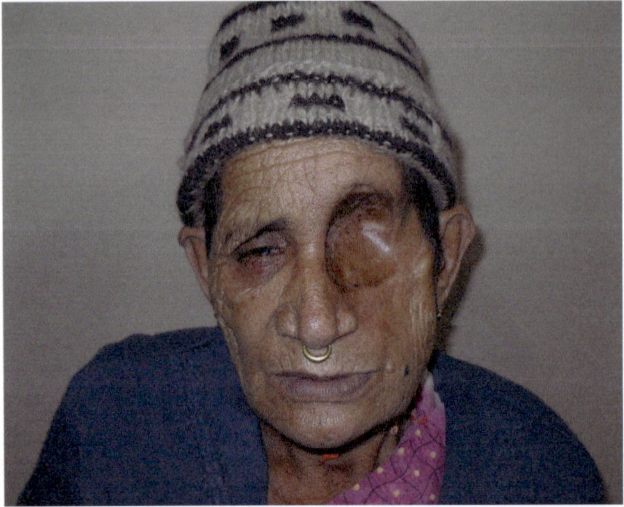

Fig. 11.89 Long-term outcome

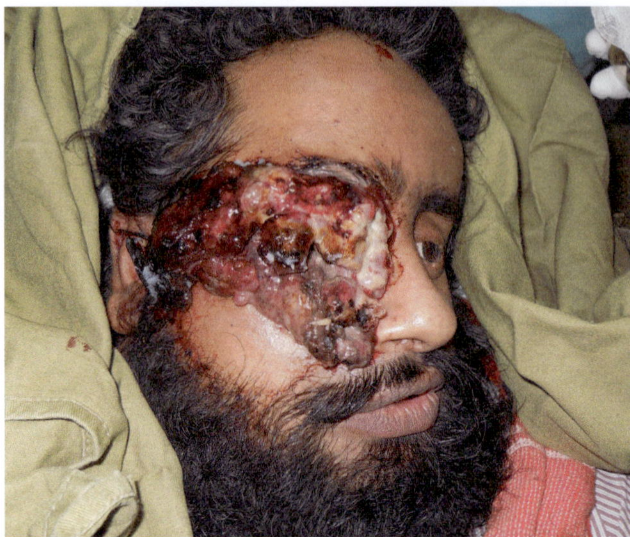

Fig. 11.90 Patient with fungating mass involving the eye

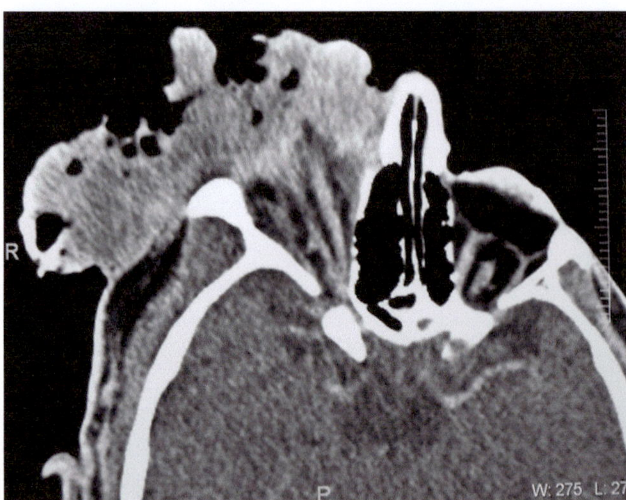

Fig. 11.91 Imaging study showing lesion involving only the eyeball and the apex is free

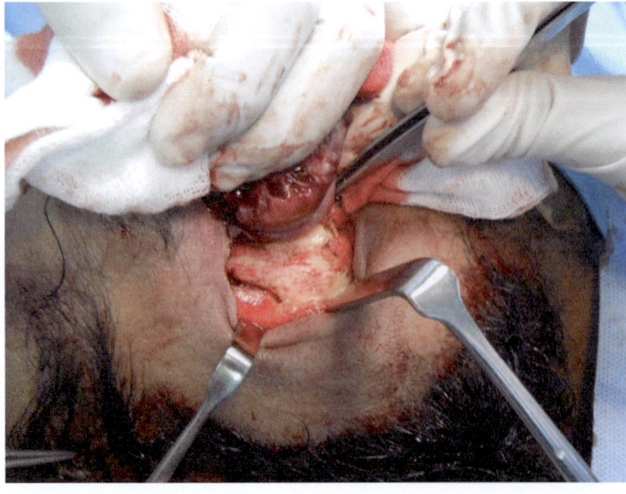

Fig. 11.92 Surrounding bone is exposed to place the necessary bone cuts

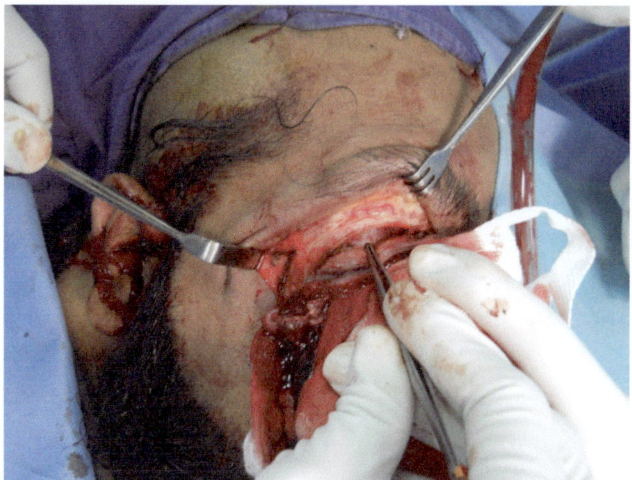

Fig. 11.93 Tumor has been freed from superior aspect

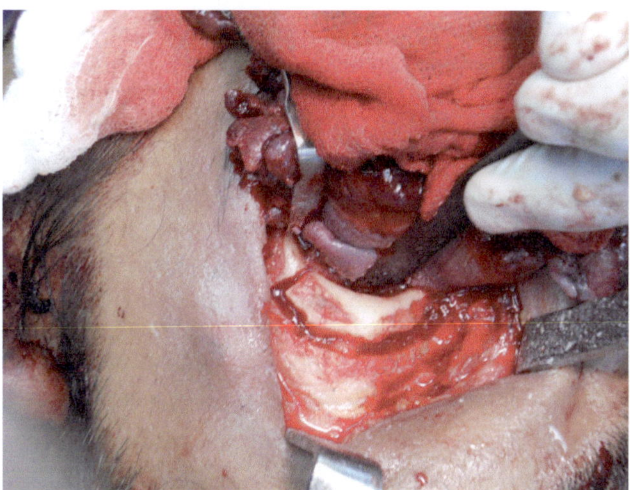

Fig. 11.94 The orbital floor is removed to have access to the apex

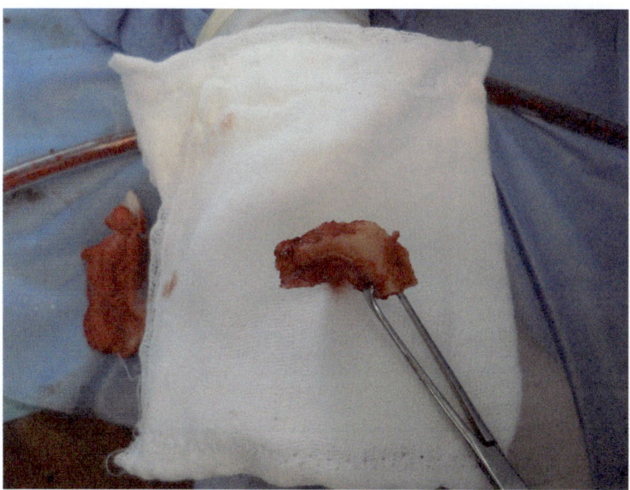

Fig. 11.95 Removed bone of orbital floor. This can be put back at the end of the procedure. This is an important step in dealing with large lesions of the eye where reaching orbital apex is difficult

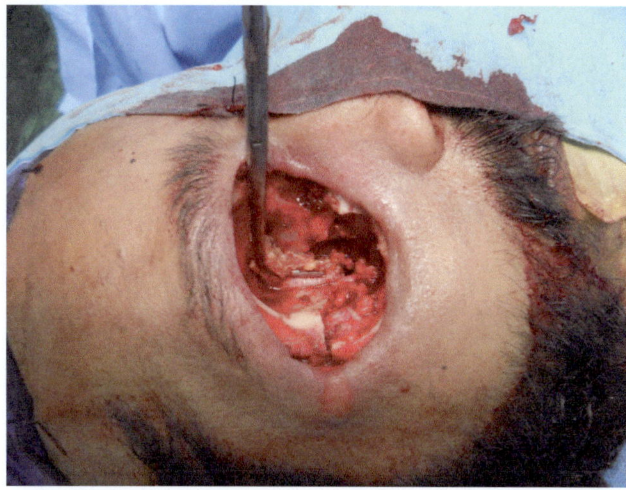

Fig. 11.96 The photograph showing clamp in position. One can see the space available in this step

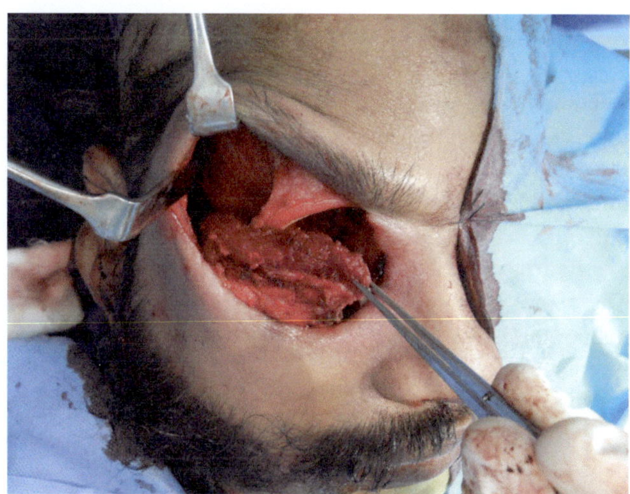

Fig. 11.97 Reconstruction is achieved by temporalis flap

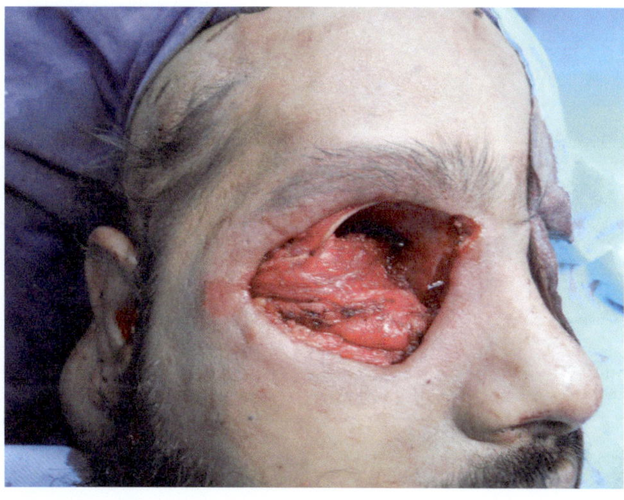

Fig. 11.98 Muscle is used to fill the maxillary and orbital cavity

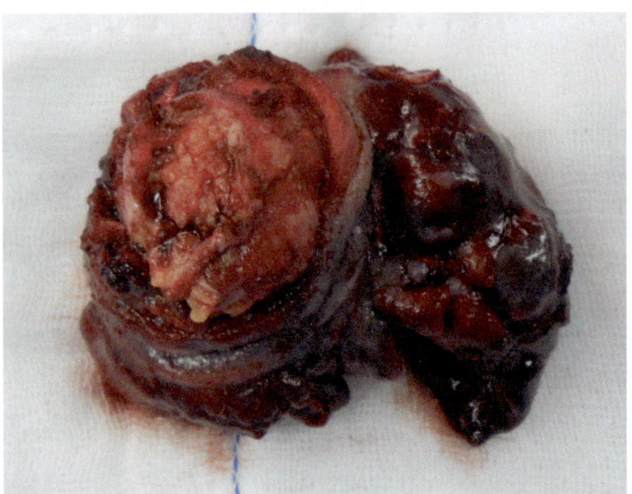

Fig. 11.99 The specimen

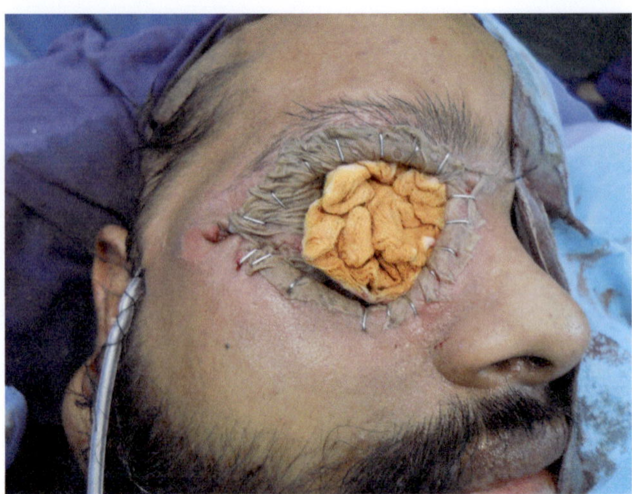

Fig. 11.100 The STG with dressing

Reconstruction

Reconstruction of maxillectomy defect is very challenging. These defects were left without any reconstruction for many years. This trend has changed with the advent of microvascular free flap for reconstruction. The surgical outcome has improved in recent years, and this has resulted in patients demanding for better quality of life. The complex anatomy and association with vital function make the reconstruction of maxillary defects very interesting.

The reconstruction algorithm can be based on two aspects – functional and cosmetic. The cosmetic outcome depends upon the preservation of zygomatic buttress and pre-maxilla. The functional outcome is related to two important components – the palate and alveolus component and the orbital floor component. One must consider these aspects while choosing reconstructive options. The general condition of patients and their comorbidity status also play a major role in selecting various options. Figure 11.3 demonstrates reconstructive options for various defects. The functional outcome is given an utmost importance in deciding which option to use. The palatal obturator can be provided by an obturator in dentate patient or by a soft tissue flap. The bone flap is used for pre-maxilla reconstruction or in a patient who wants dental implants. The orbital floor support can be provided with titanium mesh or vascularized bone flap (preferred in setting of adjuvant radiotherapy). There are many options for reconstruction of total maxillectomy defect ranging from soft tissue flaps to vascularized bone flaps. The soft tissue flaps can be used to reconstruct lower half of the defect, and orbital floor support can be achieved by titanium mesh or coronoid process with temporalis muscle. These defects can also be reconstructed with scapula, iliac crest, or fibula free flaps depending upon the needs of the patient and expertise of the surgeon.

12 Skull Base Tumors

Surgical Anatomy

The treatment of cranial base tumors is very challenging due to the complex anatomy of the region and its relation to important structures like the brain, eye, and cranial nerves. The space is limited at skull base and proper understanding of anatomy and extent of disease spread forms basis for skull base surgery. It is important to achieve three-dimensional clear margins even for skull base tumors, and a variety of surgical approaches have been described to achieve that. It is advisable to combine trans-facial approach with transcranial approach to have adequate exposure for three-dimensional clearance tumor.

Figure 12.1 shows schematic anatomy of the anterior skull base. The skull base bone forms dividing line between the cranial and facial sections. The dura and brain form a cranial component while nose and PNS with the eye forms the facial component. The cranial nerves and vessels passing through various foramina provide channels for communication between the two compartments, and the tumor can pass through any of these channels to adjacent area.

The cranial base area can be divided into five sections for ease of discussion:

1. Anterior cranial base
2. Anterolateral cranial base
3. Lateral cranial base
4. Central cranial base
5. Posterior cranial base

The central and posterior cranial base tumors are mainly addressed by neurosurgeons and are beyond the scope of this book. The remaining areas are discussed in this chapter in detail.

N. Trivedi, *Atlas of Head and Neck Cancer Surgery: The Compartment Surgery for Resection in 3-D*,
DOI 10.1007/978-81-322-2050-3_12, © Springer India 2015

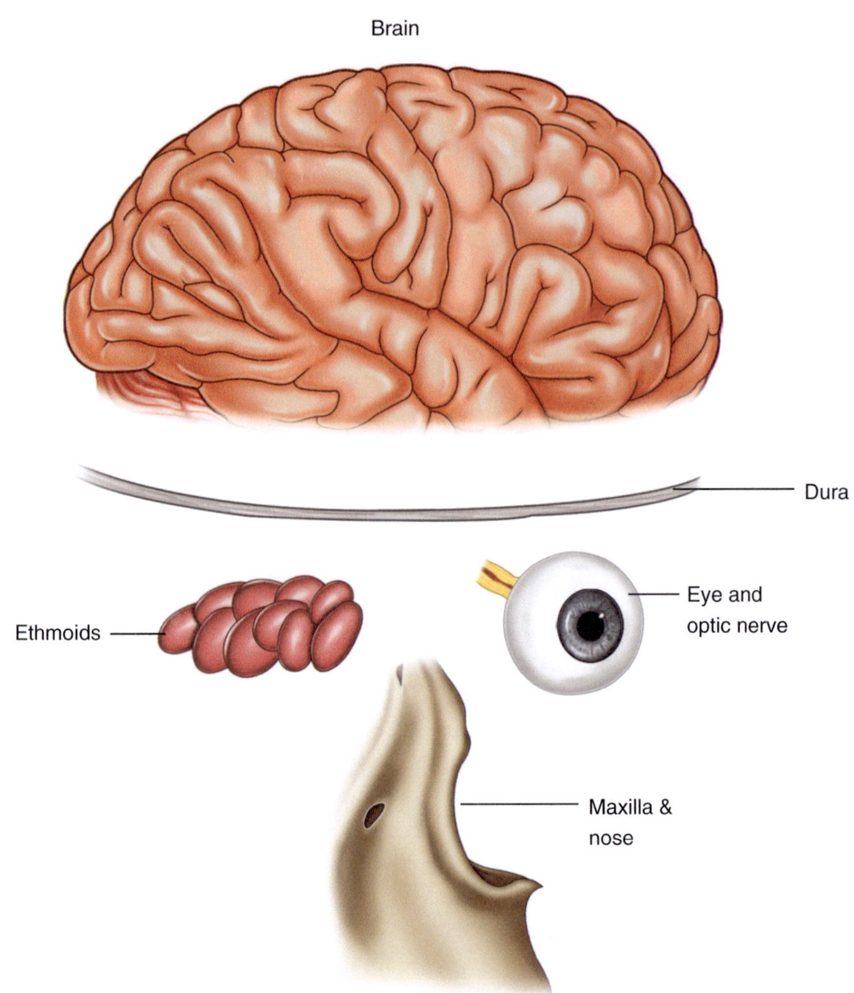

Fig. 12.1 Schematic diagram of skull base anatomy

Surgical Pathology

The tumors at the skull base mostly arise from adjacent structures and wide variety of lesions can be encountered in this region. This can range from benign tumors to aggressive malignant lesions, and establishing tissue diagnosis is essential to plan appropriate treatment. The IHC studies are often helpful to establish the final diagnosis. Imaging studies help in identifying the structure of origin and its relation to the surrounding areas, and this can add in achieving the final diagnosis.

Figure 12.2 is a schematic representation of various skull base areas and its relation to areas from where the tumor spread. Anterior cranial base is the most frequently involved skull base area, and tumors arising from the nose and paranasal sinuses are the main culprits. The lesions arising from nose and maxilla traverse the ethmoid sinus and involve cribriform plate and dura. The olfactory neuroblastoma, minor salivary gland neoplasms, and various other neoplasms are also not uncommon in this area. The anterolateral cranial base is associated with masticator space and ITF. The tumor can spread to middle cranial fossa from ITF and requires combined approaches to achieve complete clearance. The tumors arising from the oral cavity and posterior maxilla are more inclined to spread in this area. The lateral cranial base is associated with tumors arising from the ear and temporal bone. These tumors are addressed by lateral temporal bone approaches. The author doesn't have enough experience to treat these tumors. It is a specialized area and is ideal to refer a book on temporal bone resection.

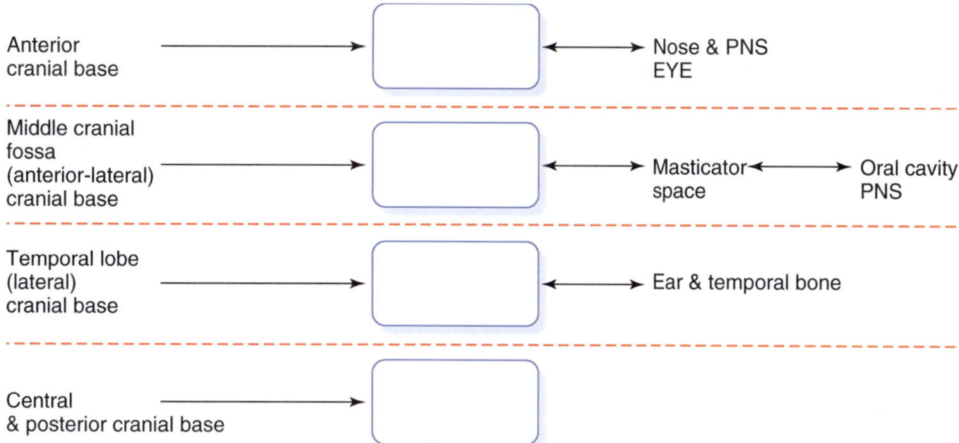

Fig. 12.2 Relations of cranial base to surrounding structures and pattern of spread

Surgical Concepts

- Figure 12.3 demonstrates the concept of combined craniofacial resection (CFR). The skull base area has limited space and is associated with vital structures. The combination of transcranial approach with trans-facial approach allows better exposure to tumor from above. This helps in identifying and preserving important structures while removing the tumor in en bloc fashion.
- Involvement of the brain and carotid artery by a tumour is generally considered sign of inoperability. The lesion can be resected if it involves a limited portion of the brain. The long-term outcome is equivocal for such group of patients.
- Involvement of the dura and skull base bone in certain areas is considered operable provided it is possible to achieve negative margins. There is hardly any role of incomplete removal of tumor or debridement in skull base surgery.
- It is difficult to achieve 1 cm disease-free margin at the skull base. The decision to sacrifice or preserve a vital structure for disease clearance is difficult in many cases. It is acceptable to preserve the structure when there is a clear tissue plane between the disease and the structure.
- Minimal invasive approaches (endoscopic skull base approach) have become popular in recent times. In order to be a good endoscopic skull base surgeon. One needs to have adequate experience in open as well as endoscopic surgery for skull base tumors. First attempt is the best attempt and no compromise on oncological clearance should be done to improve cosmetic outcome.
- Reconstructive strategy is essential for each skull base surgery, and appropriate repair of the dural defect influences the postoperative morbidity and mortality.
- These procedures are best performed in an institution with a backup team to manage unexpected complications.

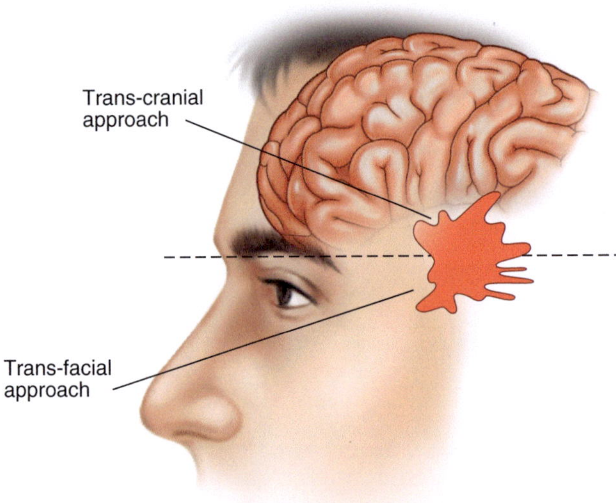

Fig. 12.3 Concept for combined CFR

Surgical Approaches

The craniofacial resection is performed by combination of trans-facial and transcranial approaches to remove skull base tumor. These approaches are used based on areas of the skull base involved by the tumor.

1. Anterior skull base:
   - Trans-facial approach – lateral rhinotomy, midfacial degloving, Weber–Ferguson, and endoscopic approach
   - Transcranial approach – bi-coronal flap with frontal craniotomy, subcranial approach (Rave's approach)
2. Anterolateral skull base:
   - Trans-facial approach – transmandibular approach, facial translocation approach, pre-auricular trans-zygomatic approach, post-auricular temporal approach
   - Transcranial approach – frontotemporal craniotomy
3. Lateral skull base:
   - Lateral temporal bone resection, subtotal temporal bone resection, and total temporal bone resection

Anterior Craniofacial Resection

This procedure is required for nose and PNS tumors involving the anterior skull base (cribriform plate, dura). The transcranial part can be performed either by conventional frontal craniotomy approach or by subcranial approach. The conventional approach is preferred for large tumors that involve the dura and brain. This approach requires brain retraction and may cause edema in postoperative period. The subcranial approach is preferred for limited lesions that extend up to the dura. It is preferred to have a large frontal sinus to perform this limited approach. It requires minimal brain retraction resulting in less postoperative morbidity. Tumor removal is rarely a problem with subcranial approach, but dura repair is challenging particularly for tumors with large posterior spread reaching up to the sphenoid sinus.

This section demonstrates two operative procedures describing technical details for conventional and subcranial approaches.

Conventional Anterior CFR

The patient has nasal mass with anterior skull base extension infiltrating dura.

These patients can ambulate in 4–5 days and can be discharged in 1 week time if no complications are observed. They are advised to clean the nose frequently to avoid post-operative crusting. Majority of patients with malignant neoplasms require adjuvant treatment.

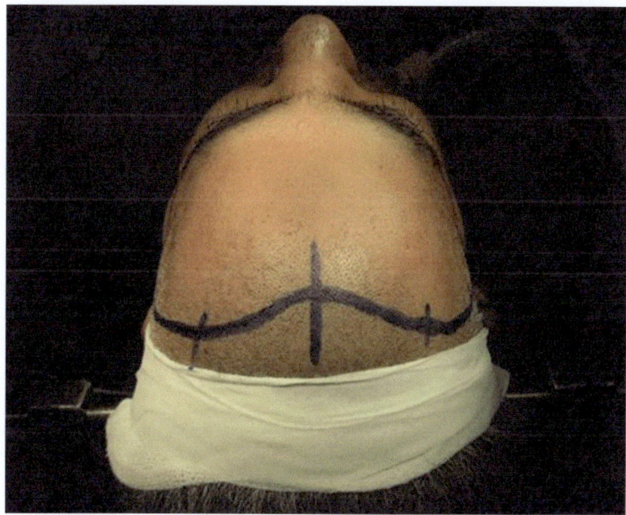

Fig. 12.4 Bi-coronal incision for raising the flap

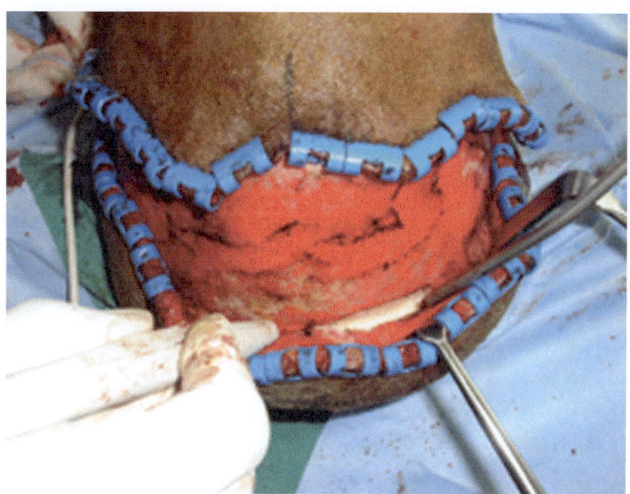

Fig. 12.5 The posterior flap is raised beyond and posteriorly to get added length for pericranial flap that can help in sealing the dural defect

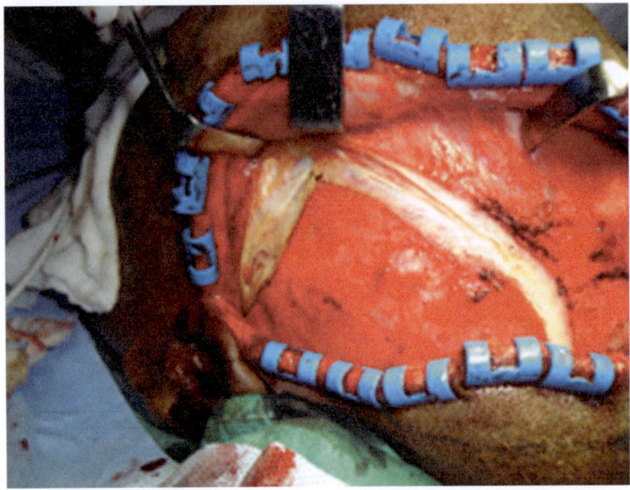

Fig. 12.6 On the lateral aspect, care is taken to avoid injury to frontal branch of facial nerve. The incision is placed on temporalis fascia and further dissection is carried out in a deeper plane

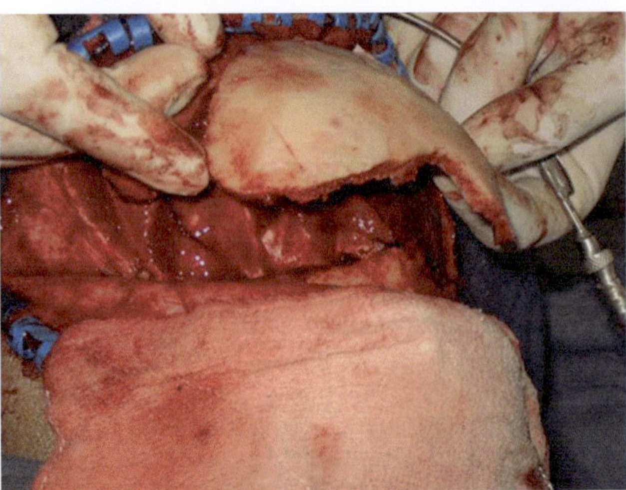

Fig. 12.8 The frontal craniotomy is performed

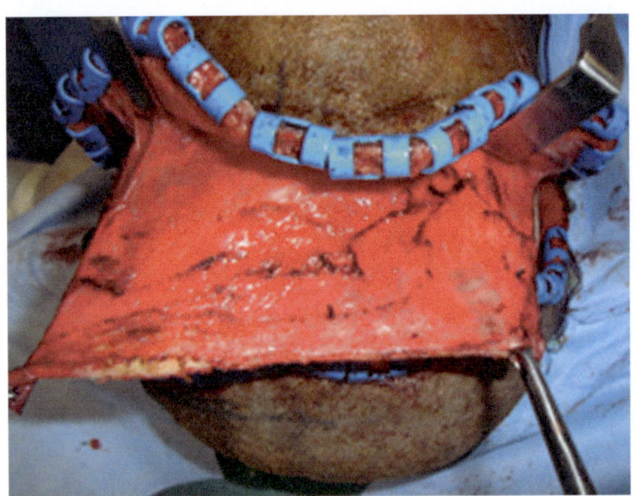

Fig. 12.7 The peri-cranial flap is raised and isolated from the skin flap. It is important to avoid button holes while raising this flap. The vascularized flap can be used for patching the dural defect

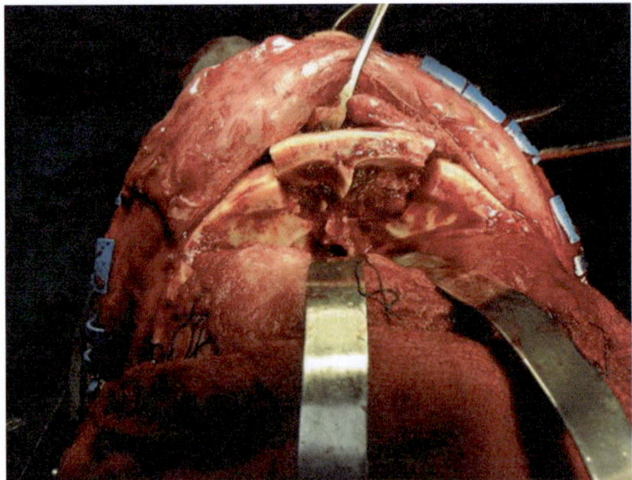

Fig. 12.9 The brain is retracted to expose anterior skull base. The dura is separated gradually from skull base bone and olfactory tracks are clamped and cut to isolate cranial cavity from the tumor. If the tumor is involving the dura, the dura is resected with adequate margins

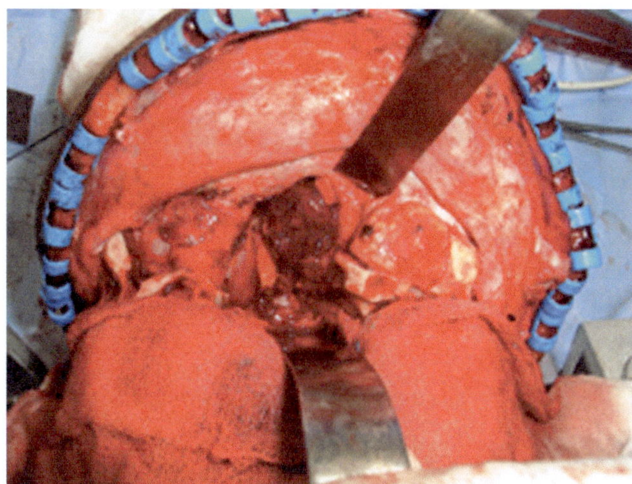

Fig. 12.10 The tumor is separated from all around. The skull base bone is cut from one side of orbital wall to another side of orbital wall and from the frontal sinus to anterior wall of the sphenoid sinus. This manoeveur pushes the tumor and skull base down and exposes the frontal and sphenoid sinuses

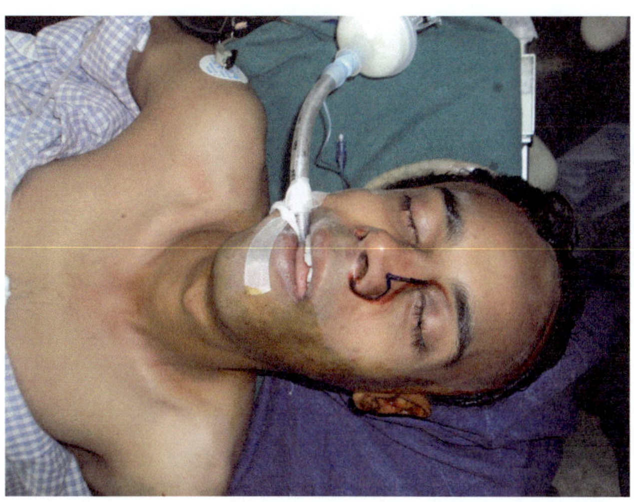

Fig. 12.11 The lateral rhinotomy approach is planned for this case

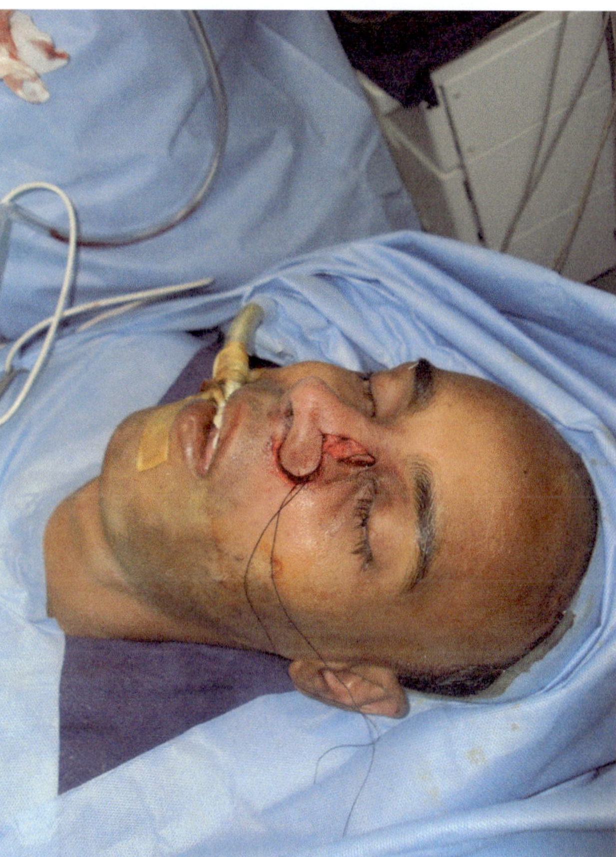

Fig. 12.12 The flaps are being raised

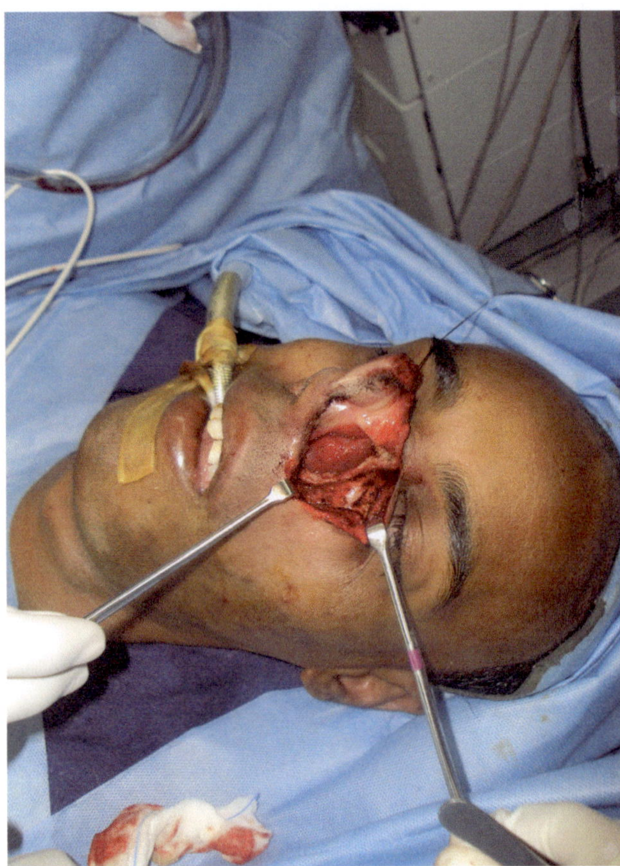

Fig. 12.13 Medial wall of the maxilla with lateral nasal wall is exposed

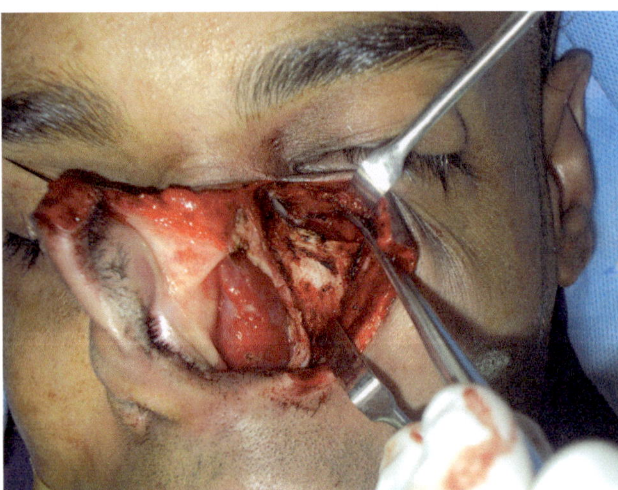

Fig. 12.14 The maxilla is exposed to perform medial maxillotomy that exposes lateral nasal wall with tumor

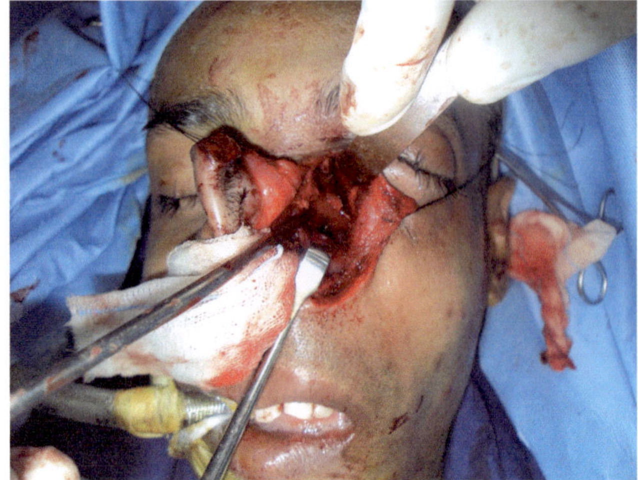

Fig. 12.15 Medial maxillotomy is performed and tumor is mobilized from below

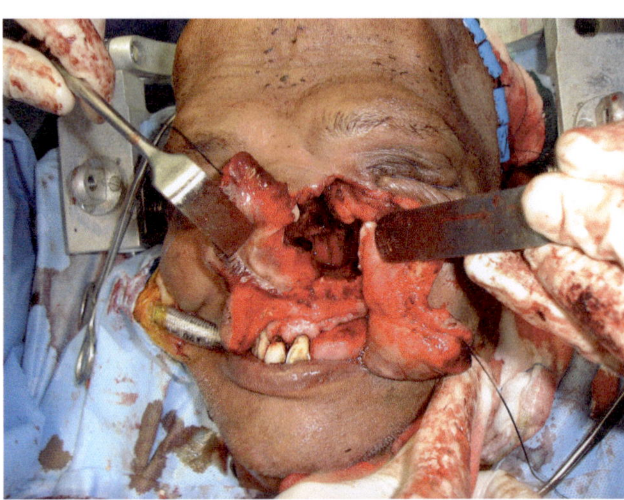

Fig. 12.16 One has to identify and secure anterior and posterior ethmoid vessels. The septum is sacrificed in posterior part in almost every case to gain exposure to the skull base. The entire ethmoid sinus is included in the specimen from one eyewall to another. The specimen is delivered from the nose

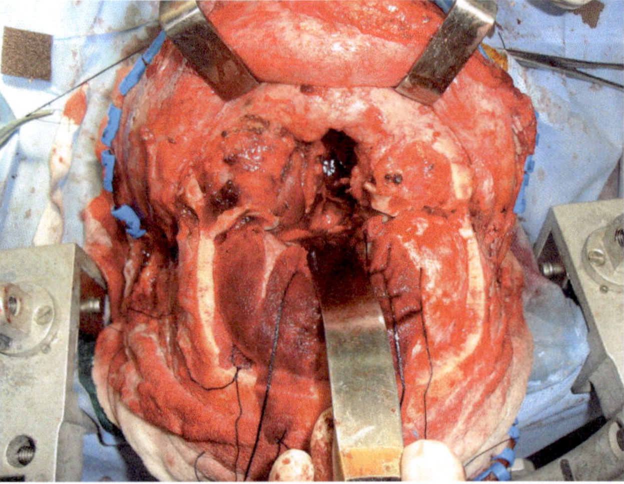

Fig. 12.17 The tumor is completely removed. One can see the exposed eyeballs on either side with complete clearence of anterior skull base

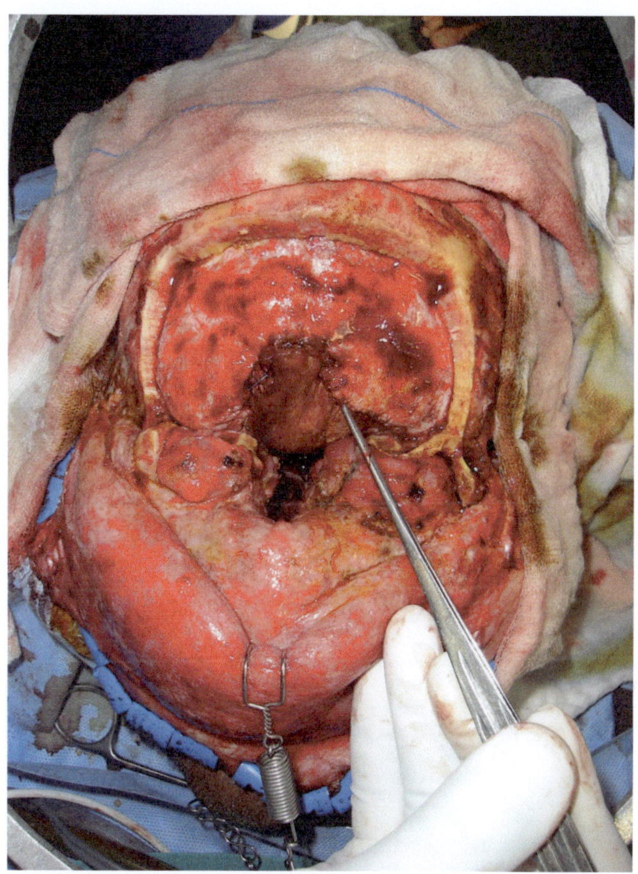

Fig. 12.18 The dural defect is patched with temporalis fascia. One can alternatively use fascia lata or pericranial flap for the same. It is ideal to perform multilayer dural closure and use fat to fill in between layers

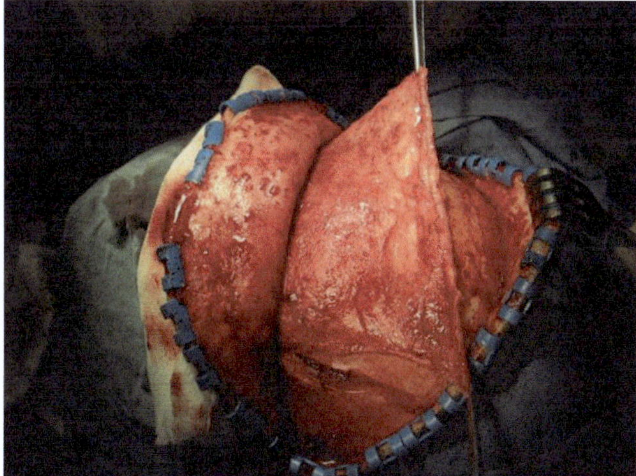

Fig. 12.19 The vascularized pericranial flap is used as a second layer to provide additional support to dural seal

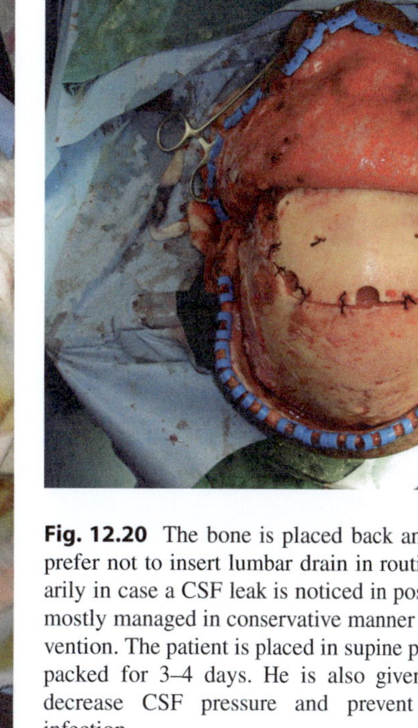

Fig. 12.20 The bone is placed back and the wounds are closed. We prefer not to insert lumbar drain in routine cases. It is placed secondarily in case a CSF leak is noticed in postoperative period. The leak is mostly managed in conservative manner and very rarely requires intervention. The patient is placed in supine position, and the nasal cavity is packed for 3–4 days. He is also given antibiotics and diuretics to decrease CSF pressure and prevent life threateing intracranial infection

Subcranial Approach

The patient has a nasal mass with limited skull base involvement. The frontal sinus is large and posterior extension of tumor is limited in this case. This is an appropriate case for subcranial approach.

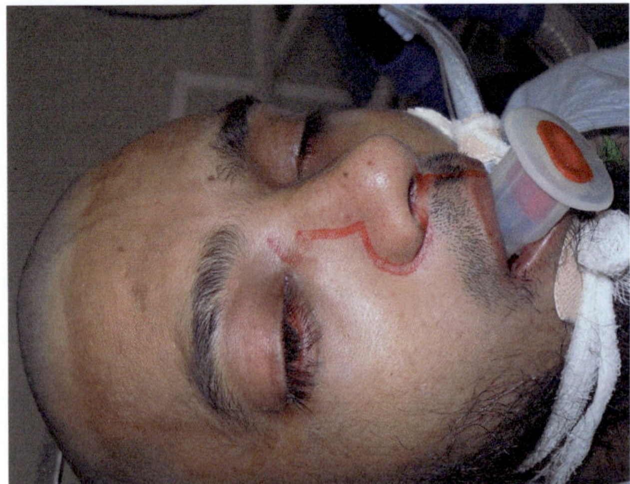

Fig. 12.21 The lateral rhinotomy incision with lynch extension

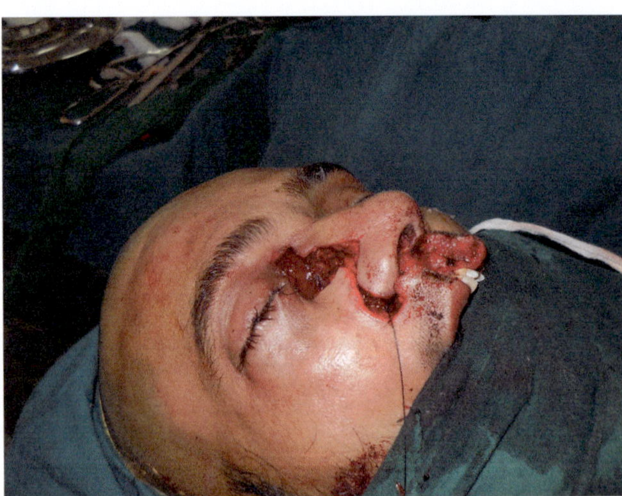

Fig. 12.22 Incision is placed and the flap is raised

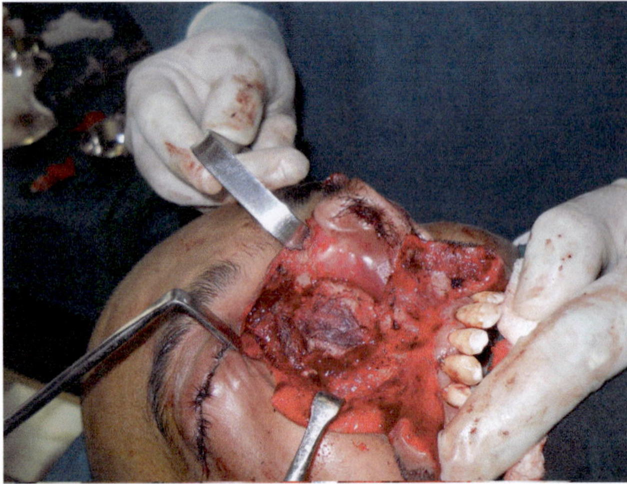

Fig. 12.23 The tumor is exposed

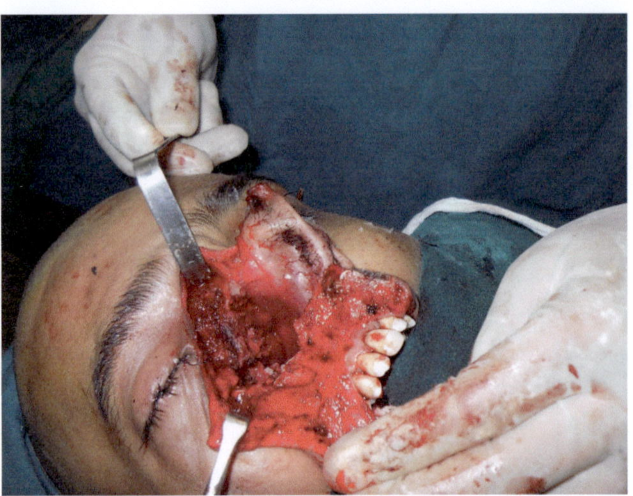

Fig. 12.24 Medial maxillotomy is performed and tumor is separated from the eyeball and nasal floor

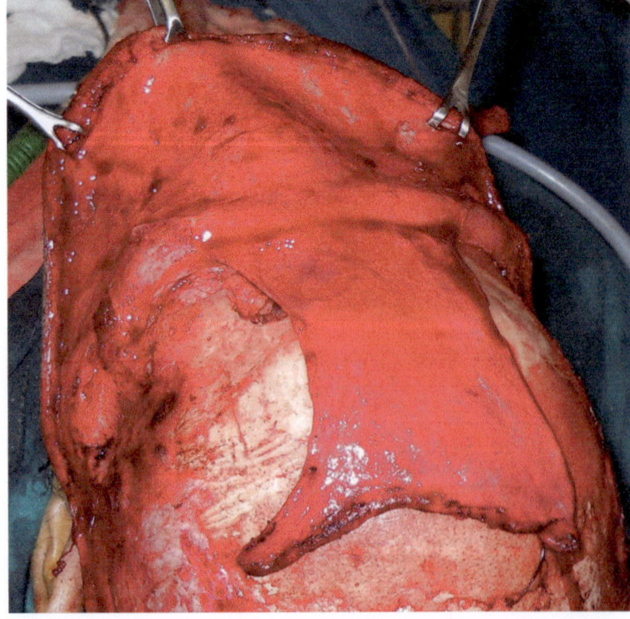

Fig. 12.25 Bi-coronal flap is raised and pericranial flap is isolated

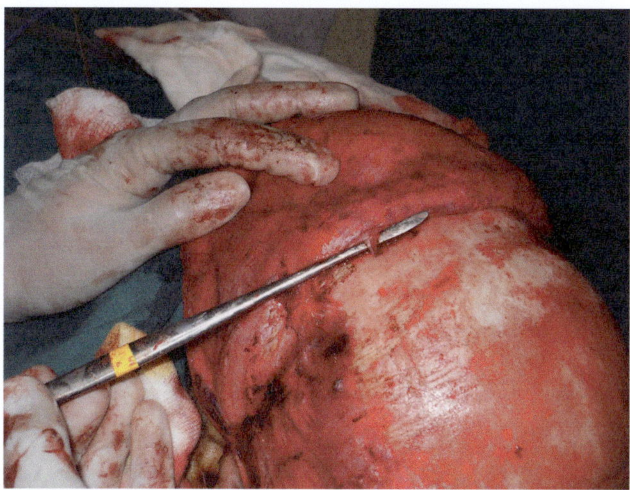

Fig. 12.26 The supratrochlear and orbital vessels being freed from the groove

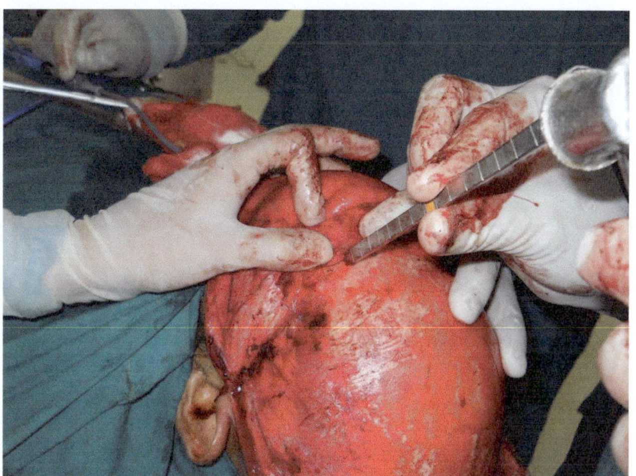

Fig. 12.27 Vessels are being freed from the groove and care should be taken not to injure them

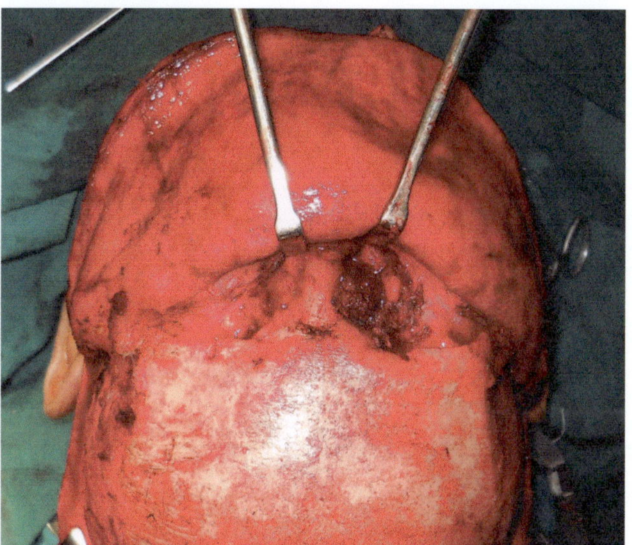

Fig. 12.28 Flap is raised till lower border of nasal bone. The tumor can be seen in orbital cavity medial to eyeball

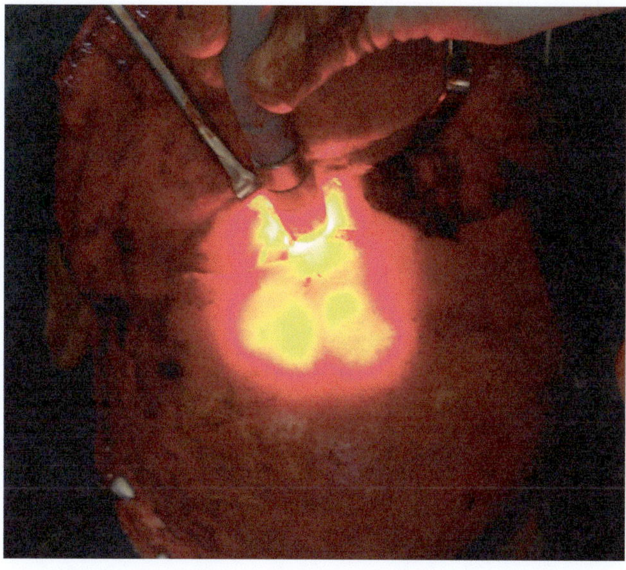

Fig. 12.29 This is a novel way of identifying the extent of frontal sinus. The light illuminates the sinus cavity and borders are marked

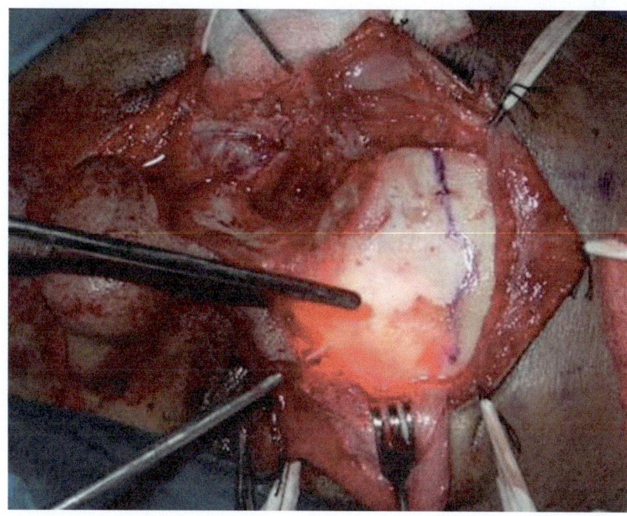

Fig. 12.30 The boundaries can be exactly marked with this simple method

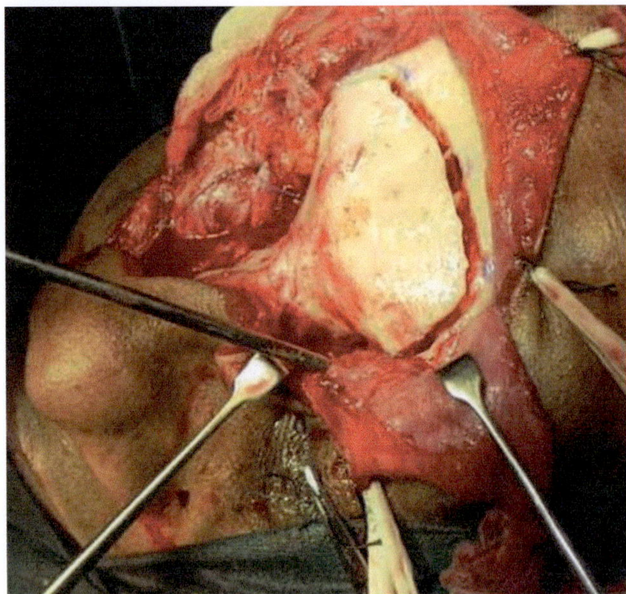

Fig. 12.31 The anterior wall of frontal sinus is removed to expose the frontal sinus. Care must be taken not to go beyond the marked boundaries

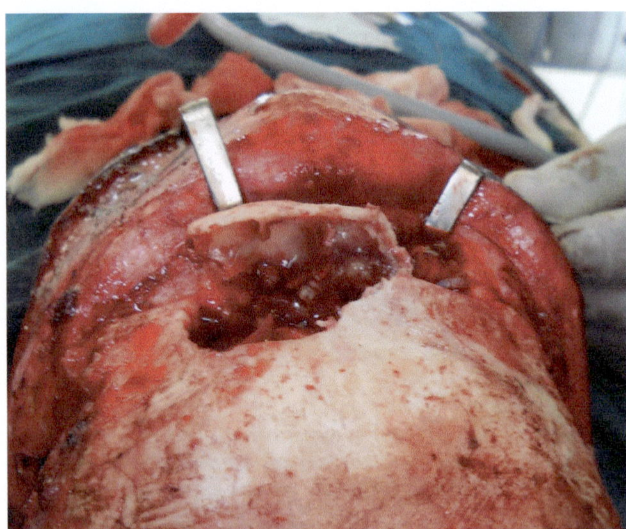

Fig. 12.32 Anterior wall of sinus is removed and the tumor can be seen in the sinus

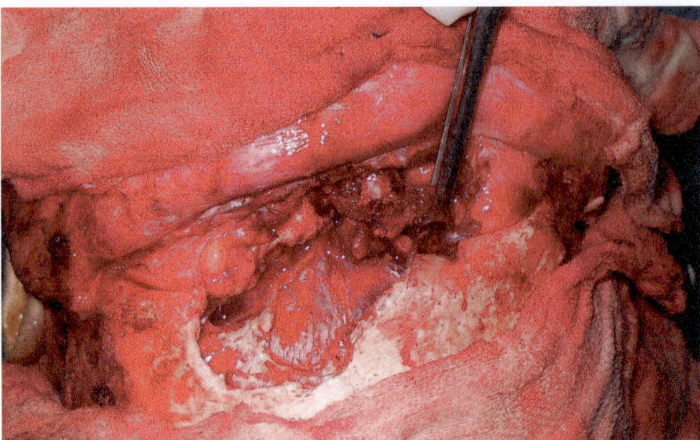

Fig. 12.33 Posterior wall of sinus is drilled to cranialize the cavity. The tumor involves the dura and wide margin is of dura is removed for clearance. Further dissection is carried out in similar fashion as described in previous procedure

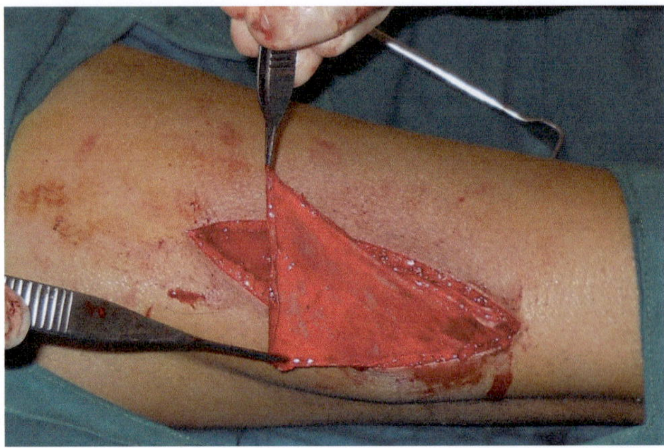

Fig. 12.34 Fascia lata is harvested for dural closure

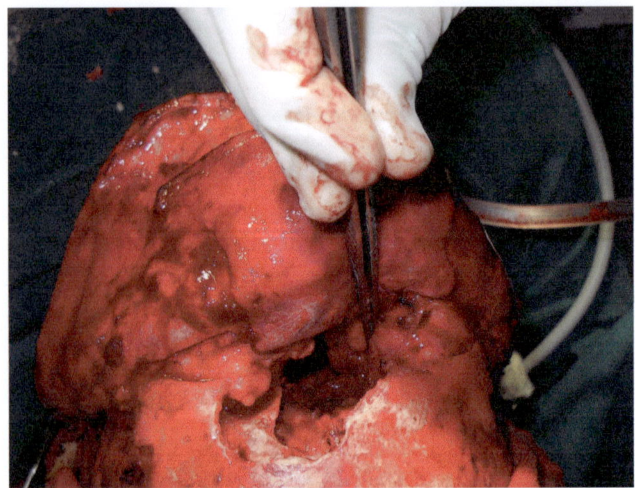

Fig. 12.35 The primary layer of dural closure is complete. We prefer to have a multilayer closure

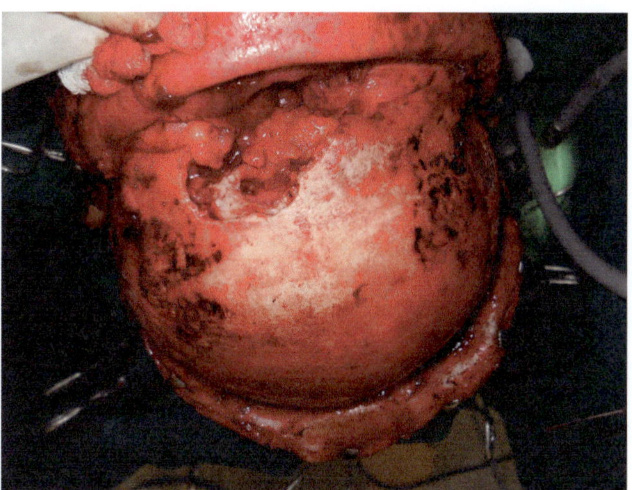

Fig. 12.36 The second layer is made of free fat graft. This is very important to provides water tight seal and provides vascularity to the first layer. The third layer is formed by previoulsy isolated pericranial slap

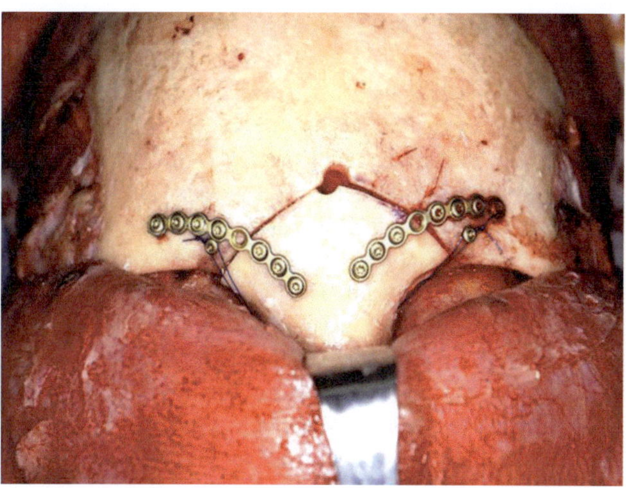

Fig. 12.37 The bone flap is put back. One can see prolene sutures in place to tag medial canthal ligament. This is an important step for cosmetic outcome. Postoperative care remains similar to the previous procedure

Anterolateral Craniofacial Resection

The tumor extending from ITF to middle cranial fossa needs this surgical approach. ITF has a complex anatomy and is connected to intracranial compartment with various foramina that transfer cranial nerves and vessels. The oral cavity and maxillary tumors with infiltrative pattern are more likely to spread to these areas. Involvement of internal carotid artery and cavernous sinus is a difficult surgical problem, and it is often difficult to clear the tumor completely in this situation. The decision to operate is often taken based on the pathology of the tumor, and more aggressive approach is reserved for low-grade malignancies. There are two trans-facial approaches commonly used to address the tumor in infratemporal fossa. The transmandibular approach is reserved for lesions situated below the occlusal plane, while facial-translocation approach is reserved for tumors situated above the occlusal plane. These trans-facial approaches are combined with frontotemporal craniotomy to address middle cranial fossa lesion.

Two surgical procedures are demonstrated in this chapter:

- Frontotemporal craniotomy
- Facial-translocation approach

The transmandibular approach described in the chapter addreses infratemporal fossa tumors.

Frontotemporal Craniotomy

This procedure shows steps to perform frontotemporal craniotomy to address squamous cell cancer involving the skin of the, eye and skull bone.

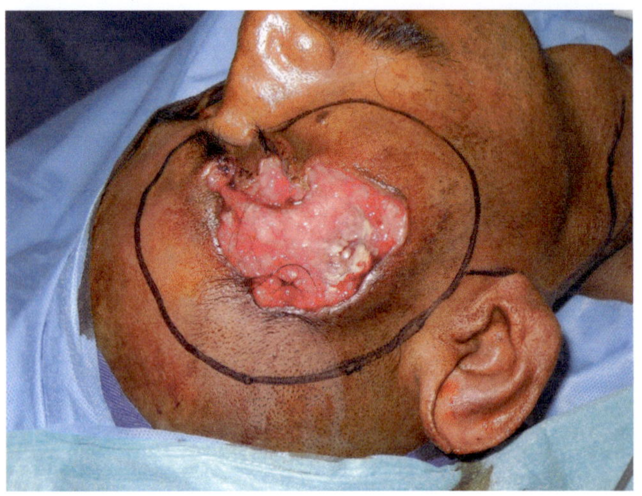

Fig. 12.38 The tumor involving the skin of the face near the eye and forehead with involvement of the underlying bone and eye. The proposed incision provides adequate margins and allows space for craniotomy and neck dissection

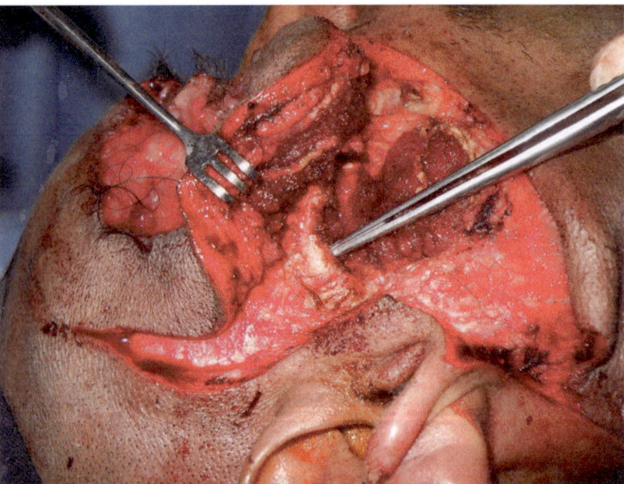

Fig. 12.39 Skin flaps are raised to expose the zygoma. The muscles of mastication are divided and the bone is exposed to perform osteotomy

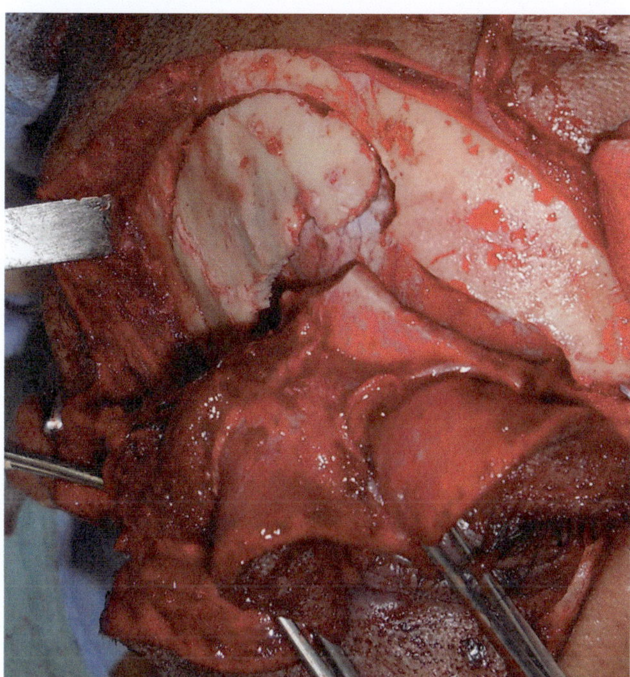

Fig. 12.40 The tumor is involving the underlying termporal bone, zygomatic bone and part of frontal bone. Appropriate bone cuts are put. There is a separate craniotomy bone cut in frontotemporal area. This allows for en bloc removal of the tumor along with the skull bone

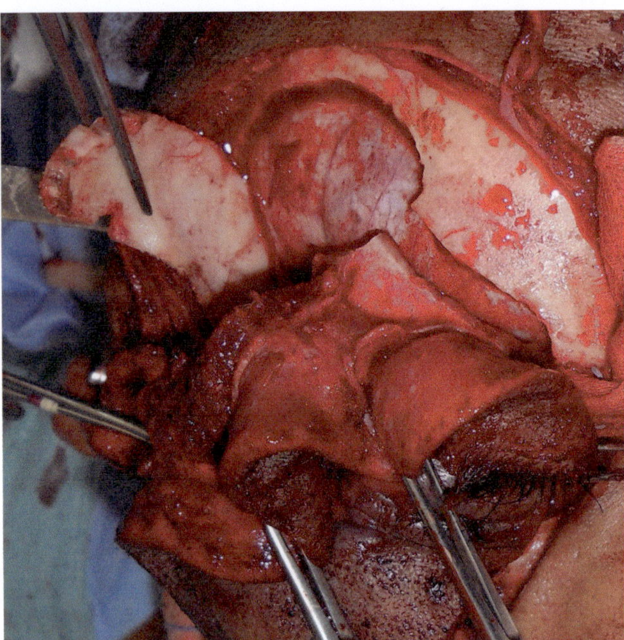

Fig. 12.41 The craniotomy bone flap is raised

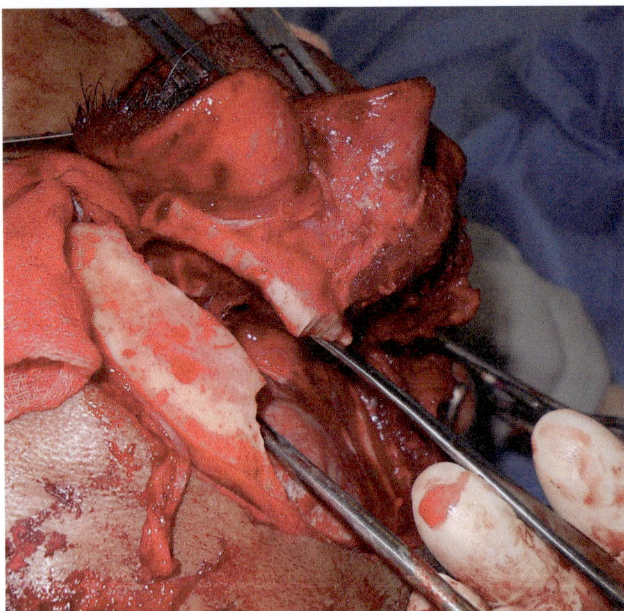

Fig. 12.42 The tumor is lifted off to expose orbital apex from the cranial side

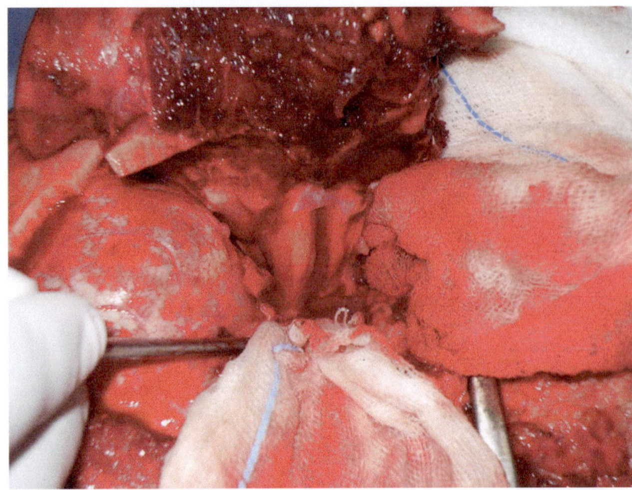

Fig. 12.43 The orbital apex is exposed. The entire tumor is mobilized anteriorly and deep margin is free

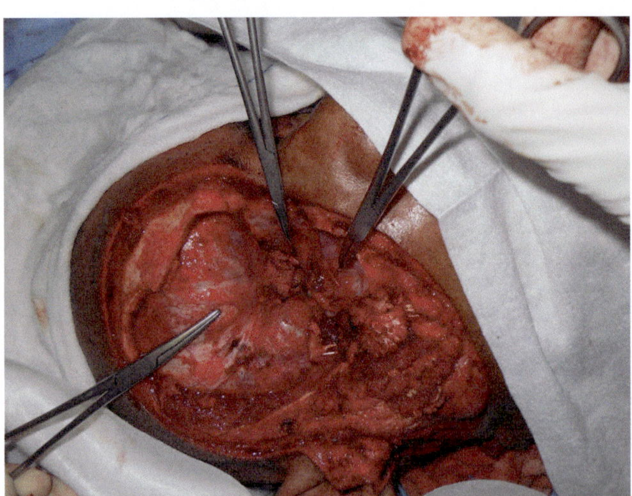

Fig. 12.44 The resection is complete. Wide excision with en bloc removal of the eye, suprastructure maxilla bone, and skull bone is complete

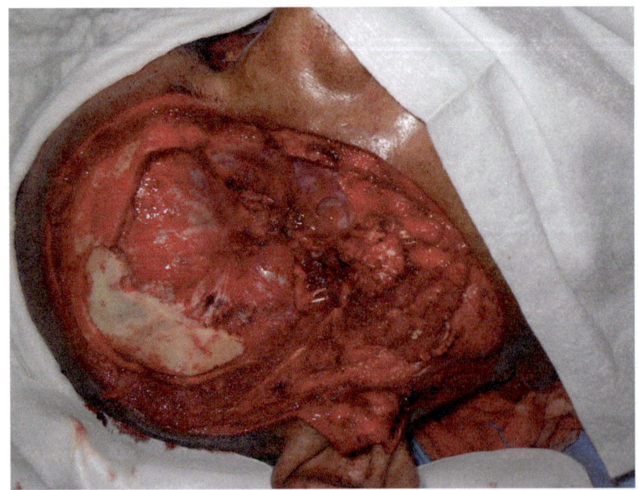

Fig. 12.45 The bone flap is put back

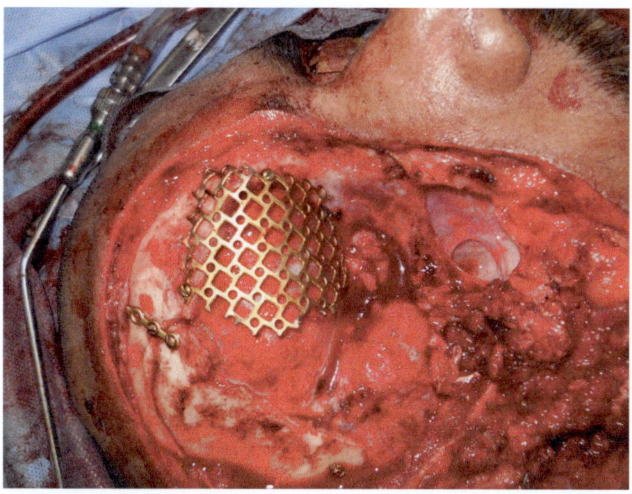

Fig. 12.46 Titanium mesh is used to cover the bone defect in the eye region

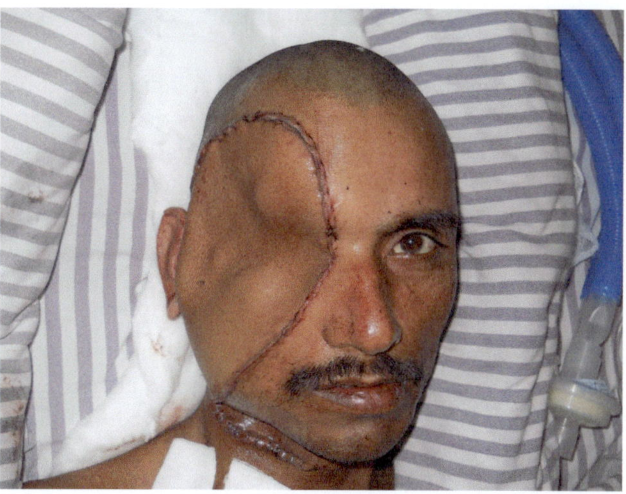

Fig. 12.48 The final outcome on the 8th postoperative day. Wounds are healed and patient has acceptable cosmetic outcome

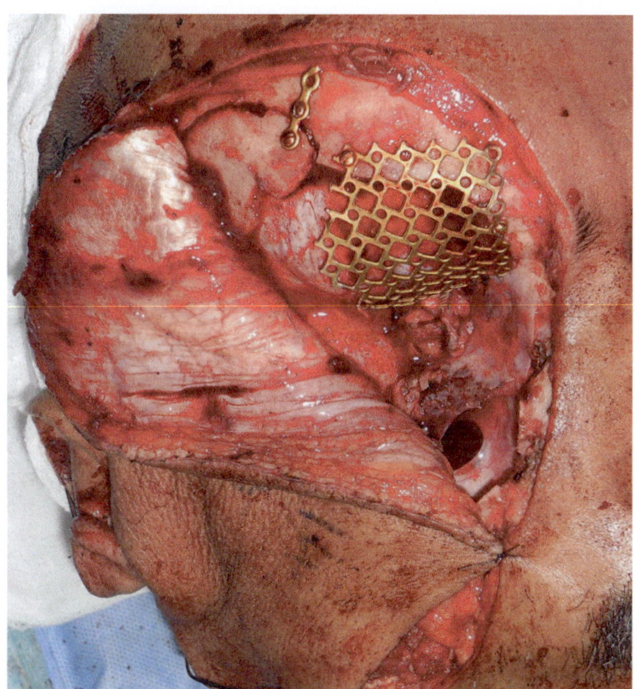

Fig. 12.47 Anterolateral thigh flap is used to reconstruct the skin defect

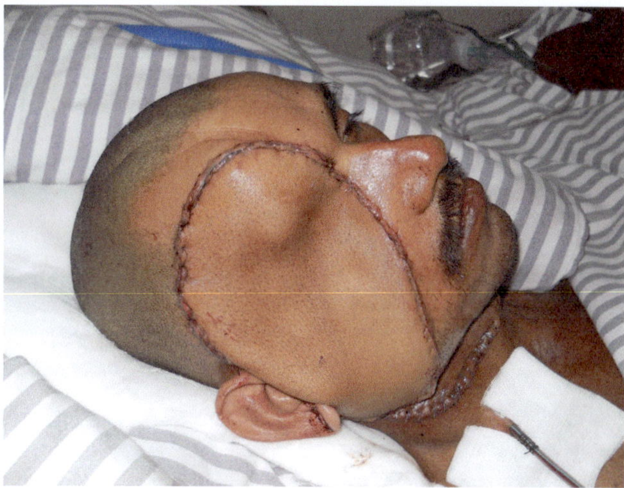

Fig. 12.49 Photograph showing another view of reconstructed defect

Facial-Translocation Approach

This approach was initially described by Jenecka in 2002. The concept is based on the theory of modular disassembly. The face is divided into subunits that have separate neurovascular supply. These subunits can be dismantled preserving their blood supply to expose areas that cannot be visualized otherwise. These units can be assembled at the end of the procedure without any long-term consequences.

This approach is particularly useful to address tumors in nasopharynx area with involvement of intracranial compartment. The maxilla with overlying skin can be lifted off to expose these areas. The blood supply to maxillary bone is provided by the overlying skin, and the entire unit can be put back at the end of the procedure to retain normal function and cosmesis.

These approaches can be broadly classified into:

- Limited facial-translocation
- Standard facial-translocation
- Extended facial-translocation

The standard facial-translocation procedure is described in this section.

Standard Facial-Translocation

This procedure is often used to address tumors in nasopharynx area. The recurrent nasopharynx cancers and recurrent angio-fibromas are common indications for this procedure.

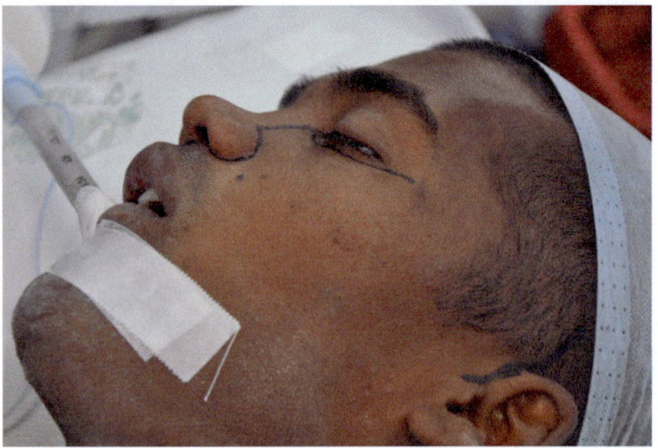

Fig. 12.50 Patient with recurrent angio-fibroma. The incision is Weber–Ferguson with pre-auricular extension for zygomatic bone cut

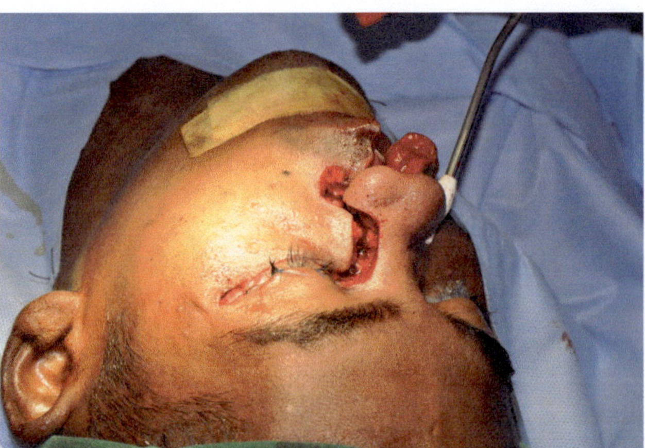

Fig. 12.51 The incision is deepened to expose the bone for osteotomy. The bone is exposed just enough so that pre-plating can be done. It is very important to remember not to raise skin flap too much as skin is left attached to underlying maxilla bone and this preserves blood supply for the bone

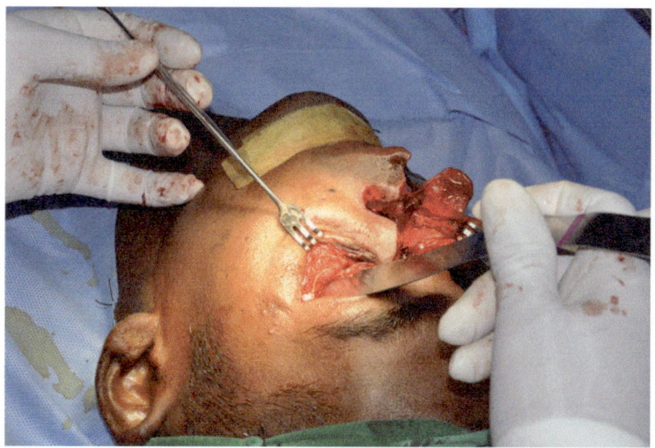

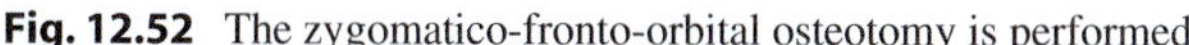

Fig. 12.52 The zygomatico-fronto-orbital osteotomy is performed

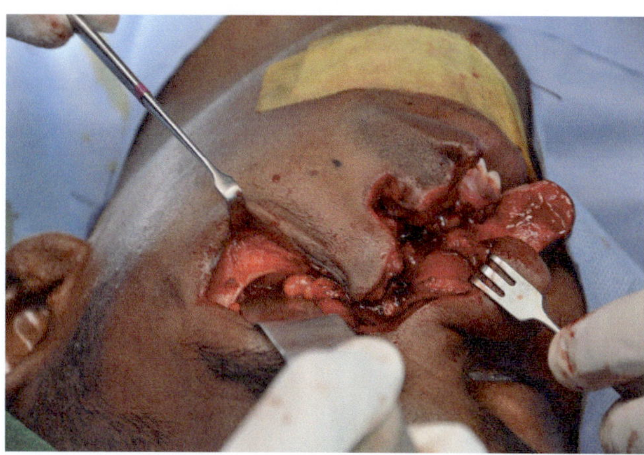

Fig. 12.53 The eyeball is separated from orbital floor

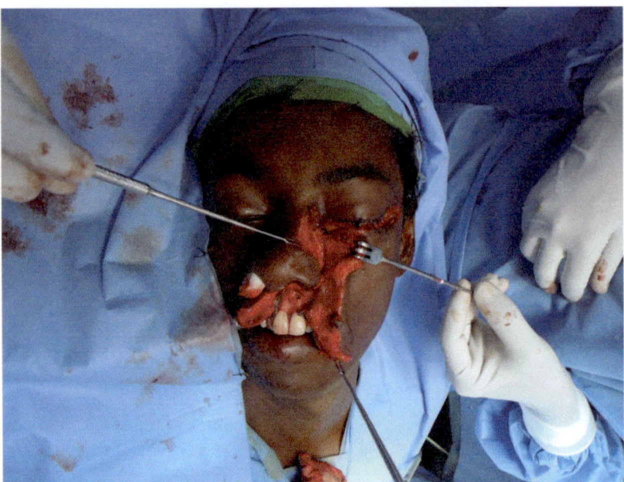

Fig. 12.54 Pre-plating is done at nasal bone

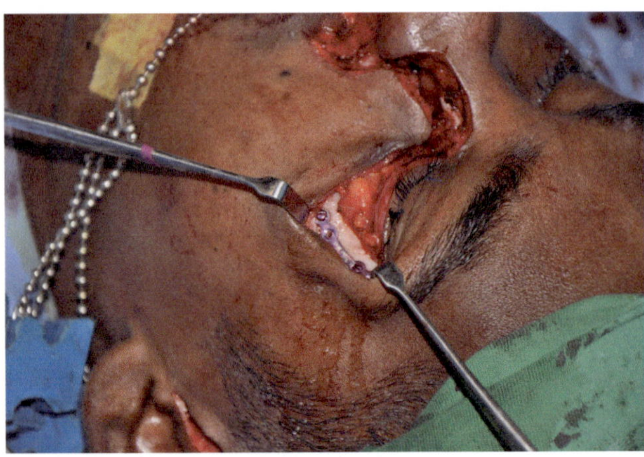

Fig. 12.55 The plate is fixed at fronto-orbital suture

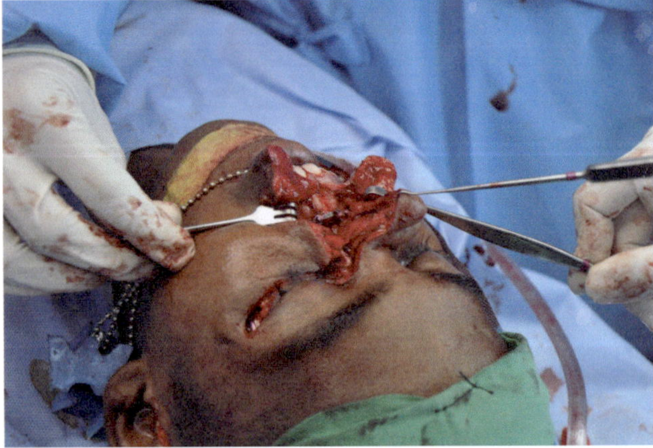

Fig. 12.56 The plate is fixed at pre-maxilla. These plates are removed to facilitate bone cuts and are put back at end of procedure to retain maxilla in occlusion

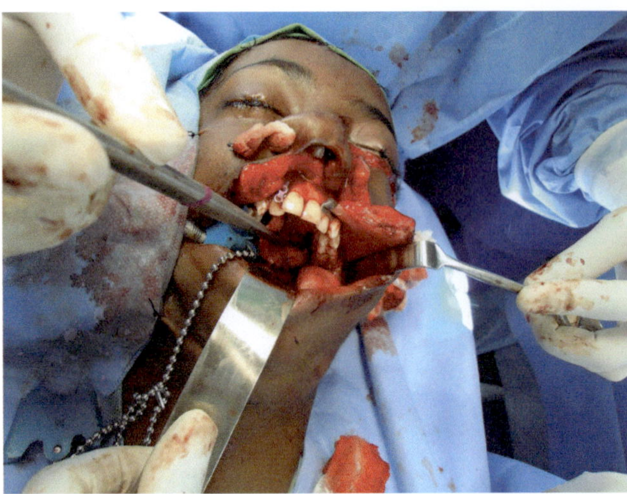

Fig. 12.57 The mucoperiosteal palatal flap is separated from underlying bone

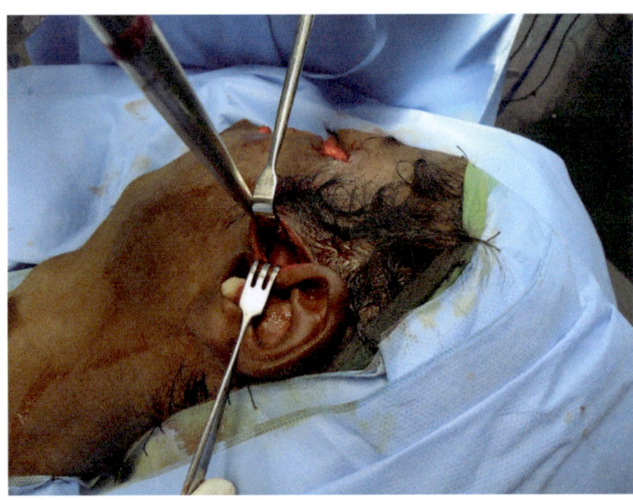

Fig. 12.58 Pre-auricular incision is placed to expose Zygoma to place the bone cut. Try and avoid damage to frontal branch of facial nerve

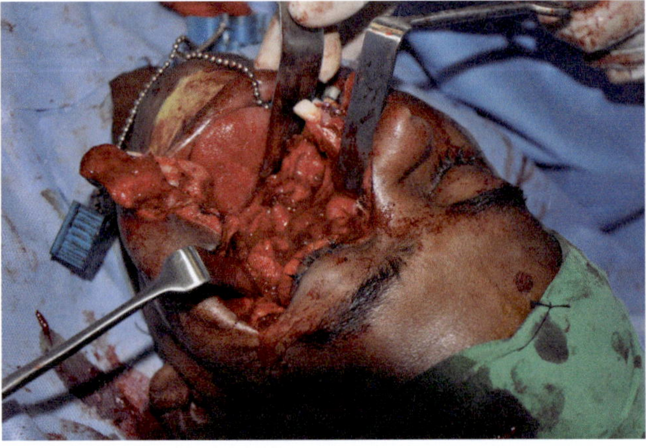

Fig. 12.59 The entire maxilla with overlying skin is shifted laterally to expose posterior nasopharynx area

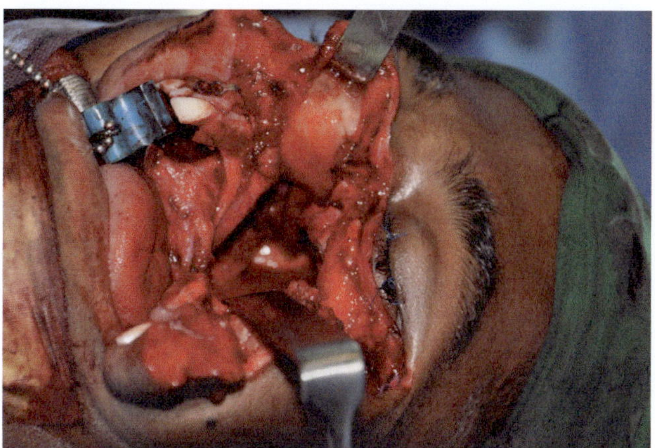

Fig. 12.60 The tumor is mobilized and removed. Care is taken not to injure internal carotid artery and eustachean tube serves here as a guide. The artery is located posterior to eustachean and dissection should be done carefully in this area

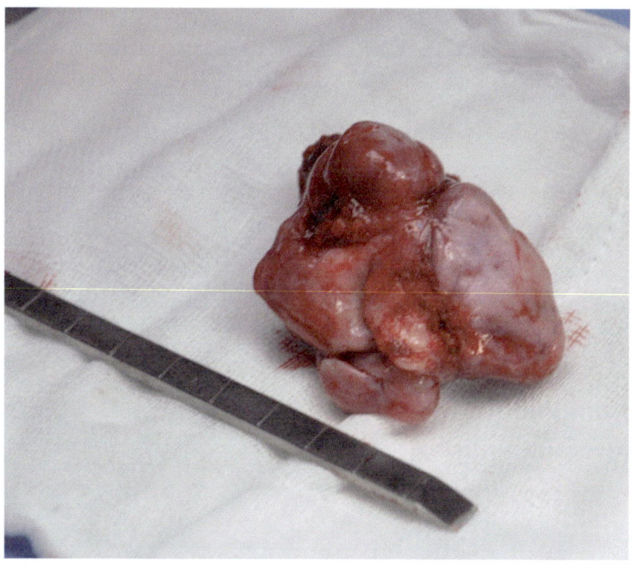

Fig. 12.61 The tumor is completely removed

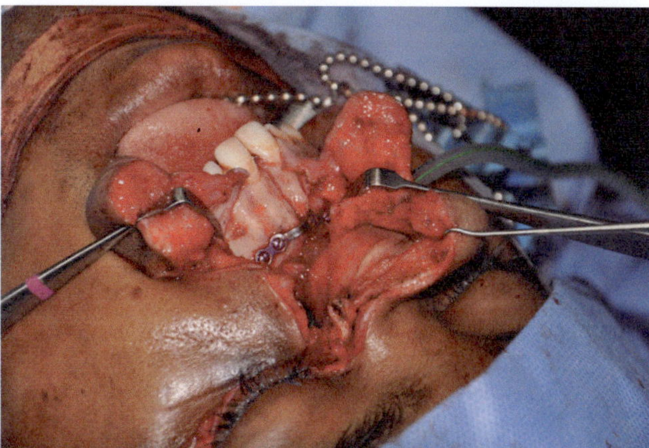

Fig. 12.62 The bone flap is put back in position and plates are fixed in position

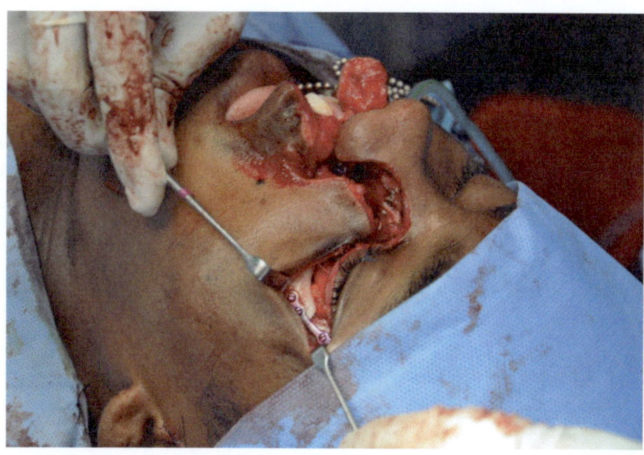

Fig. 12.63 It is important to keep maxilla in occlusion while fixing these plates. The plates need to be fixed appropriately to avoid extrusion at a later date

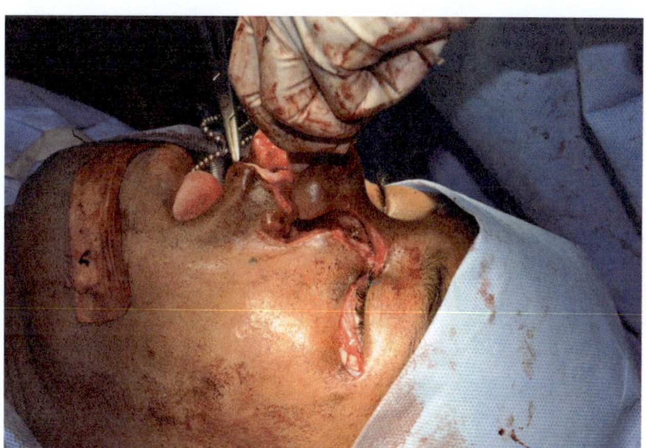

Fig. 12.64 The palatal flap is sutured back and skin closure is performed

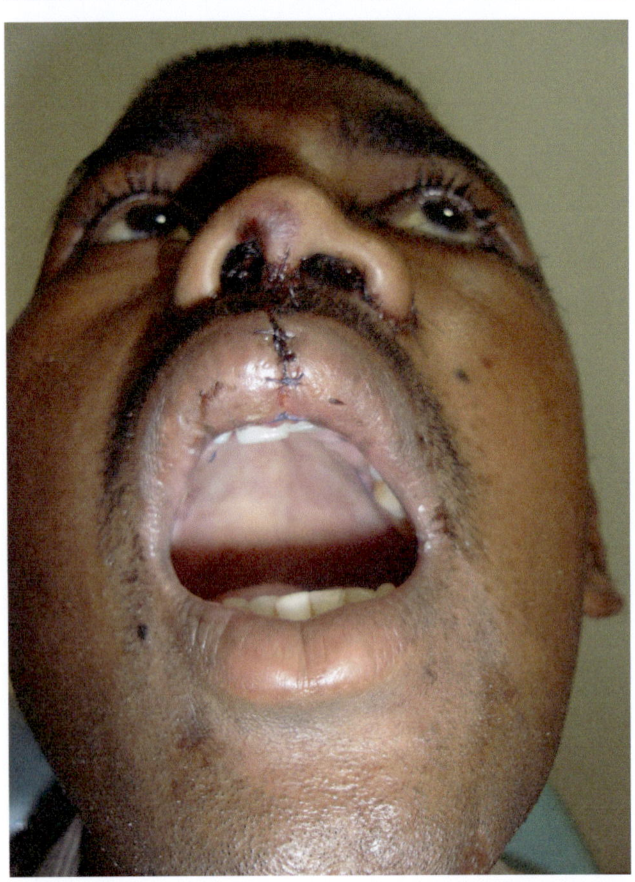

Fig. 12.65 The healed palatal flap is shown in photograph

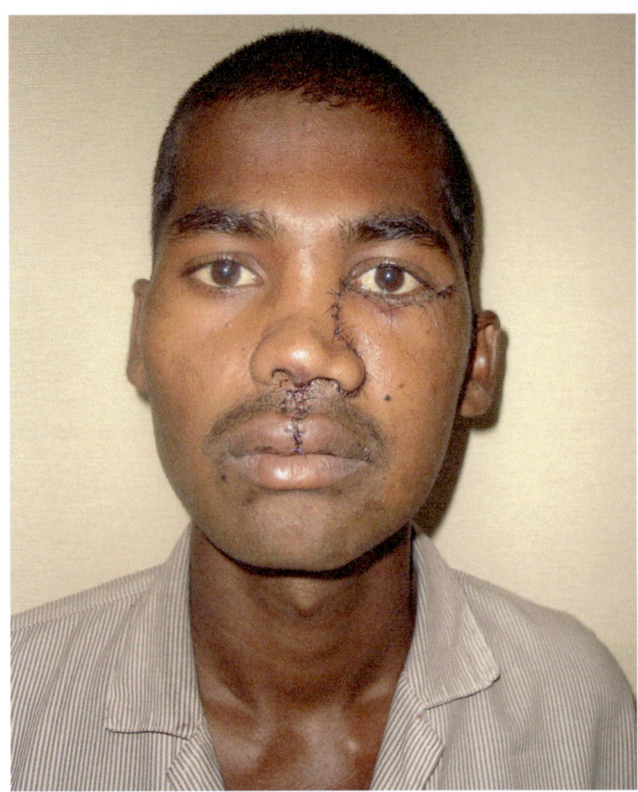

Fig. 12.66 Photograph of patient showing outcome on 6th post-operative day

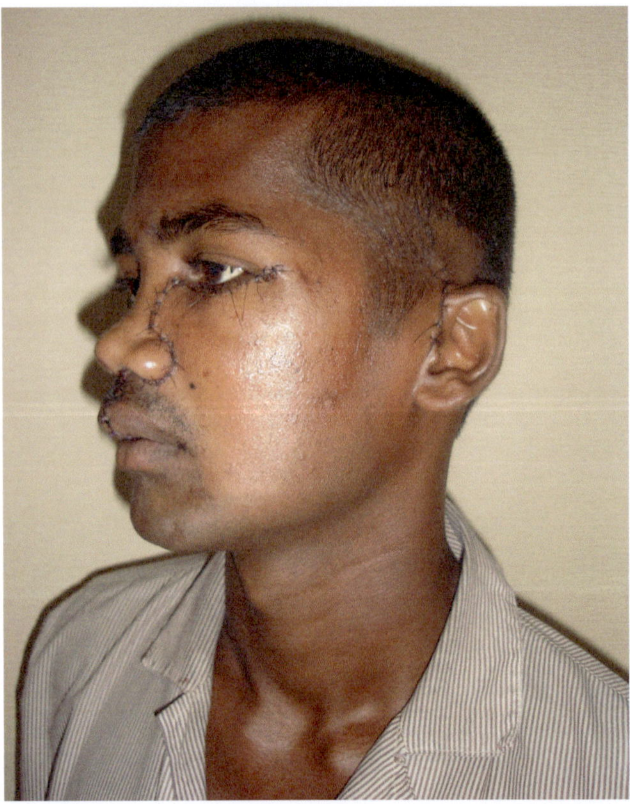

Fig. 12.67 The facial edema has subsided and wounds have healed well

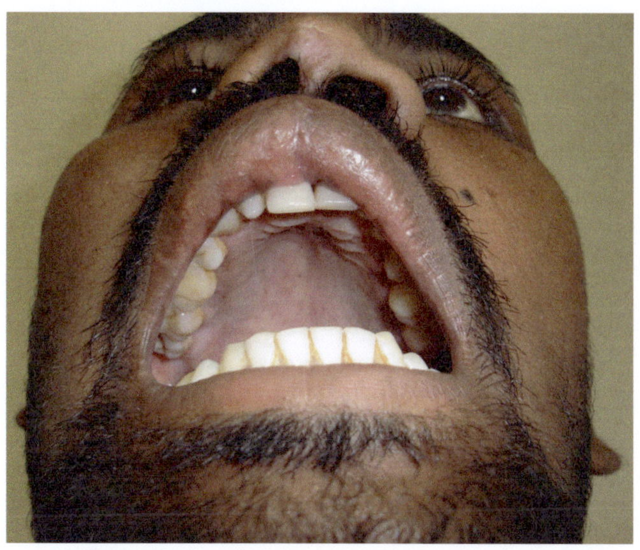

Fig. 12.68 The completely healed palate after few months of procedure

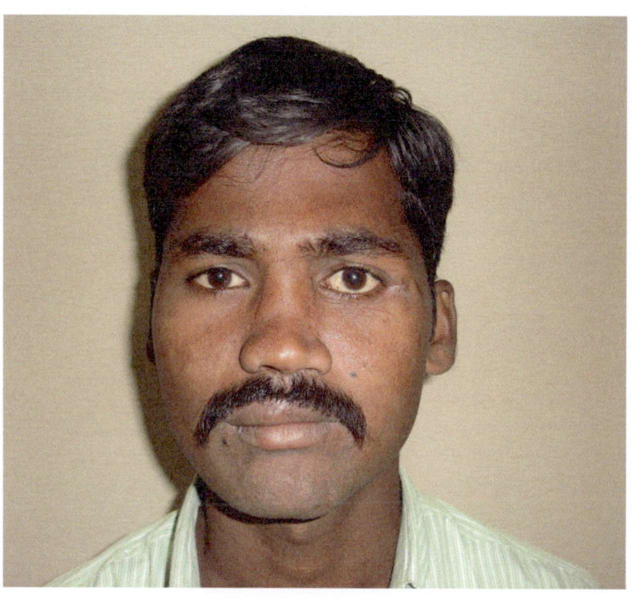

Fig. 12.69 Photograph is showing long-term cosmetic outcome of the patient. The outcome of these procedures is very acceptable if basic principles are maintained in appropriate way

Reconstruction of Skull Base Defects

The craniofacial resection is a complex procedure involving many vital structures. It is essential to reconstruct these defects in appropriate way to provide patient with decent afterlife.

There are basic principles for reconstruction of skull base defects are:

- To achieve effective seal for dura.
- Cranio-nasal separation and support to dura.
- Provide cover to carotid artery.
- Support to orbital contents.
- Oro-nasal separation.
- Good cosmetic and functional outcome.

The reconstruction is provided based on an algorithm that is demonstrated in Figs. 12.70, 12.71, and 12.72. The most important goal is to provide water tight seal for dural defect and provide necessary support for brain. The remaining reconstruction is performed based on structures removed. The reconstruction is generally carried out with combination of local flap and a free flap.

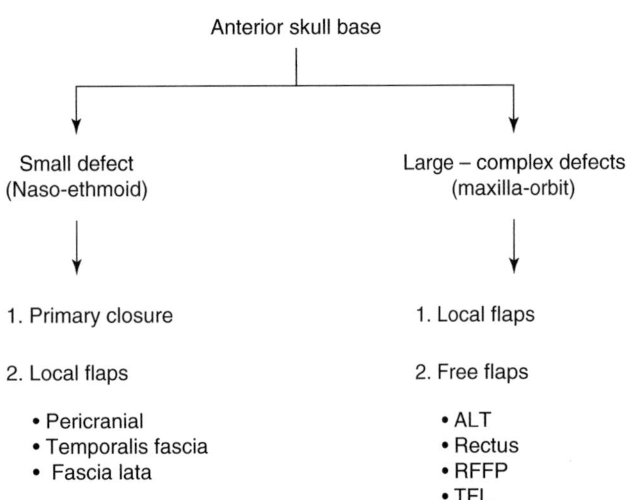

Fig. 12.70 Reconstruction algorithm for anterior skull base defects

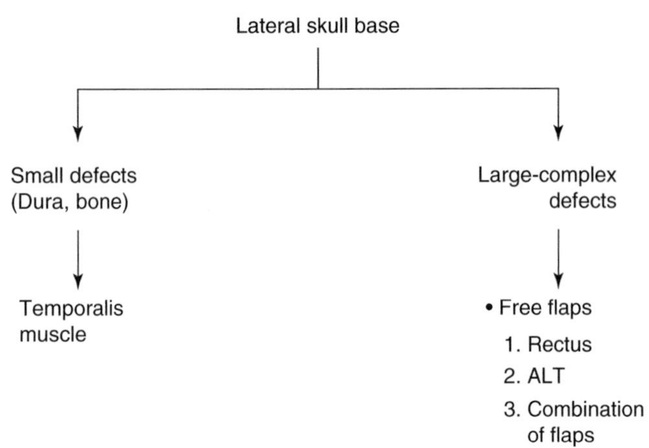

Fig. 12.72 Algorithm for lateral skull base defects

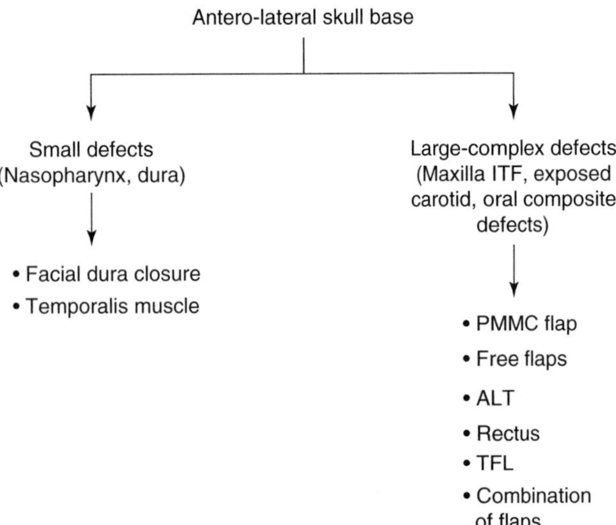

Fig. 12.71 Reconstruction for Antero-lateral skull base

13 Tumors of Infratemporal Fossa

The infratemporal fossa (ITF) has been a challenging area for clinicians for a long time. This area has complex anatomy with communications to many surrounding areas. Accurate assessment of disease spread is limited by the edema of tissue, and the area has a tendency to bleed heavily during surgery. These factors make the treatment of patient with lesion in ITF very complicated and challenging. There is very little in published literature regarding surgical approaches for ITF. This chapter focuses on various surgical approaches for ITF clearance. These approaches are based on our clinical experience of treating these cases over the past few years.

Surgical Anatomy and Pattern of Spread

Figure 13.1 is a schematic representation of the anatomy of masticator space. The masticator space includes masseter muscle, both the pterygoid muscles, temporalis muscle, ascending ramus of mandible, and pterygoid plates. The ITF consists of space medial to the mandible and masseter muscle is excluded. This area contains various neurovascular bundles and also harbours pterygoid venous plexus. The tumor can easily spread from ITF to various surrdunding areas to which it is connected (Fig. 13.2). The oral cavity tumors, particularly buccal mucosa and RMT tumors, have a high tendency to spread to masticator space due to close proximity to muscles of mastication. The ITF can also get involved by posteriorly located maxillary sinus lesions, and this poses a difficult surgical challenge. Tumors of temporal bone and orbital apex can also spread to this region. The ITF is connected to the middle cranial fossa through various foramina and lesion can spread to intracranial compartment early in its spread. Appropriate imaging studies are required to evaluate disease spread in this area.

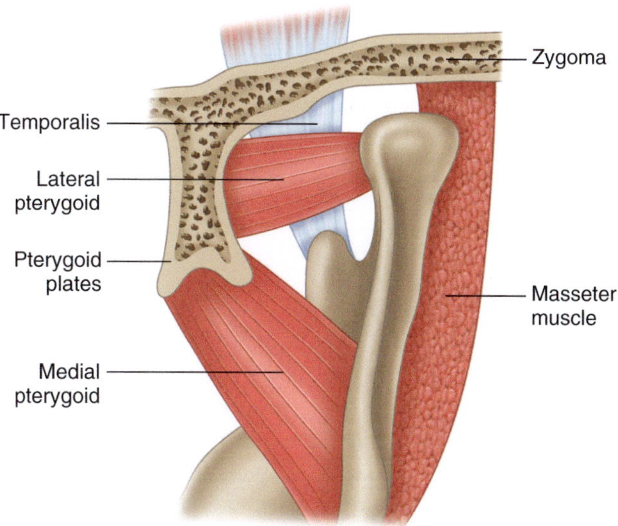

Fig. 13.1 Surgical anatomy of masticator space

N. Trivedi, *Atlas of Head and Neck Cancer Surgery: The Compartment Surgery for Resection in 3-D*,
DOI 10.1007/978-81-322-2050-3_13, © Springer India 2015

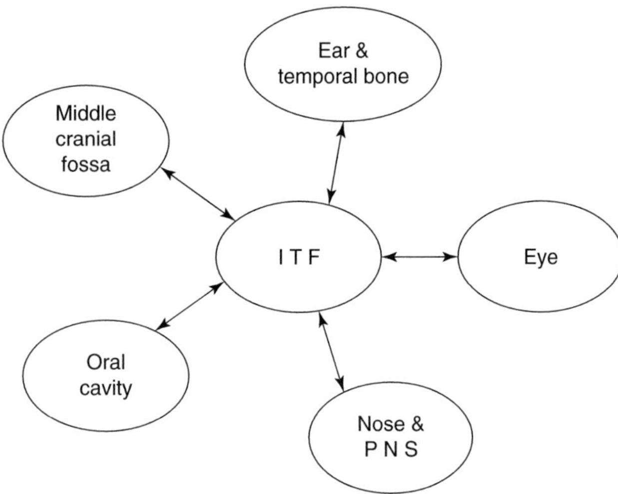

Fig. 13.2 Pattern of spread to and from ITF

Surgical Concepts

- It is advisable to remove the entire masticator space as a single unit once involved (compartment approach). There are many advantages of this approach. The bleeding is minimal as we go around contents rather than through it. The entire content is removed, and hence a chance of leaving behind the disease is minimal and error in personal judgment about the extent of disease spread and surgical resection is avoided. The functional outcome remains largely similar to conventional approach.
- The oral cancer spreading to ITF is best dealt with compartment clearance described in this chapter. We have classified these lesions to simplyfy their management. It is not ideal to group all such patients in one compartment and it is important to understand their pattern of spread.
- The maxillary sinus tumors with ITF spread are best dealt by transmandibular approaches or posterior to anterior approaches. This is the only way to remove these tumors in en bloc fashion and achieve negative margin in depth.
- The oral cavity tumors (mainly buccal mucosa and RMT) and PNS tumors involving only masticator space have fewer tendencies for distant metastasis. These tumors with extensive primary tumor spread have relatively less involvement of lymph nodes and distant organs. This warrants an aggressive surgical approach with a real possibility of curing them. This fact changes when tumor spreads to involve lateral pharyngeal wall and nasopharynx area. They present with large nodes and outcome reduces significantly for this group. If addressed surgically, it is advisable to remove parapharyngeal lymph nodes as we have found them involved in many instances.

Oral Cancer with Masticator Space Involvement (T4b)

The oral cancers that spread to masticator space are staged as T4b and are considered inoperable in majority of cases. There is a recent trend to stage these tumors as low ITF (below sigmoid notch) and high ITF (above sigmoid notch). The low ITF tumors are considered operable and are offered curative intent surgery while high ITF tumors are treated with palliative intent. However, this guideline is based on very limited data (eight cases for high ITF) and needs further evaluation [1, 2]. Buccal cancers generally involve the entire masticator space, while the tongue and oropharynx tumors tend to involve ITF.

The concept of compartment clearance for masticator was proposed by our group [3, 4]. The masticator space is essentially a soft tissue compartment containing various muscles, fats, lymphatics, and neurovascular bundles that are related closely to each other. This area is highly vascular and bleeds heavily during surgery. It is also very difficult to assess the exact extent of disease spread in this area either preoperatively or intraoperatively. These factors make conventional approach of clearance with 1 cm margin technically difficult. Removal of the entire soft tissue en bloc irrespective of the extent of spread solves many of these problems, and bleeding is minimal as dissection is around the compartment in facial planes. Initial experience with this approach was published with very satisfactory results for this group [3].

It is not ideal to group all these tumors in one as only tumors with potential to involve intracranial contents do badly. All the specimens of patients who underwent compartment surgery were studied extensively to understand the pattern of disease spread in masticator space [4]. The study correlated findings of clinical examination with findings of radiological and pathological examination to propose a classification system to form a treatment strategy.

Classification: (Fig. 13.3)

- Category I: Low ITF – involvement of medial pterygoid and masseter muscle
- Category II: Intermediate ITF – involvement of both pterygoid muscles, temporalis muscle, and pterygoid plates
- Category III: High ITF – (A) involvement of pterygomaxillary fissure and (B) involvement of intracranial compartment

Categories I and II are considered operable and show good clinical outcome. The category III is considered to have high ITF involvement and generally has variable outcome. Involvement of pterygomaxillary fissure in the lower half can have good outcome with below described procedure for high ITF clearance, and we consider it in borderline operable category. The disease extending to intracranial compartment is considered inoperable and needs further studies. The study revealed that compartment surgical approach was helpful in achieving three-dimensional negative margins in all the cases of categories I and II. When the tumor reaches beyond the compartment (probably through pterygomaxillary fissure or through cranial foramina), then there is a chance of leaving behind the residual disease. This was also reflected in very good local control rate in published studies [3, 4]. The functional outcome remains similar to conventional approach as only the extra nonfunctioning tissue in depth is removed.

The surgical procedure is described in the subsequent section.

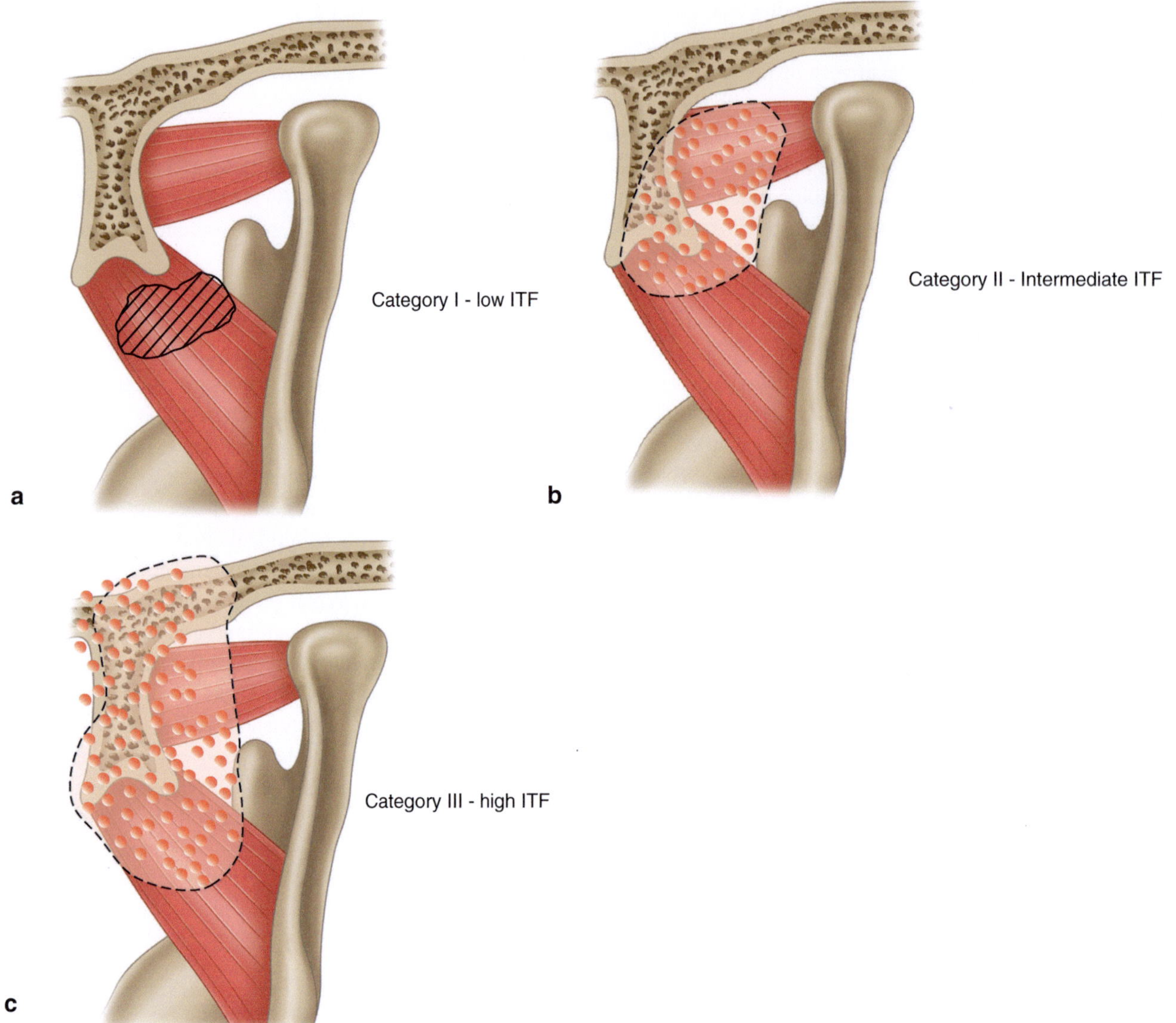

Fig. 13.3 Classification for oral cancer involving masticator space (T4b)

Compartment Surgery for Low ITF

We perform classical compartment surgery for category I and few category II cases. It is essential to remove the entire compartment also for category I lesions as that serves as an additional margin in depth. This is described in this section.

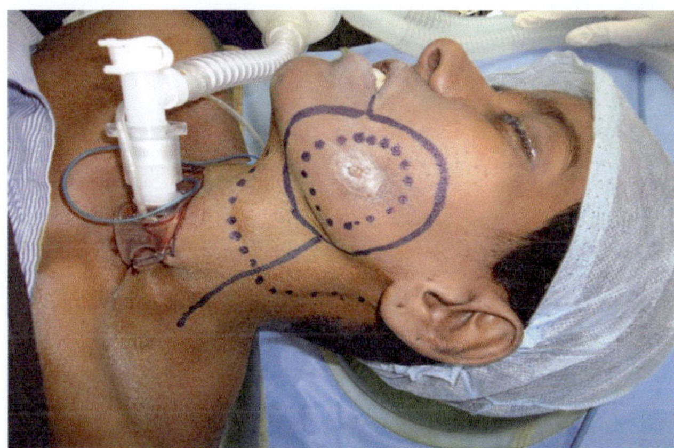

Fig. 13.4 Patient having recurrent buccal cancer involving masticator space. The lesion involves medial pterygoid muscle (category I) and causes complete trismus. The incision is planned with adequate skin margins. It is advisable to palpate for induration and edema and include all in resection margins

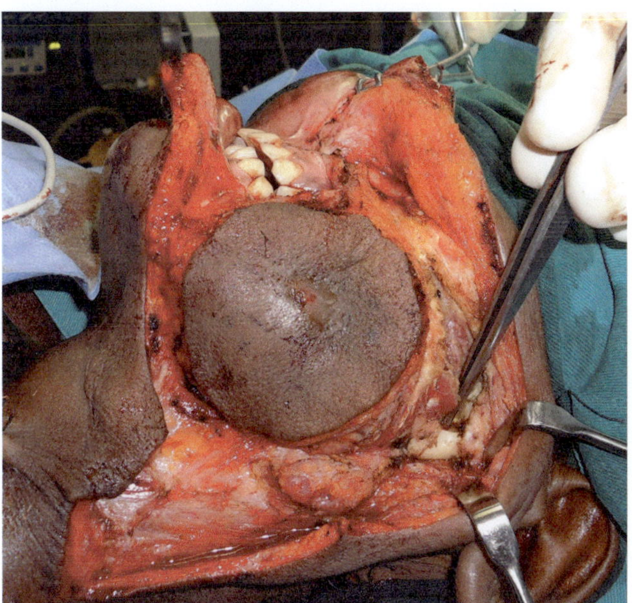

Fig. 13.5 Flaps are raised in conventional way exposing the zygoma and maxilla above and mandible below. The sigmoid notch is exposed posteriorly

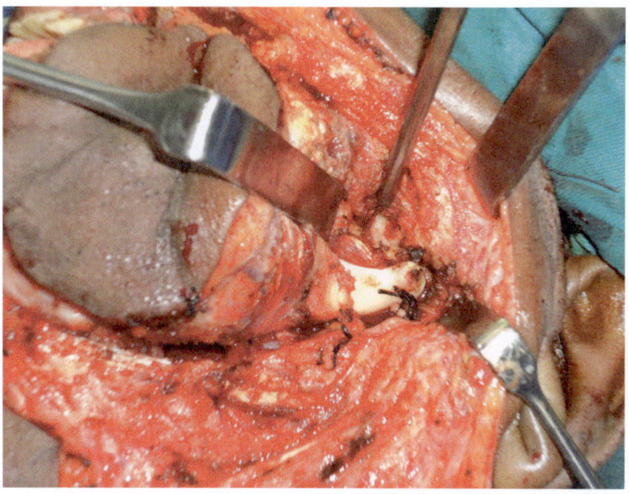

Fig. 13.6 The masseter and temporalis muscles are transacted to expose the skull base. The photograph shows exposed sphenoid wing of the skull base, lateral pterygoid muscle, and condyle

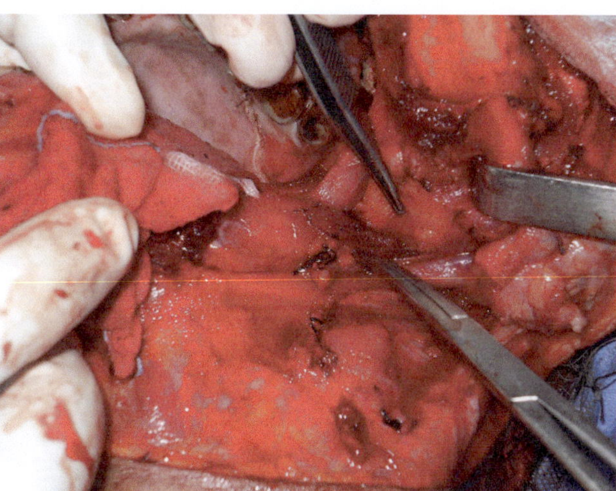

Fig. 13.7 The other steps to address buccal component are similar to conventional composite resection. This photo shows anatomy of prestyloid parapharyngeal space. The muscles attached to styloid process serve as entry place for parapharyngeal space and fat pad is clearly evident in this photograph

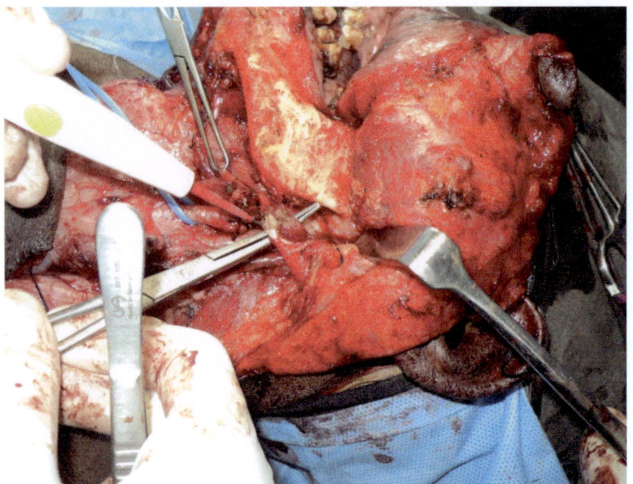

Fig. 13.8 In case where lesion is going posteriorly to involve oropharynx and lateral pharynx, one needs to enter the space and expose the internal carotid artery in the entire length. The posterior belly of digastric muscle is identified, divided along with styloid muscles for that purpose. This step is not needed when dealing only with masticator space

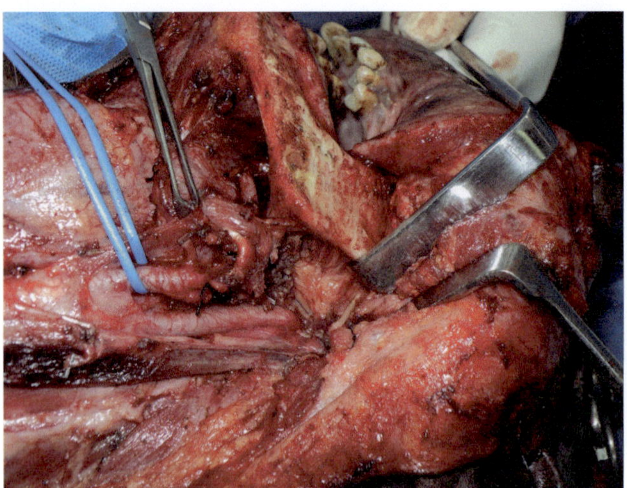

Fig. 13.9 The relation of medial pterygoid muscle to parapharyngeal fat plane is visible in this photograph

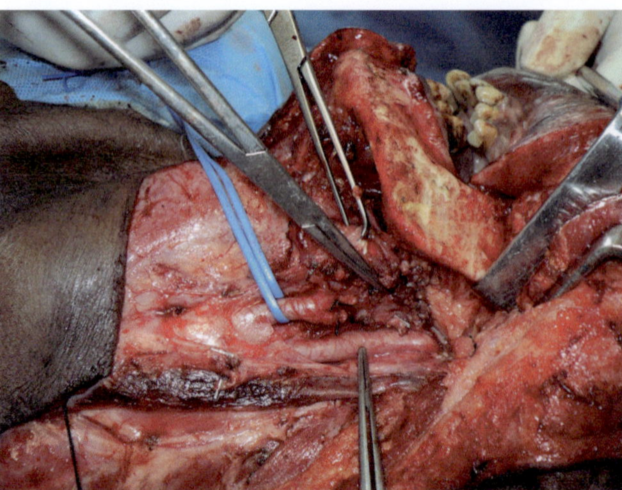

Fig. 13.10 The mandible is mobilized anteriorly by dividing stylomandibular ligament. The internal and external carotid arteries are exposed to demonstrate anatomy

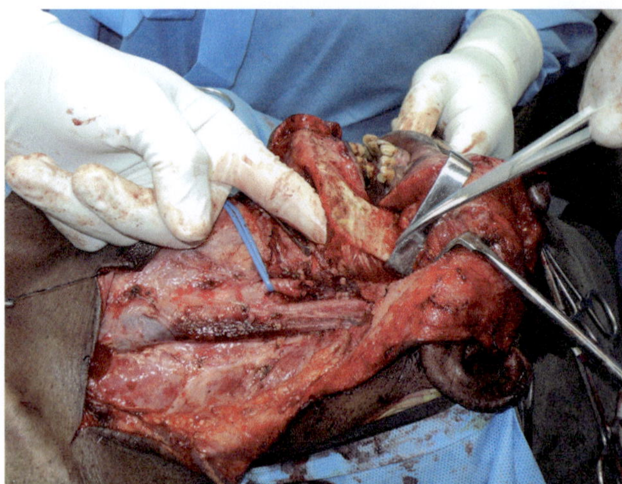

Fig. 13.11 The medial pterygoid muscle is lifted from parapharyngeal space just by inserting finger. This is an avascular plane from where skull base and lateral pterygoid plate can be palpated. This process mobilizes the entire masticator compartment posteriorly. The internal carotid artery is safe below the deep fascia

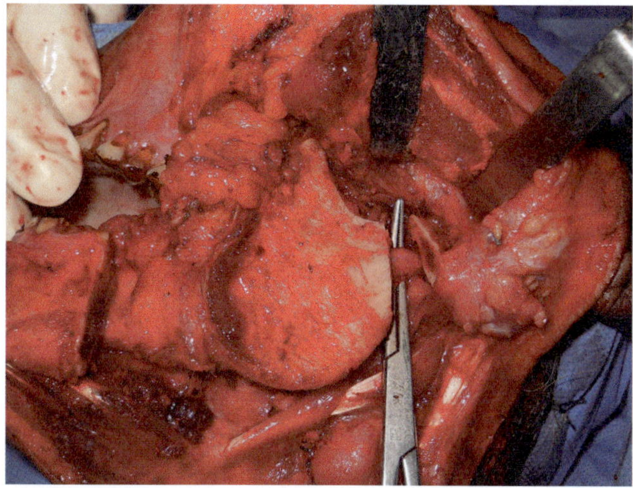

Fig. 13.12 The bone cuts are placed appropriately. The posterior mandible cut is made at sigmoid notch level preserving condyle to expose internal maxillary artery that can be ligated

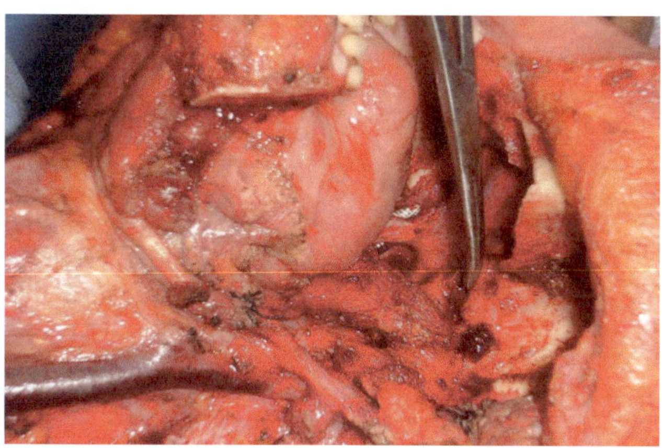

Fig. 13.13 The lateral pterygoid muscle and temporalis muscle are resected from skull base bone. This dissection is done by hugging the skull base bone and this is the single most important step in this process. The dissection is carried out from posterior to anterior direction. There are two areas that bleed heavily. The one is foramen ovale and the other is pterygomaxillary fissure. It is advisable to keep the blood pressure low (80 mmHg) while doing this process, and this really helps in reducing blood loss. We also use bone wax and gelform appropriately to control the bleeding. The bleeding stops immediately once the specimen is removed completely. The bone cuts on maxilla are placed to include both pterygoid plates from its root in the specimen. The photograph shows complete infratemporal fossa clearance with exposed skull bone, pterygomaxillary fissure, and root of pterygoid plates. The carotid artery is rarely at risk as the masticator compartment is mobilized from parapharyngeal space and the artery is safe behind the fascia all the time

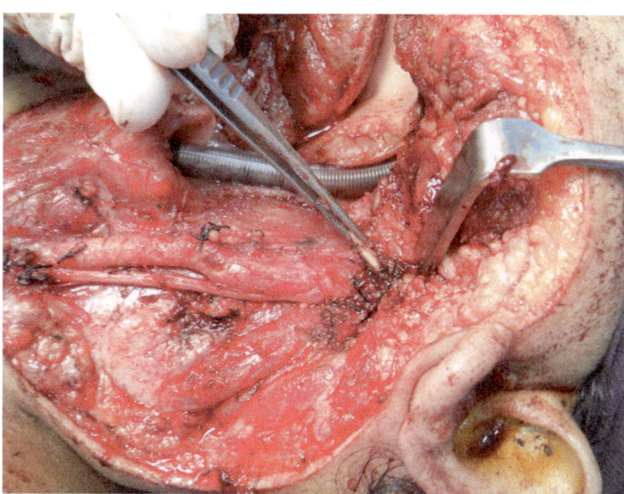

Fig. 13.14 This photograph shows a case where part of the oropharynx and lateral pharyngeal wall was removed. The internal carotid artery passes behind the styloid process and should be isolated at beginning of the procedure

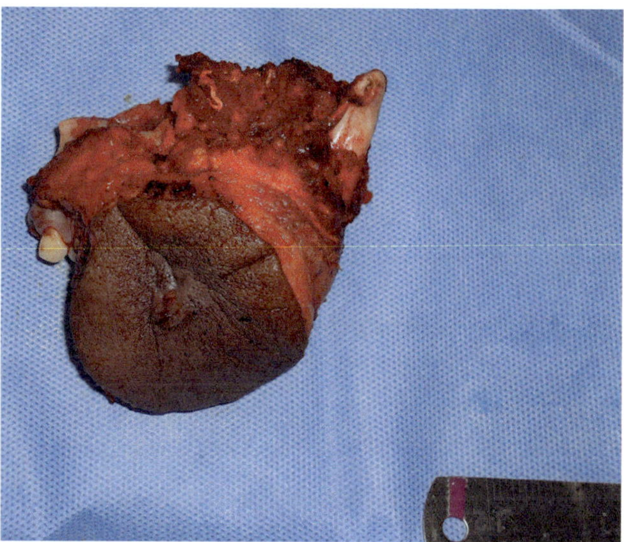

Fig. 13.15 The specimen shows en bloc resection of ITF tissues. One can achieve extra soft tissue margin in ITF for category I tumors that ensures very good local control for this group

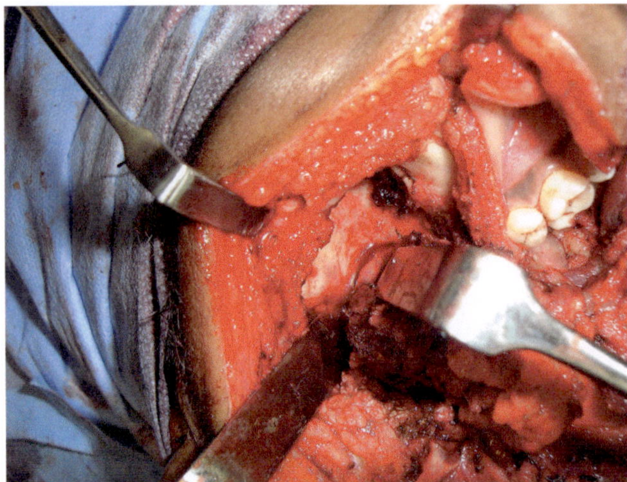

Fig. 13.16 The photograph shows a case where the tumor involved inferior alveolar nerve while entering the foramen ovale. This merits a formal temporal craniotomy to clear the middle cranial fossa but scans showed limited involvement of nerve only in extradural compartment

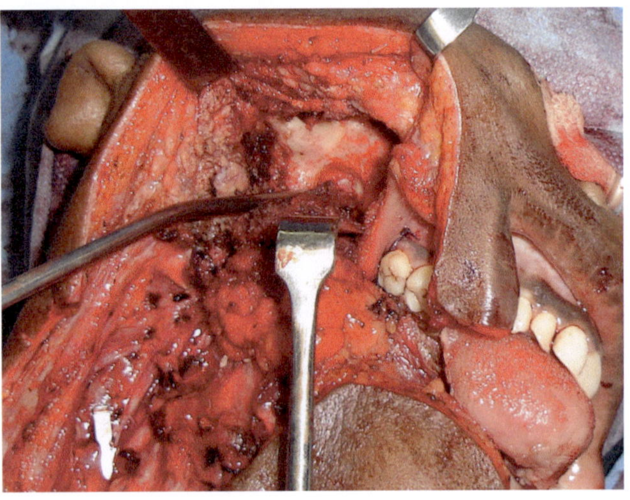

Fig. 13.17 A mini-craniotomy with diamond burr was planned to remove the extradural part of nerve. The margin was sent separately and a clip is left attached at this site for radiation planning

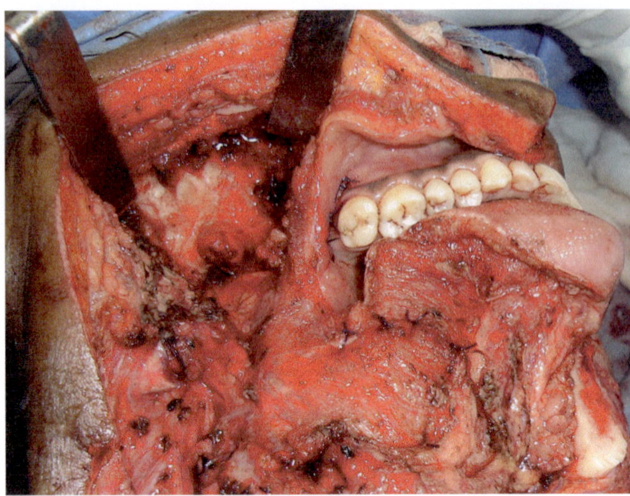

Fig. 13.18 The photograph shows complete resection with no CSF leak. This approach reduces postoperative morbidity and helps in early recovery. The neurosurgeon also prefers this approach for limited spread in intracranial compartment, and exposure is almost always sufficient for them to perform mini-craniotomy

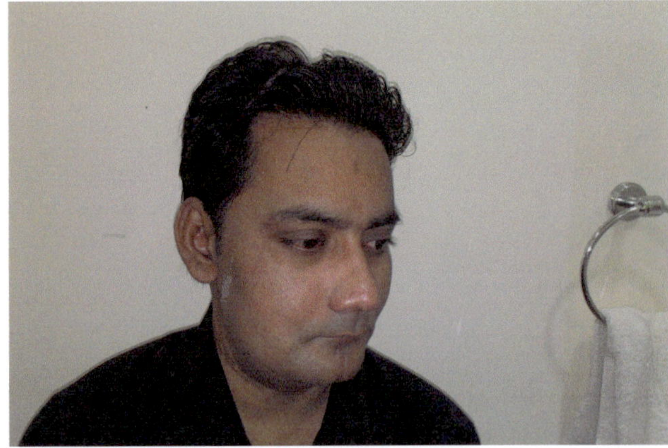

Fig. 13.19 The photograph shows good recovery from such procudure in another patient. The reconstruction was achieved with PMMC flap and functional and cosmetic outcome is quite acceptable. We prefer to use soft tissue flap as most of these patients have trismus

Compartment Surgery for High ITF

This approach is suitable for the majority of category II cases where lateral pterygoid muscle, temporalis muscle, and pterygoid plates are involved. We have tried this approach for category III-A) tumors and have found decent outcome (about 50 % local control in 22 patients). We offer category III-A) patients this surgical procedure but it is advisable to have a good imaging study to rule out intracranial extension.

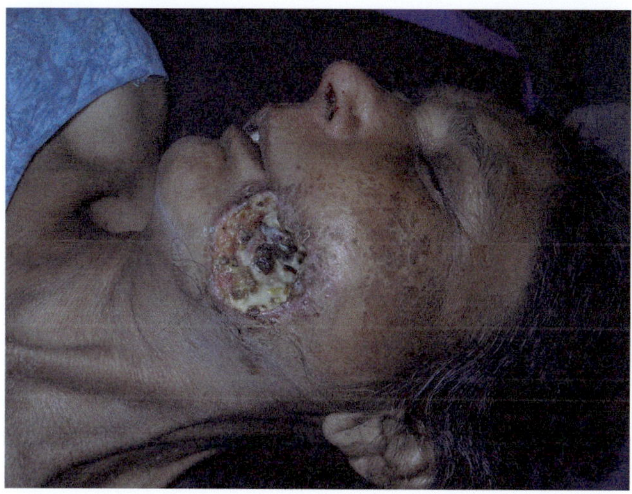

Fig. 13.20 Photograph showing extensive buccal mucosa cancer with category II involvement of masticator space. It is interesting to note that The neck is NO even for such large primary tumour. This points towards a disease pattern that favours local spread compared to distant spread. These patients need aggressive surgical approach and have realistic chance of cure with three-dimensional clearance

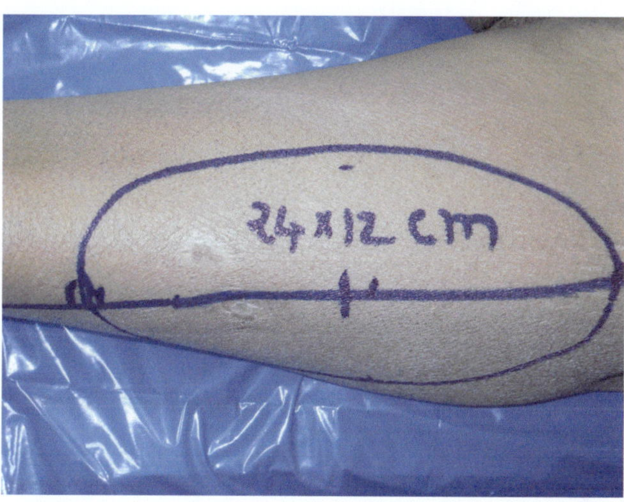

Fig. 13.22 The ALT flap is marked. This flap is most suited for such complex defects. Alternative is to perform double flap reconstruction that may not be feasible in majority of centers. Sometimes these defects can also be reconstructed with spiral PMMC flap

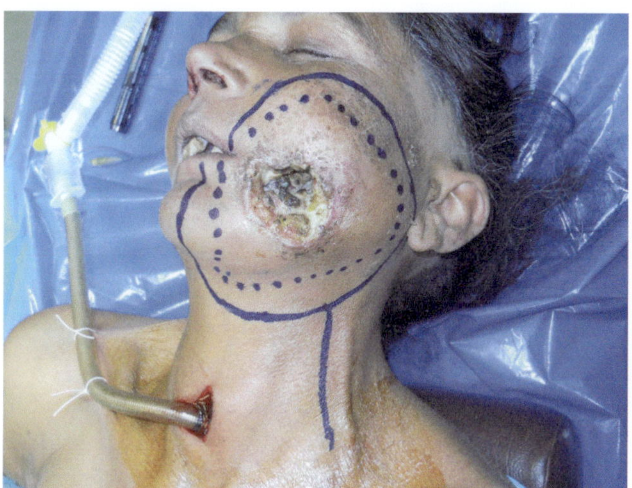

Fig. 13.21 Tumor induration and edema are always included in resection margins as a policy

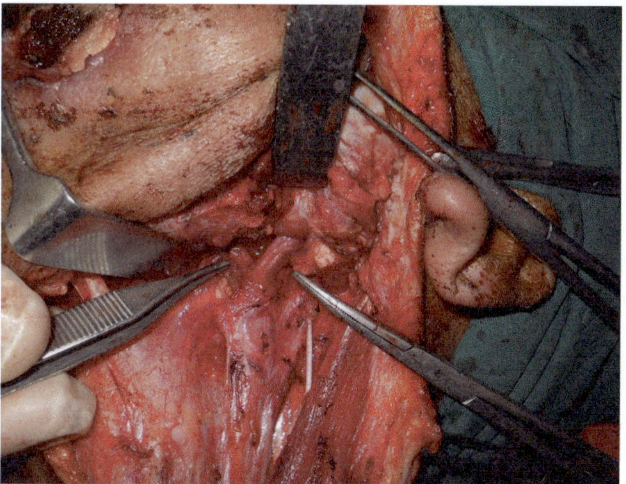

Fig. 13.23 The initial steps are similar to the procedure described for low ITF. This photograph shows external carotid artery entering deep lobe of parotid and also shows mobilization of masticator compartment from parapharyngeal space. It is advisable to preserve external carotid artery if possible to preserve superficial temporal artery. The forehead flap can be of great use in case of flap failure and can be used in combination with PMMC to salvage the situation. These are complex cases and one should have a backup plan ready for all situations

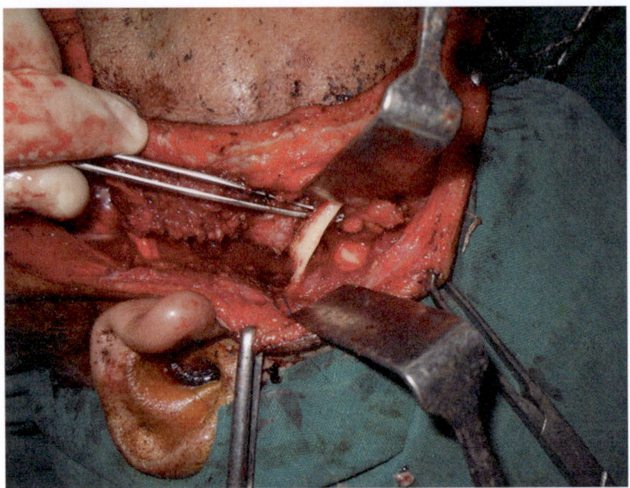

Fig. 13.24 The upper extent of ITF resection goes above the zygoma in this instance. The zygoma is exposed, taking care not to damage the eye branch of facial nerve. The nerve is sacrificed if skin infiltration needs resection of that area. This can be rehabilitated with simple procedures like gold weight implants if needed. The osteotomy is placed at the proposed site

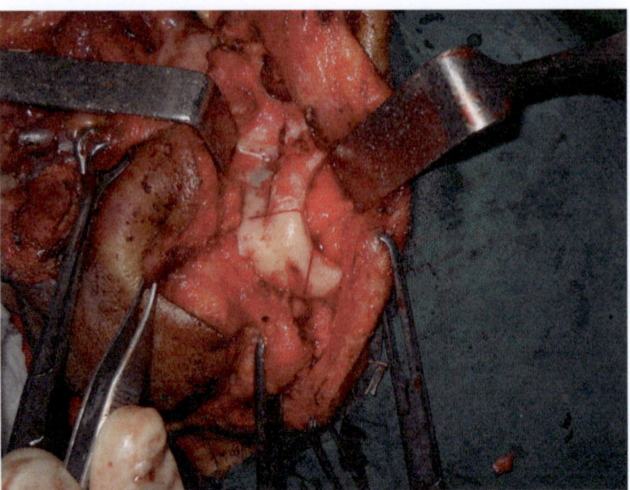

Fig. 13.26 The remaining osteotomies are performed like infrastructure maxillectomy procedure. This way one can preserve almost the entire orbital floor with rim but can include inferior orbital fissure and lower half of pterygomaxillary fissure in specimen

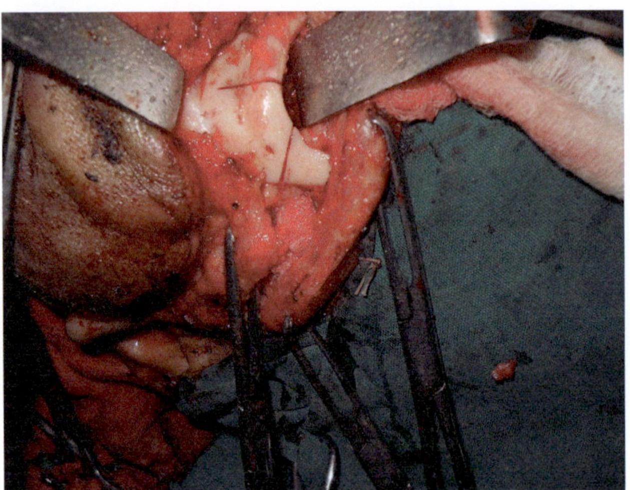

Fig. 13.25 These osteotomies are placed at fronto-orbito-zygomatic suture and in orbital floor. The osteotomy in orbital floor runs through the inferior orbital fissure

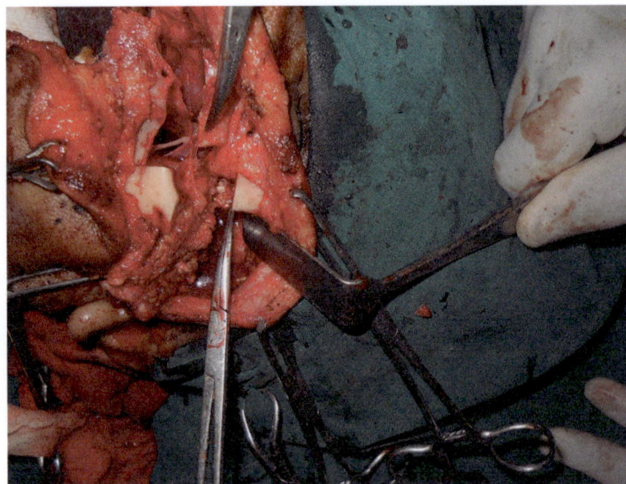

Fig. 13.27 The maxilla is pulled down to expose temporalis muscle that is transected at the level of sphenoid bone

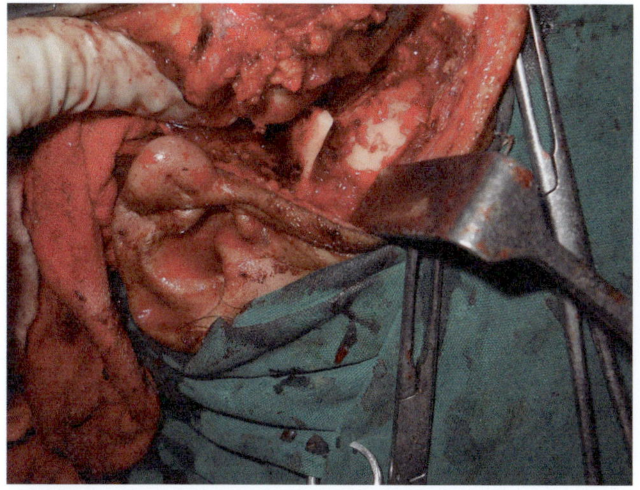

Fig. 13.28 The sphenoid bone is exposed completely by separating the temporalis first and then the lateral pterygoid muscle. One can expose the root of pterygoid plates with this mobilization and osteotomy is placed here

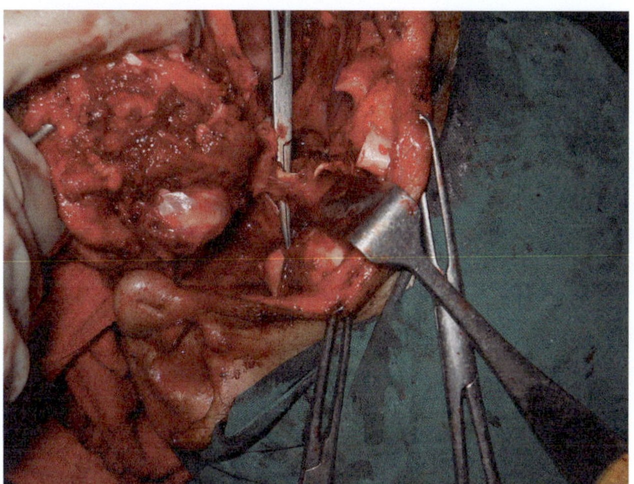

Fig. 13.29 The osteotomy passes through pterygomaxillary fissure including the entire pterygoid plates in specimen. The photograph shows contents of fissure that passes through infraorbital fissure. These are sent separately to understand margin clearance and clips are placed for adjuvant radiotherapy boost. The carotid artery enters the skull base about 1 cm posterior to foramen ovale and if one can stay anterior to foramen ovale, the artery remains safe during entire procedure. The inferior alveolar nerve entering this foramen serves as good guide to anatomy

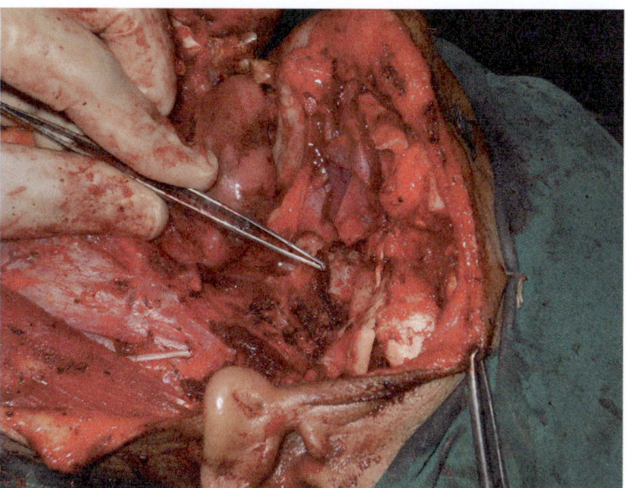

Fig. 13.30 The photograph shows complete clearance at skull base and also shows resected root of pterygoid plates

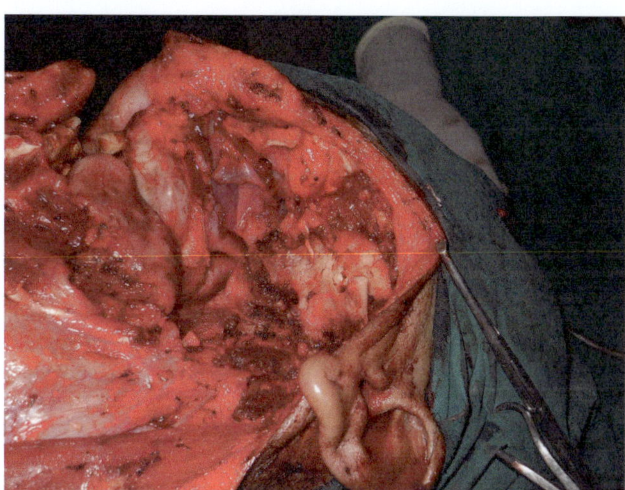

Fig. 13.31 The photograph shows complete clearance of the entire skull base. The tumor will recur only if it has spread in intracranial compartment through one of the fissures or foramens

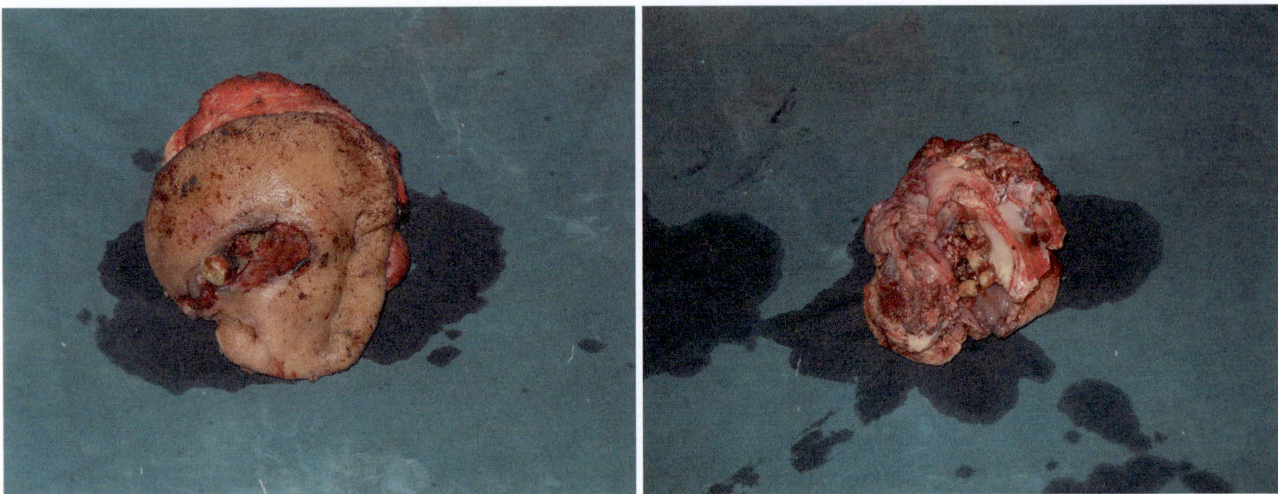

Figs. 13.32 and 13.33 The resected specimen shows adequate margins

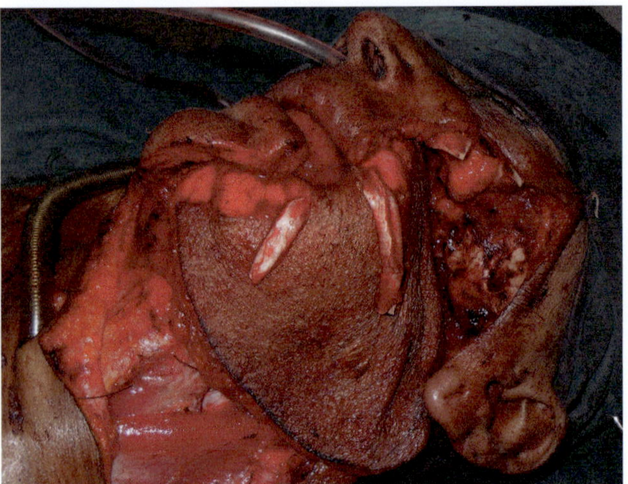

Fig. 13.34 The reconstruction was achieved by bi-paddled ALT flap. Sling of fascia lata was used to reconstruct angle of the mouth

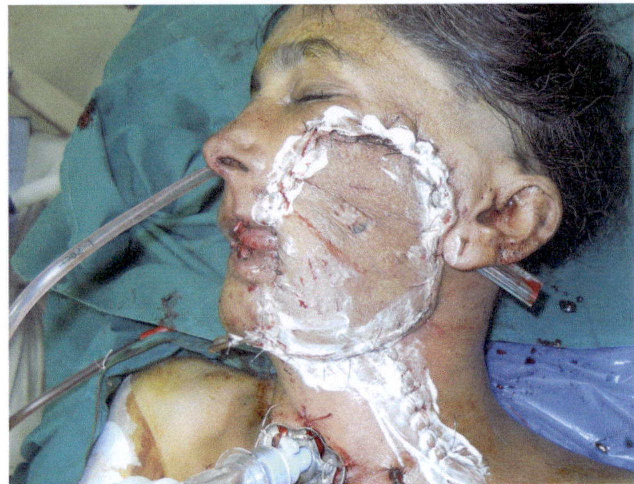

Fig. 13.35 The immediate postoperative picture. This procedure was carried out in a rural clinic in India with basic facilities and no postoperative ICU facility. It is important to realize that if surgical concepts are understood, this is a relatively safe procedure and can be performed in any environment

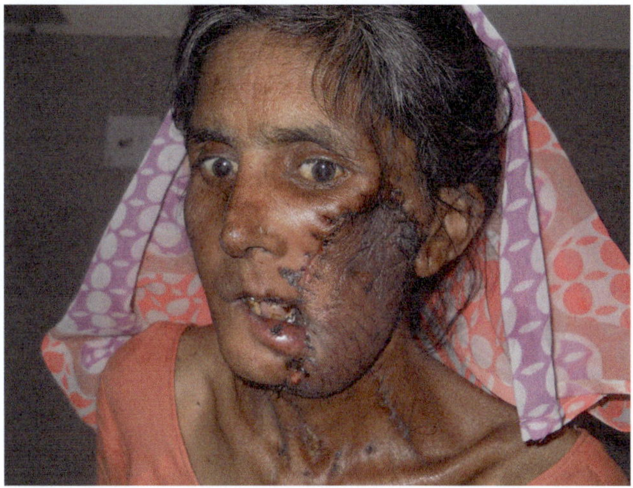

Fig. 13.36 Patient after 15 days of surgery. The feeding tube is out and she has started taking oral semisolid foods. These patients recover quickly as defect is lateralized and doesn't interfere with swallowing or speech function

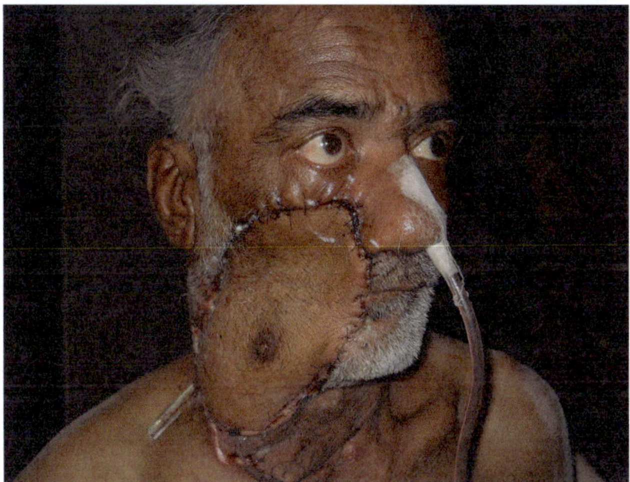

Fig. 13.37 Similar patient with spiral PMMC flap reconstruction

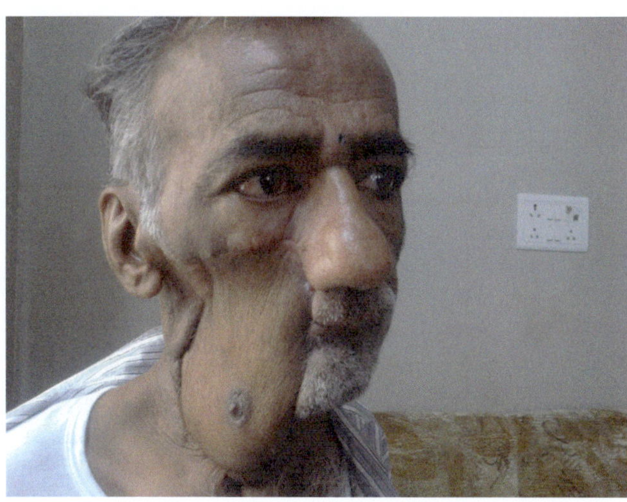

Fig. 13.38 The same patient after 1 year of completion of treatment. This is not the most ideal reconstruction but nevertheless a very simple, reliable, and functionally effective way of reconstruction. This is quite cost-effective and can be used in limited setting

Maxillary Sinus Cancer with ITF Involvement

The cancer involving posterior part of the maxilla has tendency to pierce posterolateral wall and spread into pterygoid muscles (Fig. 13.39). It is very difficult to approach these tumors anteriorly and the tumor often comes out in pieces. This results in leaving behind gross residual disease in many cases. The posterior or transmandibular approach is better suited for these cancers and provides an opportunity to achieve en bloc three-dimensional resection. This approach is again in accordance with compartment approach where the aim is to remove the entire ITF compartment along with the maxilla.

It is essential to perform transmandibular approach to clear posterior soft tissue in ITF. The paramedian mandibulotomy approach has been developed for this purpose and provides good exposure. However, this approach is associated with postoperative complications like severe trismus and plate exposures. We have developed angle mandibulectomy concept that is similar in concept but aims to remove small lateral segment of mandible to avoid abovementioned complications.

- Mandibulotomy approach
- Angle mandibulectomy approach

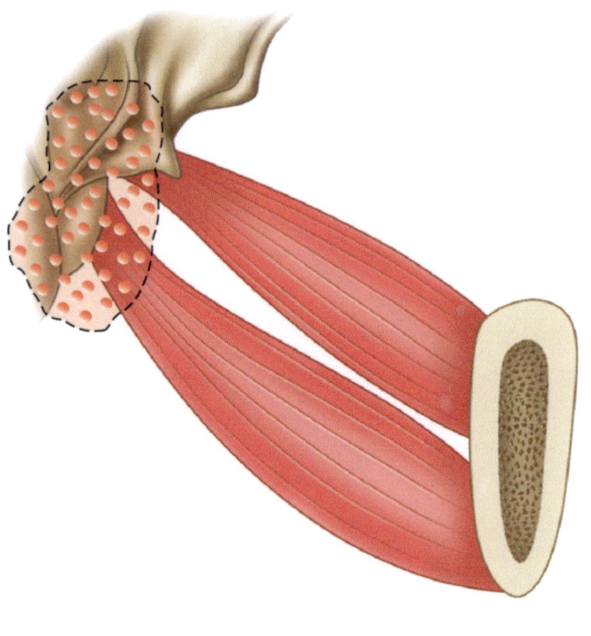

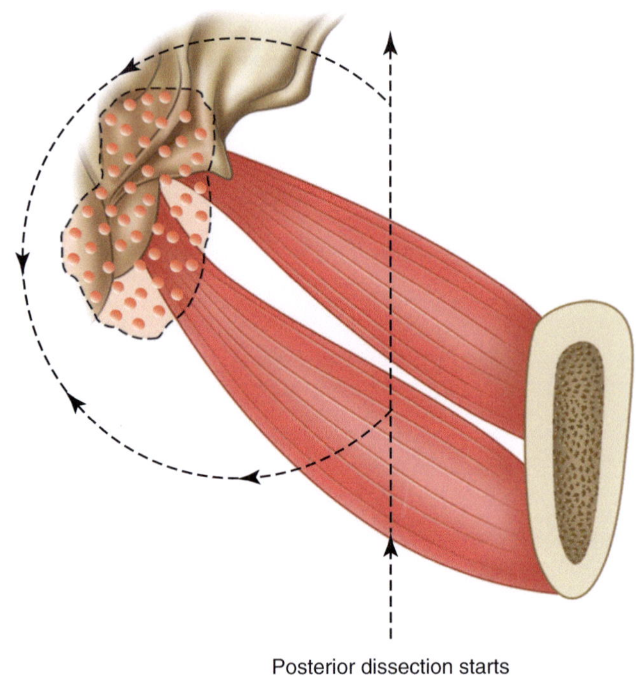

Fig. 13.39 Maxillary sinus cancer with ITF involvement

Mandibulotomy Approach

We prefer to perform selective neck dissection in all cases as the neck is already exposed. The reconstruction can be achieved by radial forearm free flap in such cases, and mandibulotomy can be closed by miniplates. The cosmetic outcome is generally very acceptable. These patients receive adjuvant radiotherapy and have a chance of developing severe trismus and sometimes plate-related complications.

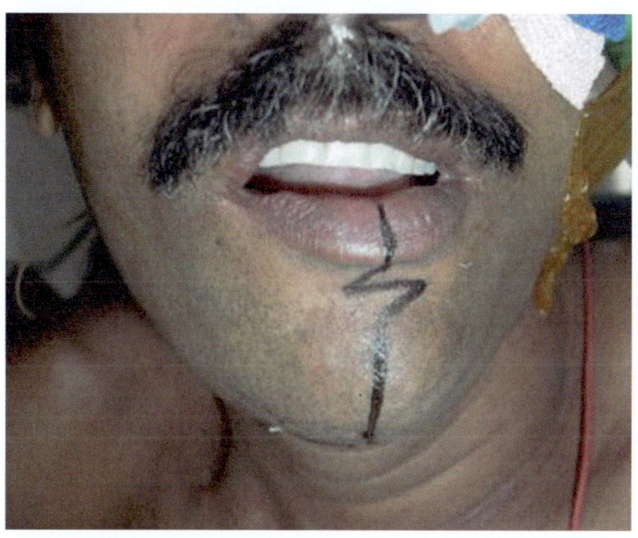

Fig. 13.40 The photograph shows planned midline lip split approach. The incision can be placed with or without step-plasty

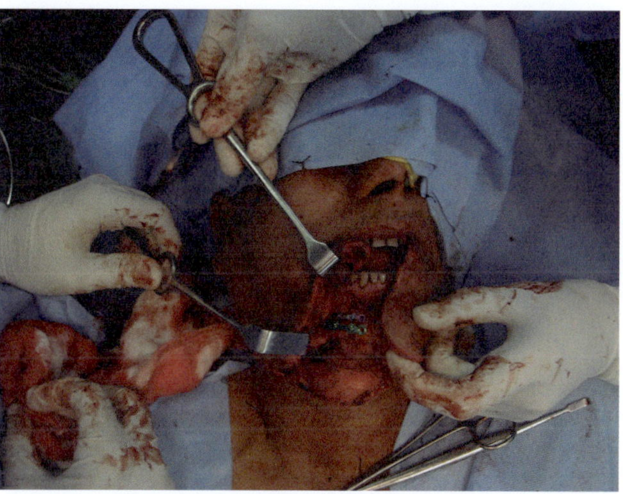

Fig. 13.42 The flap is raised only to expose paramedian mandibulotomy site. Miniplates are preadapted at proposed osteotomy site. One has to be careful not to raise the entire cheek flap to preserve blood supply to the mandible

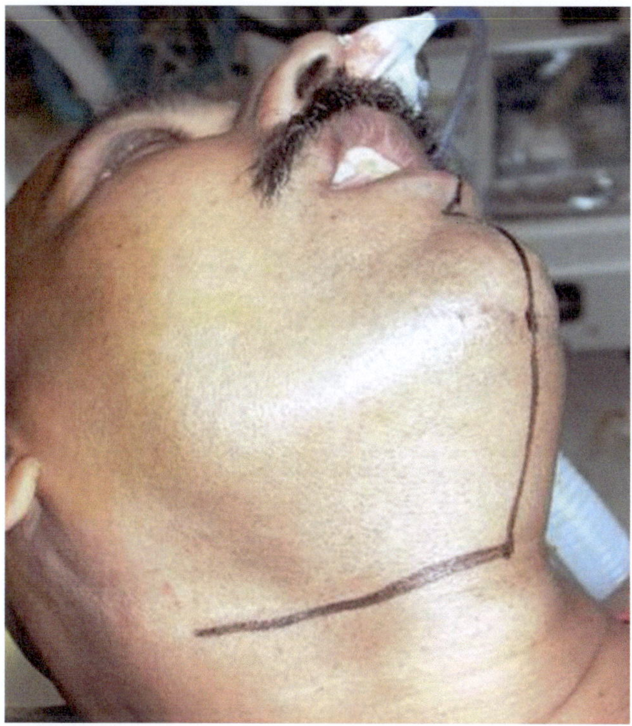

Fig. 13.41 The photograph shows transverse extension of the incision

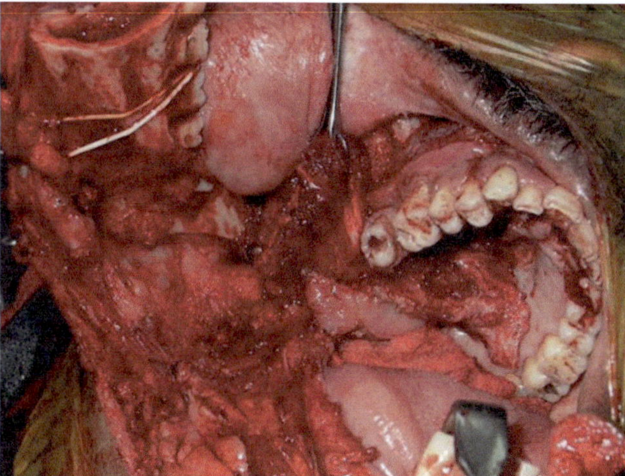

Fig. 13.43 Mandibulotomy is done and the mandible is swung out. The mylohyoid muscle is transected and mucosal cuts are placed to achieve this. The lingual nerve serves as a guide to incision placement and should be preserved in the entire length. The medial pterygoid muscle is separated from the mandible in posterior part. The inferior alveolar nerve is identified and preserved in the entire length

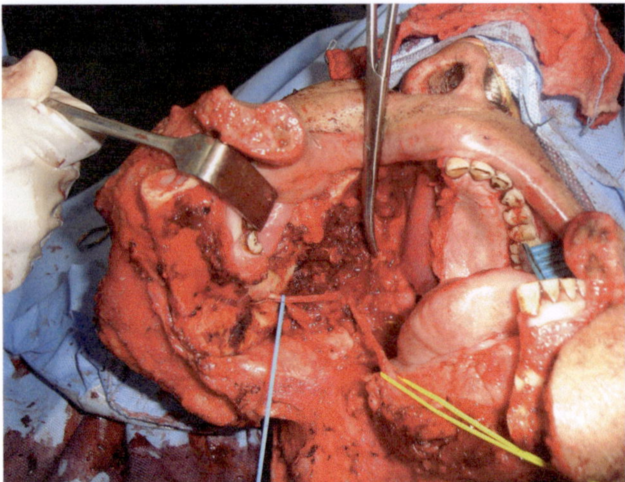

Fig. 13.44 The photograph shows a completed resection. The pterygoid muscles are transected from the mandible, and both the lingual nerve and inferior alveolar nerves can serve as a guide to this. All the muscles anterior to these nerves are included in the specimen, and dissection goes till skull base and foramen ovale as shown in this picture. The internal maxillary artery is identified between pterygoid muscles and ligated early in the procedure to reduce bleeding. The entire posterior compartment is mobilized first before placing appropriate maxillectomy cuts. The pointer is showing resected portion of pterygoid plate

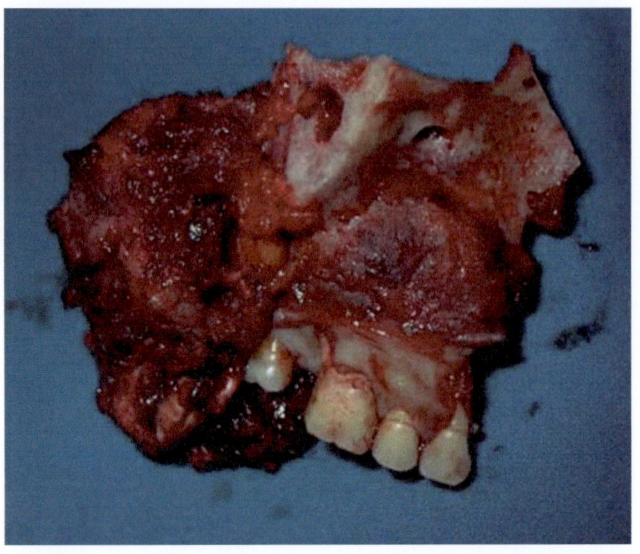

Fig. 13.45 This is an en bloc resection with complete posterior clearance. It is not possible to achieve such clearance with anterior approach

Angle Mandibulectomy Approach

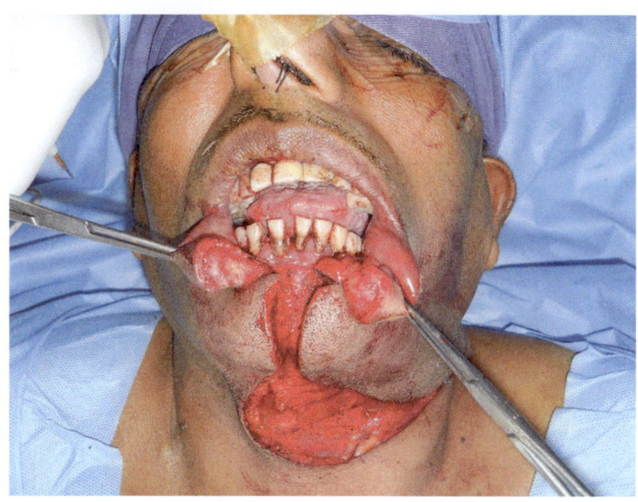

Fig. 13.46 The midline lip split incision is placed

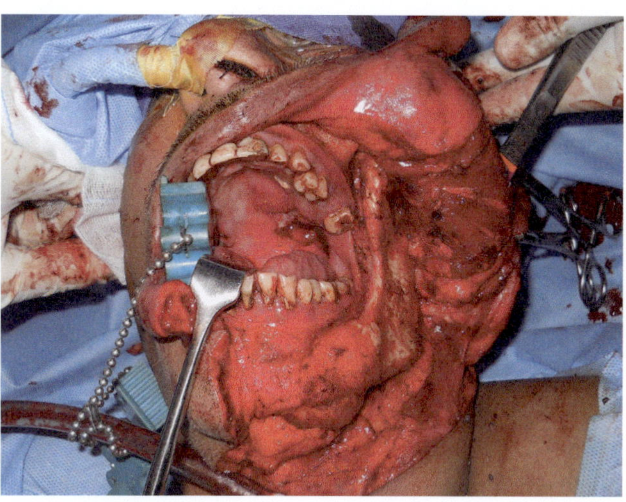

Fig. 13.49 The patient had severe trismus and the posterior maxillary lesion was not visible clearly preoperatively. One can see the lesion more clearly in this photograph

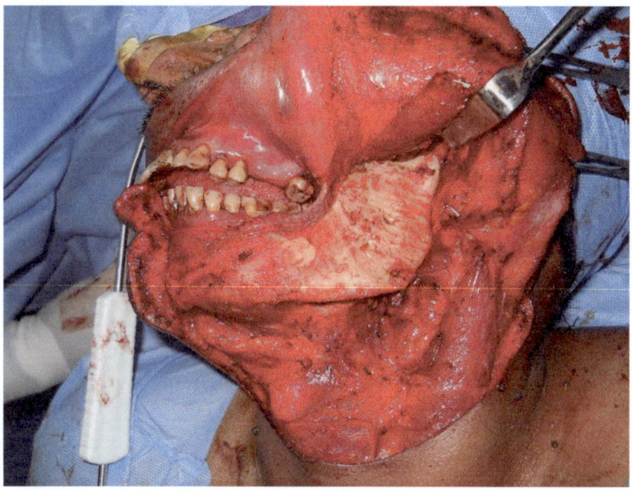

Fig. 13.47 The cheek flap is raised in the entire length to expose the angle of mandible and sigmoid notch. The masseter muscle is included in the flap. This provides exposure for limited segmental resection at the angle

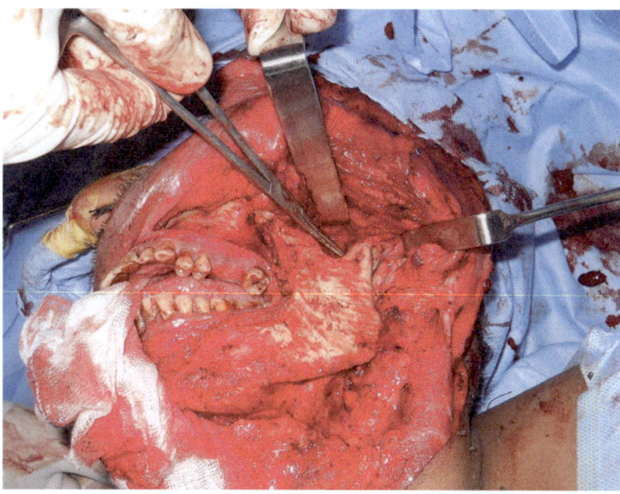

Fig. 13.50 The proposed site for osteotomy, the condyle is preserved

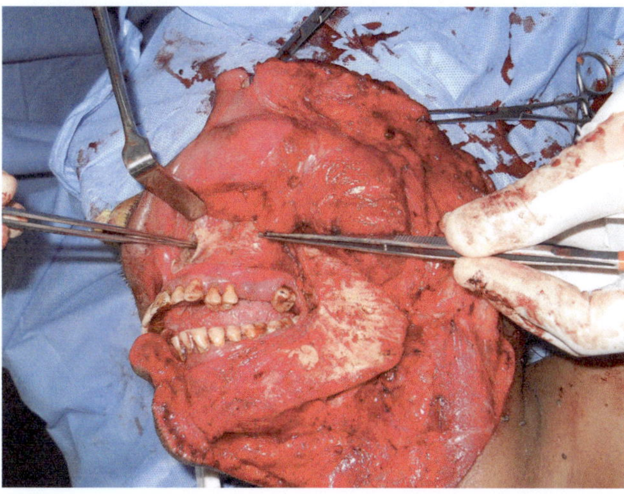

Fig. 13.48 The cheek flap is raised further to expose the maxilla

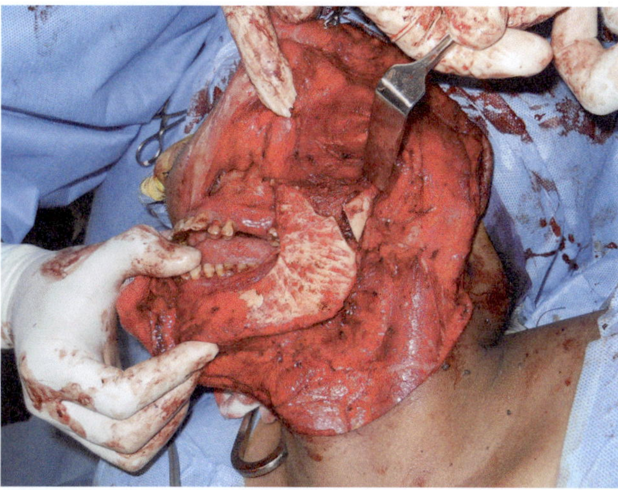

Fig. 13.51 The subcondylar osteotomy is completed

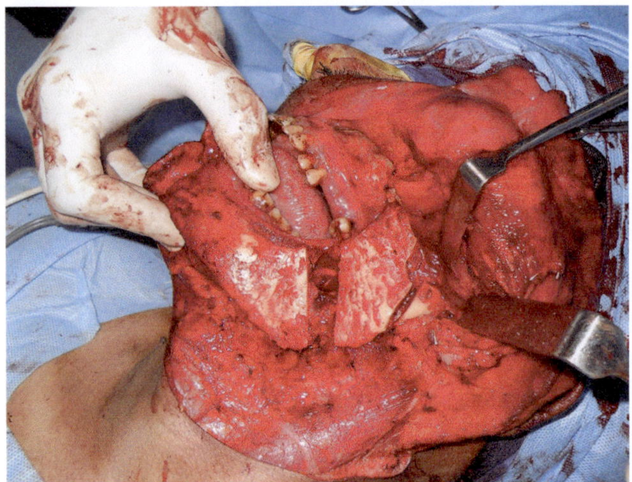

Fig. 13.52 The other osteotomy is performed to include 1–2 cm segment of the mandible including the coronoid process. This works as a pathological fracture and prevents postoperative trismus without compromising severely on occlusion

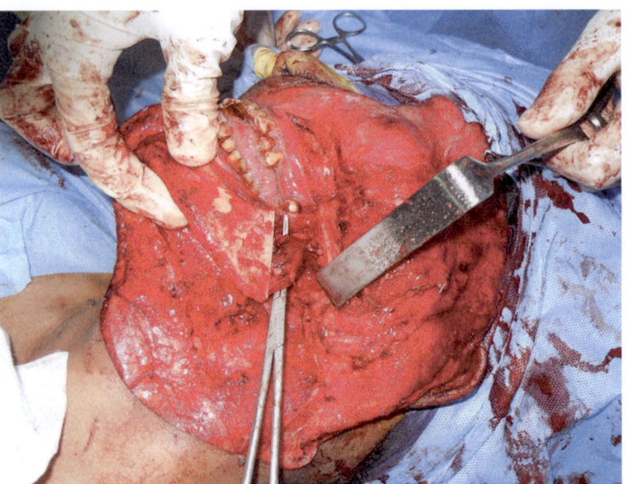

Fig. 13.53 The medial pterygoid muscle is divided

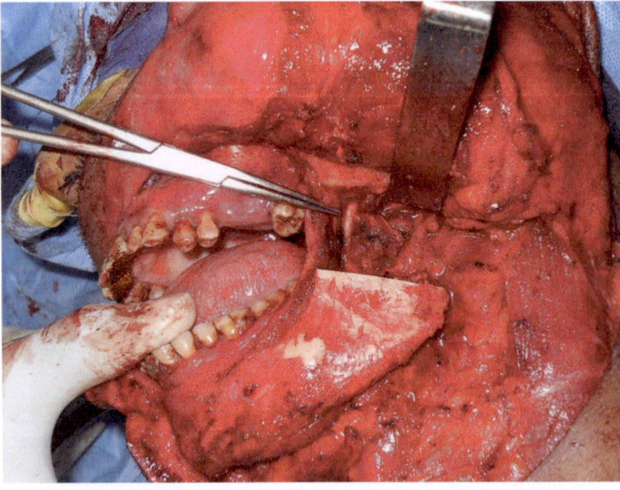

Fig. 13.54 One can see the inferior alveolar nerve and that is traced further up till the foramen ovale

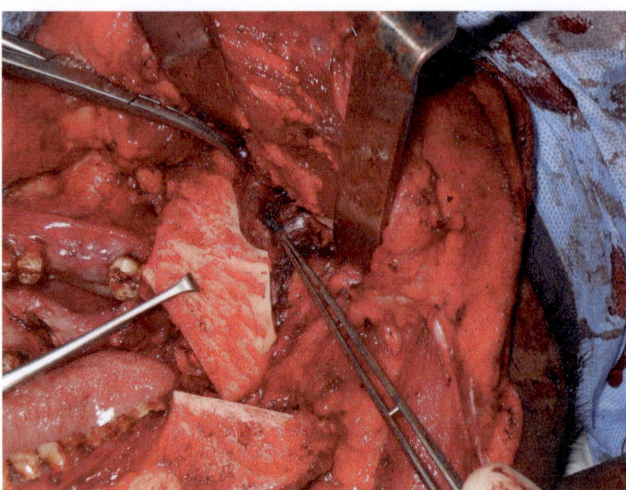

Fig. 13.55 A ligated internal maxillary artery and exposed lateral pterygoid muscle

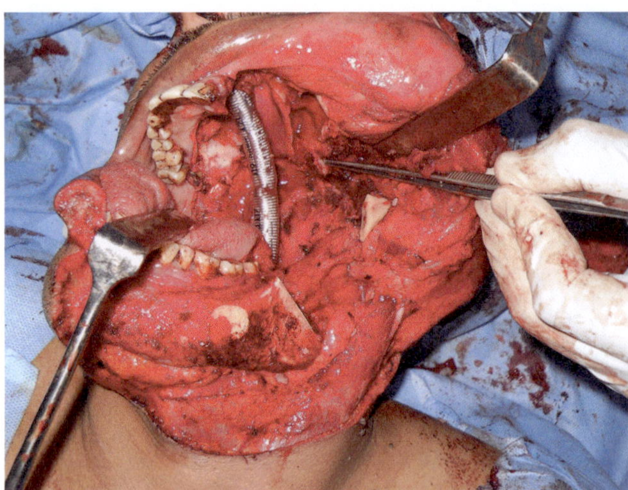

Fig. 13.56 The entire ITF is cleared in a similar manner as described in this chapter. The dissection is carried out next to the skull and all the tissue anterior to the foramen ovale is included in the specimen. The maxillectomy cuts are placed last to deliver complete specimen

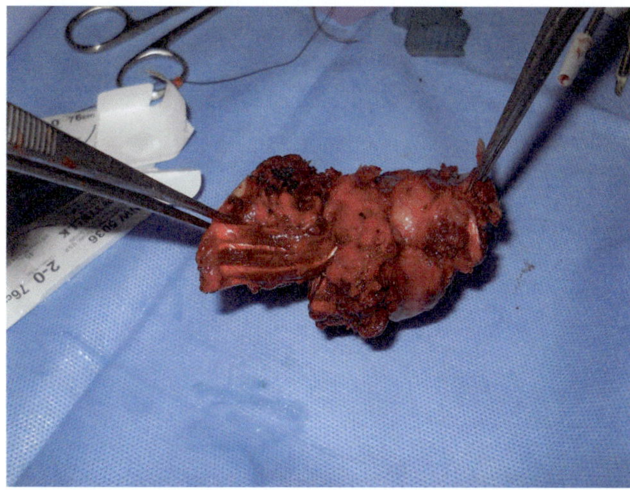

Fig. 13.57 The photograph shows the posterior maxilla containing the tumor where pterygoid muscles are inserted. We can also see the pterygoid muscles in entire length till its insertion in the mandible. This approach gives best posterior clearance that is necessary for such lesions

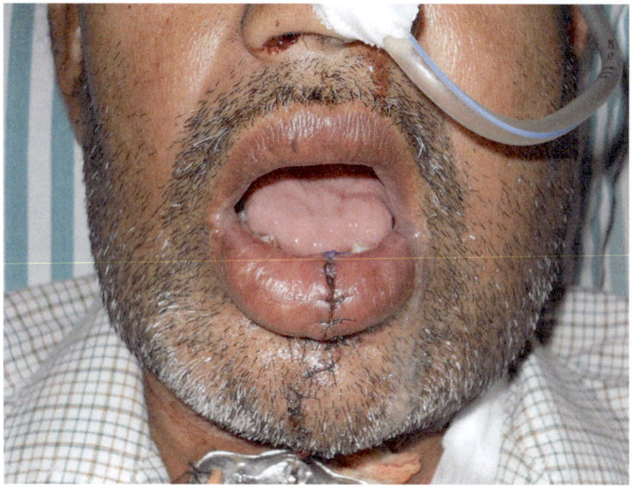

Fig. 13.58 The postoperative photograph showing good mouth opening

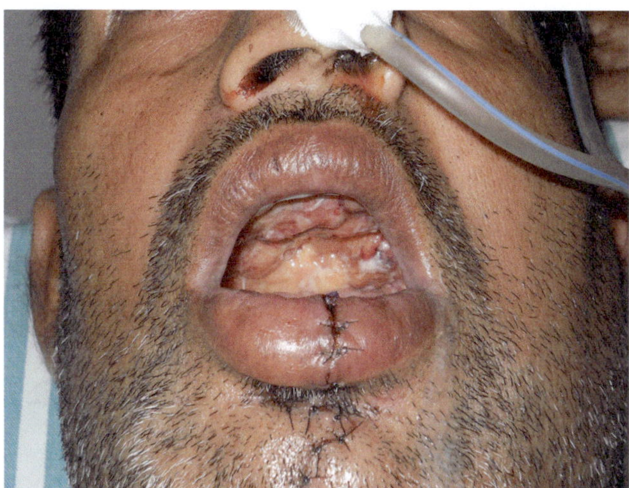

Fig. 13.59 Reconstruction was achieved with fascia only ALT flap

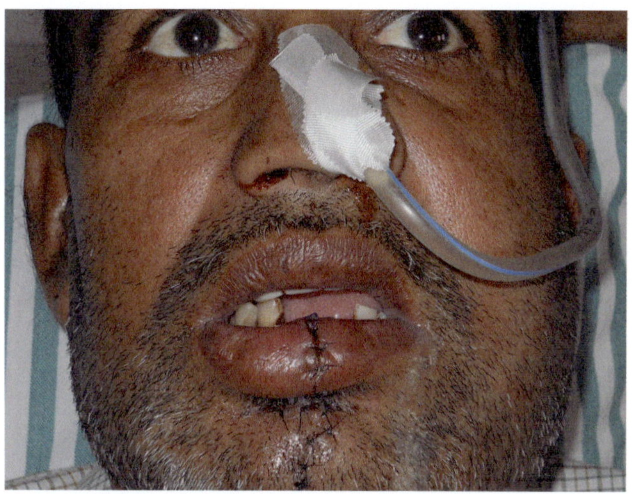

Fig. 13.60 The photograph shows good occlusion without significant jaw deviation

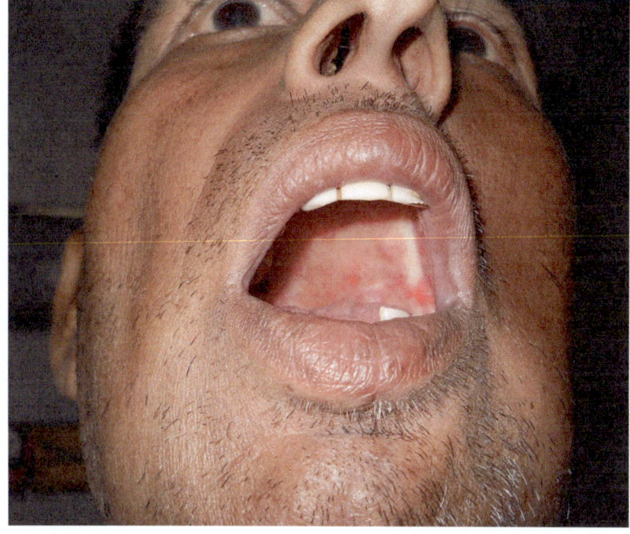

Fig. 13.61 Result after 1 year of completion of the entire treatment. Completely healed flap with very good mouth opening is seen in this photograph

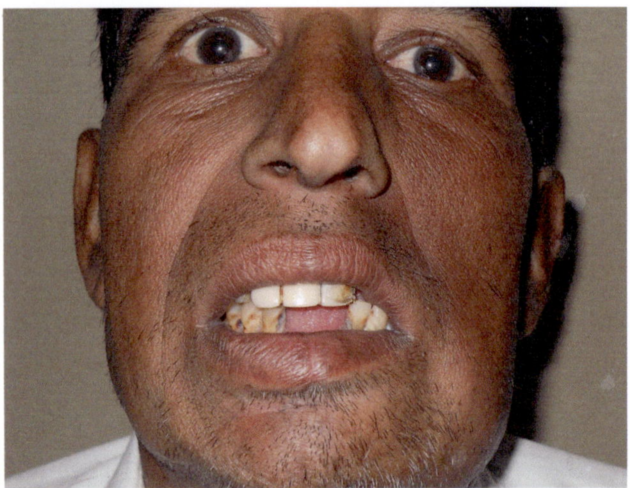

Fig. 13.62 The occlusion is quite acceptable. This patient can eat hard food without any problem

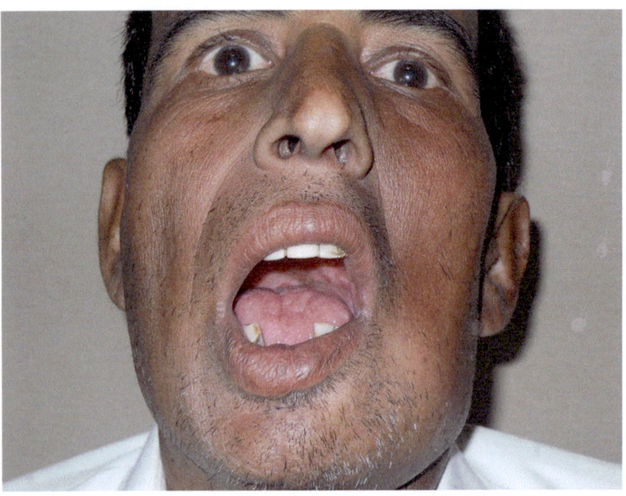

Fig. 13.63 The photograph is showing adequate mouth opening even after adjuvant CTRT. There is a slight jaw deviation when the mouth is opened, but this doesn't hamper the function in anyway. Avoiding trismus is a major challenge and we routinely prefer this over the paramedian mandibulotomy approach in current practice

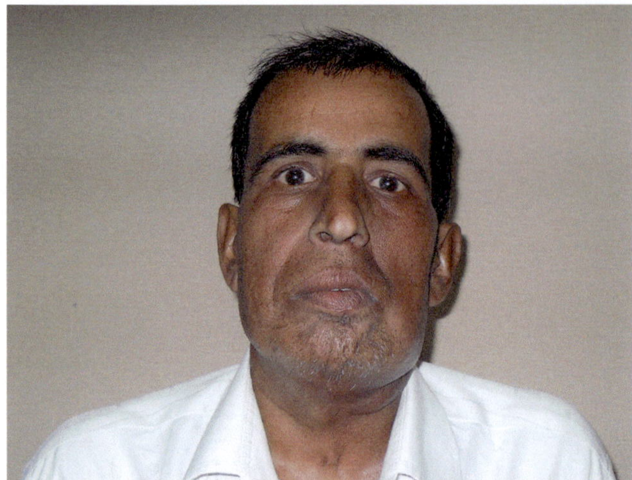

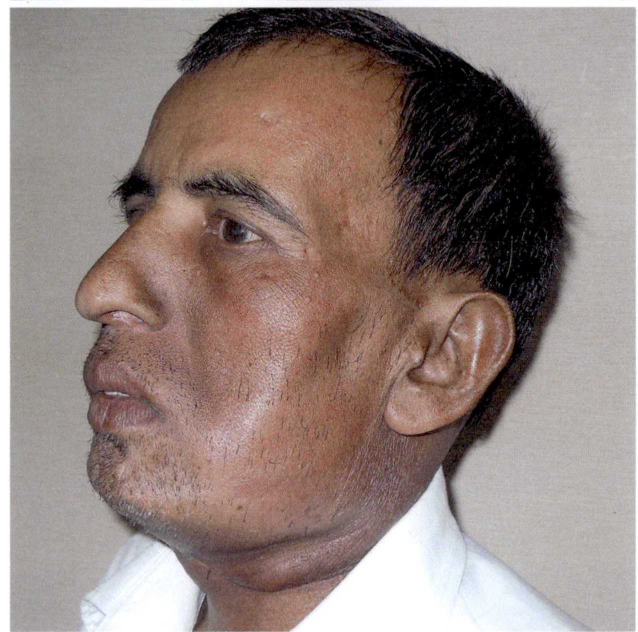

Figs. 13.64 and 13.65 The final cosmetic outcome is also quite acceptable

References

1. Calabrese L, Giugliano G, Bruschini R, et al. Compartmental surgery in tongue tumours: description of a new surgical technique. Acta Otorhinolaryngol Ital. 2009;29(5):259–64.
2. Calabrese L, Bruschini R, Giugliano G, et al. Compartmental tongue surgery: ong term oncologic results in the treatment of tongue cancer. Oral Oncol. 2011;47(3):174–9.
3. Trivedi NP, Kekatpure V, Kuriakose MA. Radical (compartment) resection for advanced buccal cancer involving masticator space (T4b): our experience in thirty patients. Clin Otolaryngol. 2012; 37(6):477–83.
4. Trivedi NP, Kekatpure V, Kuriakose MA, et al. The pathology of buccal mucosa cancer involving masticator space. (Accepted for publication in IJC).

14 Treatment of Very Advanced Stage Head and Neck Cancer

Approximately 50–60 % cases of head and neck cancer present in advanced stage in developing world. The conventional TNM staging considers only limited factors, and it is not feasible to group every advanced cancer in the same group. There are various factors that predict biological behavior that can be of great help in treating these tumors. The treatment of such cases needs clear philosophy, and choices need to be rational to avoid catastrophic outcome. These patients are often miserable due to constant pain, fungation, and bleeding and deserve good care. Majority of these patients are treated with palliative intent considering them either inoperable or borderline operable without actually considering possibility of cure. It is also essential to realize that these patients are actually at very advanced stage and surgery remains the only realistic chance of cure. Any other treatment including chemoradiotherapy essentially remains a palliative option. We have developed a rational approach to treat these patients that is discussed in this chapter.

Guidelines for Very Advanced Cases

The conventional classification system stages all cases of T4 in one group, and this doesn't help in treatment decision planning. It is important to assess these patients individually and also to have some rational guidelines to maintain consistency in treatment. We follow the guideline demonstrated in Fig. 14.1. The aim is to assess biology of disease and prognosis of patient before deciding on treatment options. The cases that present de novo have best prognosis, while patients with recurrent disease have inferior outcome. Many patients present with inappropriate first treatment and they actually fare better compared to recurrent disease that came back after complete treatment. The primary tumors can be broadly classified in two sections. The one class of patients has large primary disease with very limited nodal disease (gingivobuccal sulcus, PNS), and this indicates aggressive disease at local site with limited tendency to distant spread. We prefer to offer aggressive surgical option to this group and have obtained very good long-term results. The other group with large nodal disease has high tendency for regional and distant failure, and this fact should be kept in mind while making treatment selection. The palliative surgery has an important role for select group of patients who has limited local disease that is affecting their quality of life (QOL) and can be addressed by simple surgical procedure. It is important to remember what you wish to palliate while making such choice.

N. Trivedi, *Atlas of Head and Neck Cancer Surgery: The Compartment Surgery for Resection in 3-D*, DOI 10.1007/978-81-322-2050-3_14, © Springer India 2015

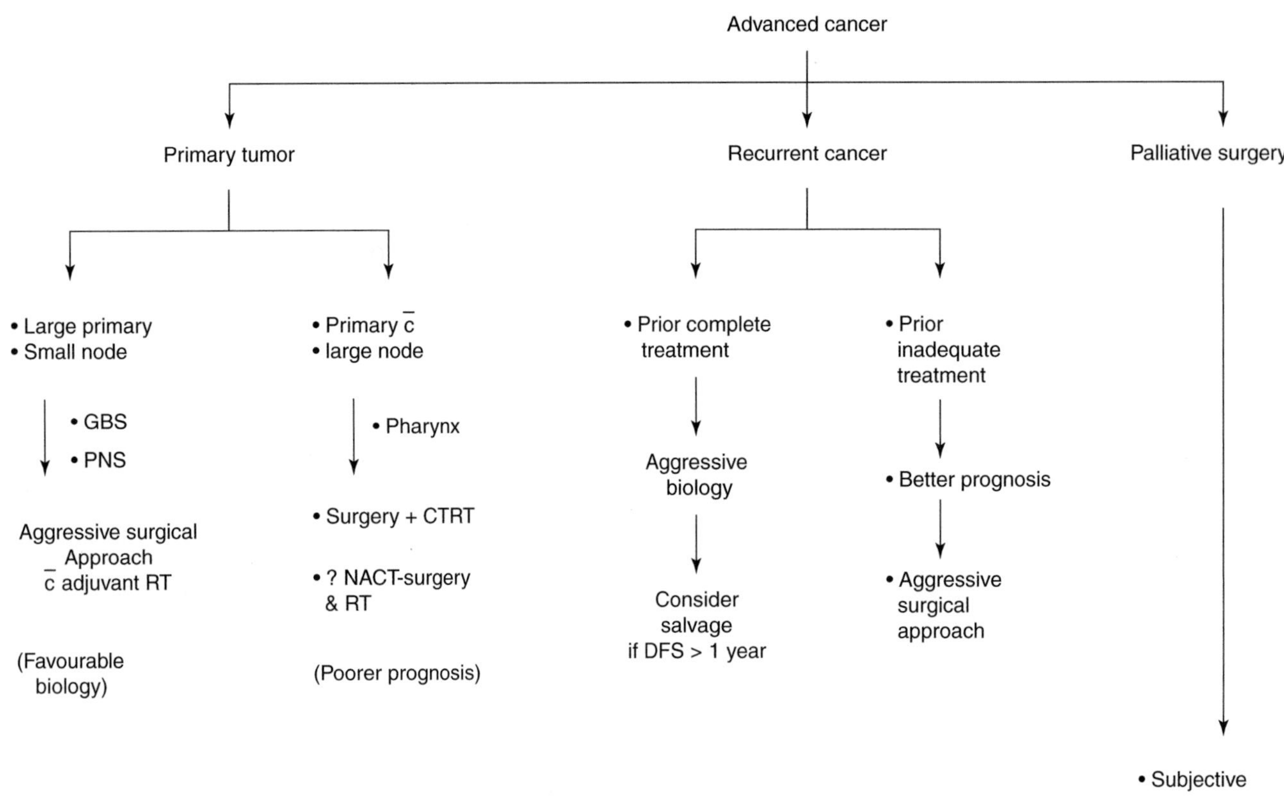

Fig. 14.1 Advanced head and neck cancer – concepts for treatment approach

Tumors Without Previous Treatment

These patients have the best prognosis among all advanced cancers. They can be grouped broadly into two, one of which has favorable biology than the other. Few subsites like gingivo-buccal sulcus cancer and PNS cancer have a tendency to grow locally with limited nodal spread, and these patients have good outcome if local treatment is adequate. The other group where large nodal mass is the main presentation has high rate of regional and distant failure and one needs to have rational approach for their treatment. Even with their comparably poor outcome, surgery remains the mainstay treatment for truly advanced cancers.

Achieving negative three-dimensional margins remains the most important prognostic factor for patients receiving surgery. This holds true even for very advanced cancers. The concept of compartment surgery applies for these tumors as discussed in this book. This concept has added consistency in achieving negative margins for large tumors involving soft tissue at depth. All the surgeons treat cases like these in their practice and have reasonable results. They would treat them more aggressively and consistently if an approach delivers negative margins regularly. The aim of any surgery is to achieve good local control and if one can remove all cells with potential to harbour cancer cells, this can be achieved. The concept of compartment resection has been practiced for about 5 years in our institute, and we feel confident about achieving good local control in majority of these cases. Improved options for reconstruction with microvascular technique have made these approaches more feasible.

The treatment of advanced and complex cases needs different considerations for each site. These are discussed in subsequent sections:

- Buccal mucosa and alveolus cancer
- Tongue and floor of mouth cancer
- Oropharynx cancer
- Neck cancer

Buccal–alveolus complex cancer

- Cancer with extensive skin infiltration and surrounding edema
- High ITF with extensive skin involvement
- Patient requiring double flap reconstruction

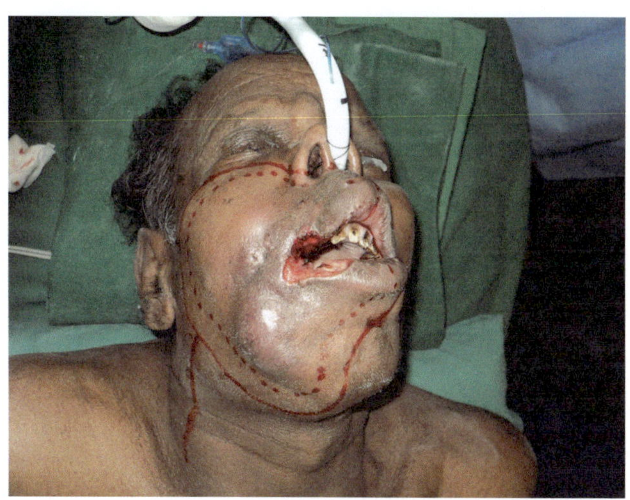

Fig. 14.2 Patient with extensive skin infiltration, involving the entire upper and lower lip with surrounding edema. This is an inoperable case for majority of centers. It is interesting to note that it doesn't involve any structures that are strictly nonremovable and he has no neck nodes. If we can remove the entire tumor with negative margins, we may have good outcome

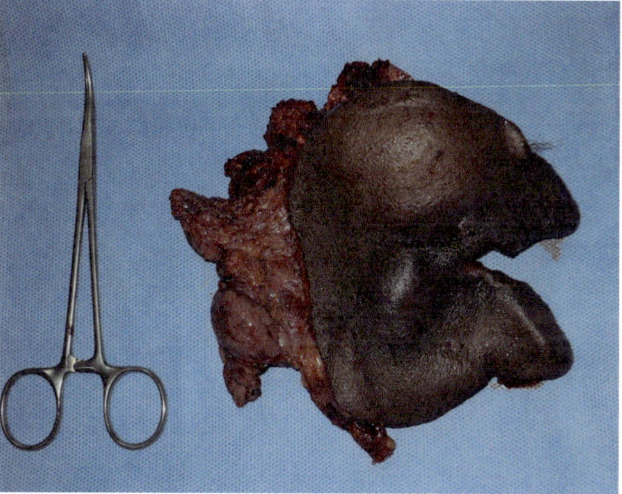

Fig. 14.3 Resected specimen with adequate skin margins. Always try to include surrounding edema and redness in resection margin

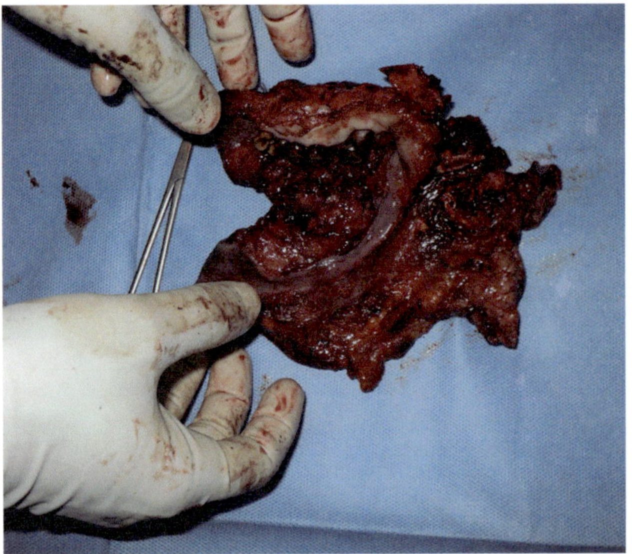

Fig. 14.4 Adequate mucosal margins are shown in the specimen

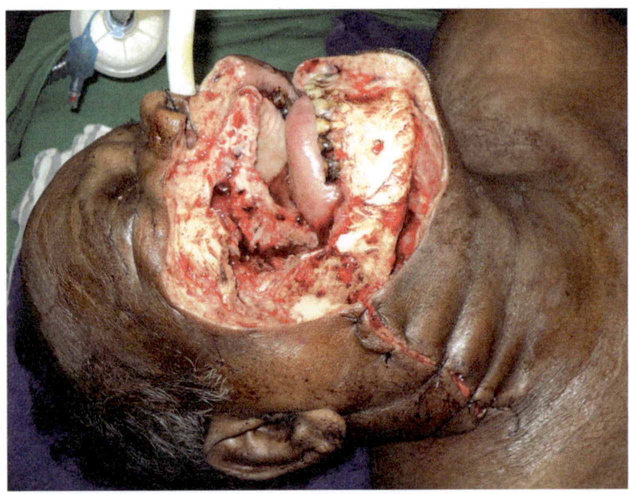

Fig. 14.5 Photograph shows completed resection

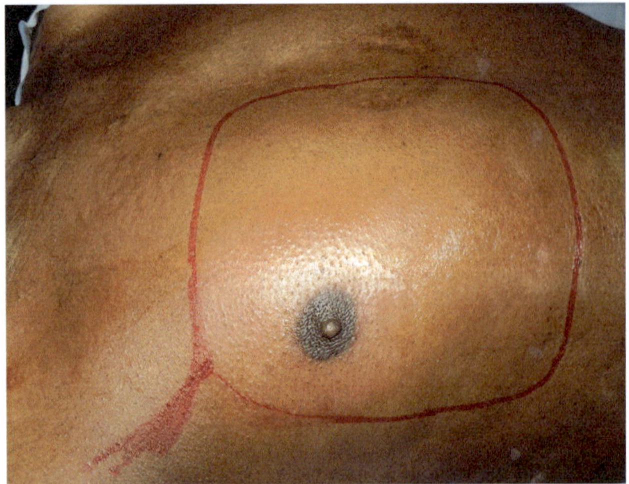

Fig. 14.6 Proposed PMMC flap. The donor site would need STG

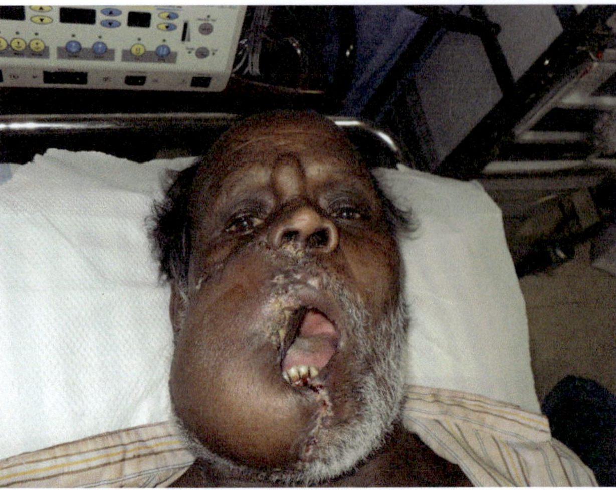

Fig. 14.7 Outcome after 10 days of procedure. The feeding tube is out and the patient can take semisolid food

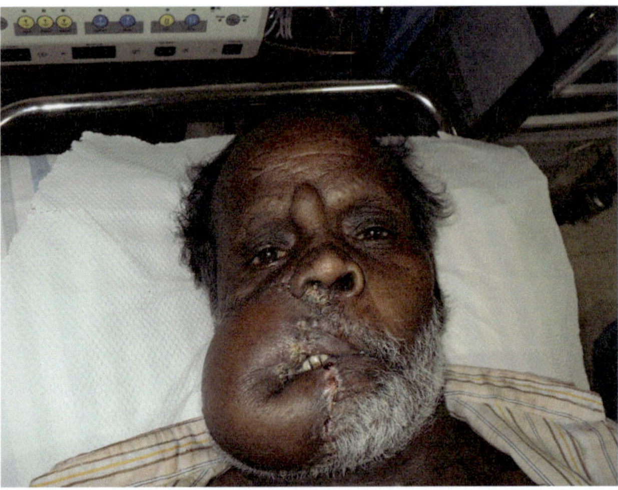

Fig. 14.8 Oral continence is acceptable for such disease. This patient is disease free for 1 year (last follow-up). There is a chance that these patients may develop skin nodules, but the incidence is very rare in patients who have not received any treatment before. The incidence of distant metastasis for N0 neck is also not very high

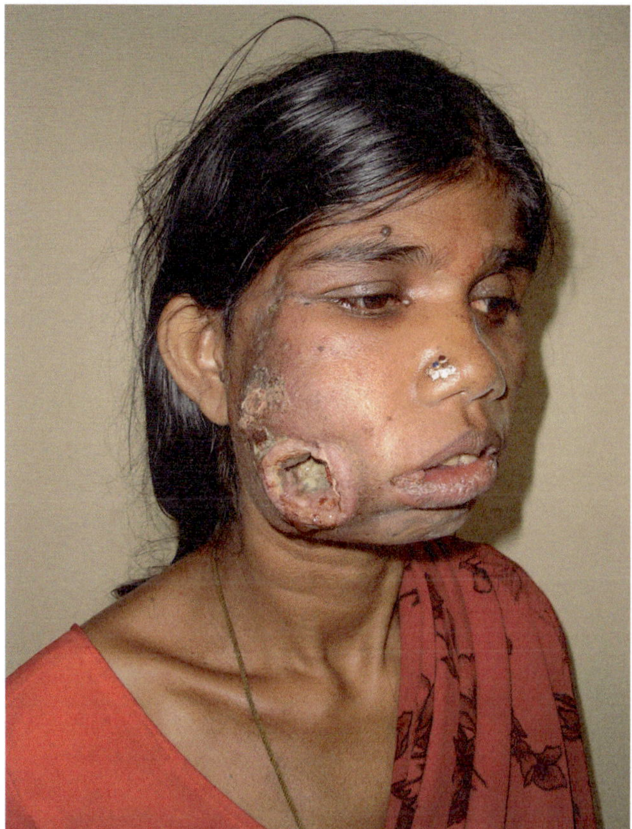

Fig. 14.9 A case with extensive skin fungation, disease going beyond the zygoma and involving high ITF

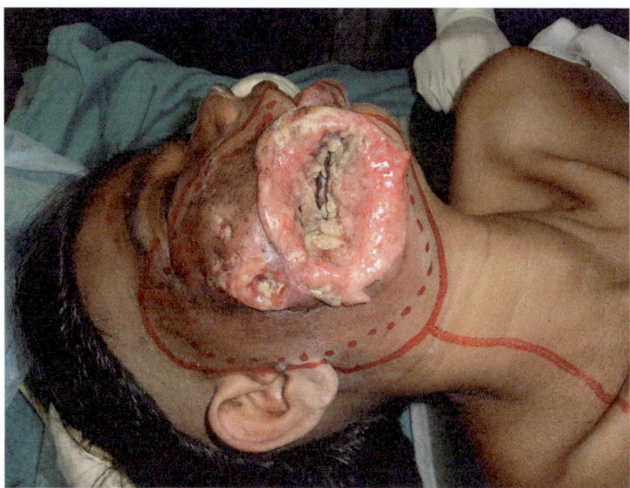

Fig. 14.10 Proposed resection with adequate margins. Intracranial involvement and involvement of prevertebral fascia and carotid artery are the only contraindications for us not to offer treatment to any patient

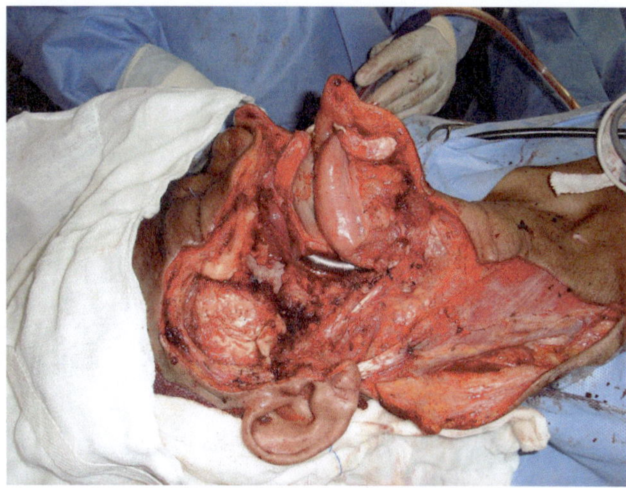

Fig. 14.11 Compartment resection with clear margins

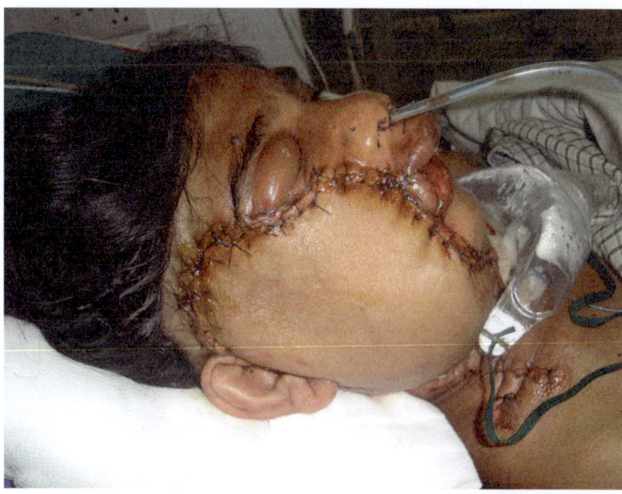

Fig. 14.12 ALT flap reconstruction. She defaulted for adjuvant radiotherapy (RT) and developed opposite node after 6 months and died of distant metastasis. She didn't have local recurrence till she died and had good QOL

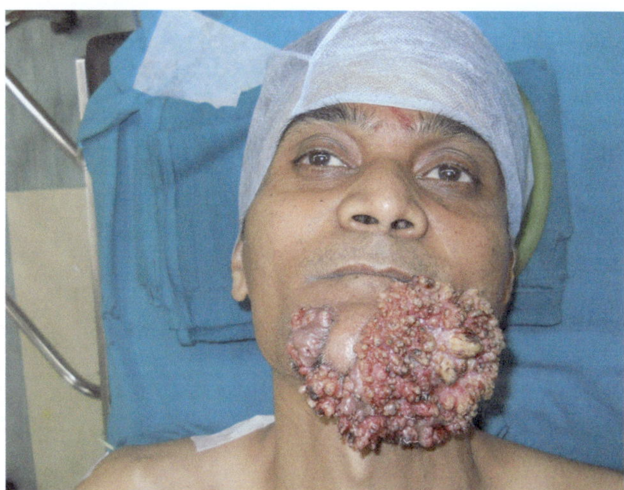

Fig. 14.13 A verrucous type of cancer involving extensive skin and anterior arch of the mandible. He requires two flap reconstruction

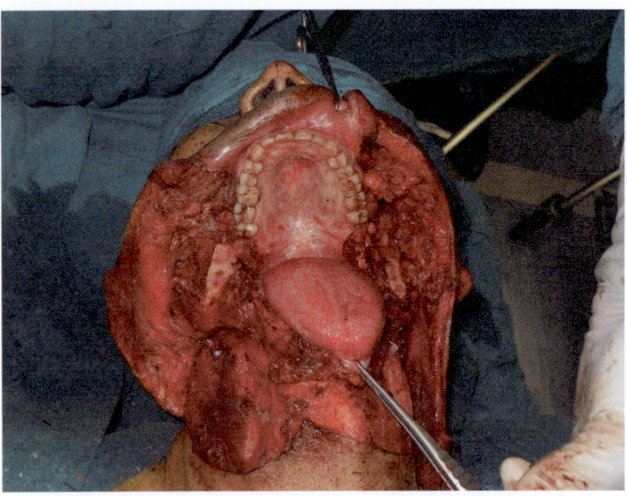

Fig. 14.14 The resection includes angle to angle mandible with skin. The focus of reconstruction would be to provide support to anterior tongue and FOM

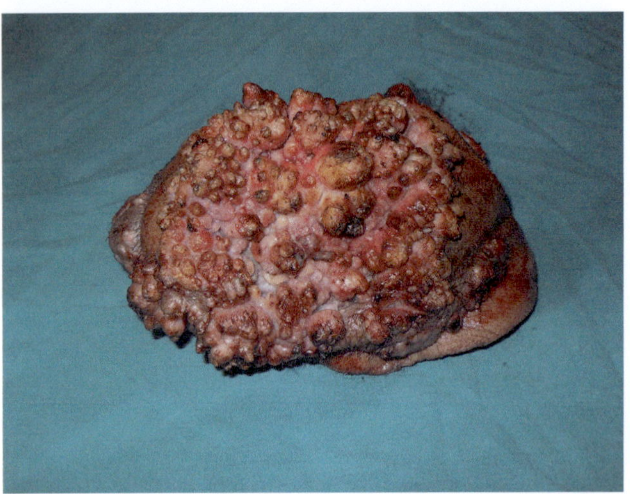

Fig. 14.15 The resected specimen showing adequate margins

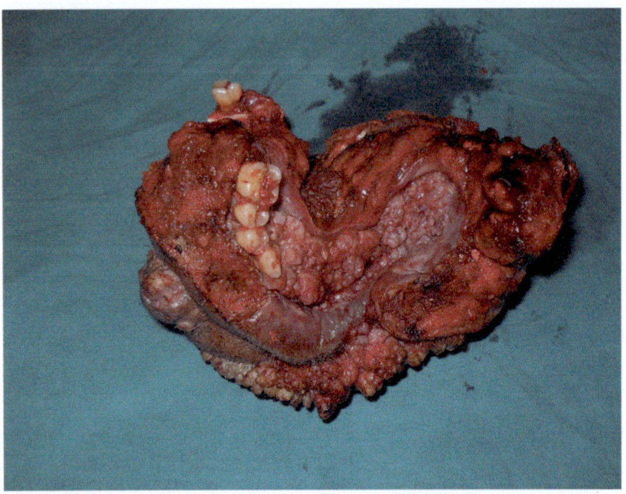

Fig. 14.16 The specimen with adequate mucosal margins

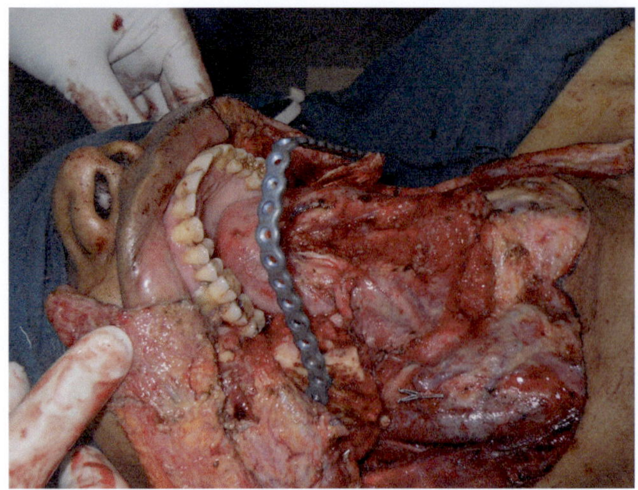

Fig. 14.17 The preadapted plate is fixed maintaining occlusion

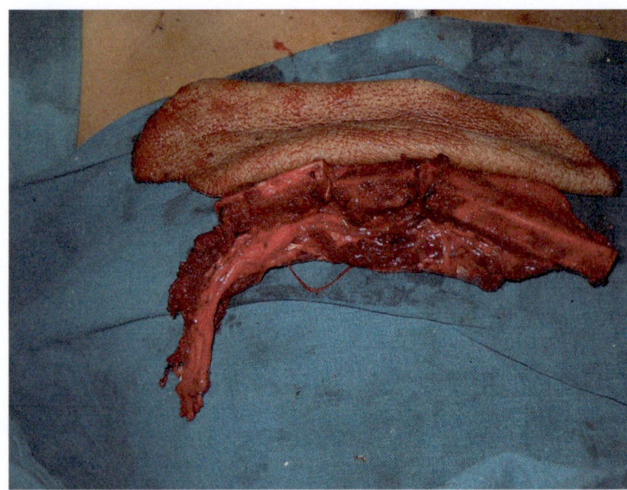

Fig. 14.18 The fibula flap with appropriate osteotomy and vascular pedicle

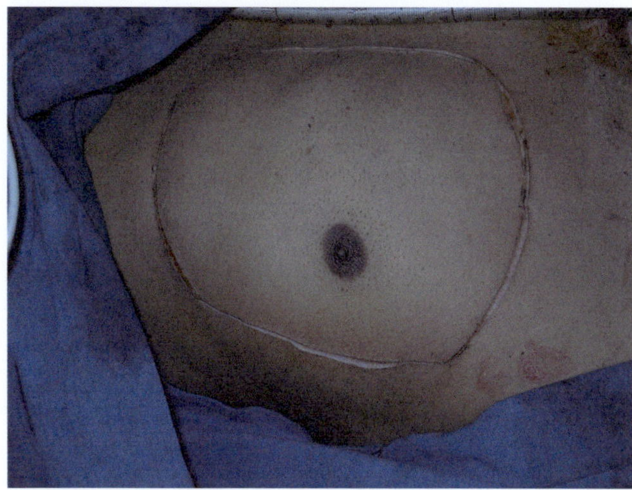

Fig. 14.19 The PMMC flap is marked for external cover. This flap should be raised on the opposite side where microvascular anastomosis is planned

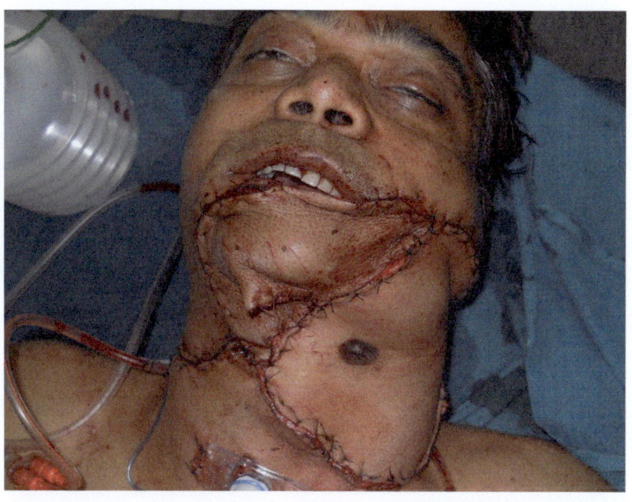

Fig. 14.20 Both flaps are inserted. The muscle of the fibular flap is used for inside lining. The tongue muscle is sutured to the plate of fibula for support. The skin of fibula flap and PMMC flap is used to cover large external defect

Tongue and FOM

The large tumors of tongue and FOM can spread anteriorly to the mandible or posteriorly to the larynx and oropharynx. These tumors generally have significant lymph node volume as well, but surgery remains the only realistic chance of cure.

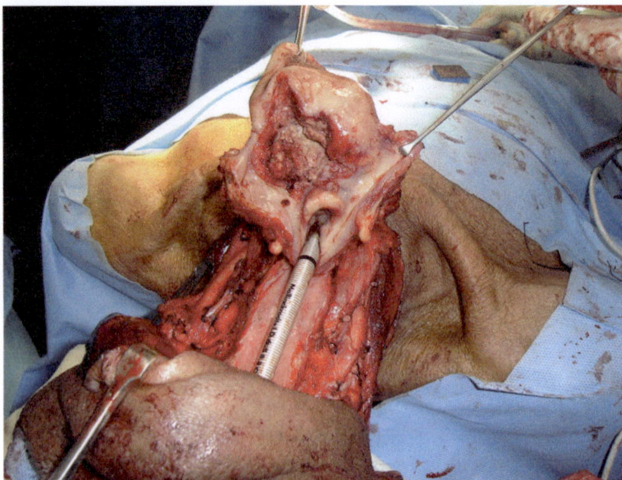

Fig. 14.21 The photograph shows large-volume posterior tongue tumor involving vallecula and pre-epiglottic space. Total glossectomy with laryngectomy is performed that achieve good local clearance

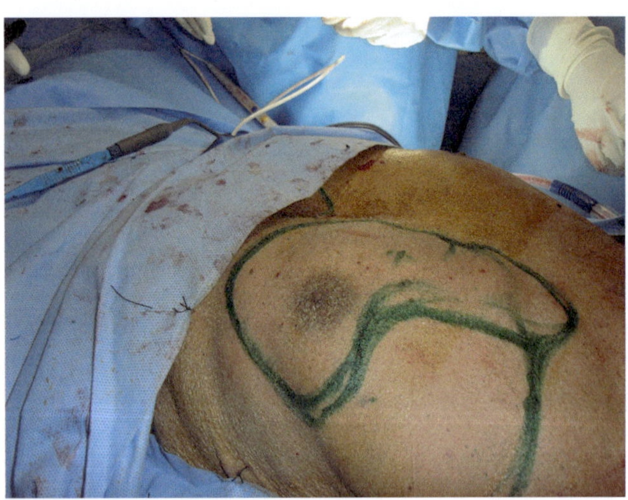

Fig. 14.22 The proposed PMMC flap. One can use ALT flap as well for such defect

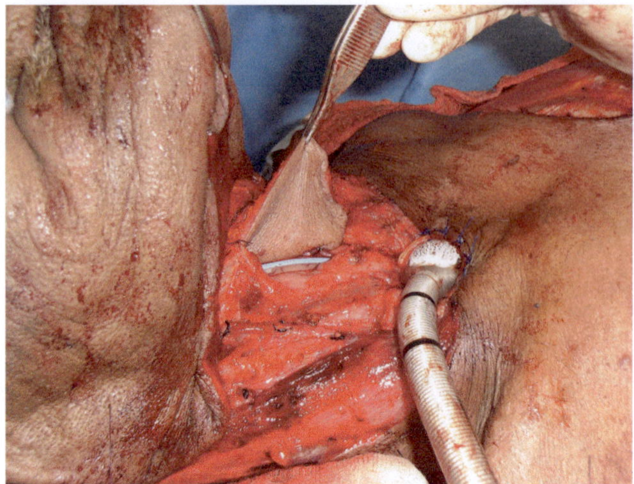

Fig. 14.23 The flap suturing is carried out using skin paddle for pharyngeal and tongue defect

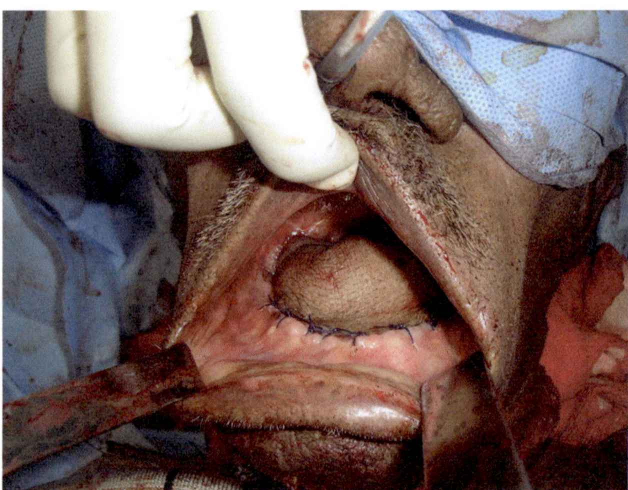

Fig. 14.24 The photograph shows completely reconstructed defect. These patients can swallow semisolids, can do all physical activity, and can live a very normal life. The esophageal speech can be developed to manage their routine communication in few words

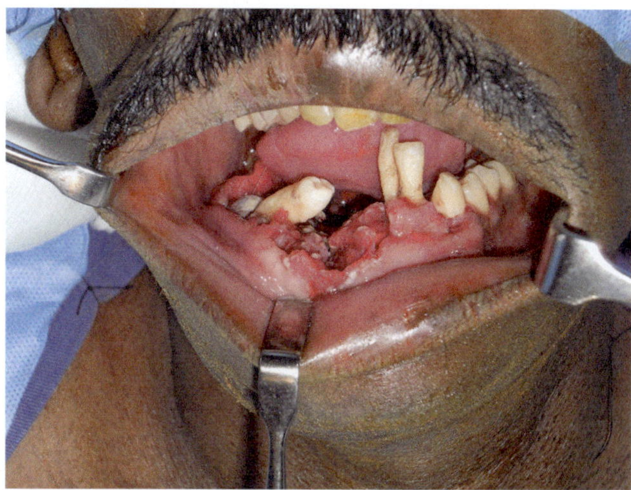

Fig. 14.25 Tongue lesion with pathological involvement of mandible

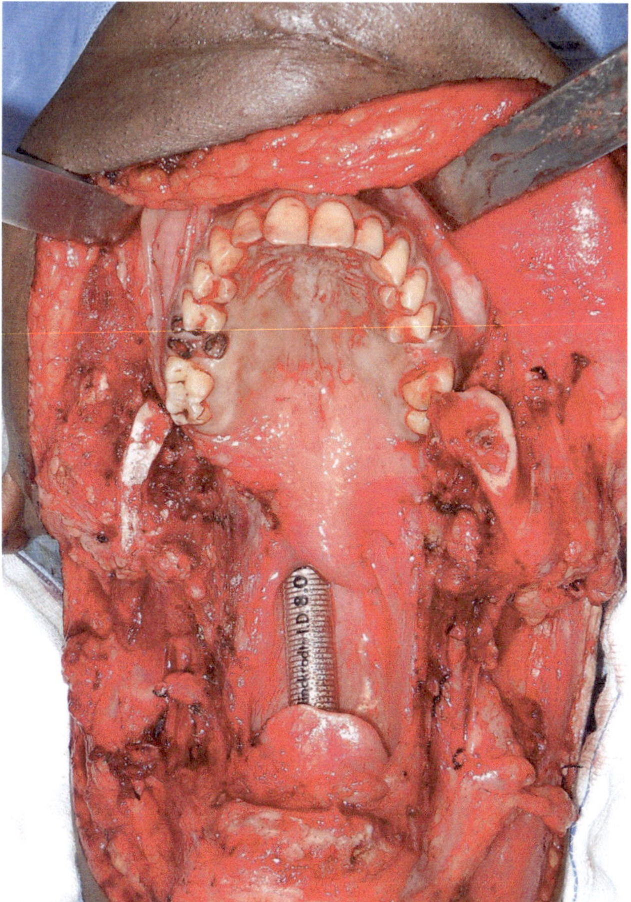

Fig. 14.26 The patient had total glossectomy with angle to angle mandibulectomy as described in the previous chapter

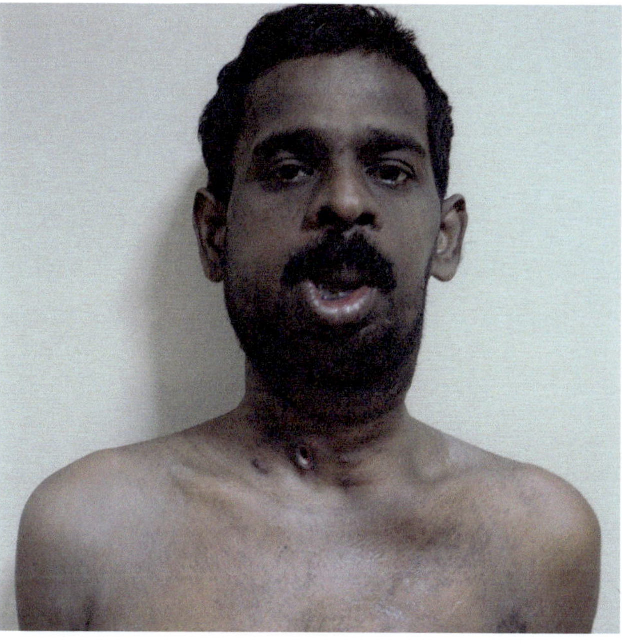

Fig. 14.27 The patient after appropriate two flap reconstruction. This is the best possible way of cure and best palliative care if disease biology is poor

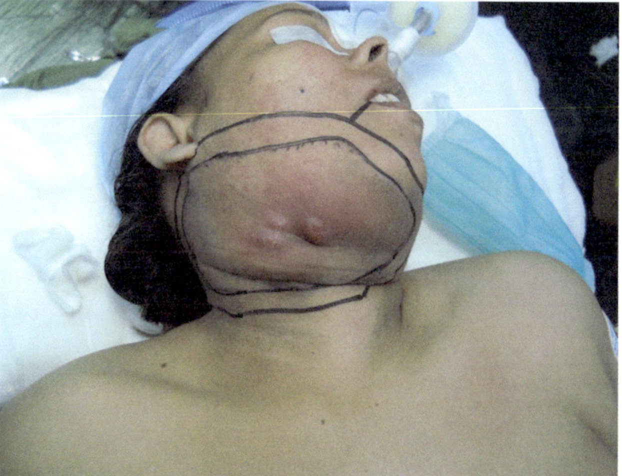

Fig. 14.28 A case of FOM with extensive skin infiltration

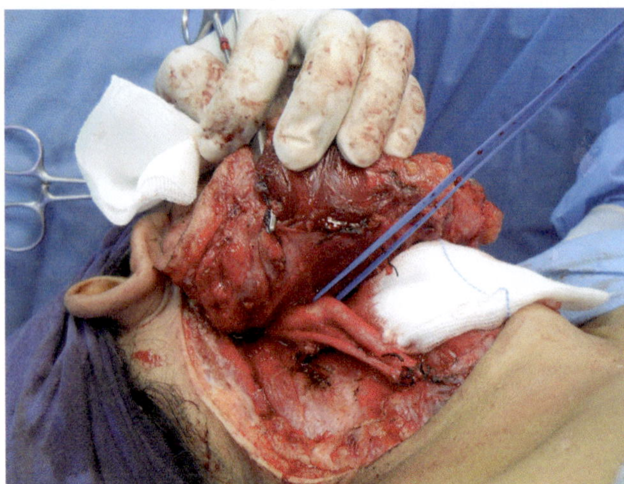

Fig. 14.29 The internal carotid artery is separated from the mass

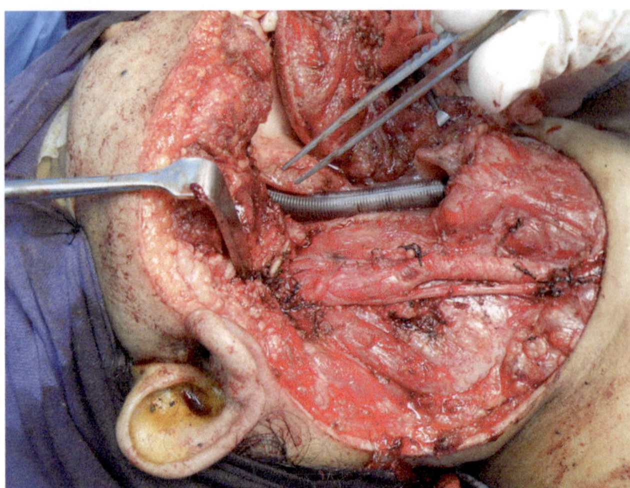

Fig. 14.31 The photograph shows complete clearance of the disease. It is important to note that this is a systemic resection from hyoid to skull base and from internal carotid artery to midline

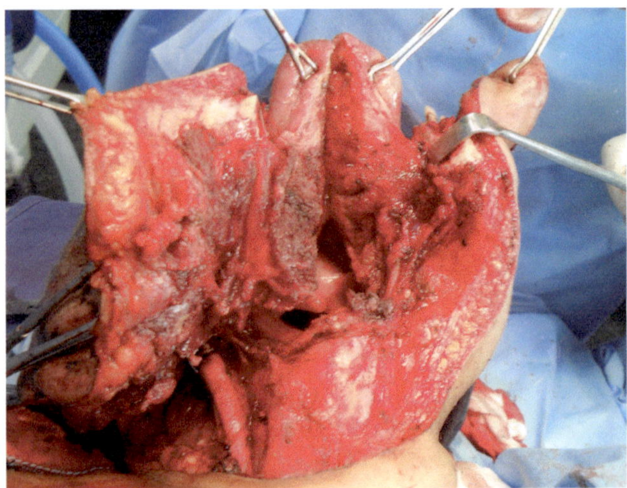

Fig. 14.30 The surgery is carried out with the concept of compartment resection

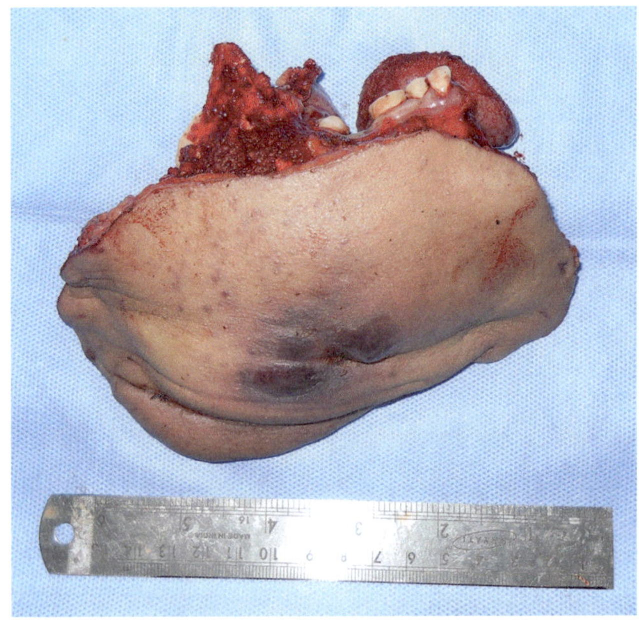

Fig. 14.32 The resected specimen with good margins

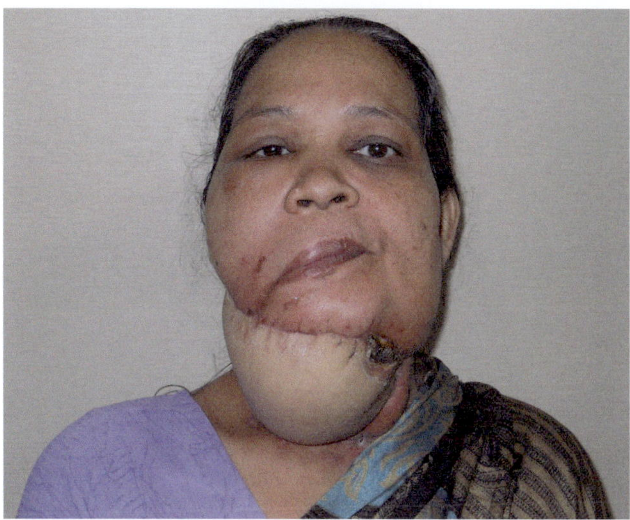

Fig. 14.33 Reconstruction is achieved with ALT flap. The vessels for micro-vascular anastomosis are are used from opposite side of the neck as ipsilateral external carotid artery is ligated from its origin

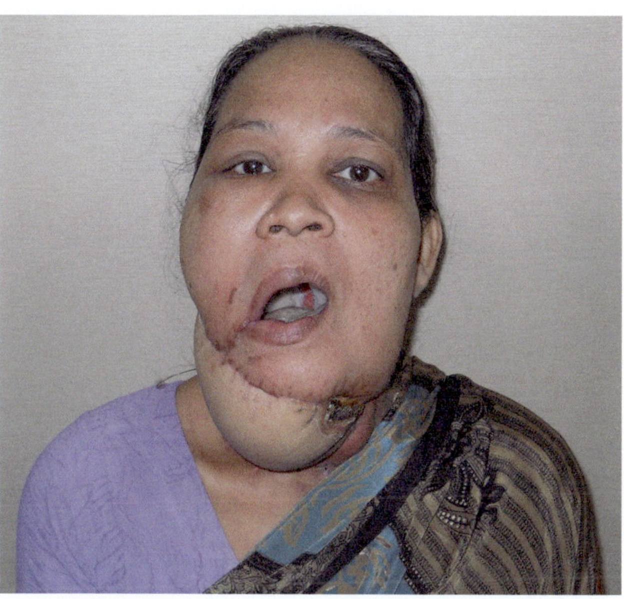

Fig. 14.34 The photograph shows intraoral flap healing. The patient can take semi-solid food

Oropharynx Tumor

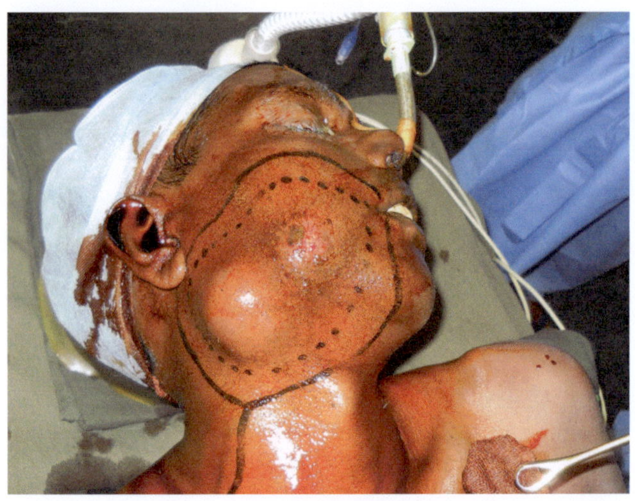

Fig. 14.35 Advanced oropharynx cancer with enlarged lymph node. The vast majority of oropharynx cancers in our part are tobacco-related tumors, and very advanced cancers do well with upfront surgery rather than chemoradiation

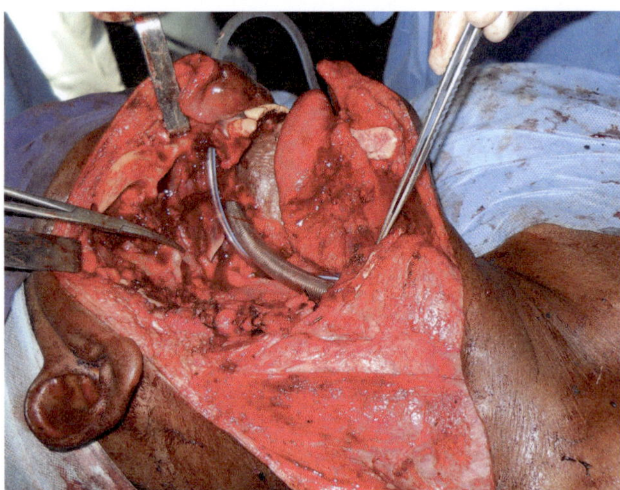

Fig. 14.36 The resection is carried out from hyoid to skull base in compartment resection approach. All the margins are clear

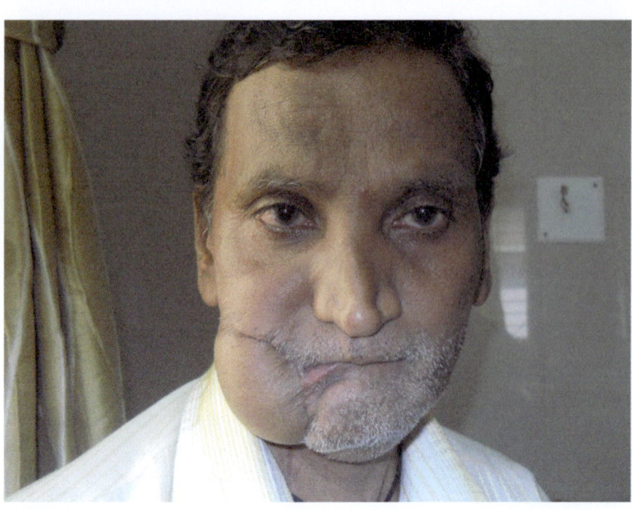

Fig. 14.37 The long-term result with ALT flap. The patient is living normal life after 3 years of treatment

Neck Mass

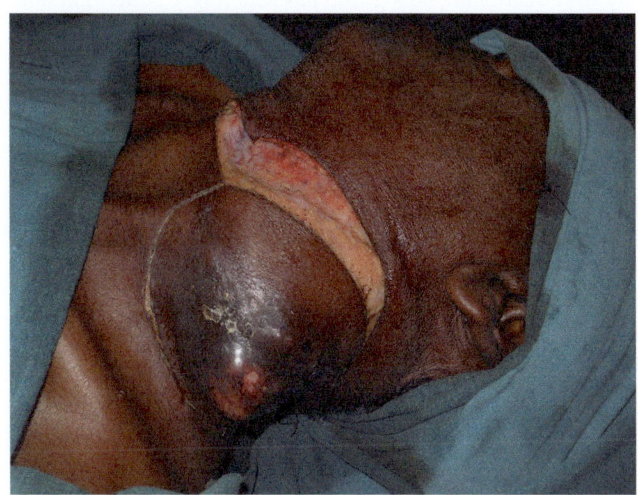

Fig. 14.38 Advanced neck mass involving the carotid artery. Involvement of prevertebral fascia is the only absolute contraindication for surgery. The carotid artery can be either ligated (after establishing contralateral circulation is adaquate) or can be replaced with vascular graft. This is only carried out if primary tumor is under control; patient is healthy and has potential for reasonable life

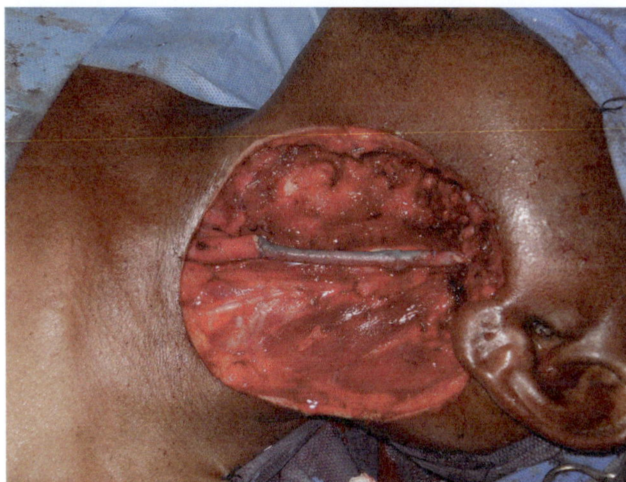

Fig. 14.39 The carotid artery is resected and saphenous vein graft is used to replace it

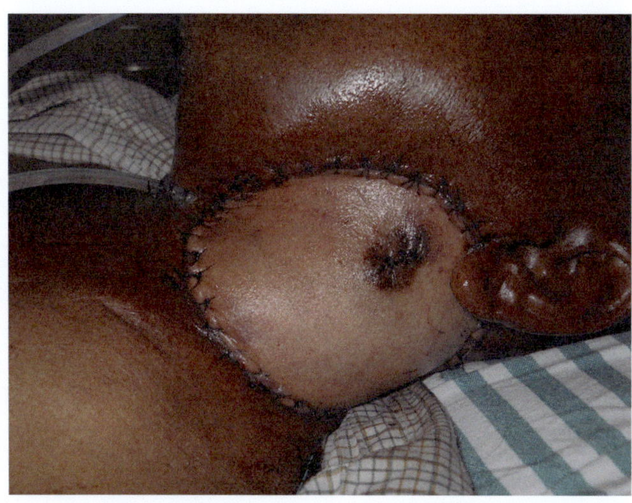

Fig. 14.40 The reconstruction is achieved with PMMC flap

Recurrent Disease (Salvage Surgery)

These cases are very challenging and all the surgical skill and experience of a surgeon helps in making appropriate decisions. It is essential to make rational decisions to avoid catastrophic postoperative complications. The recurrent tumors can be divided into two groups. The first group consists of patients who received incomplete or inappropriate first treatment. This group has seemingly better outcome as disease recurrence is probably due to incomplete previous treatment. Salvage surgical procedure can end up in catastrophic life-threatening complications of infection and bleeding due to vessel rupture. It is essential to do as minimal as possible and keep it as simple as possible.

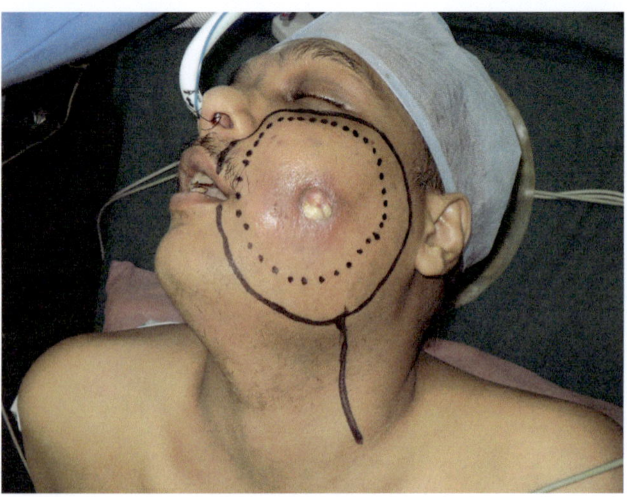

Fig. 14.41 This patient received three cycles of chemotherapy elsewhere. He gave history of tumour regression but there was no objective documentation. This is inappropriate treatment and we advise to include all tissue-disease with surrounding induration and oedema into resection specimen

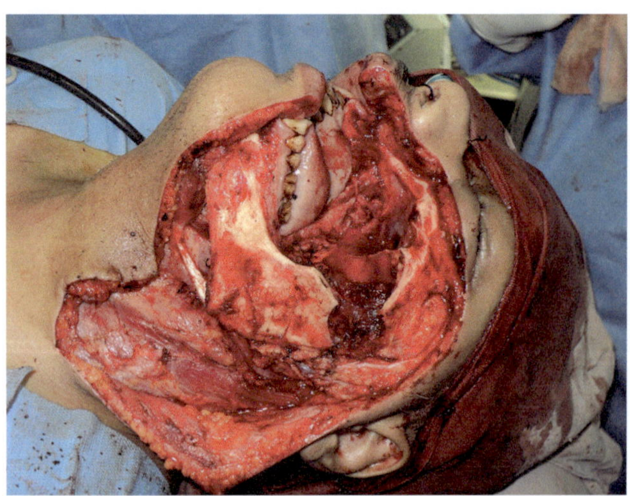

Fig. 14.42 The resection is complete with compartment surgery approach

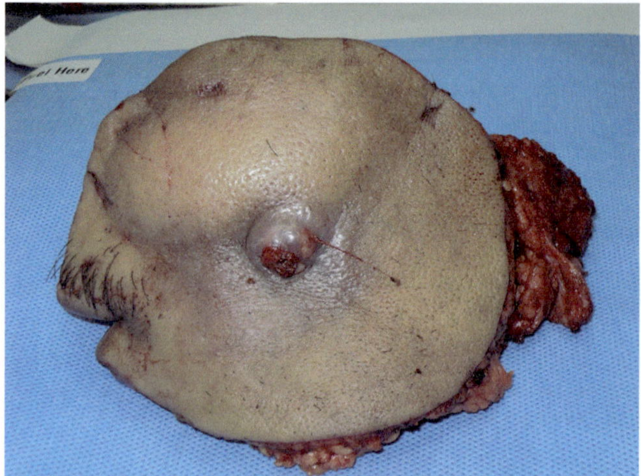

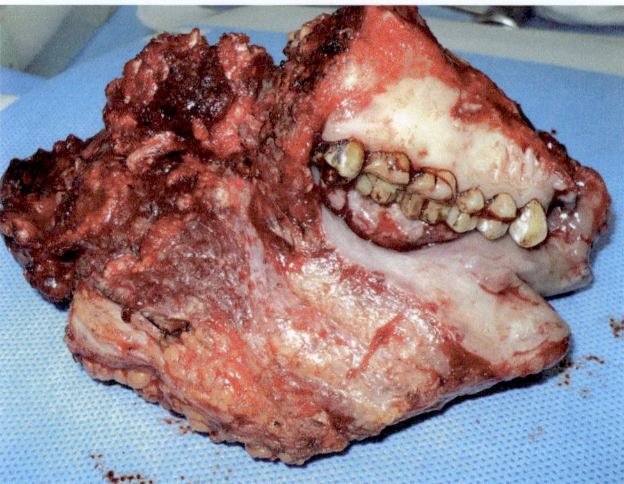

Figs. 14.43 and 14.44 The resection specimen shows adequate margins

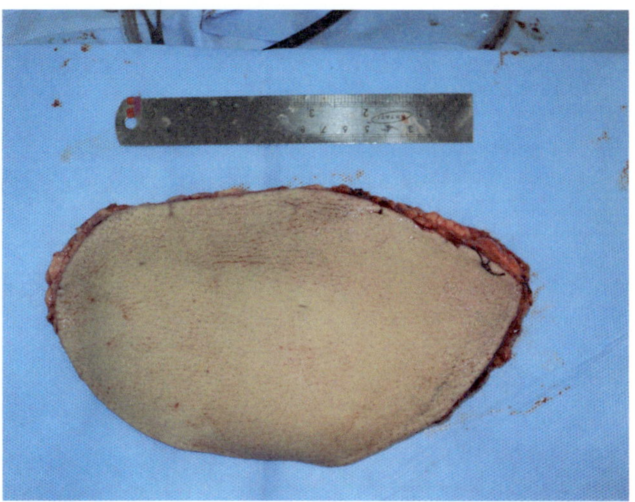

Fig. 14.45 ALT flap is raised for reconstruction

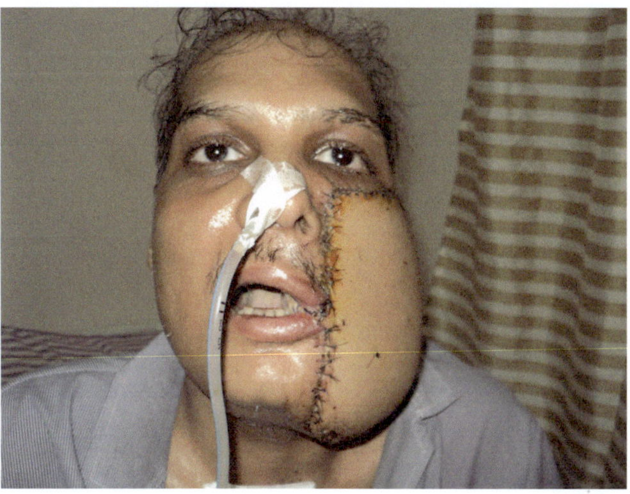

Fig. 14.46 The patient on the seventh postoperative day. This patient is disease free and doing well after 3 years of treatment

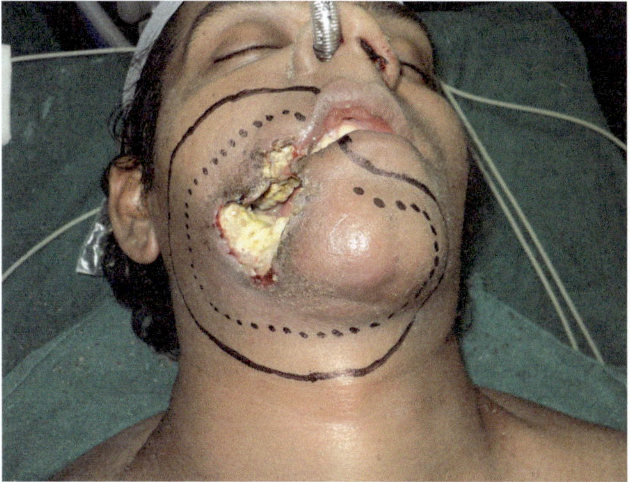

Fig. 14.47 A young patient with residual buccal cancer who received chemoradiation as first-line treatment. This is an inappropriate first-line treatment for advanced oral cavity cancer, and the salvage surgery has become much more complicated

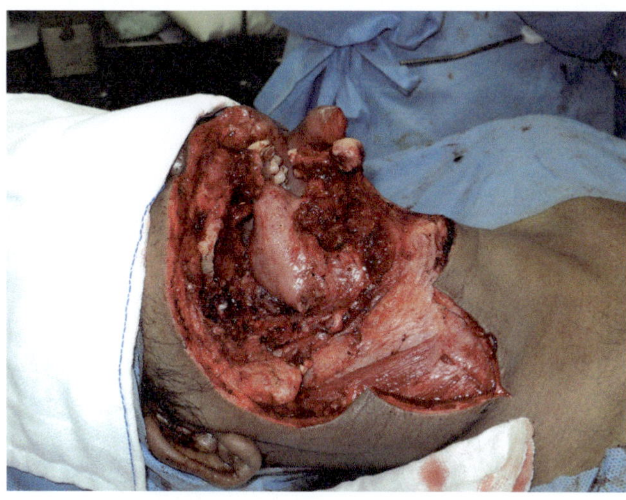

Fig. 14.48 The resection is complete

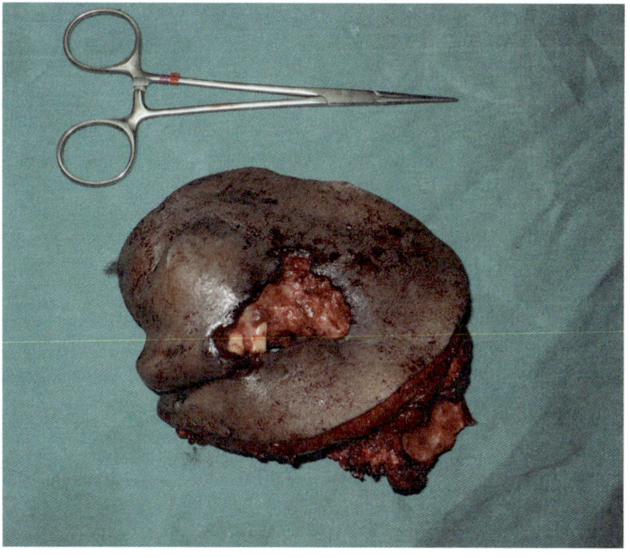

Fig. 14.49 The specimen shows adequate margins are achieved

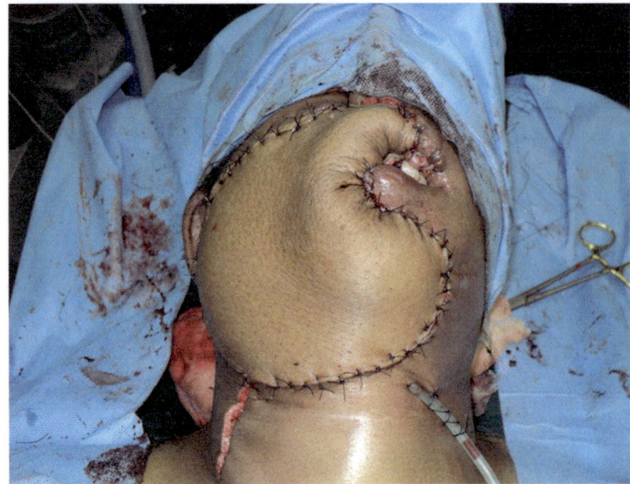

Fig. 14.50 Reconstruction is achieved with ALT flap. The patient developed dermal metastasis within 4 months of treatment. This is one of the most common mode of disease failure in patients who have received previous radiotherapy

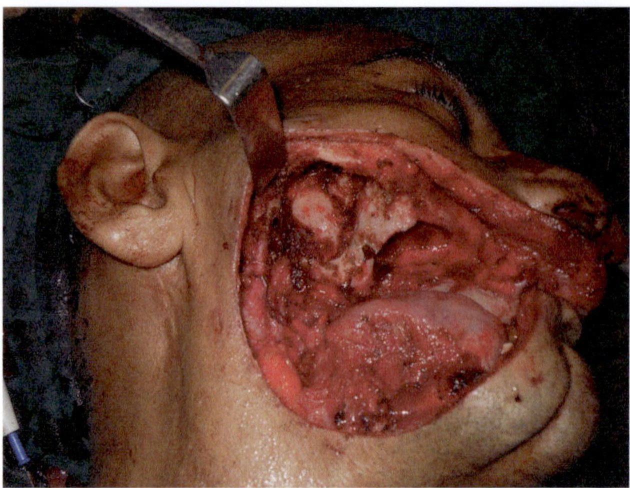

Fig. 14.52 The resection is complete with compartment ITF clearance. One can see the entire skull base devoid of any tissue. The reconstruction is planned with forehead flap. It is essential to preserve external carotid artery and superficial temporal artery in dissection to preserve blood supply for forehead flap. Another alternative is to do an ALT flap with anastomosis to opposite side vessels. This case was carried out in a rural clinic with limited facility where free flap facility was not available

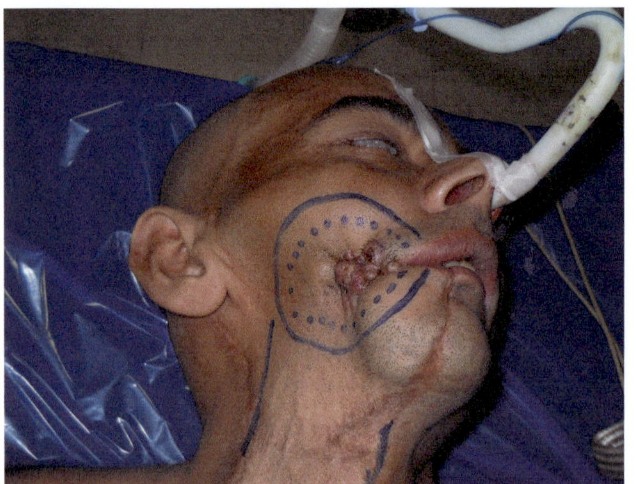

Fig. 14.51 This is another patient with recurrent buccal mucosa cancer. This patient had received surgery 1½ years ago, and good disease-free interval suggests favorable biology. There are two challenges in this case. The disease is extending into ITF and it is a vessel depleted neck due to previous surgery where PMMC flap was used

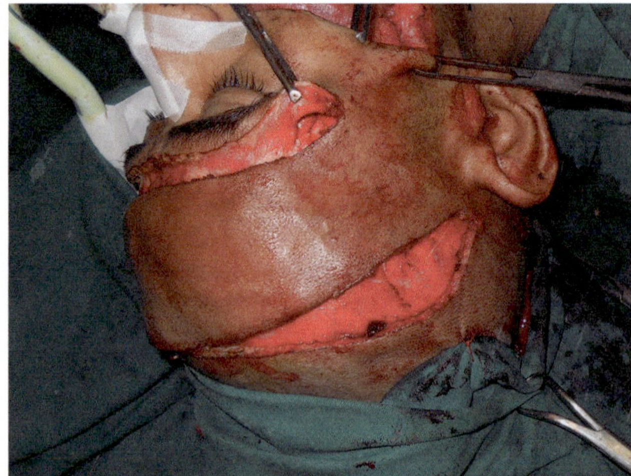

Fig. 14.53 The flap is raised

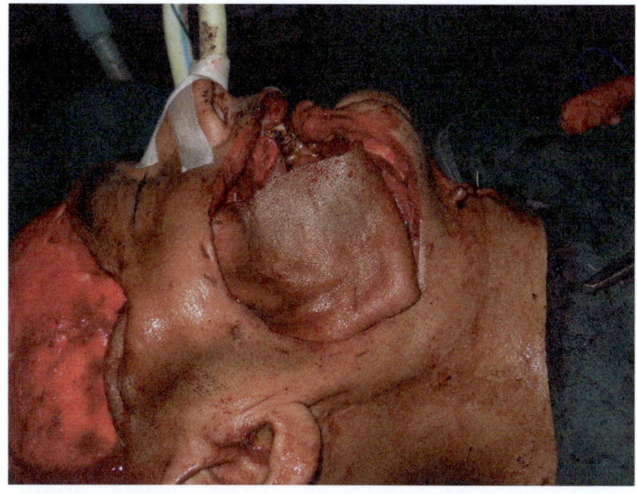

Fig. 14.54 The flap is tunneled below the skin, over the zygoma and bi-paddled to achieve double-layer closure

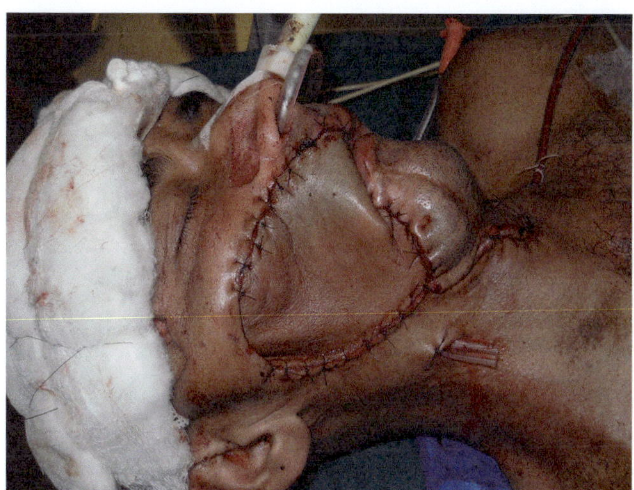

Fig. 14.55 The closure is complete

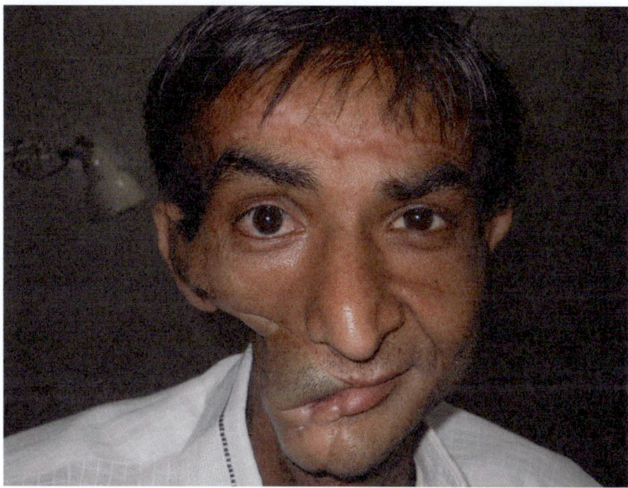

Fig. 14.56 The patient after 1 year of treatment. He takes semisolid diet and carries all his routine work without any problems

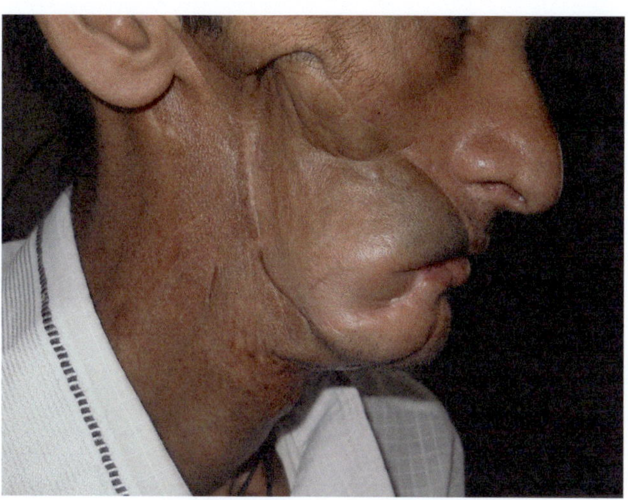

Fig. 14.57 The photograph shows completely healed flap

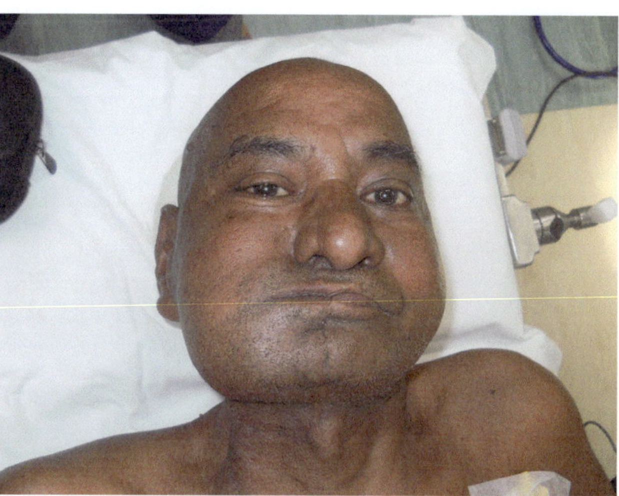

Fig. 14.58 This is a case of recurrent buccal mucosa cancer that has failed after ITF. This is a common pattern of failure for posteriorly located buccal cancer

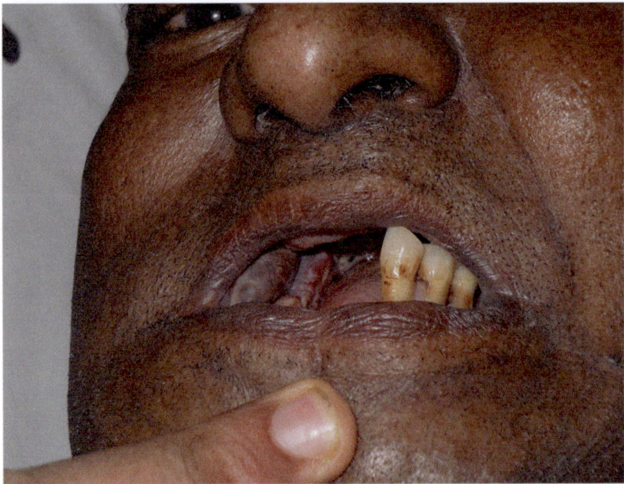

Fig. 14.59 The photograph shows local recurrence with involvement of PMMC flap. One has to include the entire flap in resection in case there is a large-volume disease

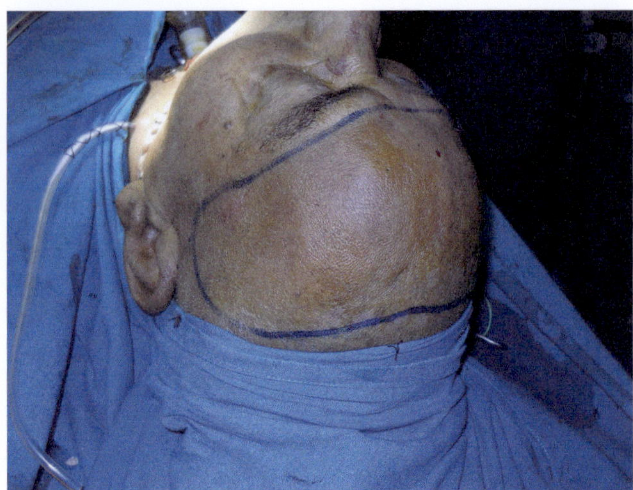

Fig. 14.61 The planned forehead flap. The PMMC flap was already used in this case and microvascular flap was not possible in operative setup. It is important to remember that it is the oncological clearance that determines the long-term outcome and even regional flap can provide decent functional outcome

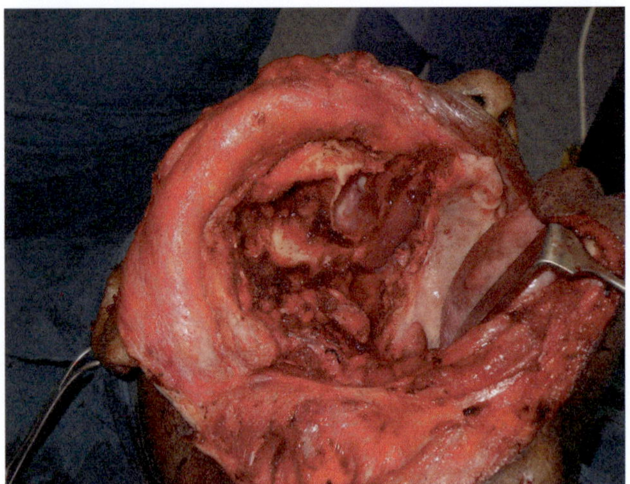

Fig. 14.60 The photograph shows high ITF clearance

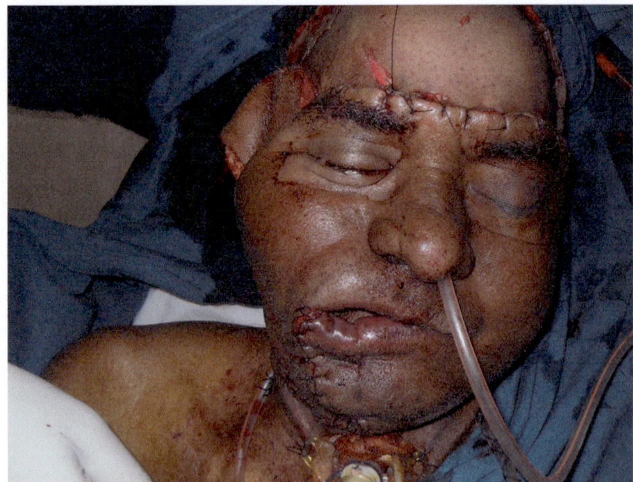

Fig. 14.62 The intraoperative photograph showing completed reconstruction

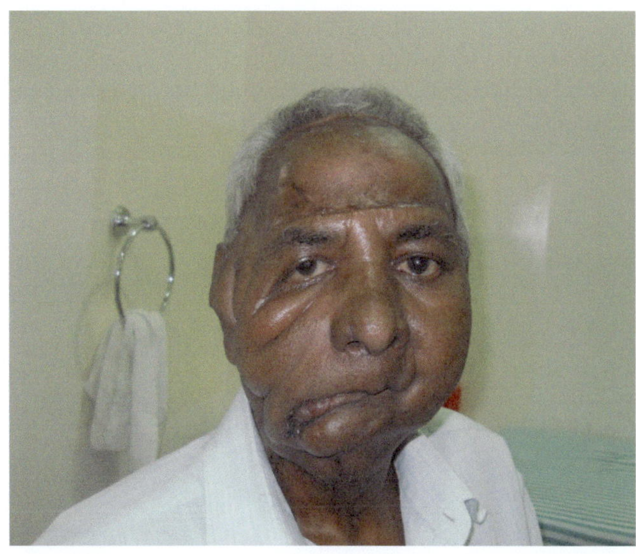

Fig. 14.63 The patient after 2 years of treatment manages to live routine life

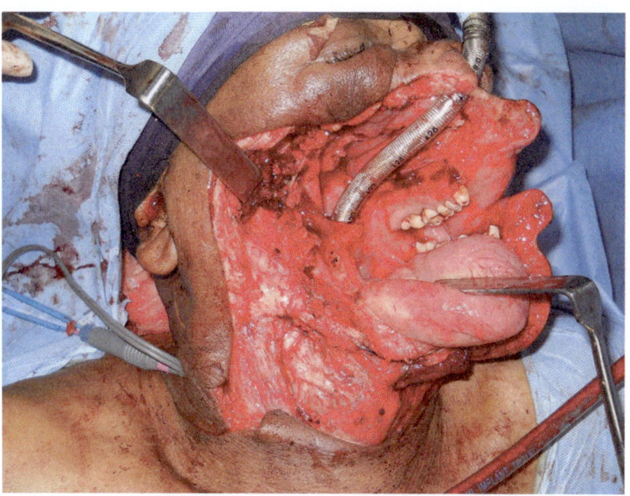

Fig. 14.65 The resection is complete

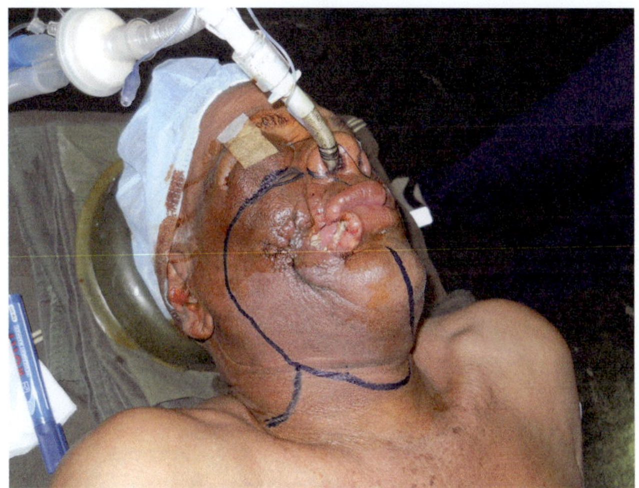

Fig. 14.64 This patient had received surgery and radiotherapy 4 months back, and this case falls under poor prognosis category. It is advisable to explain prognosis to patient and relatives before attempting surgical salvage

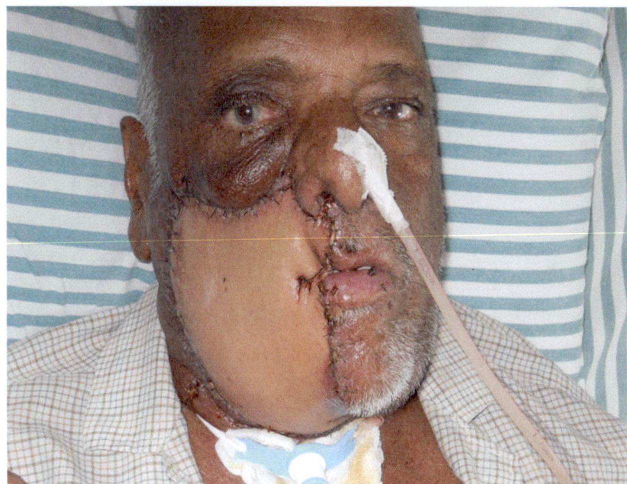

Fig. 14.66 Reconstruction was achieved with ALT flap. This patient developed dermal metastasis in 6 months time

Palliative Surgery

This is a very subjective topic and decisions need to be made on individual basis. We do offer palliative surgery to patients in whom we can improve their quality of life. It is essential that surgical procedure is relatively simple, recovery is quick and the patient is relatively healthy. Not only good quality of life but good and dignified death is equally important.

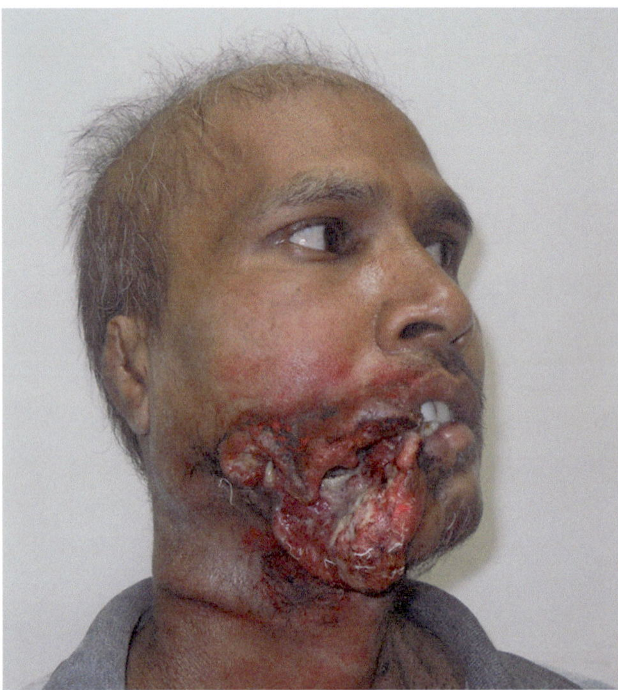

Fig. 14.67 Patient with advanced and recurrent buccal cancer with lung metastasis

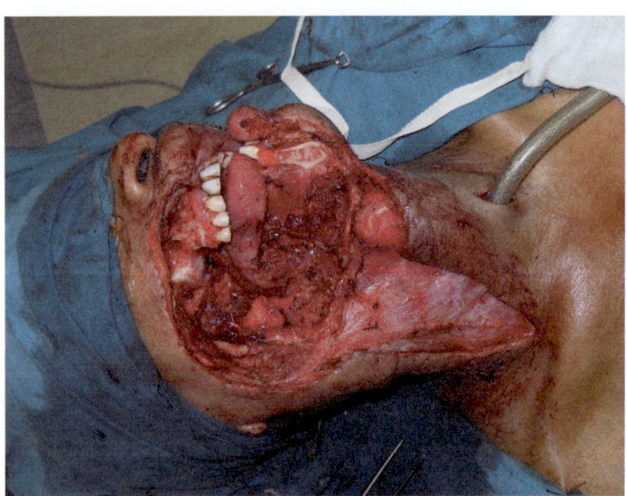

Fig. 14.68 The resection is complete. We were reasonably confident of achieving negative margins and decent local control in this patient before the procedure

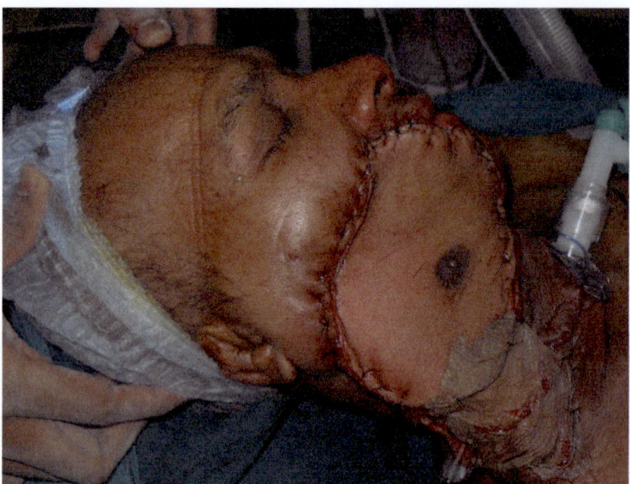

Fig. 14.69 The reconstruction was achieved with spiral PMMC flap. We prefer to keep the procedure as simple as possible

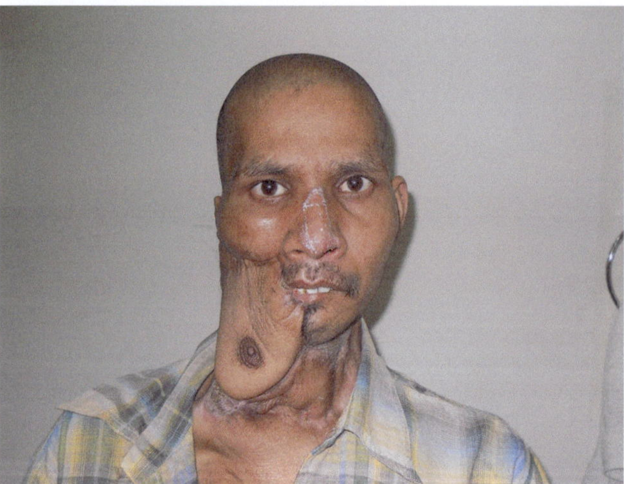

Fig. 14.70 The patient after 1 month of surgery. He survived for 7 months after surgery without local disease and had relatively good QOL

15 Head and Neck Cancer Surgery in Resource Constrained Setup

Head and neck cancer is a major health challenge in developing world. The habit of tobacco chewing and smoking is quite prevalent in this part of the world, making head neck cancer as one of most common cancers. Many people live in socioeconomically compromised situation and they present at a very advanced stage of the disease (50–60 % of all patients). This makes their treatment complicated and costly. The treatment facilities are diverse in large developing countries and many patients are treated in centers with basic infrastructure. It is difficult to maintain consistency in treatment delivery, and many patients receive compromised care.

It is essential to understand the infrastructure available in a center where one is working. This helps in deciding treatment approaches that are feasible in that setup. It is advisable to form a guideline that is feasible in the center and deliver consistent treatment [1]. It is possible to perform most complicated and challenging surgery with basic setup if the surgeon is well trained and experienced enough to work in that environment [1–3].

The operative room setup is similar to any other general surgery and otolaryngology surgery theater. One needs to have a cautery machine, drill and saw system with plating kit, and suction machine as basic requirements. The anesthetist should have experience in managing difficult airway or one has to perform tracheostomy in majority of cases for induction. We also prefer to perform elective tracheostomy in postoperative period as intensive care unit (ICU) facilities are very basic in most part. It is also feasible to perform microvascular free flap reconstruction in such setup if microscope is available [3]. It is also possible to do anastomosis with loops, and this can increase feasibility of this procedure in remote location.

The aim of this chapter is to demonstrate that almost any complicated procedure is possible with proper planning. We prefer to use regional flaps for reconstruction as far as possible as this is safer, less intensive, quick, and cost-effective. Patients recover earlier and postoperative care is easy. The extent of resection remains the same, and this helps in maintaining oncological outcome at par with other centers. There has been a conscious effort all throughout this book to demonstrate reconstruction with regional flaps to highlight that all the surgical concepts described in this book are feasible in all setup. Many cases of advanced cancers treated with compartment surgery concept that are demonstrated in this book were performed in a rural clinic. This chapter contains few challenging clinical situation that were solved in a simple manner with available resources.

N. Trivedi, *Atlas of Head and Neck Cancer Surgery: The Compartment Surgery for Resection in 3-D*,
DOI 10.1007/978-81-322-2050-3_15, © Springer India 2015

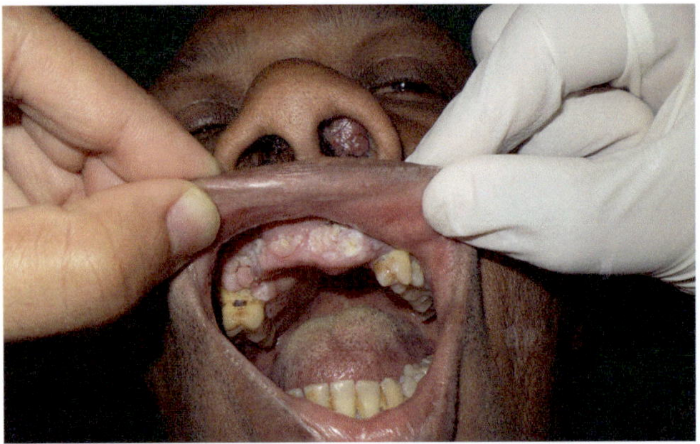

Fig. 15.1 A patient with cancer involving central arch maxilla with extension onto hard palate and bilateral maxillary sinus. The reconstruction is the major challenge and ideally requires vascularized bone flap. This patient had many comorbidities and it was not possible to perform such reconstruction in a limited setup by a single surgeon

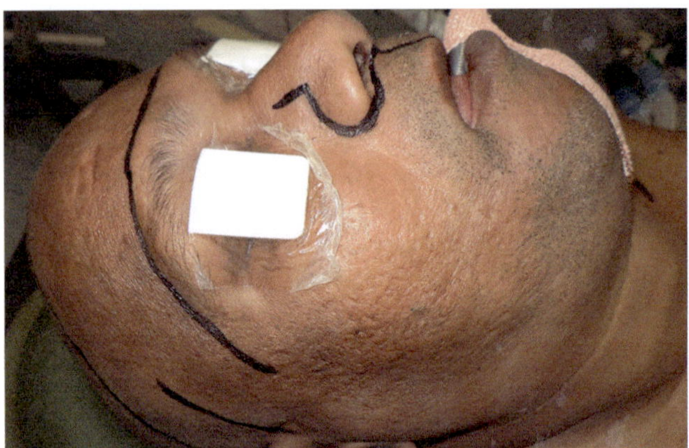

Fig. 15.2 A lateral rhinotomy incision with planned forehead flap

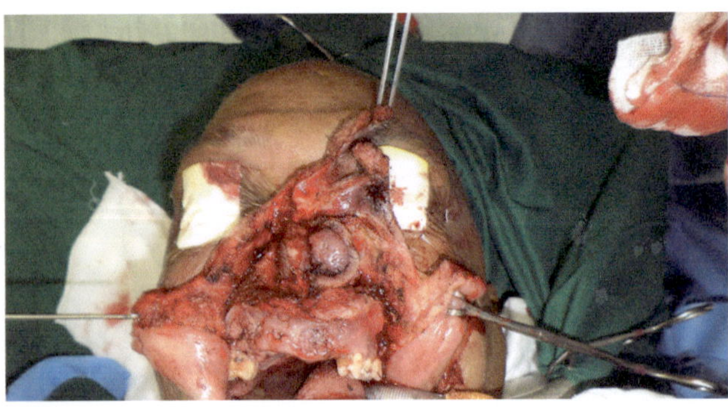

Fig. 15.3 Photograph showing adequate exposure for resection

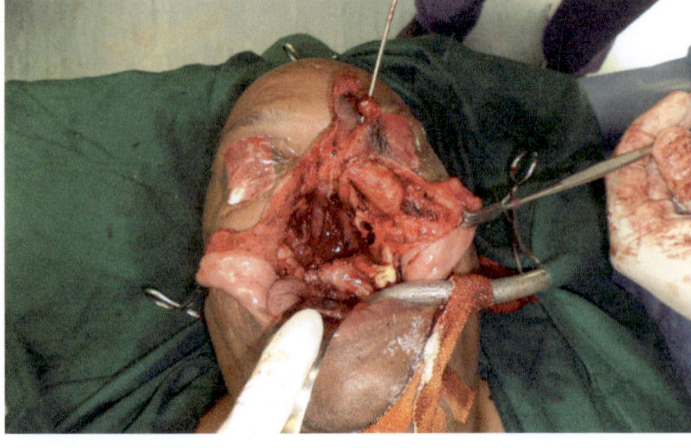

Fig. 15.4 The resection is complete

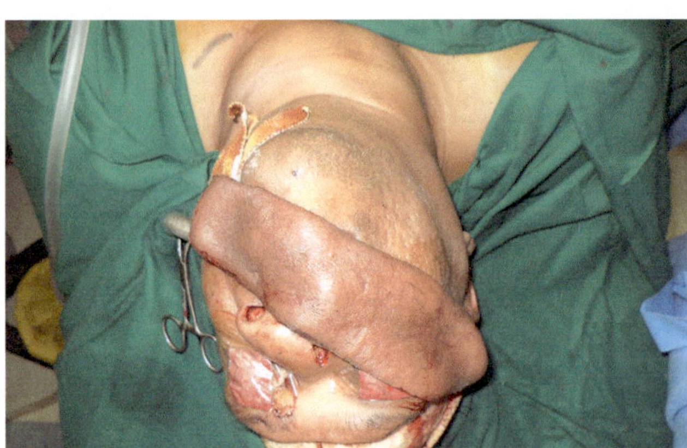

Fig. 15.5 The forehead flap is raised

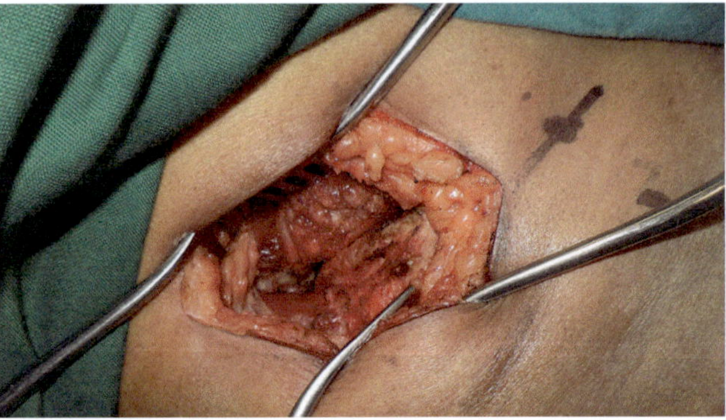

Fig. 15.6 The iliac crest bone graft is harvested

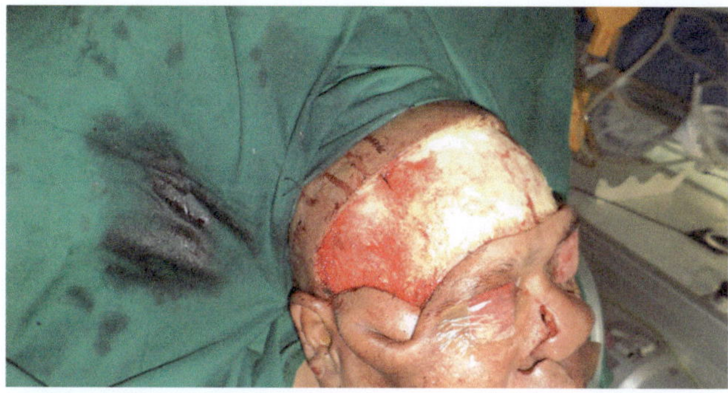

Fig. 15.7 The flap is tunneled below the skin

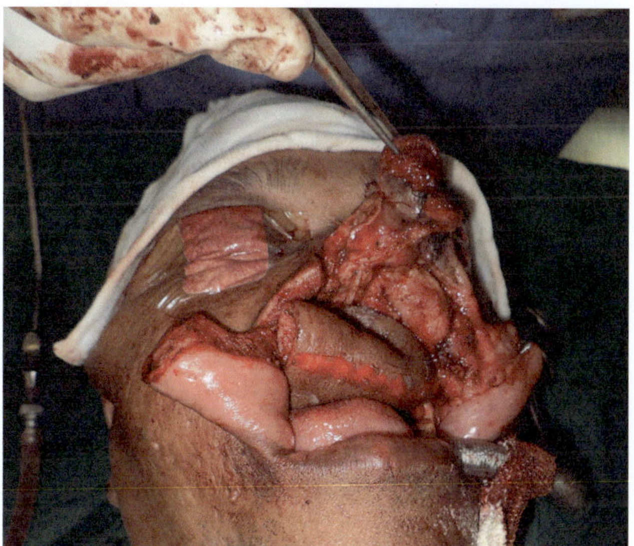

Fig. 15.8 The flap is sutured to palate and de-epithelized for lip portion

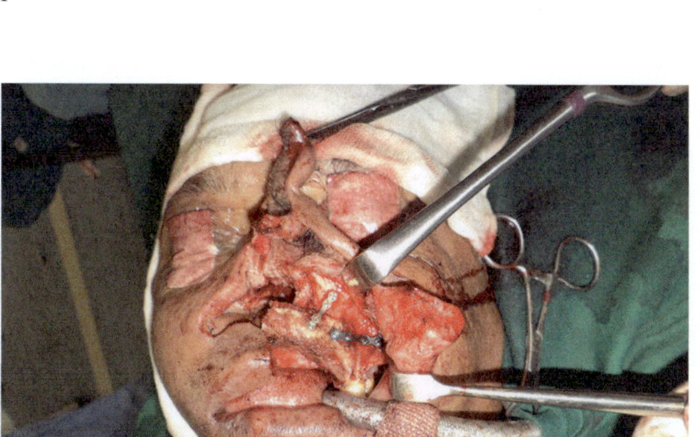

Fig. 15.9 The bone graft is plated to provide support to the nose

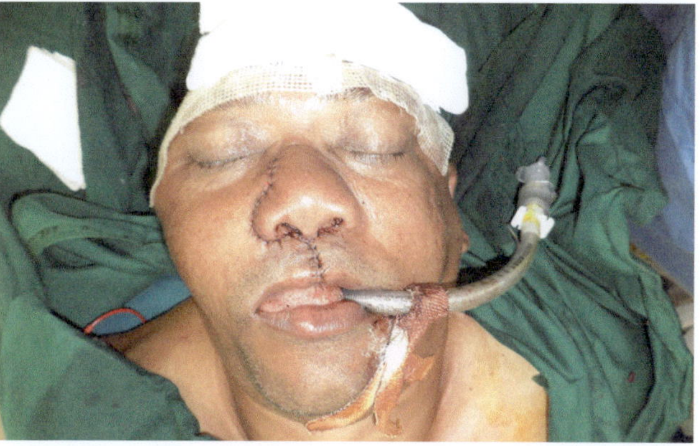

Fig. 15.10 The forehead flap would cover the bone in all direction. This will minimize possibilities of bone extrusion after radiation therapy

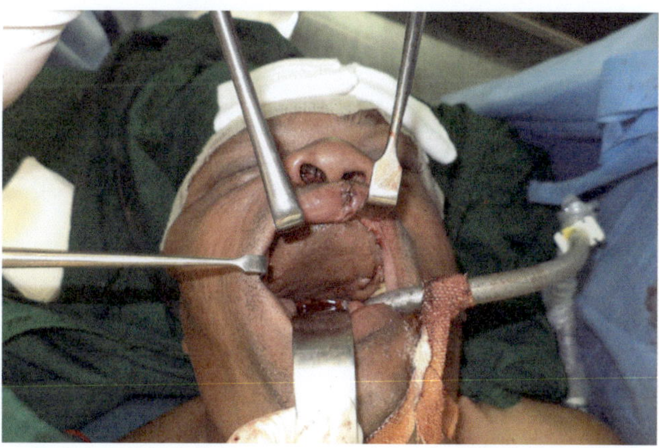

Fig. 15.11 The photograph showing palatal reconstruction

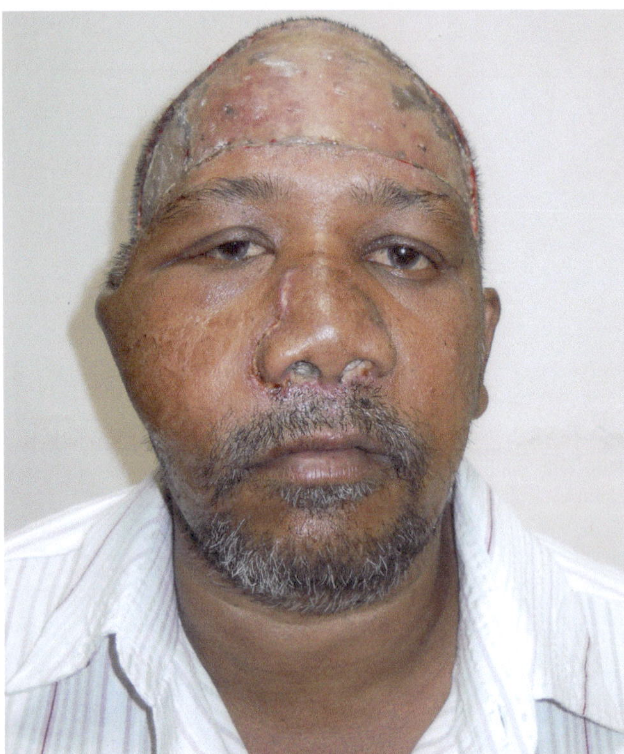

Fig. 15.12 Photograph of patient on the seventh postoperative day with healed wound. The flap will be divided after 4–6 weeks and this will further improve cosmetic outcome. The STG takes up very well on forehead area and color match is not too bad for dark individuals

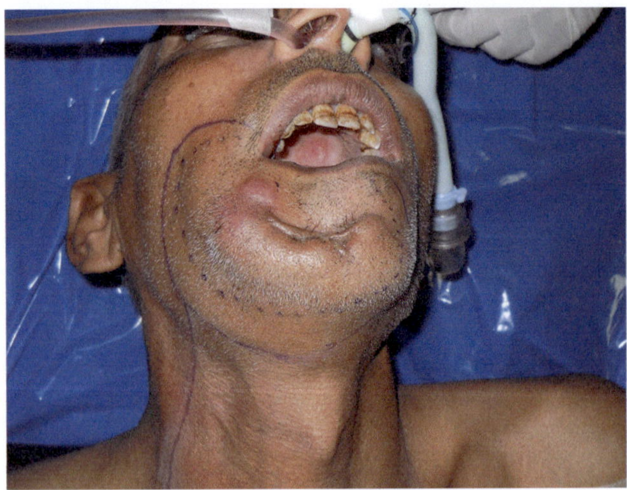

Fig. 15.13 A patient with tumor involving the floor of the mouth and central arch mandible and lower lip with the skin

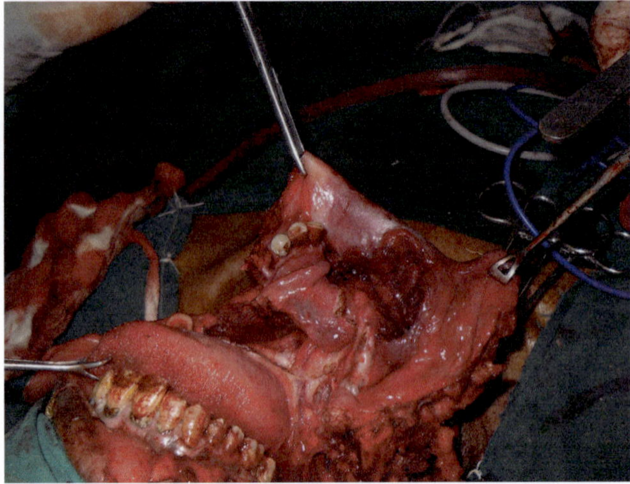

Fig. 15.14 The resection is achieved with adequate margins

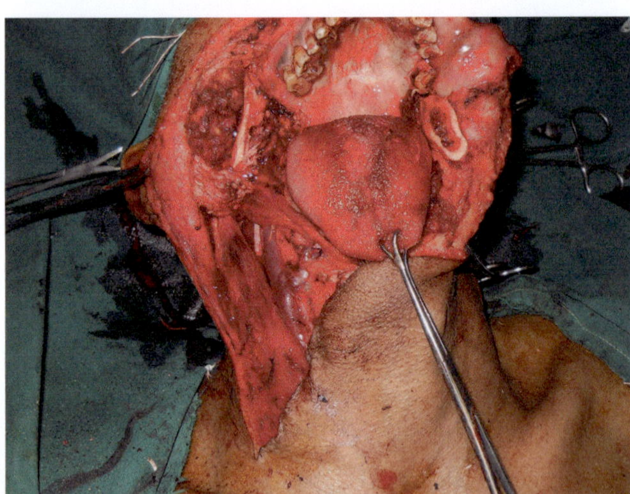

Fig. 15.15 The resulting defect shows the need for two flap reconstruction. Ideally a fibula flap for bone reconstruction and an ALT flap for skin and lip reconstruction. This was not feasible in our setup

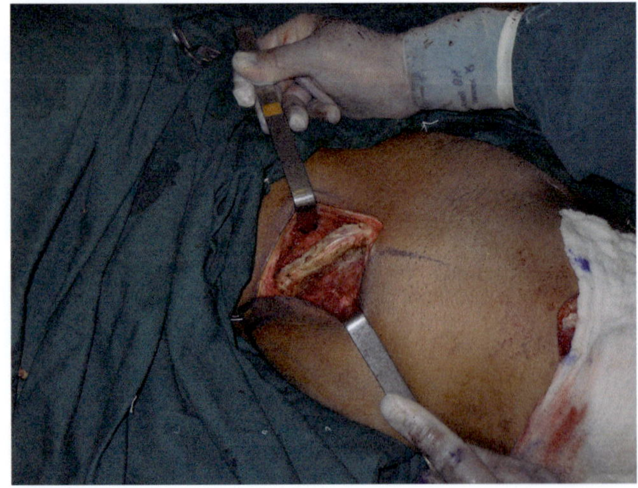

Fig. 15.16 An iliac crest bone graft is harvested

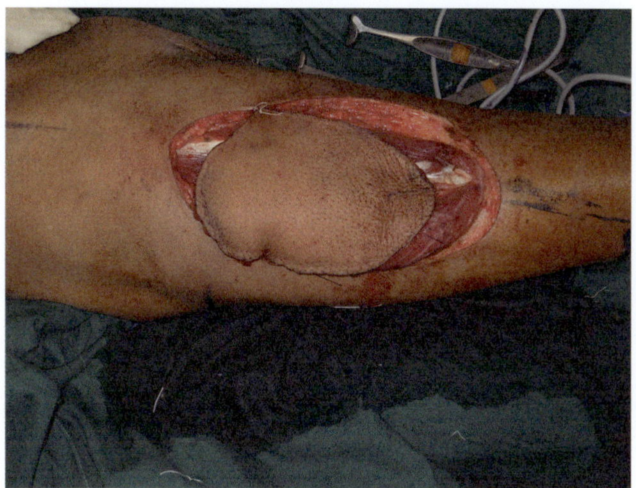

Fig. 15.17 ALT flap is raised for reconstruction

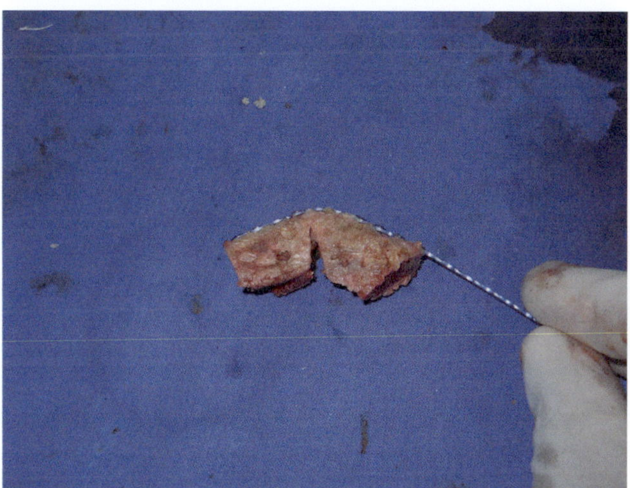

Fig. 15.18 The bone graft is plated for central arch reconstruction

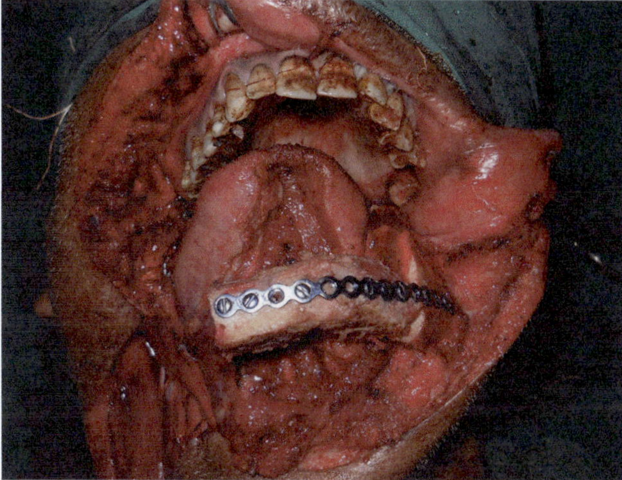

Fig. 15.19 It is plated to create the support base for anterior floor of the mouth muscles

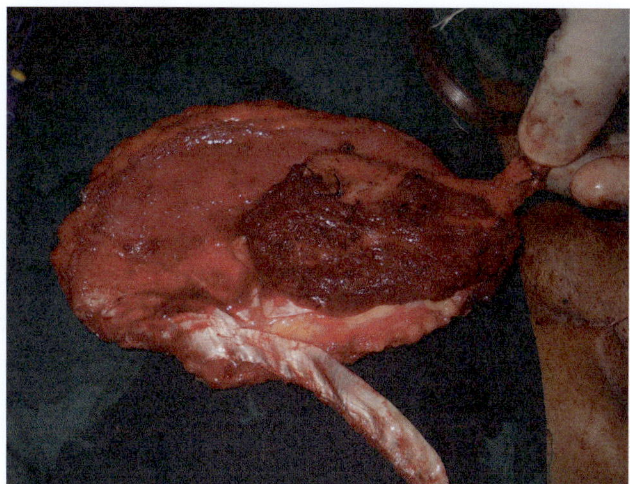

Fig. 15.20 ALT flap lata fascia with sling for reconstruction of lower lip

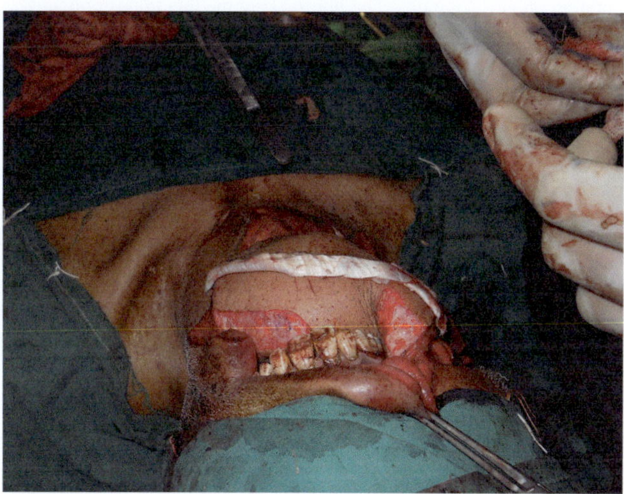

Fig. 15.21 The flap is anastomosed and the lower lip has been reconstructed as described earlier in this book. All sides of the bone graft needs to be covered so that it is not extruded out during radiation therapy

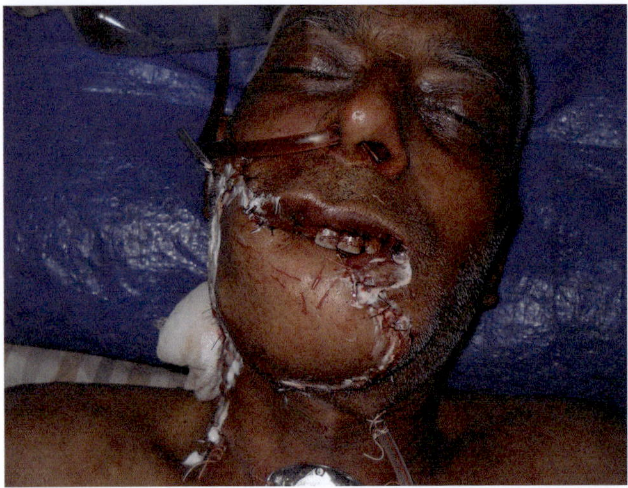

Fig. 15.22 The final outcome is quite acceptable. This patient was on oral feeds and survived for 18 months after the procedure. He developed a sinus in flap after radiation therapy and gradually the bone came out after about 12 months. The fibrosis kept the flap in position and he continued to have oral feeds till he died

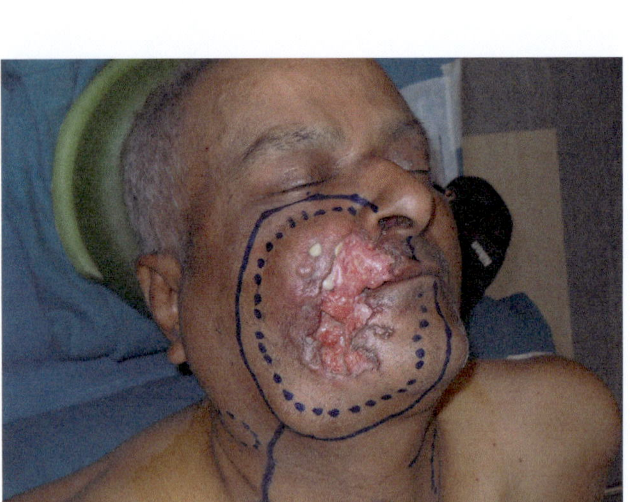

Fig. 15.23 This patient had very advanced buccal mucosa cancer with bilateral nodes

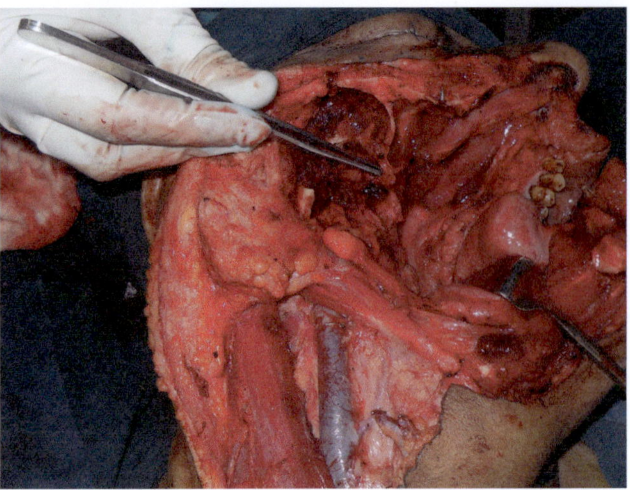

Fig. 15.24 The resection was carried out with compartment surgery concept clearing the entire high ITF

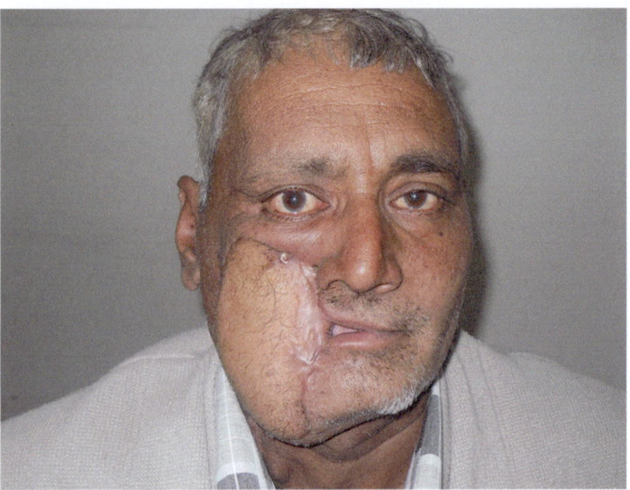

Fig. 15.25 Same patient after 1 year of treatment. The reconstruction was achieved with bi-paddled PMMC flap

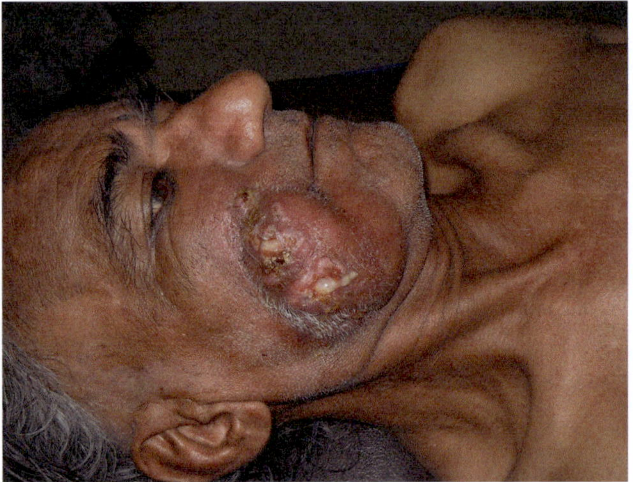

Fig. 15.26 A patient with extensive buccal mucosa cancer. He underwent similar procedure as described above

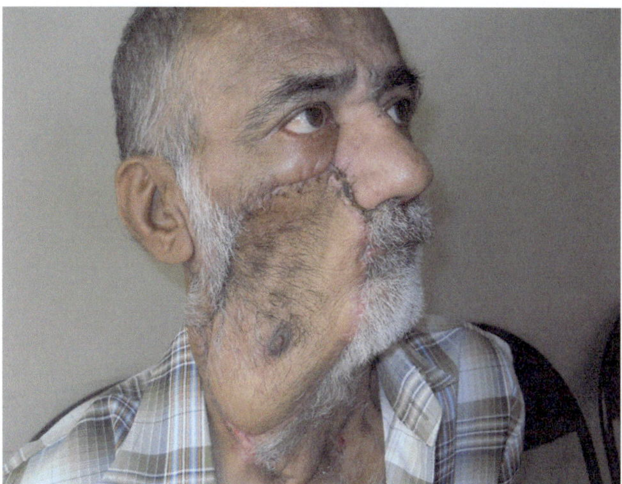

Fig. 15.27 The reconstruction was achieved with spiral PMMC as bi-paddled flap was not feasible. The patient is living well after 18 months of treatment

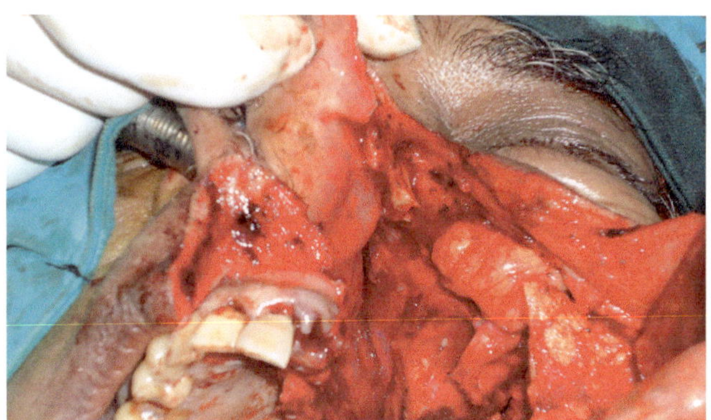

Fig. 15.28 The reconstruction of total maxillectomy defect is quite challenging and may need vascularized bone flap

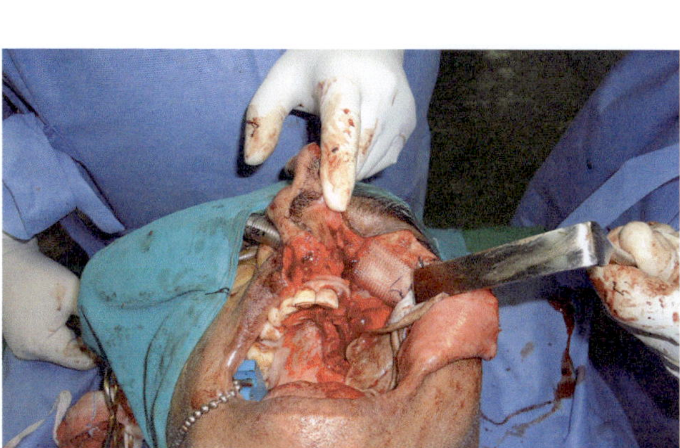

Fig. 15.29 We use prolene mesh used for inguinal hernia repair and reconstruct inferior defect with a temporalis flap

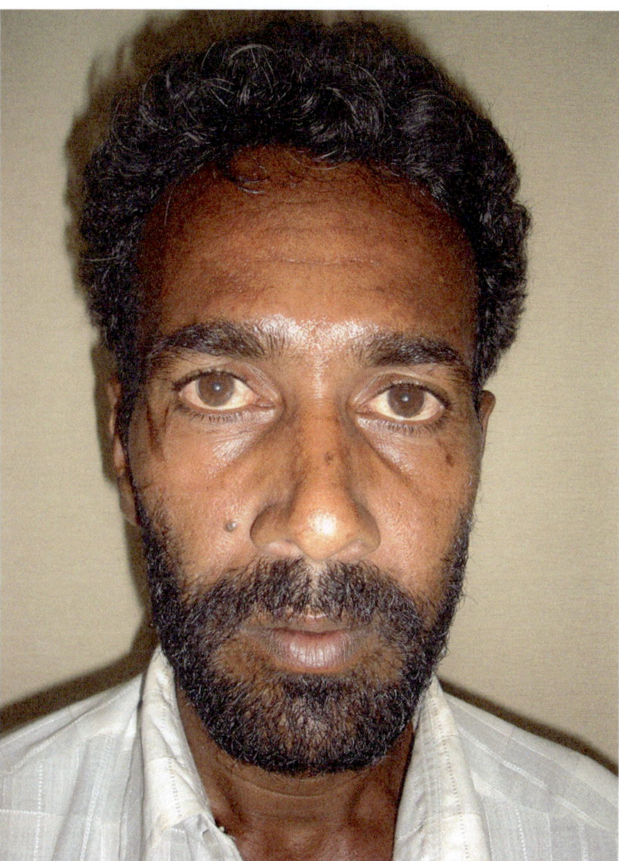

Fig. 15.30 The final outcome after 1 year of procedure shows good eye support

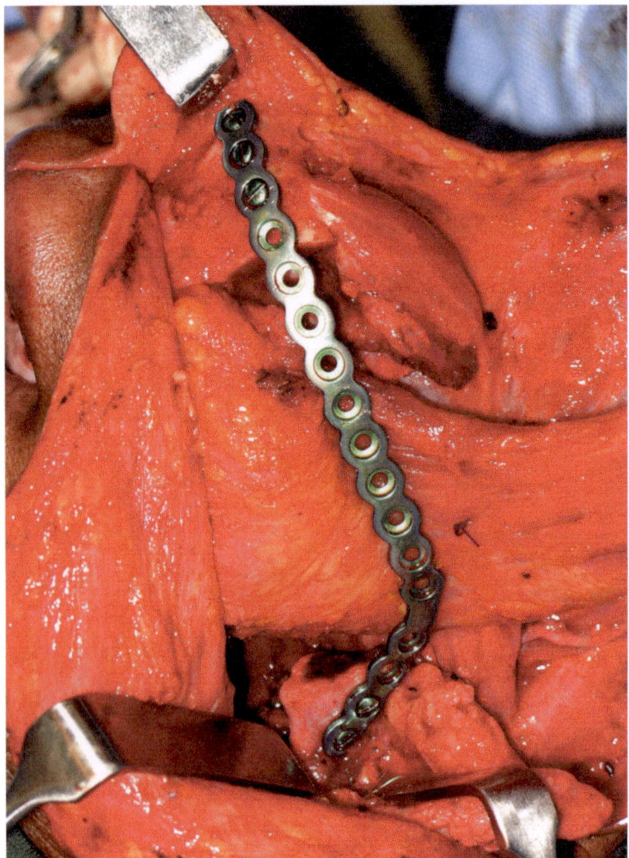

Fig. 15.31 Plate with PPMC flap was a common mode of reconstruction for segmental mandible defect. We don't do it that frequently and do not recommend it. It can be used for a very limited lateral segment defect and the plate needs to be covered with flap in all direction. There are high chances that plate will come out after radiotherapy

References

1. Trivedi NP, et al. Head and neck cancer in India: need to formulate uniform national treatment guideline? Indian J Cancer. 2012;49(1): 6–10.
2. Trivedi NP, Trivedi NN, et al. Optimizing multimodality treatment for head and neck cancer in rural India. Indian J Cancer. 2012;49(2):225–9.
3. Trivedi NP, et al. Microvascular free flap reconstruction for head and neck cancer in a resource constrained environment in rural India. Indian J Plast Surg. 2013;46(1):82–6.

16 Flaps

The flap reconstruction is an integral part of head–neck cancer surgery. The reconstruction has evolved greatly in the last few decades and that has enabled oncosurgeons to resect more advanced and complex tumors. The PMMC flap has been used as a mainstay of reconstruction for decades. The microvascular reconstruction has evolved lately and is becoming the standard of care for head and neck reconstruction. The algorithm for reconstruction of various subsites is already discussed in individual chapters. This chapter essentially focuses on flap raising technique, and only those flaps that are used frequently in our practice are described.

The following flaps are described in this chapter:

1. Pectralis major myocutaneous flap
2. Temporalis flap
3. Infrahyoid flap
4. Forehead flap
5. Anterolateral thigh flap
6. Fibula flap
7. Rectus abdominis flap
8. Radial forearm flap

N. Trivedi, *Atlas of Head and Neck Cancer Surgery: The Compartment Surgery for Resection in 3-D*,
DOI 10.1007/978-81-322-2050-3_16, © Springer India 2015

The Pectoralis Major Myocutaneous Flap

This flap has been the mainstay for head–neck reconstruction for a very long time and continues to be an important component even today. It is very simple to raise and is a very safe flap. It is based on pectoral branch of thoraio-acromial artery.

Possibilities for PMMC Flap Reconstruction

- Buccal mucosa–alveolus reconstruction: lining or for bi-paddled reconstruction
- Tongue–FOM reconstruction: for hemiglossectomy, total and extended glossectomy as a single flap or in combination with other flaps
- Oropharynx reconstruction: muscle only for small defects and composite flap for complex defects
- Larynx–pharynx reconstruction: as patch or tube reconstruction after laryngectomy and pharyngectomy. For salvage laryngectomy
- Neck–parotid reconstruction: for large skin cover after composite resection involving the skin
- Salvage surgery: reconstruction of choice for majority of salvage surgery
- Resource constrained setup: reconstruction of choice for majority of defects

Limitations

- Reach not enough for maxilla and skull base defects
- Difficult to cover defects above the zygoma
- Flaps drags down in some cases due to its weight

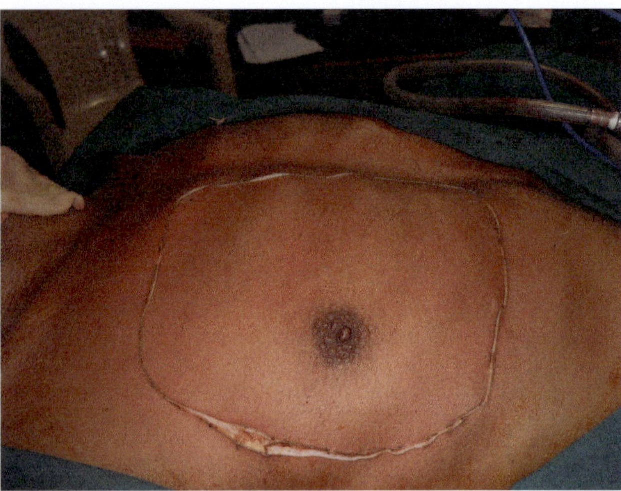

Fig. 16.1 The surface marking for large skin paddle. This is the area from where one can take skin paddle of varying sizes. The area below and medial to the nipple is preferred for small- to medium-sized defects. This donor site needs skin grafting but majority of other defects can be closed primarily. One needs to be extra careful while raising the flap in female and try to preserve as much breast tissue as possible while taking sufficient care not to harm the blood supply to skin paddle

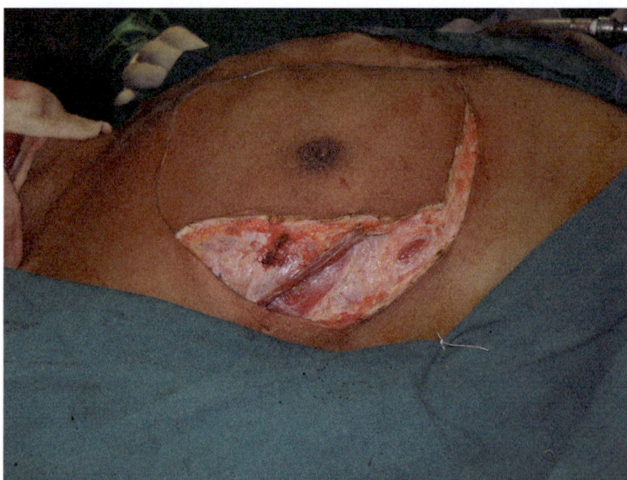

Fig. 16.2 Identifying the lateral border of pectoralis major muscle is the first step in this procedure. This gives complete orientation about further dissection

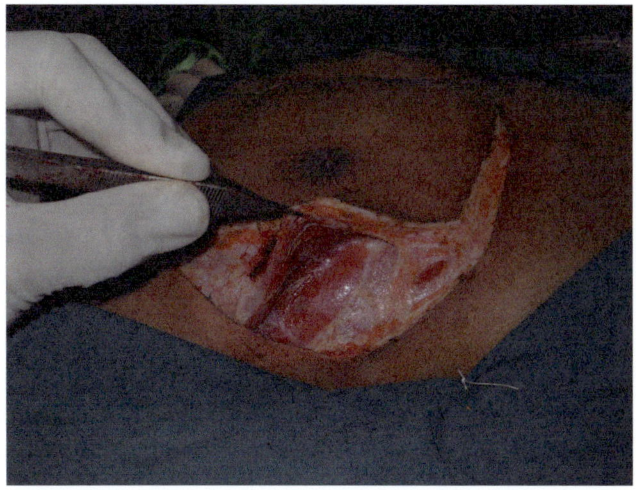

Fig. 16.3 The flap is raised separate from pectoralis minor muscle

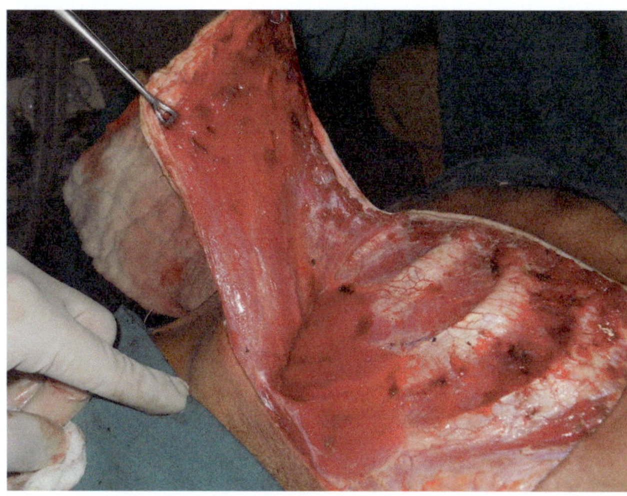

Fig. 16.6 The muscle is raised separate from the rib and pectoralis minor muscle. Try and leave periosteum over the rib for better graft uptake

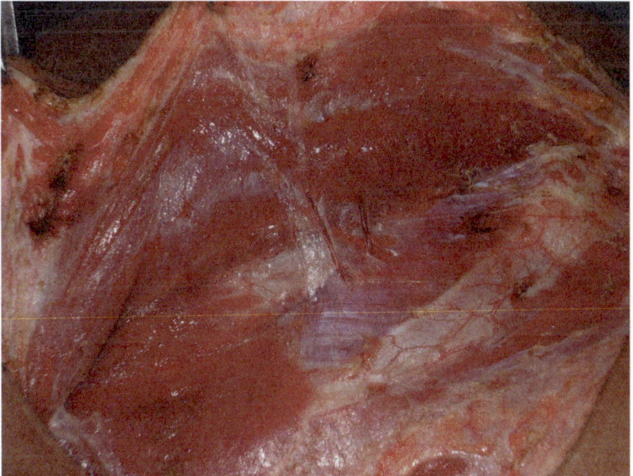

Fig. 16.4 The small perforator vessels are seen at deep surface of the muscle

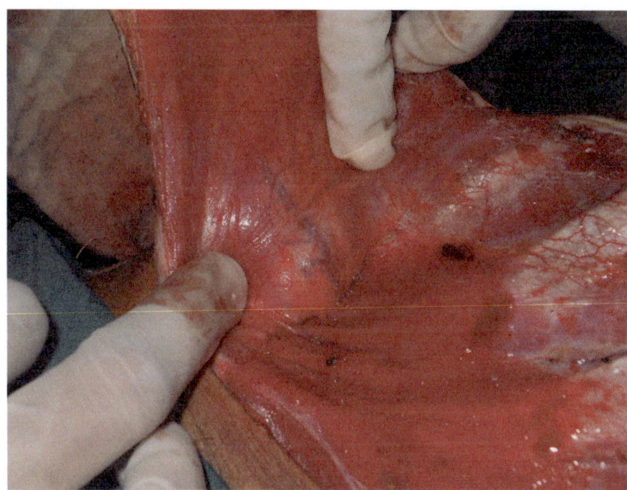

Fig. 16.7 The pedicle is seen as flap is raised further. Be careful in preserving the deep fascia over pedicle to avoid accidental injury. Further dissection is always carried with pedicle in view

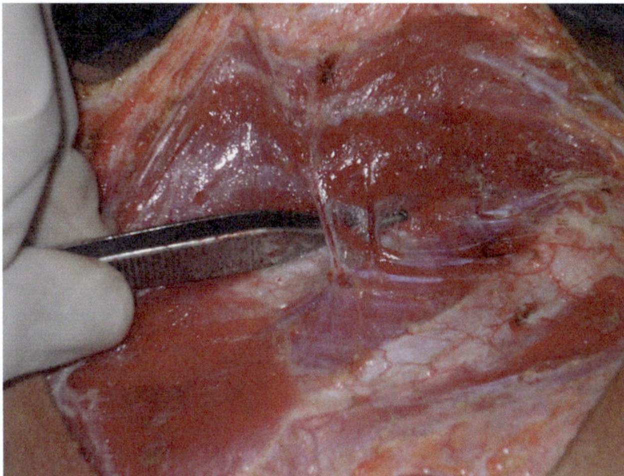

Fig. 16.5 It is important to secure these perforators to avoid postoperative hematoma

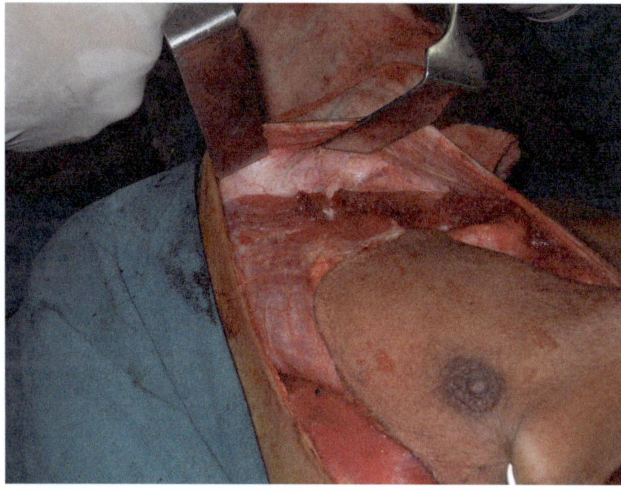

Fig. 16.8 The skin flap above is raised to tunnel the flap into the neck

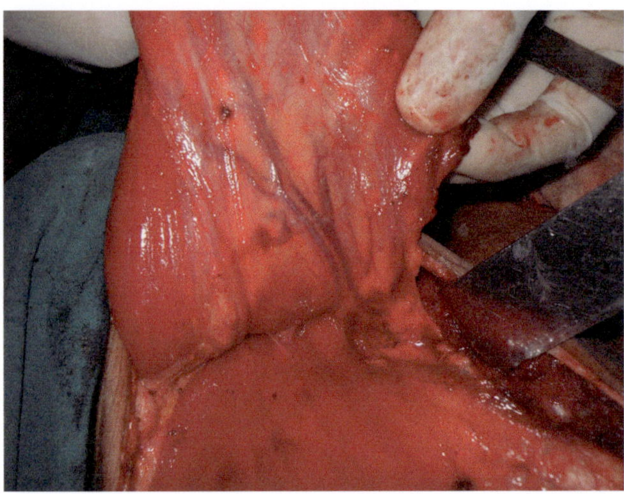

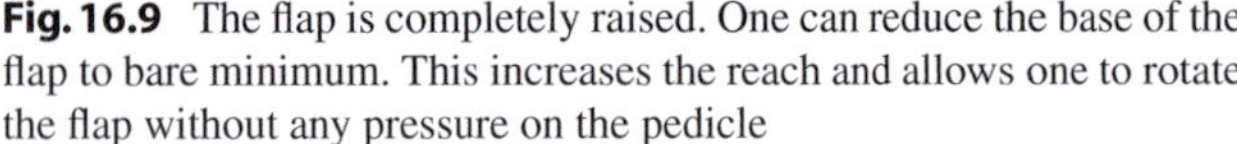

Fig. 16.9 The flap is completely raised. One can reduce the base of the flap to bare minimum. This increases the reach and allows one to rotate the flap without any pressure on the pedicle

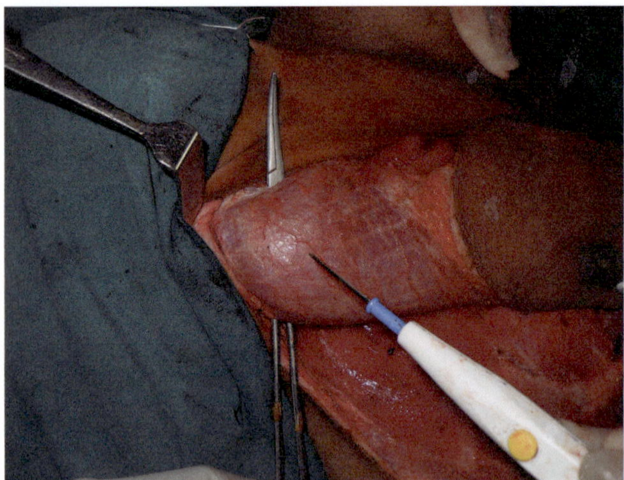

Fig. 16.10 The lateral muscle fibers are divided to increase the reach of the flap

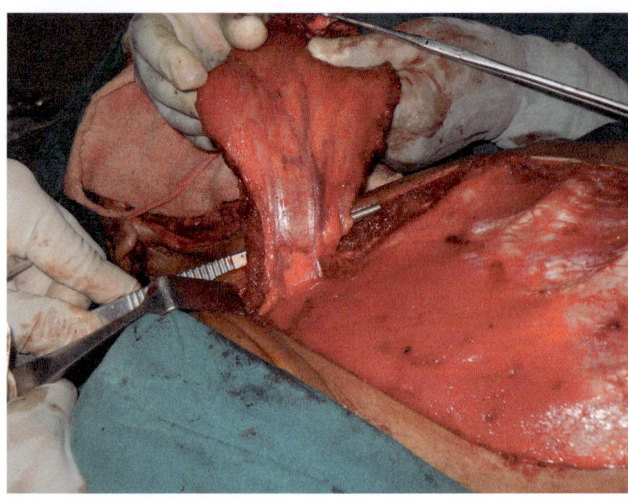

Fig. 16.11 The flap is completely raised. The base is kept bare minimum just to support the pedicle

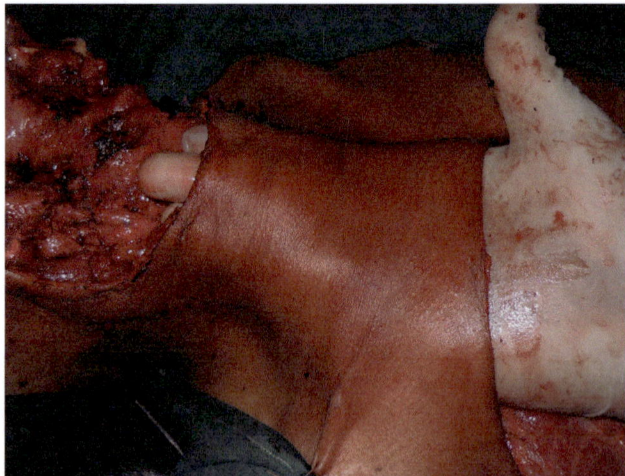

Fig. 16.12 The tunnel is complete and adequate in size. One must make the tunnel large enough for safe and tension free passage of the muscle. When there is any doubt regarding the tension over the pedicle, one has to promptly increase the size of the tunnel or put releasing incisions over the skin

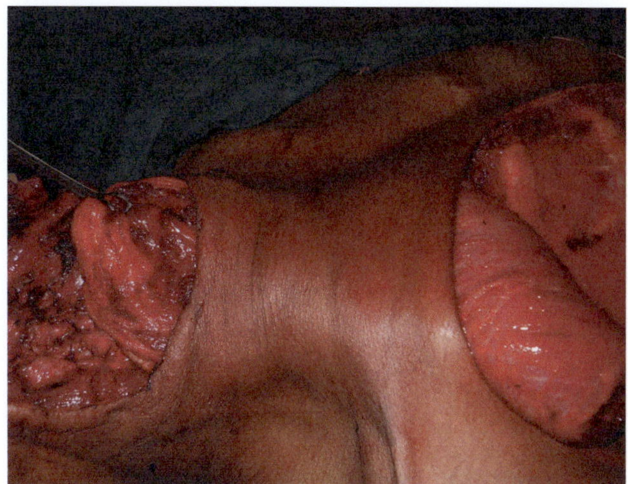

Fig. 16.13 The flap has been tunneled into the neck. It is important to avoid any twist of the pedicle particularly when the skin is required for defect of the neck. Most of the flaps are lost due to venous congestion because of the twist or pressure over the pedicle and every attempt should be made to avoid these problems

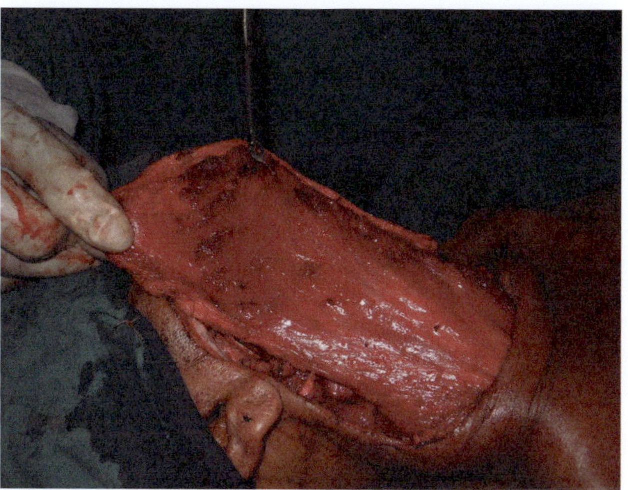

Fig. 16.14 The flap has covered the defect with ease and is tension free one must remove neck extension before raising the flap. One can remove the neck extension to increase the reach while suturing the flap. The PMMC can reconstruct majority of defects of the oral cavity and larynx–pharynx. This flap is very versatile and can be used as muscle only or large bi-paddle myocutaneous flap

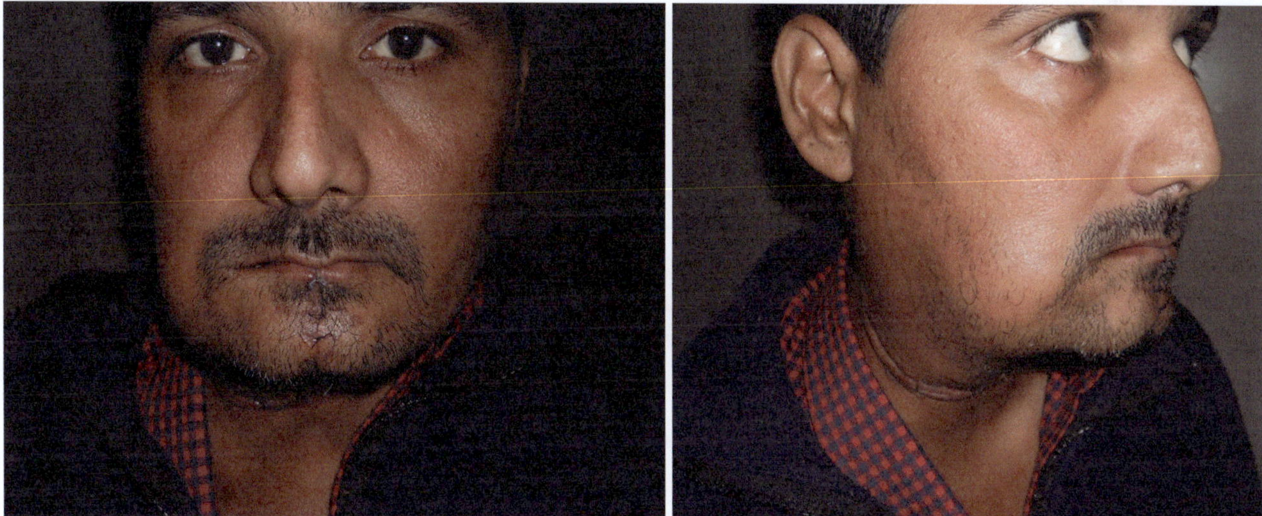

Figs. 16.15 and 16.16 The cosmetic outcome is quite acceptable in majority of patients with proper flap orientation

Temporalis Muscle Flap

The temporalis flap is a simple and safe flap for reconstruction of maxillary defects.

Possibilities for Temporalis Reconstruction

- Infrastructure maxillectomy defects
- Orbital floor reconstruction with temporalis and coronoid process
- Lateral skull base defects
- Orbit reconstruction

Limitations

- Patients develop trismus in postoperative period after oral cavity reconstruction.
- Cosmetic dip over the temple can be profound in some cases.

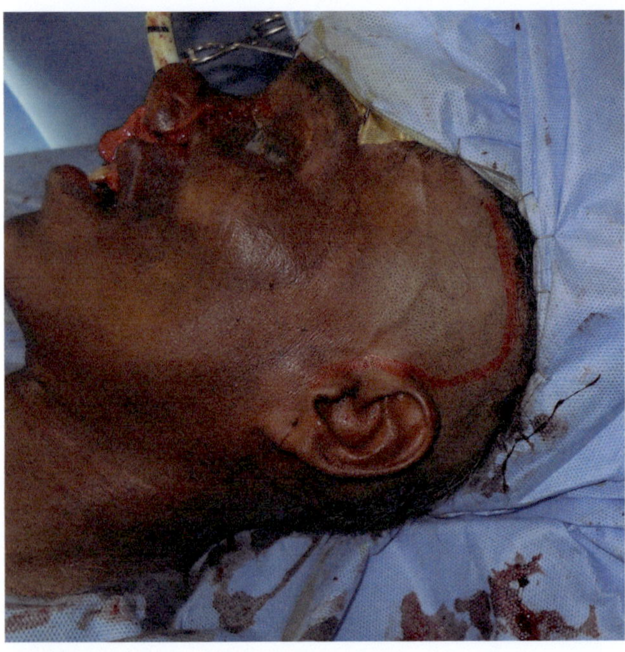

Fig. 16.17 The skin is marked to raise the flap

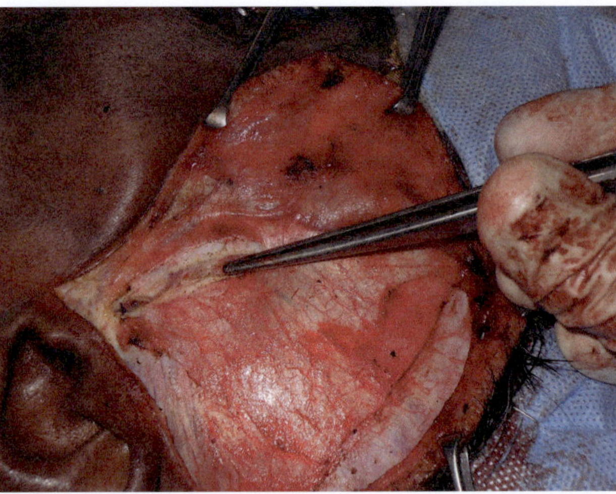

Fig. 16.19 The superficial layer of temporalis fascia is divided and fat plane is exposed for anterior dissection. This process automatically prevents injury to frontal branch of facial nerve as it runs above the superficial layer of temporalis fascia

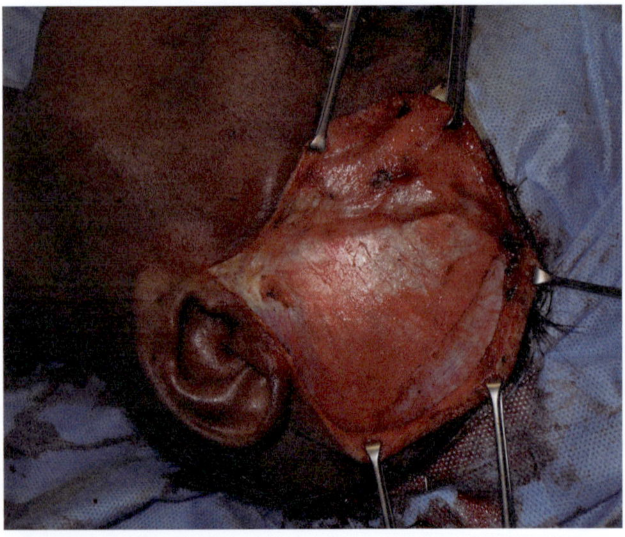

Fig. 16.18 The skin flap is raised over temporalis fascia. Care is taken not to go too anterior to avoid injury to the facial nerve

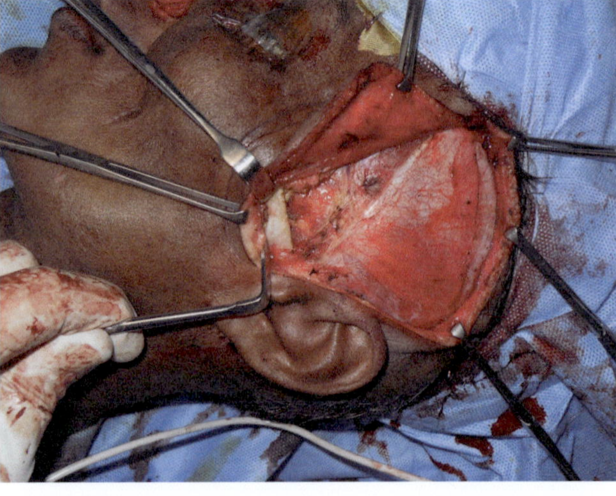

Fig. 16.20 The zygoma is exposed and temporalis muscle is freed from below

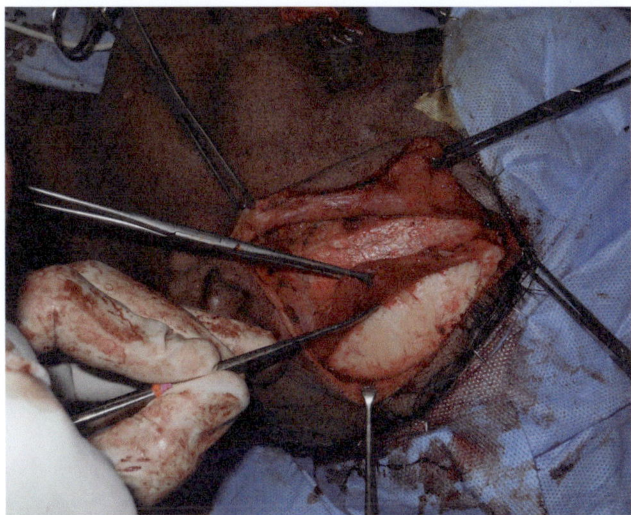

Fig. 16.21 The muscle is separated from the skull. It is important to include more muscle in the posterior part and also to include the fascia beyond muscle to increase its reach. It is advisable to use periosteum elevator instead of cautery to avoid injury to deep branches of maxillary artery particularly in the lower half

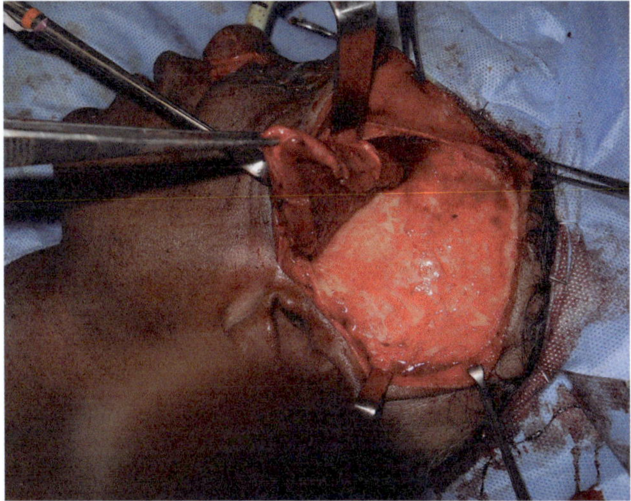

Fig. 16.22 The muscle is freed all around

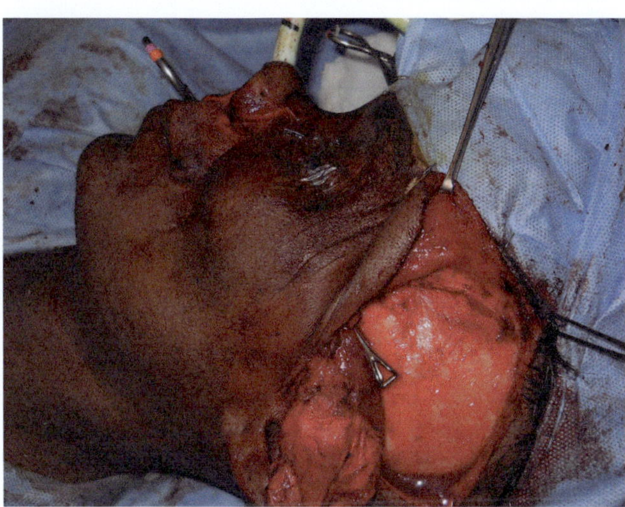

Fig. 16.23 The forceps is tunneled below the zygoma to bring the muscle into the maxillary cavity. This flap is useful when upper alveolus with maxillary tuberosity is removed. There is adequate space for flap rotation without any struggle and tension in such situation

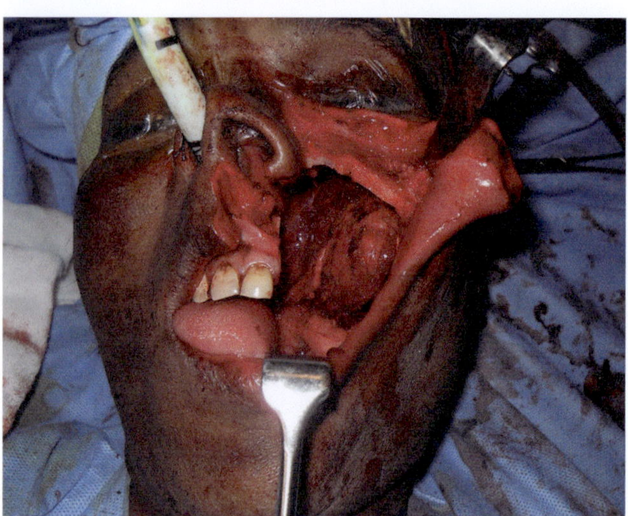

Fig. 16.24 The flap is in the cavity and can be sutured to complete the procedure. It is important to secure the medial insertion over the palate. We prefer to have holes in the palate and use nonabsorbable sutures in this region to have added strength. We also avoid placing suture on the buccal aspect to avoid tension on palatal aspect

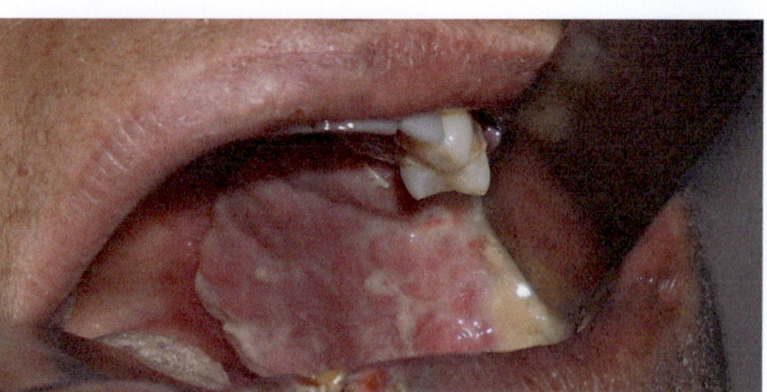

Fig. 16.25 The photograph shows healed-healthy flap in few days

Infrahyoid Flap

This is a local flap that we use quite often to reconstruct small defects of the oral cavity. We prefer this flap over submental and nasolabial flap because of its better oncological safety over submental flap and better cosmesis over nasolabial flap. This flap is reliable if care is taken not to damage the venous drainage.

Possibilities for Infrahyoid Flap Reconstruction

- Small tongue and FOM defects are ideal for this flap.
- Small base of tongue defects can be reconstructed with this flap.
- Small buccal mucosa defect with marginal mandibular resection can also be reconstructed with this flap.

Limitations

- Upper reach is limited.
- The venous drainage is a concern and can cause flap loss.

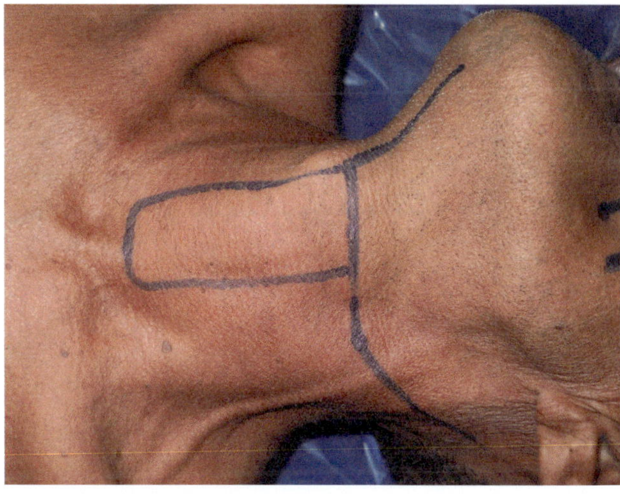

Fig. 16.26 The flap is marked over the neck. The skin width can be about 3–4 cm and the length can be from hyoid to clavicle. It is better for thin and long individuals compared to patients with short neck

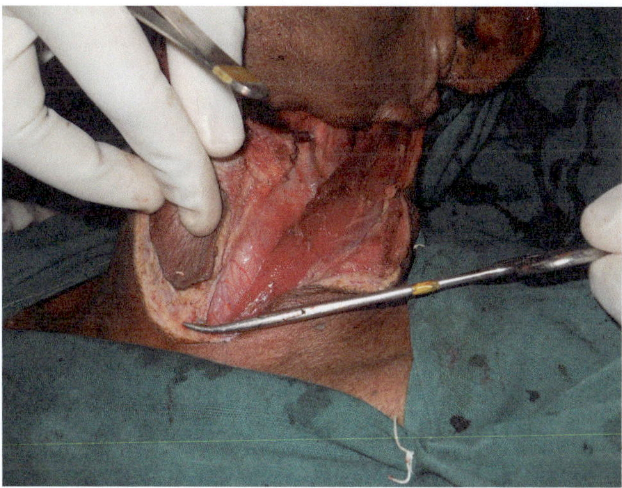

Fig. 16.28 The anterior jugular vein is ligated to expose the strap muscles

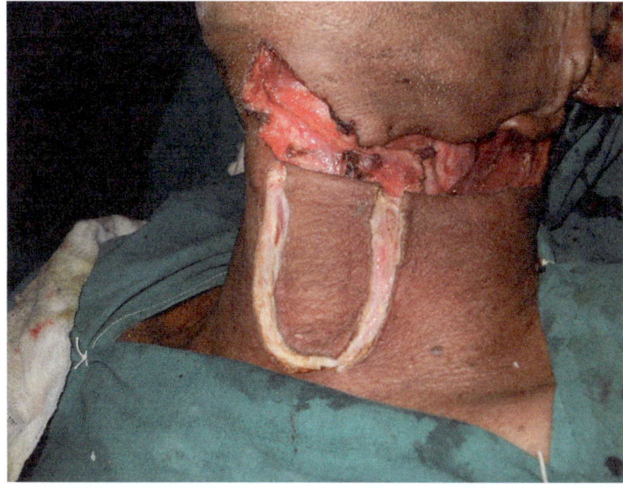

Fig. 16.27 The neck dissection is complete. It is important to avoid dissecting the area medial to IJV near the superior thyroid veins

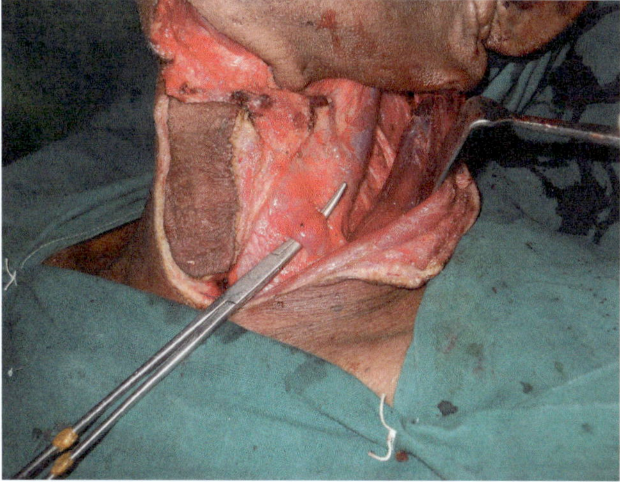

Fig. 16.29 The omohyoid muscle is divided to expose IJV

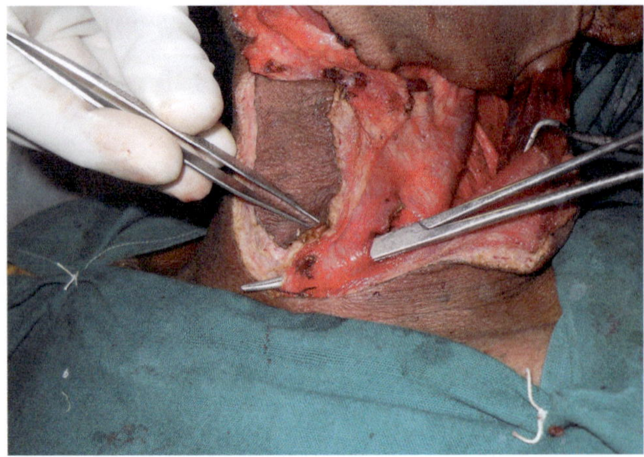

Fig. 16.30 The strap muscles are divided in the lower end

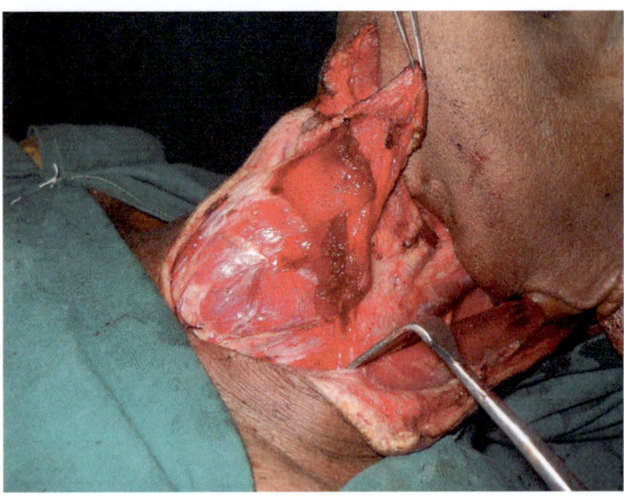

Fig. 16.31 The flap is raised from below on the surface of thyroid gland

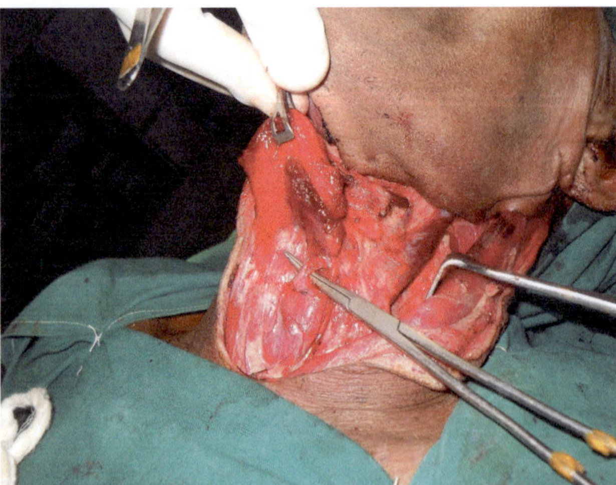

Fig. 16.32 The superior thyroid pedicle is identified and is included in the flap. The strap muscles receive their supply from small perforating branch from superior thyroid artery

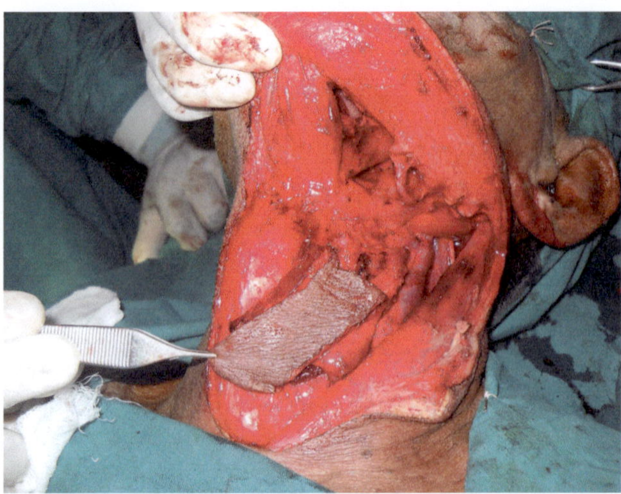

Fig. 16.33 The strap muscles are divided from their upper attachments

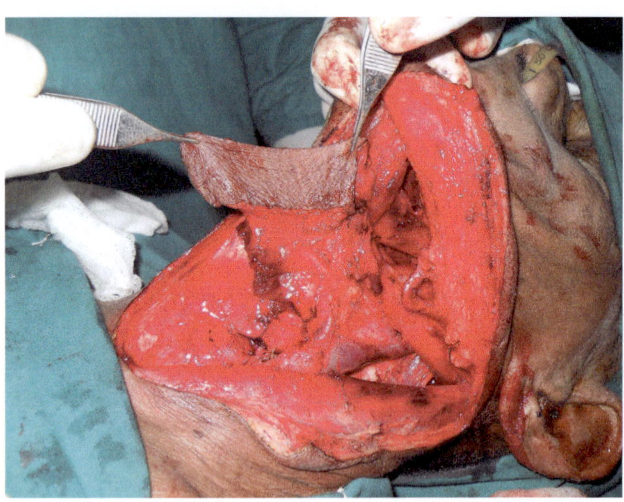

Fig. 16.34 The flap is raised. It is important to preserve facial covering over its pedicle and avoid any dissection in this area. This flap has very marginal venous drainage and its survival will solely depend upon the preservation of bunch of veins coming from IJV

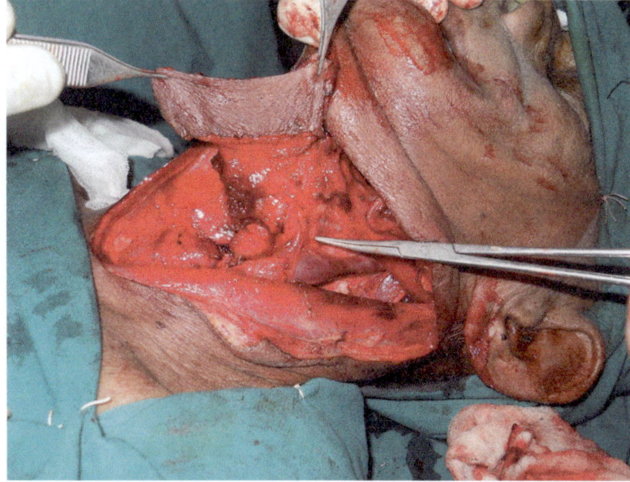

Fig. 16.35 The photograph shows a vein with surrounding facial attachments

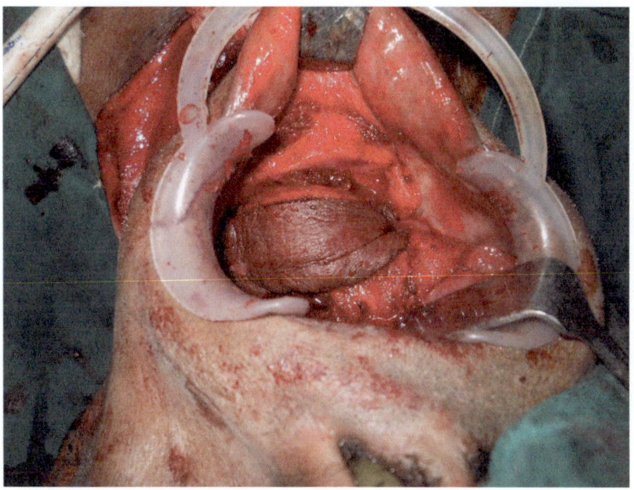

Fig. 16.36 The flap is tunneled intra-orally for coverage of anterior floor of the mouth defect

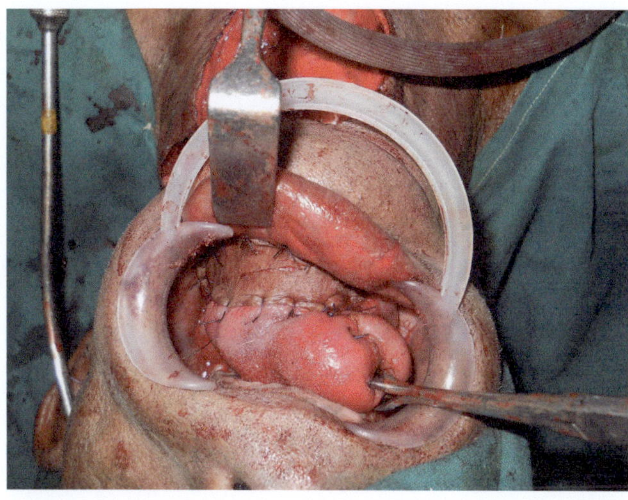

Fig. 16.37 The flap suturing is complete. This flap remains in a state of congestion throughout but generally survives if due care is taken while raising it

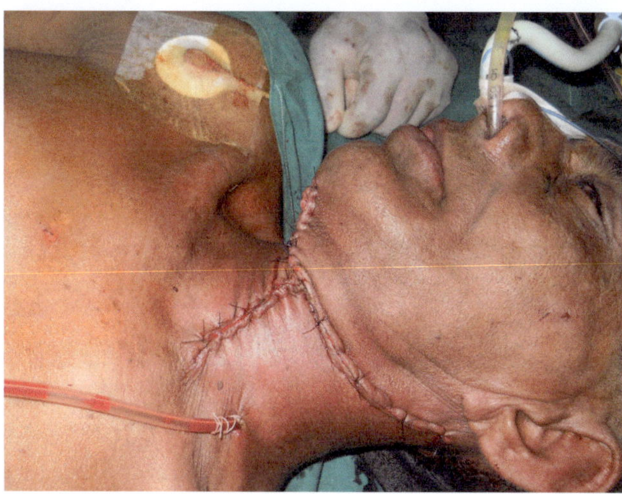

Fig. 16.38 The neck defect can be closed primarily without tension in majority of cases. Release incision is necessary in short neck patients to release the tension and improve postoperative scar

Forehead Flap

This flap is very rarely used in head–neck reconstruction in current scenario. We use this flap in salvage surgery where other conventional options are exhausted and in resource constrained setup for composite maxillary defect reconstruction. It is a very safe flap and provides very large pliable skin cover.

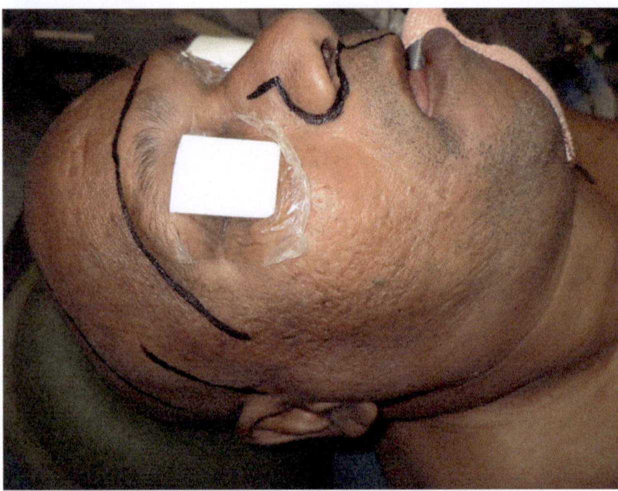

Fig. 16.39 The flap is marked for bilateral anterior maxillectomy for patients in a rural clinic where it was not possible to perform microvascular surgery. It is based on an anterior branch of superficial temporal artery

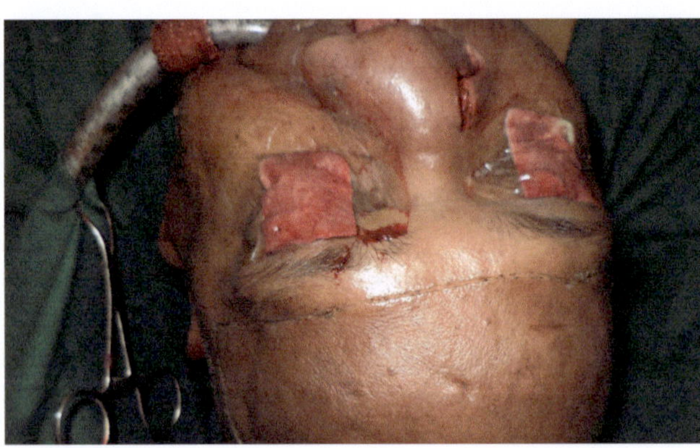

Fig. 16.40 Entire forehead can be used for reconstruction. The width can be increased by taking more scalp skin

Possibility for Forehead Flap

- Salvage surgery where other options are exhausted
- Complex maxilla and buccal mucosa defects in resource limited setup

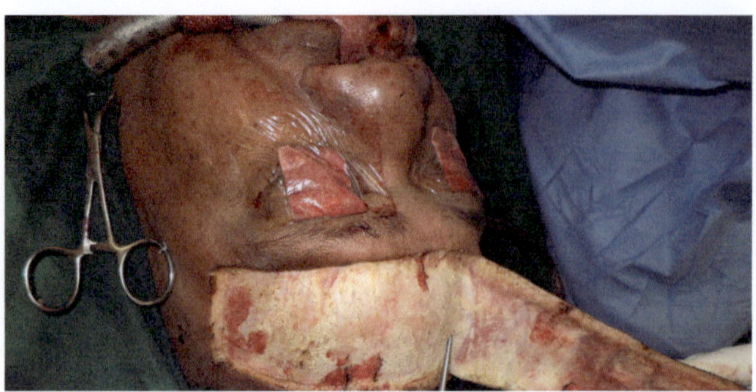

Fig. 16.41 The flap is raised leaving periosteum on skull

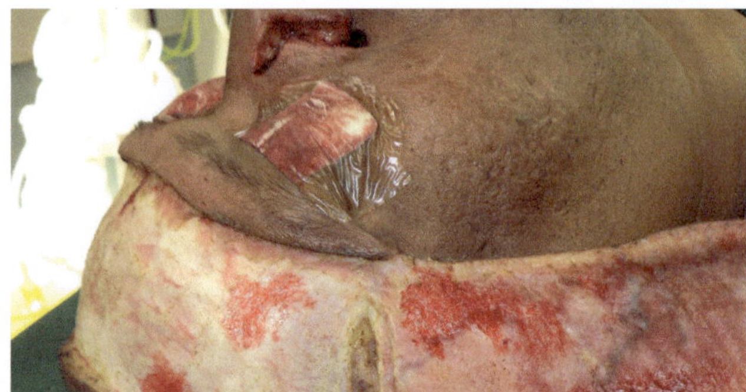

Fig. 16.42 The superficial layer of temporalis fascia is divided, and dissection goes below to protect the vessel near the base of the flap. This is an important step and ensures flap safety

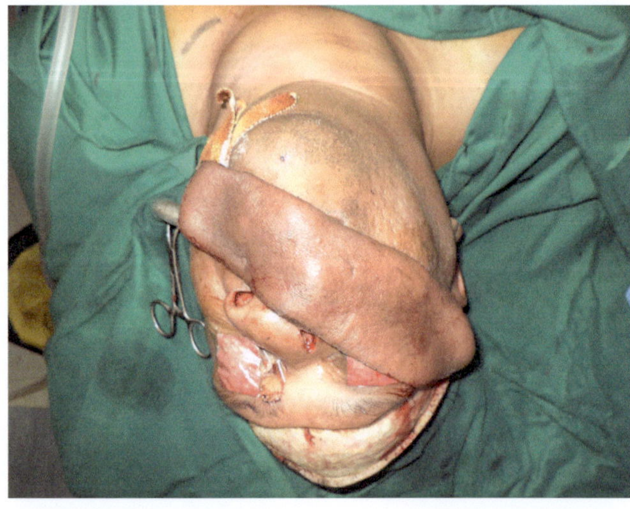

Fig. 16.43 Photograph shows that flap has excellent reach

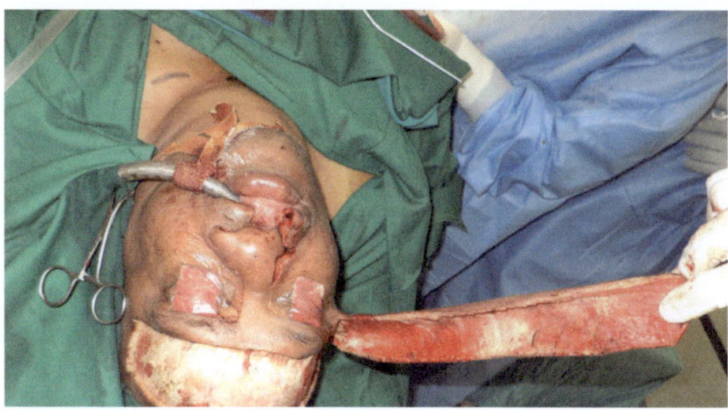

Fig. 16.44 The flap is ready for insertion. It is important to dissect adequately for tunneling flap above the zygoma

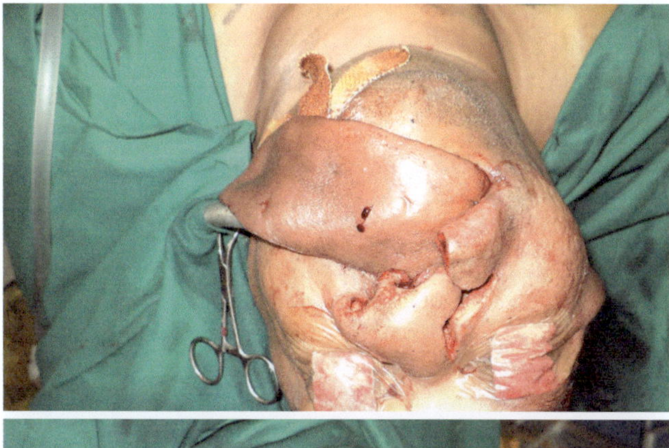

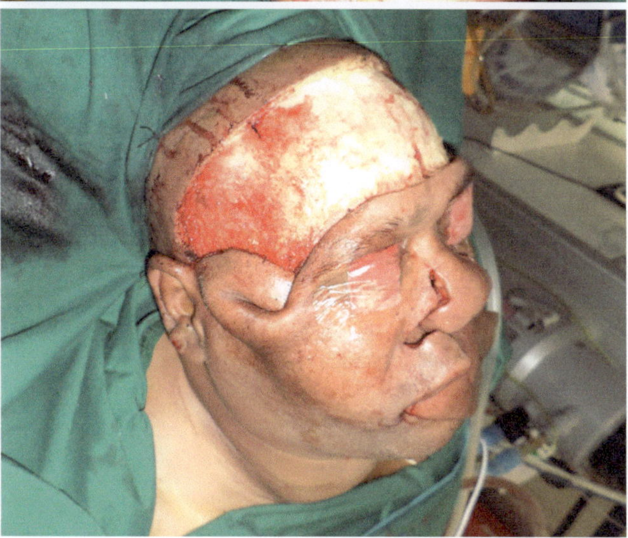

Figs. 16.45 and 16.46 The flap is tunneled into the anterior maxillary defect. This was supported by the iliac crest bone graft. The flap can be used in the same way for complex buccal defects as shown in the previous chapter

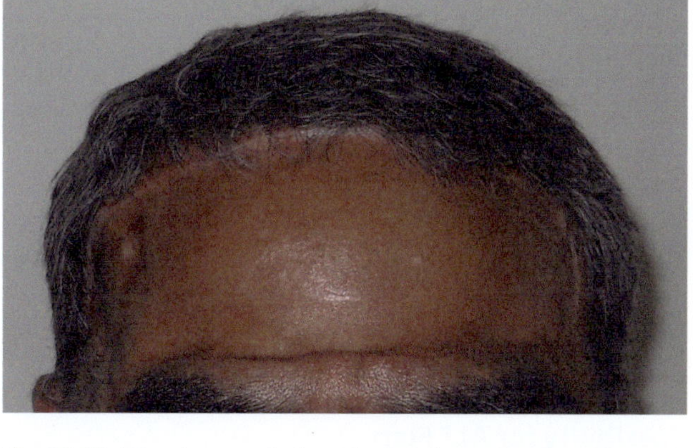

Fig. 16.47 The photograph shows healed donor site after skin graft. The color match is actually quite acceptable in dark individuals. This flap is not ideal in today's era but very effective in dealing with some tricky situations

Anterolateral Thigh Flap (ALT Flap)

The ALT flap has replaced PMMC flap to a large extent in the head–neck and has become the standard of care for head–neck reconstruction. This flap is very versatile and can be used to reconstruct very large and complex defects or to reconstruct small soft tissue defects. The flap can be thinned according to needs which increases its adaptability. It has minimal donor site morbidity and simultaneous two team approach is possible. This makes it even more attractive.

Possibility for ALT Flap

- Buccal mucosa–alveolus reconstruction: complex bi-paddled reconstruction.
- Tongue–FOM reconstruction: for hemiglossectomy, total and extended glossectomy as a single flap or in combination with other flaps.
- Oropharynx reconstruction: for large and complex defects.
- Maxilla reconstruction: for large composite defects involving the skin, bone, and eye.
- Larynx–pharynx reconstruction: as tube reconstruction after total laryngectomy–pharyngectomy. This is the preferred over jejunum flap because it is safer with lower donor site morbidity and better speech and swallowing outcome.
- Neck, parotid reconstruction: for large skin cover after composite resection involving the skin.
- Salvage surgery: for large complex defects where recipient vessels are available.
- For defects of scalps and region above the zygoma where other regional flaps cannot reach.

Limitations

- The perforator is inconsistent at times. It is important to know how to convert to TFL flap if conventional flap is not available.

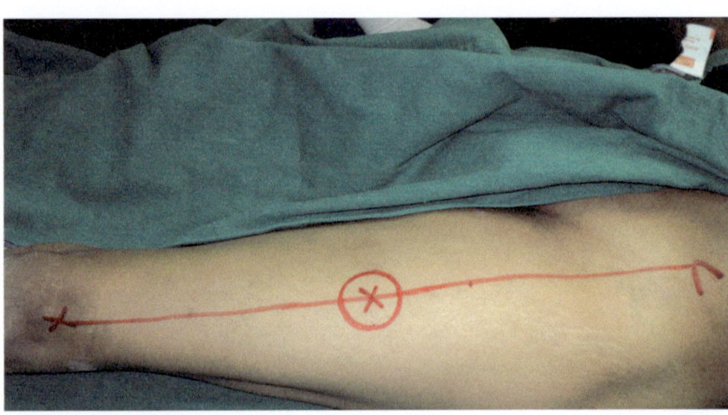

Fig. 16.48 The photograph shows surface marking for the skin perforator. A line is drawn from anterior superior iliac spine to lateral border of the patella, and the perforator approximately lies just above the midpoint of this line. One can draw a circle with 3 cm diameter, and the perforator generally falls within this

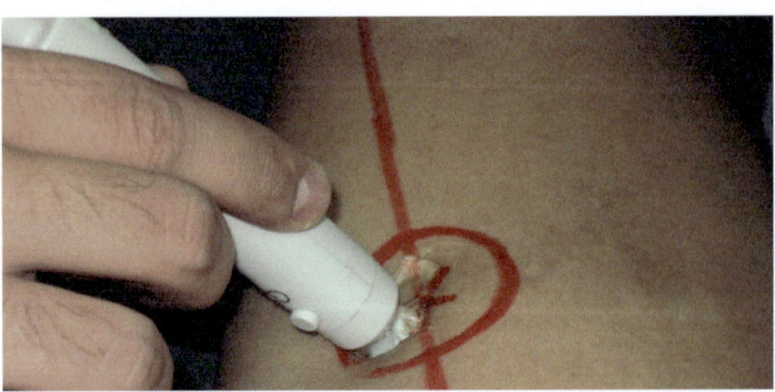

Fig. 16.49 The Doppler machine can be used to identify the perforator. This is not needed in routine cases as skin paddle is large enough that perforator will fall within this area. We use this when planning a small flap and want to be sure about its location

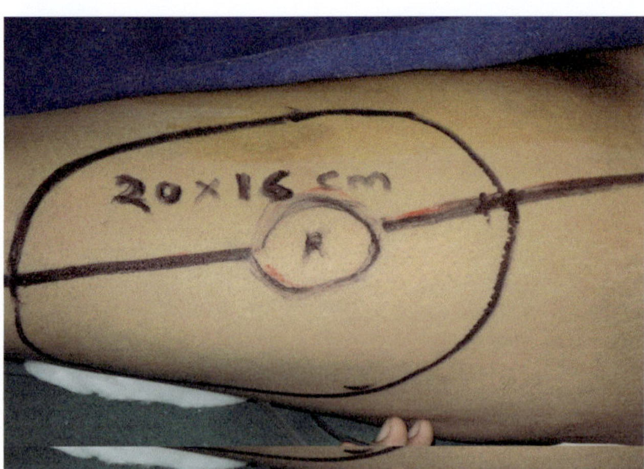

Fig. 16.50 The ALT flap size can be as large as 25–30 in length and 14–15 cm in width and can sustain on one perforator. It is important to perform anastomosis of two veins to avoid venous congestion for such a large flap

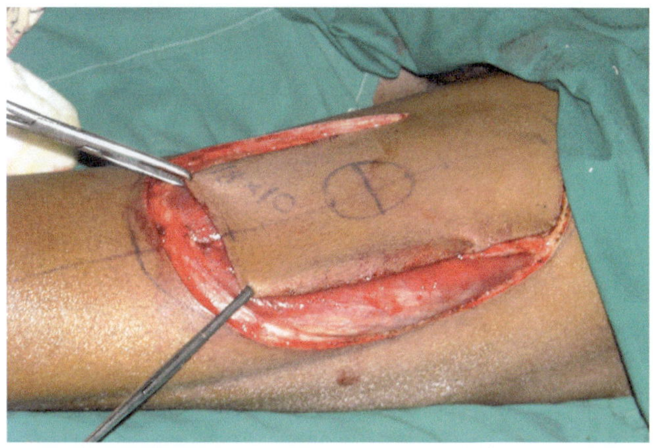

Fig. 16.51 The skin incision is placed in "U" shaped manner leaving the top-end attached. The flap can be either sutured back if perforator is not available or can be extended above and converted into a tensor fascia lata flap (TFL)

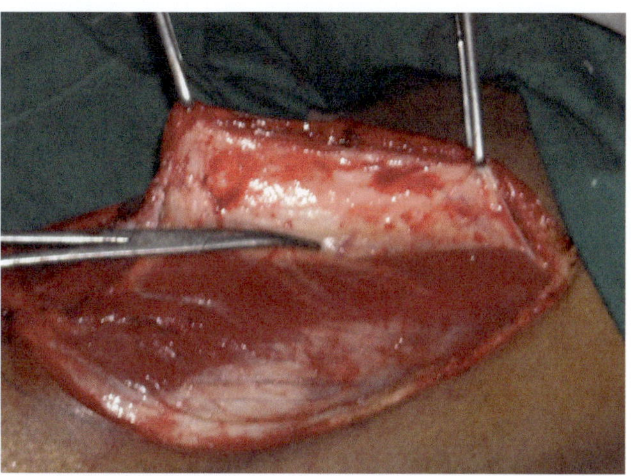

Fig. 16.53 The flap is raised over vastus lateralis muscle. The perforator can be either intramuscular or intraseptal, and further dissection proceeds accordingly. If one large perforator is not identified in the middle part, dissection is carried out in upper direction and one can generally find a TFL perforator

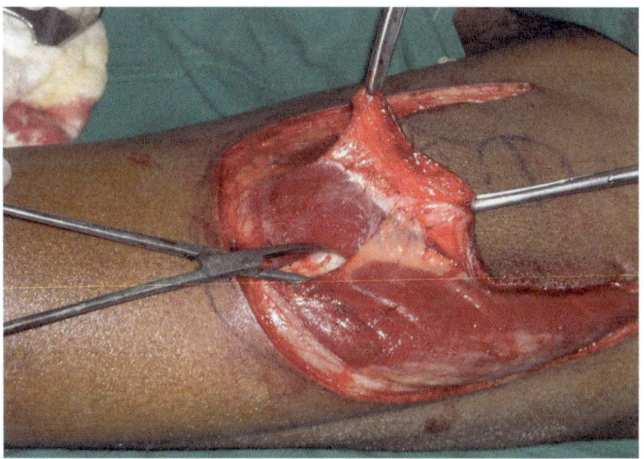

Fig. 16.52 It is better to identify the septum at lower end early in dissection. The rectus femoris muscle is medial to the septum and can be separated from the septum just with finger dissection

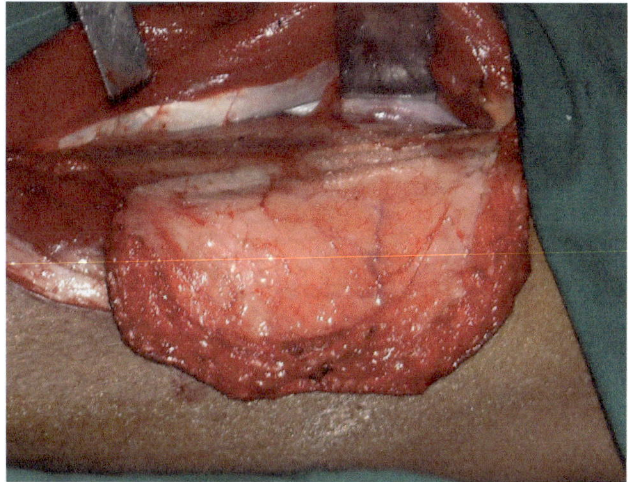

Fig. 16.54 The rectus femoris muscle is separated in the entire length to expose the main pedicle which is the descending branch of lateral circumflex artery

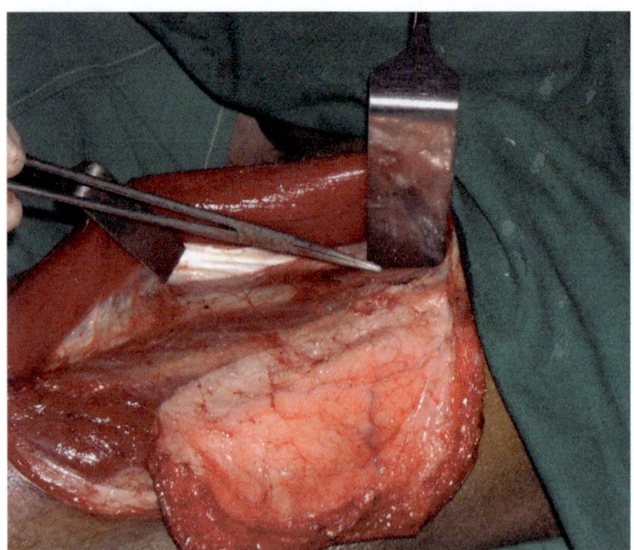

Fig. 16.55 The fascia over the pedicle is dissected to expose the pedicle in its entire length. The pedicle gives small perforators to surrounding structures and these are ligated with clips. The medial perforators are clipped early in dissection so that the pedicle can be freed from below

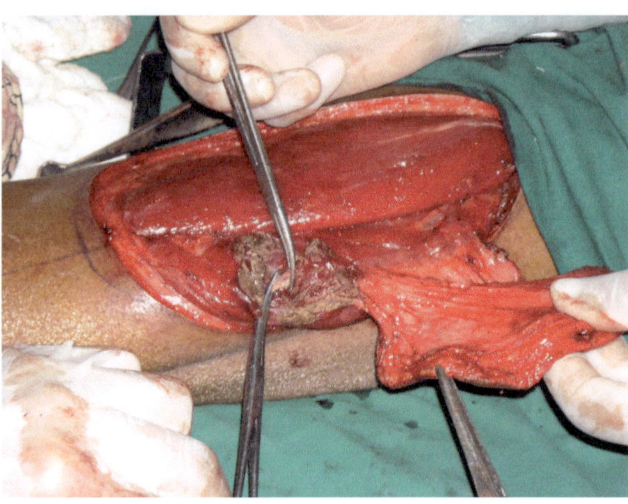

Fig. 16.57 The pedicle gives of the perforator branch and enters the vastus lateralis muscle. We prefer to have cuff of muscle around the perforator, but one can trace the perforator through the muscle. The distal end of the perforator is identified within the lateralis muscle and is ligated

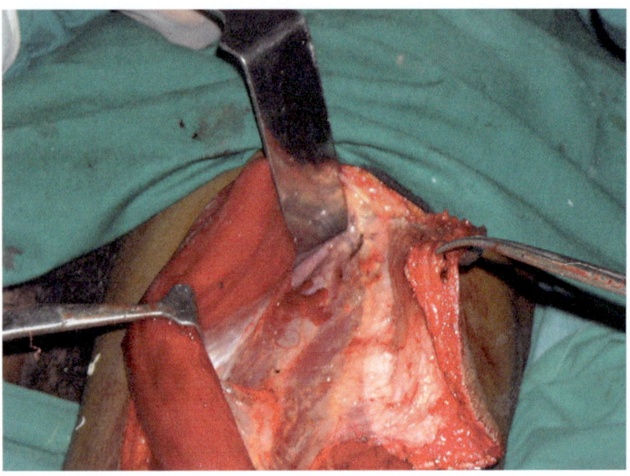

Fig. 16.56 One can see the pedicle coming down and fascia is dissected in the entire length

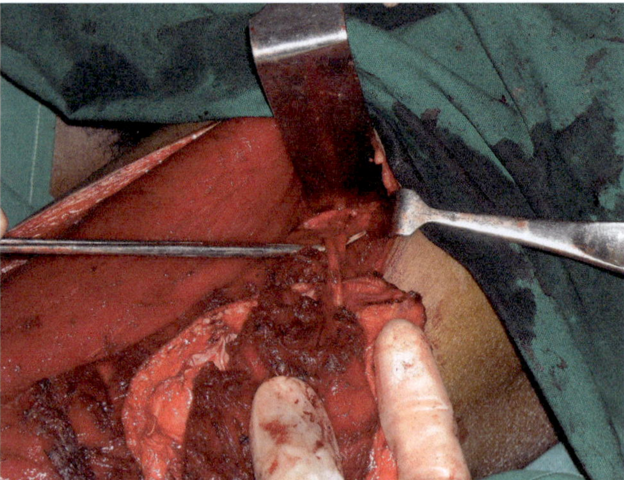

Fig. 16.58 Once the perforator is secured by dividing muscle around it, the pedicle is isolated from surrounding structure. It is advisable to trace the pedicle as high as possible to gain maximum length that helps in vascular anastomosis

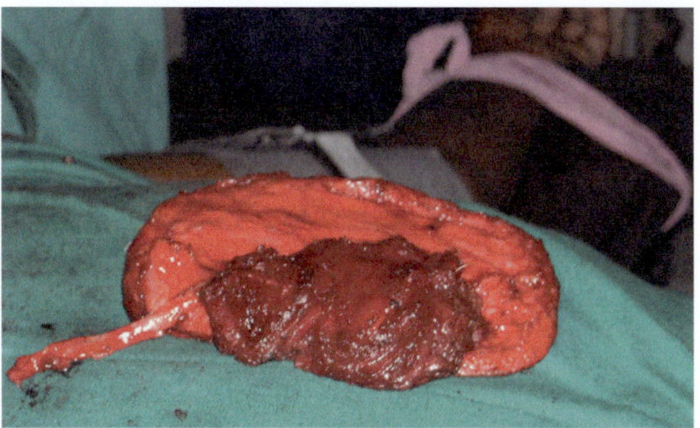

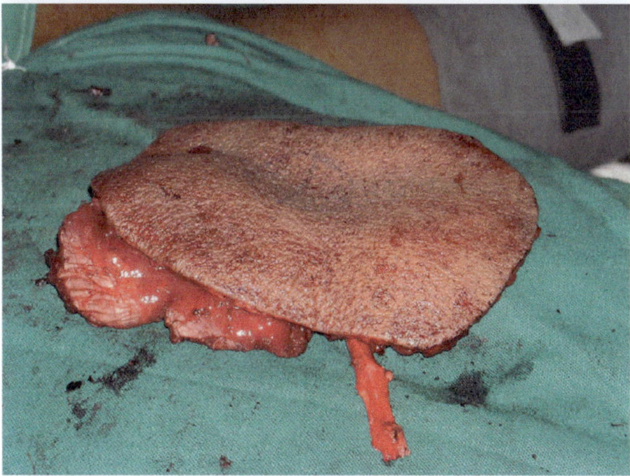

Figs. 16.59 and 16.60 The flap is raised with part of muscle and pedicle length seems adequate. Many donor site defects can be closed primarily but a few may need skin grafts. It is better to avoid closure with great tension

Fibula Flap

This is one of the most important vascular bone flaps available for reconstruction of head–neck defects. The fibula flap has many advantages over other bone flaps. The bone length is more than any other flap and large skin flap can be harvested to have a composite reconstruction. The pedicle length is long enough to perform reconstruction of relatively distal sites (maxilla, skull base). One can perform multiple osteotomies to provide accurate shape for bone reconstruction. The main disadvantage of this flap is inadequate soft tissue availability for large composite reconstruction and relatively small bone height for implant placement. The donor site morbidity for this flap is relatively less and two team approaches are easily feasible and that increases its utility in high volume centers. We very rarely perform any other bone flaps than fibula flap for head–neck reconstruction.

Possibilities for Fibula Flap Reconstruction

- Buccal mucosa–alveolus: Mandible reconstruction is the most common indication for this flap. It is a must to reconstitute the anterior arch mandible defect with vascularized bone flap, while lateral segment mandible defect can be closed with soft tissue flaps, and associated trismus plays an important role in this selection.
- Maxilla reconstruction: Reconstruction of infrastructure maxillectomy defect and total maxillectomy are other indications for fibula flap.

Limitations

- It is difficult to raise this flap compared to other flaps and has a learning curve.
- Soft tissue component is limited and is not appropriate for large soft tissue defects along with bone defects.

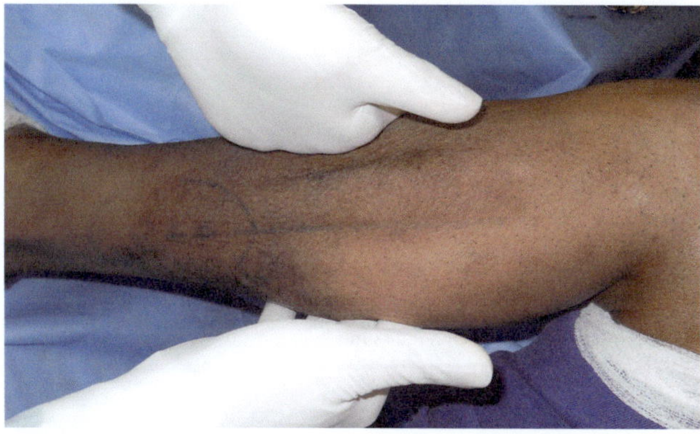

Fig. 16.61 This photograph shows ways to mark the posterior septum. It is important to remember that it is actually quite posterior to the line directly joining the two lateral condyles

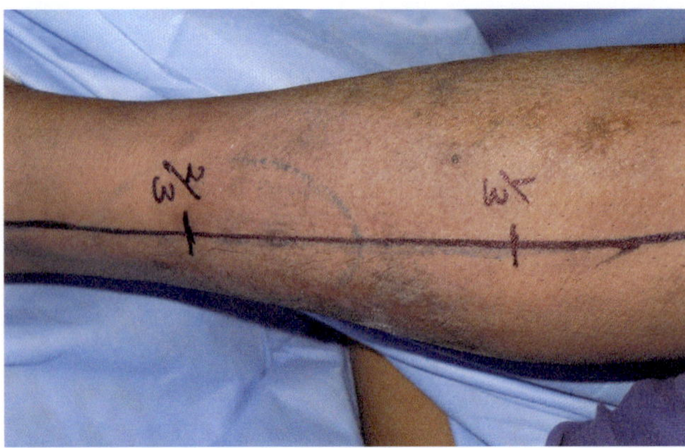

Fig. 16.62 The septum is divided into three sections in its entire length

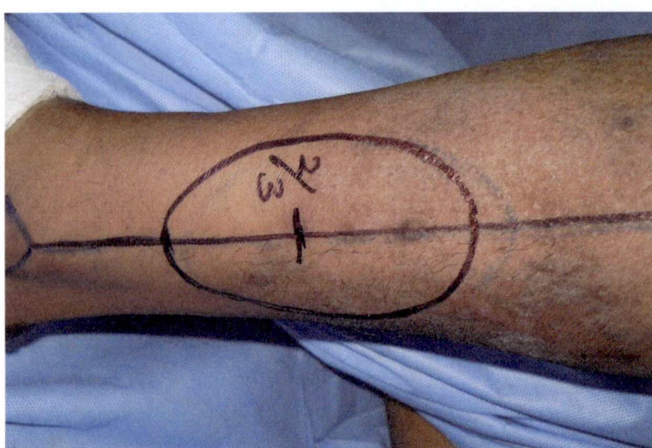

Fig. 16.63 The skin paddle is generally centered on the lower two third segment. Most of skin perforators are found in this region and it also provides long pedicle for reconstruction

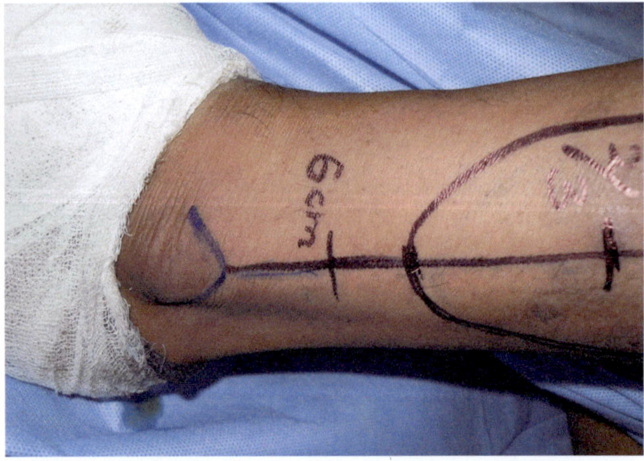

Fig. 16.64 The lower bone cut is made at least 6–8 cm above the ankle joint to provide stability to joint

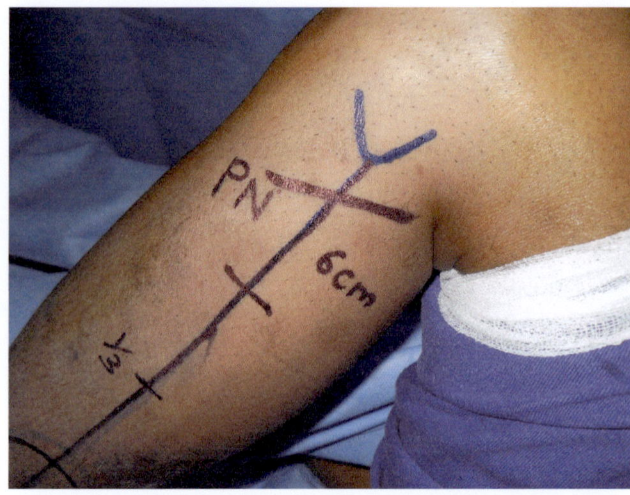

Fig. 16.65 The upper incision should not be within 6–8 cm of fibula head to prevent damage to peroneal nerve

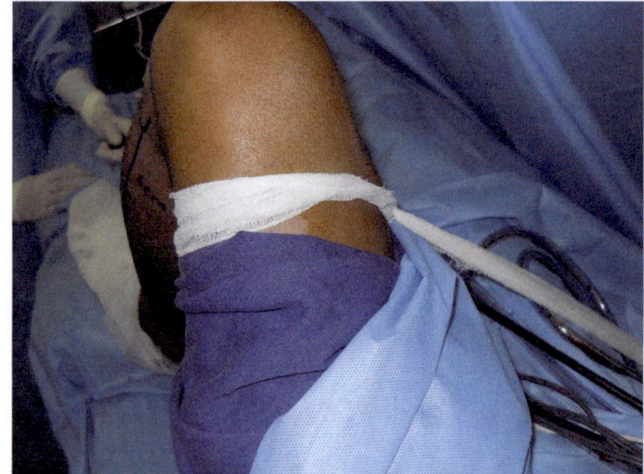

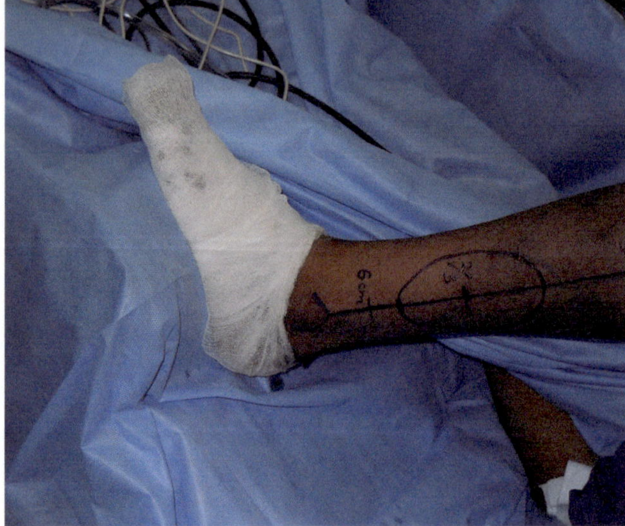

Figs. 16.66 and 16.67 This sandbag below the foot and bandage helps in keeping the leg in proper position and reduces the need for one assistant

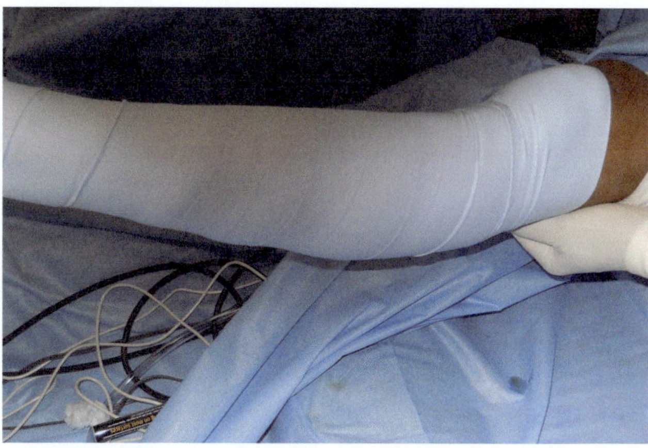

Fig. 16.68 The tourniquet is quite useful for this flap. It reduces bleeding and makes procedure clean, safe, and fast

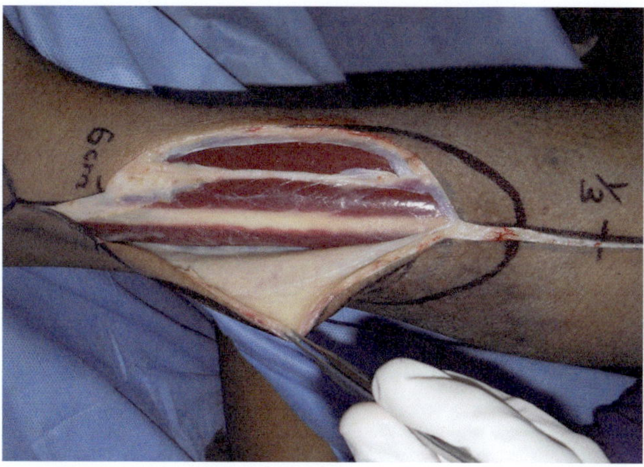

Fig. 16.71 Anterior flap is raised to expose the peroneal septum in entire length

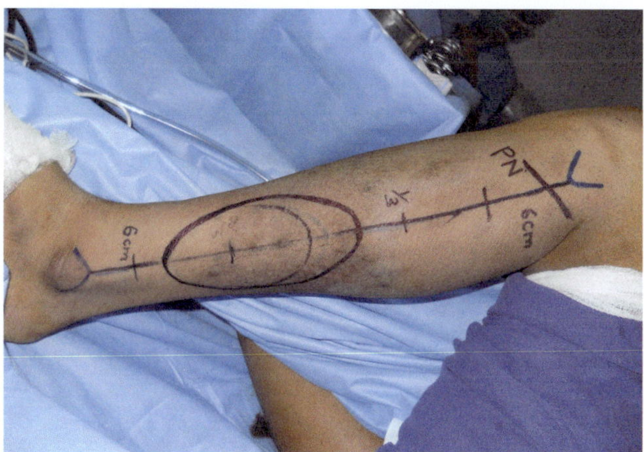

Fig. 16.69 The patient is ready for flap harvesting. It is advisable to have two assistants for this procedure for proper retraction

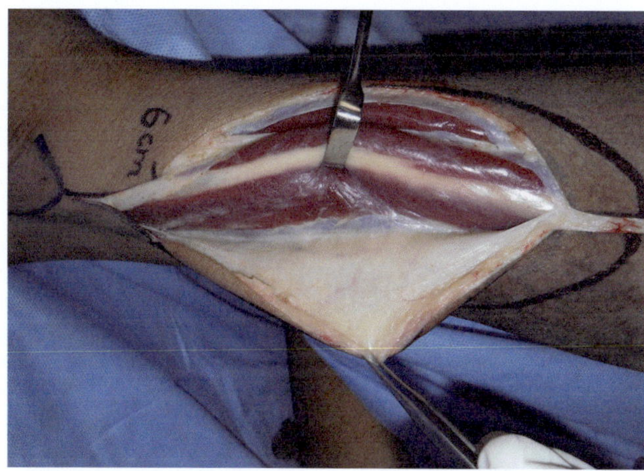

Fig. 16.72 The muscle is retracted anteriorly to identify perforator in the septum

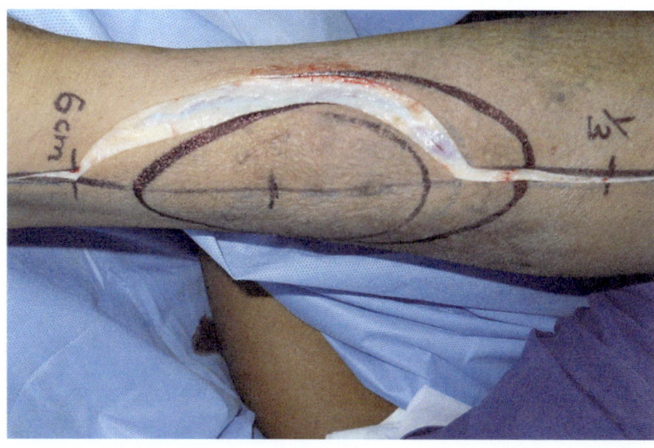

Fig. 16.70 Anterior skin incision is deep enough to include deep fascia over peroneal muscles

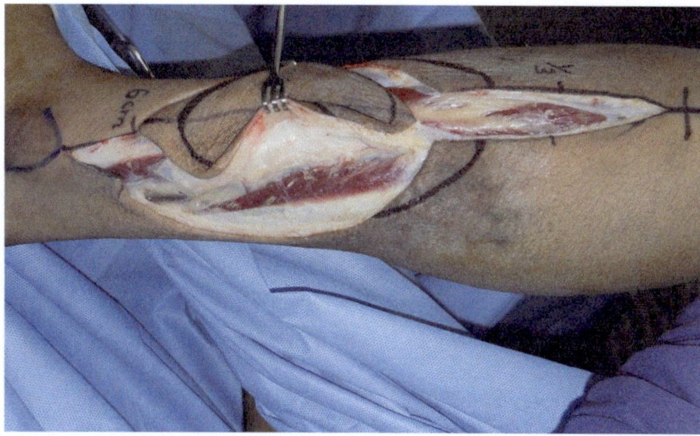

Fig. 16.73 The posterior flap is elevated anteriorly over soleus muscle

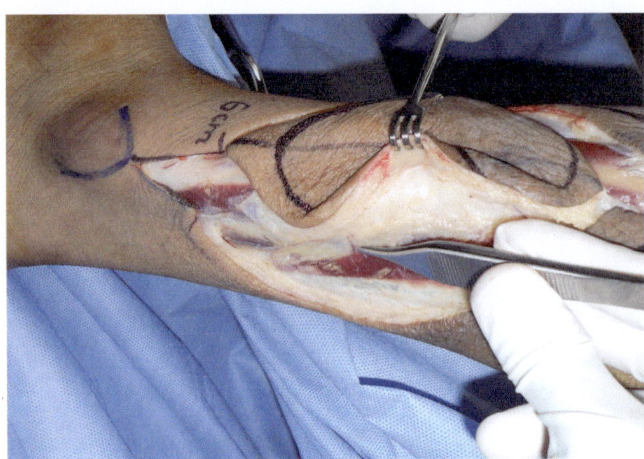

Fig. 16.74 We can see the perforator in septum and one needs to separate the soleus from septum, preserving these perforators

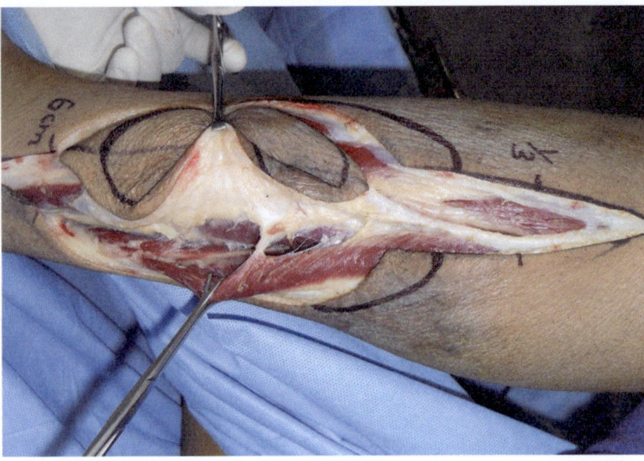

Fig. 16.75 The muscle is separated from the septum. This requires the ligation of branches to muscle, and utmost care should be taken to avoid injuring perforator to skin paddle

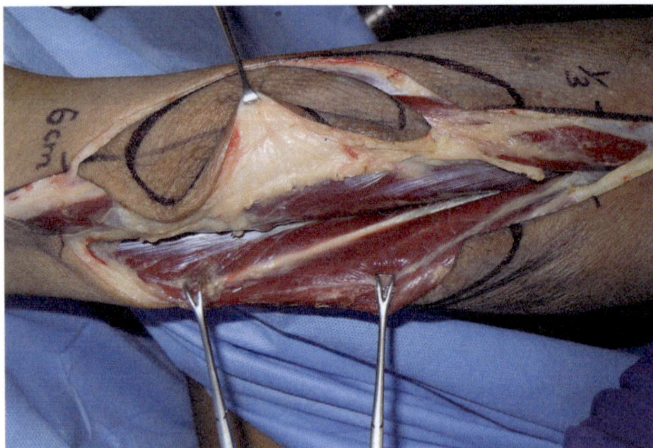

Fig. 16.76 The soleus is separated and fascia over flexor hallucis longus (FHL) is divided to release posterior compartment. This is an important step in mobilizing the fibula for anterior dissection

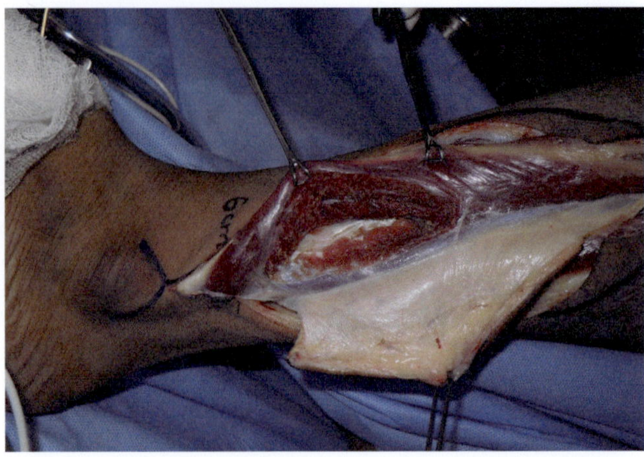

Fig. 16.77 The anterior dissection starts with detaching peroneal muscles. Cuff of the muscle is left attached to the bone to avoid injury to perforator and to preserve periosteal blood supply of the fibula

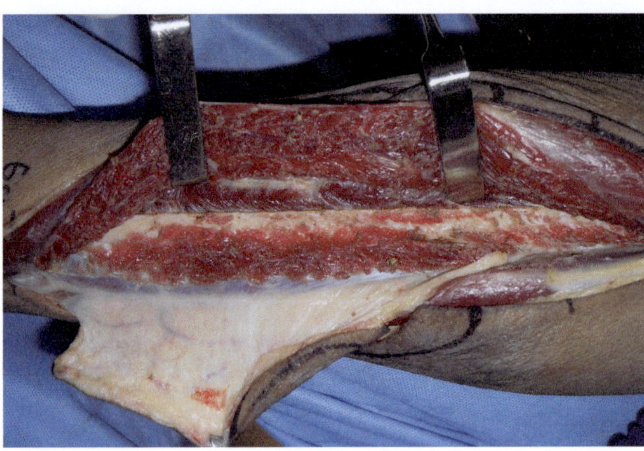

Fig. 16.78 The muscle is separated from bone the entire length and periosteum of bone is left intact. Releasing muscle in entire length also provides wider exposure for further dissection

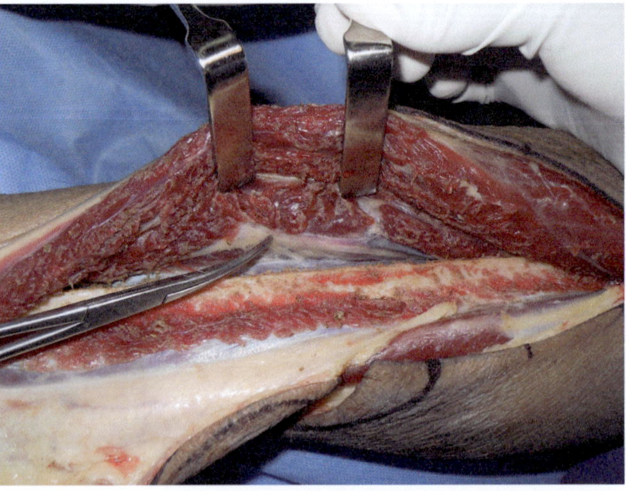

Fig. 16.79 The next muscle is extensor hallucis longus (EHL), and releasing it exposes anterior tibial vessels

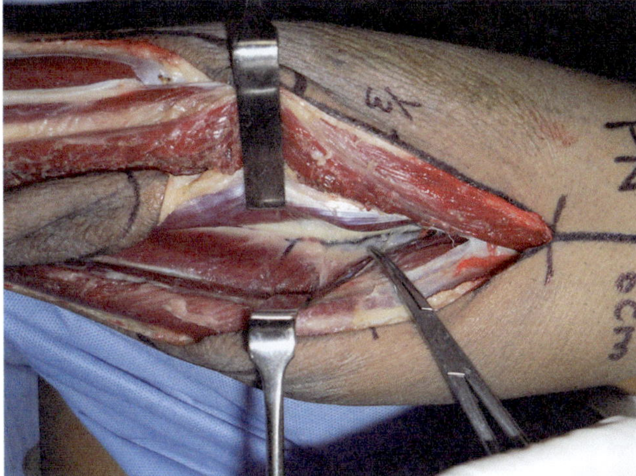

Fig. 16.80 These are posterior tibial vessels. It is very important to check the presence of these vessels before proceeding with complete flap dissection

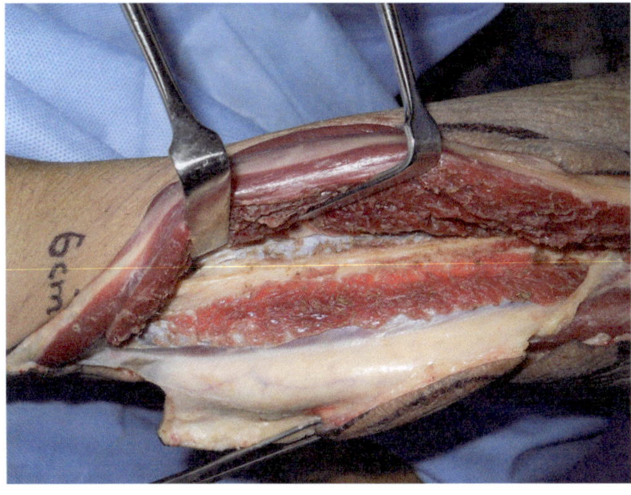

Fig. 16.81 Retraction of EHL exposes interosseous membrane and this needs to be divided in entire length

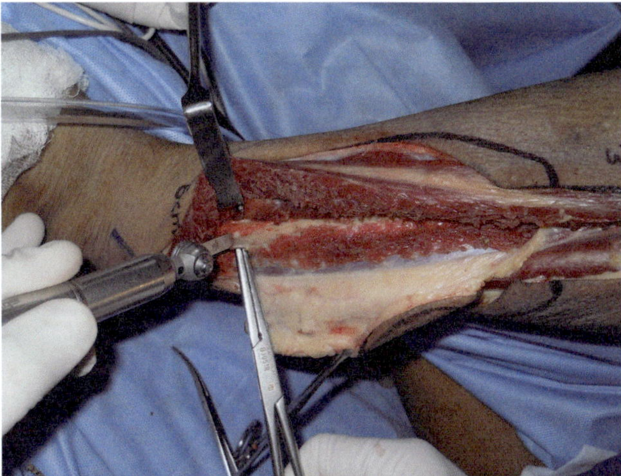

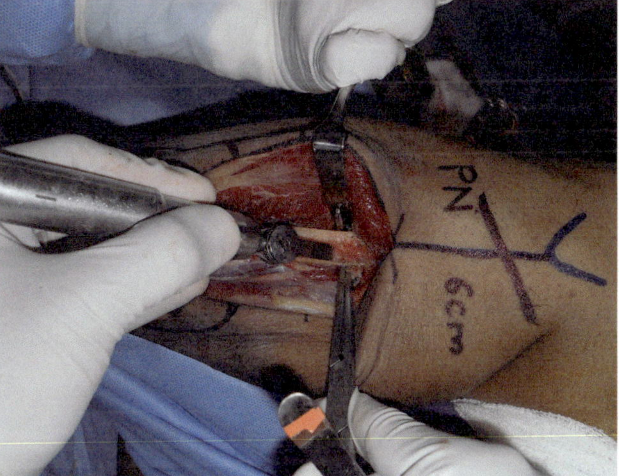

Figs. 16.82 and 16.83 The lower and upper end of bone is divided. It is important to protect the pedicle by staying very close to the bone while dividing the upper end. It is also advisable to include long bone in the upper part for ease of pedicle dissection even if small piece of bone is needed

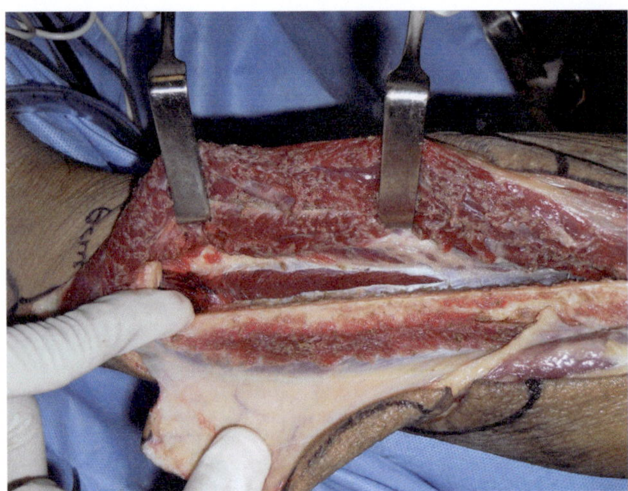

Fig. 16.84 The interosseous membrane is divided, and this releases the bone flap providing extra space for further dissection. The tibialis posterior muscle lies just beneath the membrane and peroneal vessels lies deep to this muscle

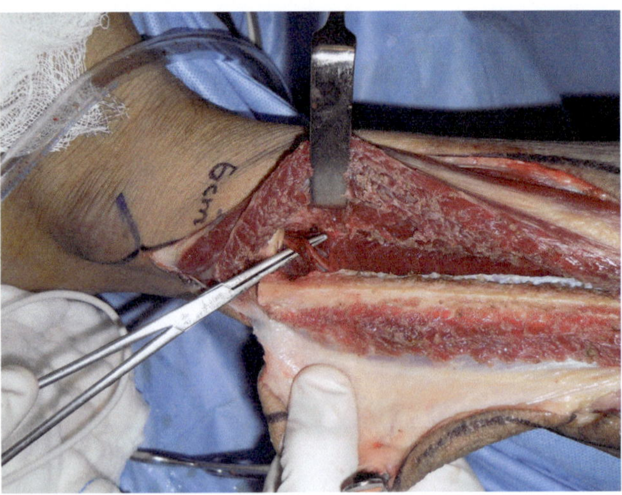

Fig. 16.85 The distal end of peroneal vessels is identified and ligated after confirming the presence of both the tibial vessels

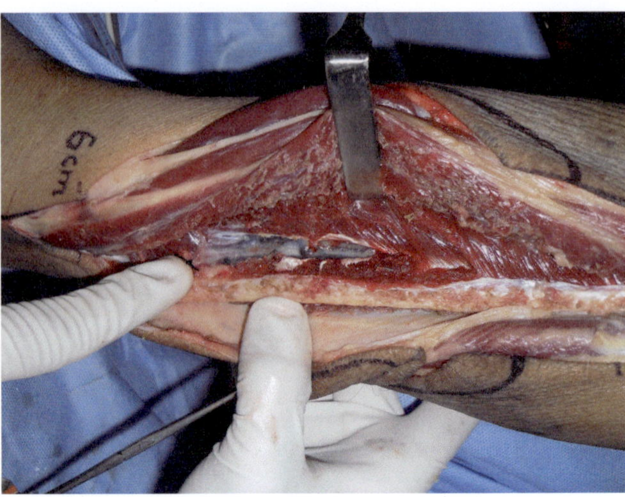

Fig. 16.86 The tibialis posterior muscle is divided to expose the pedicle. This should be done in layers clipping small muscular perforators

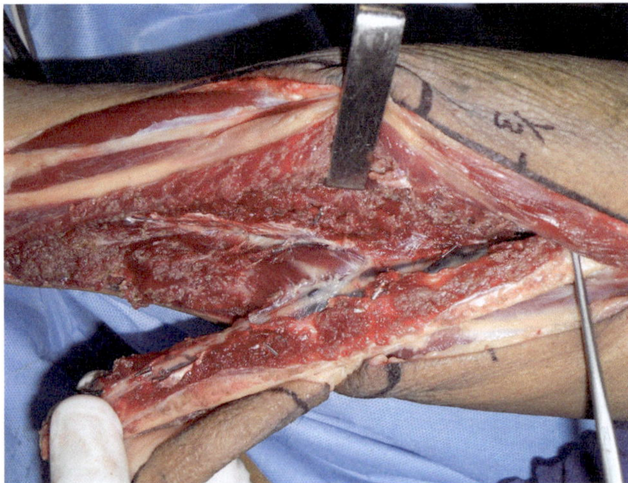

Fig. 16.87 The pedicle is separated in its entire length. The FHL muscle is either included in flap or left behind depending on the need of defect

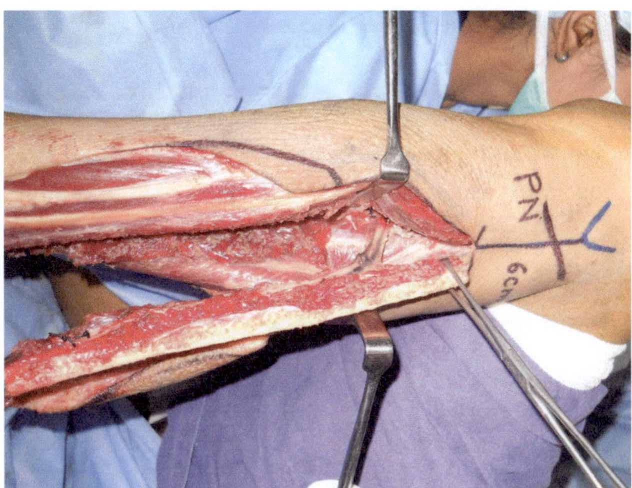

Fig. 16.88 The flap is raised in entire length. The pedicle is dissected till posterior tibial vessel is reached

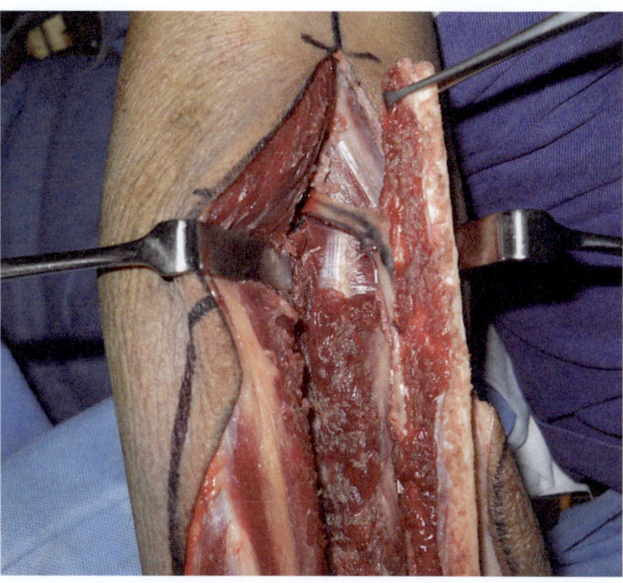

Fig. 16.89 The pedicle is dissected right till its origin. The osteotomies are performed depending upon preadapted plates. Utmost care is taken to avoid injury to pedicle while making osteotomies. The donor site defect is closed with skin graft in majority of cases. We prefer to provide plaster cast for a few days to immobilize the leg to increase skin graft take

Radial Forearm Flap

This has been the most reliable free flap used for head–neck reconstruction. This is generally the first free flap one learns in training. It is simple to harvest and easy for anastomosis. The skin is very pliable and is very useful to reconstruct small defects.

Possibilities for Radial Forearm Flap

- Buccal mucosa defect: ideal for mucosal lining for small defects
- Tongue–FOM: good choice for less than hemiglossectomy defect or for base tongue reconstruction
- Oropharynx defect: good choice for small oropharynx defects
- Maxilla: one of the choices for infrastructure maxillectomy defect
- Other: This is an ideal flap for small defects in the head and neck, and excellent pedicle length allows reconstruction of relatively distal sites with ease.

Limitations

- Donor site morbidity with graft loss is relatively high.
- Limited skin availability restricts its use for smaller defects.

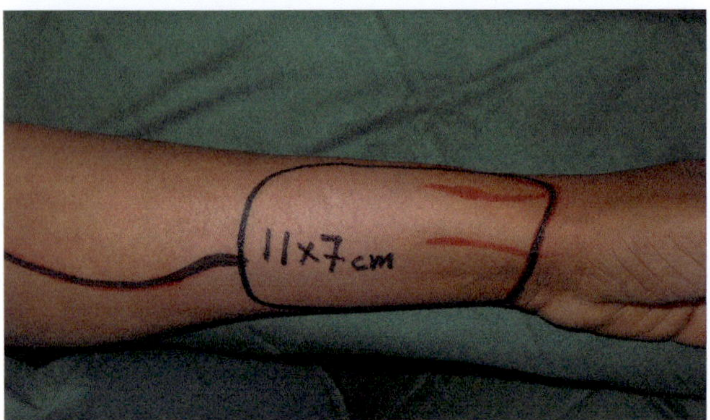

Fig. 16.90 The flap is marked in this photograph. The radial artery and cephalic vein form the mainstay of this flap, and the flap is designed to include both these within the flap substance

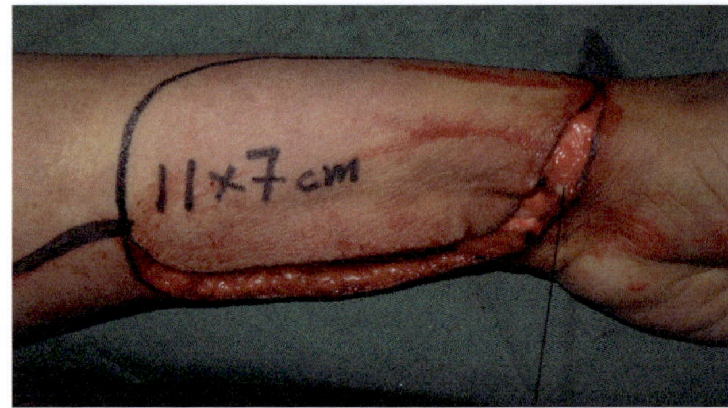

Fig. 16.92 The lateral skin incisions are placed. The cephalic vein is generally included in flap and raised along with flap harvest. Care is taken to preserve branches of radial nerve while dissecting in this area to preserve sensations in dorsum of the hand

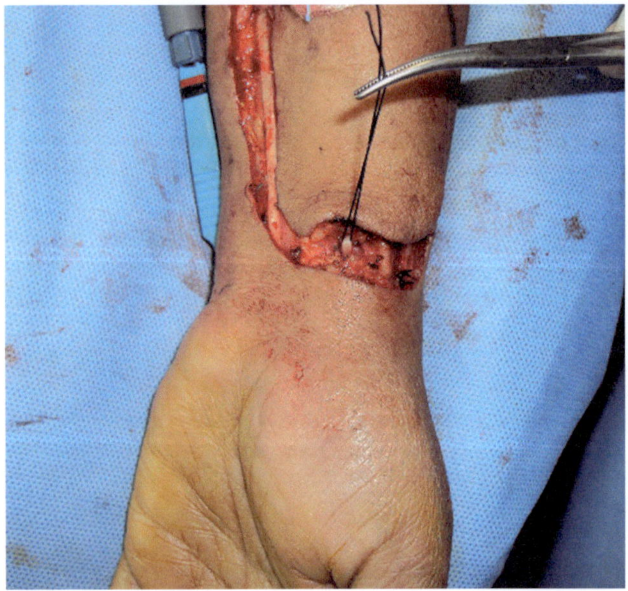

Fig. 16.91 The first step is to identify radial artery in the distal end. This gives idea for depth of pedicle and this orientation helps in further dissection

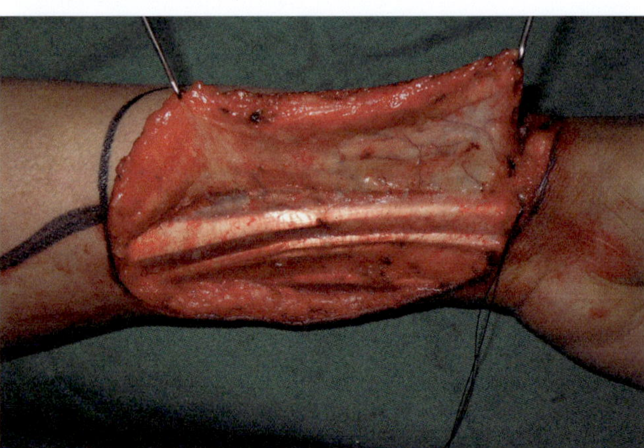

Fig. 16.93 The dissection begins from ulnar side till intermuscular septum is reached. This is achieved by elevating the fascia of flexor compartment muscles, and dissection ends when flexor carpi radialis is exposed. It is important to preserve para-tenon for better skin graft take

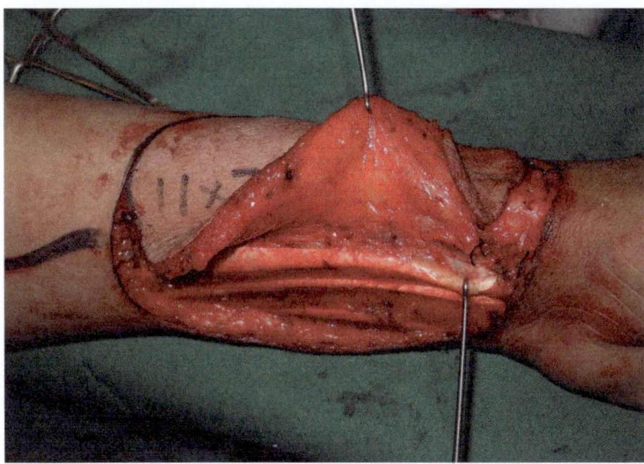

Fig. 16.94 The ulnar side dissection is done till it reaches intermuscular septum when border of brachioradialis is reached. Once this is achieved, dissection is carried forward by retracting flexor group of muscles laterally to isolate radial artery pedicle. If palmaris longus muscle is present, this can be harvested along with flap and can be used as facial sling

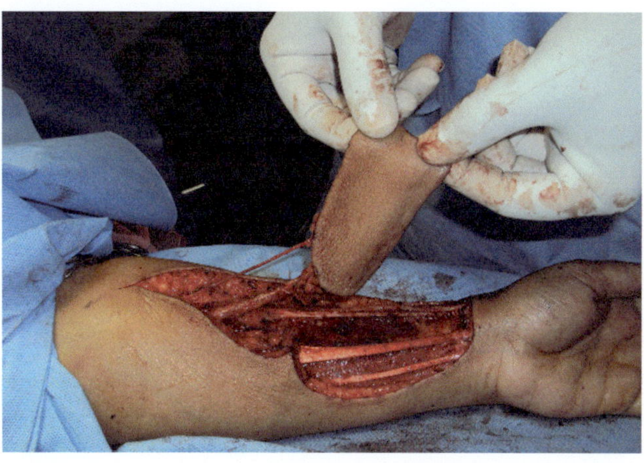

Fig. 16.97 The photograph shows isolated cephalic vein in the entire length. The size of the vein is quite large and serves as a good option for second vein anastomosis

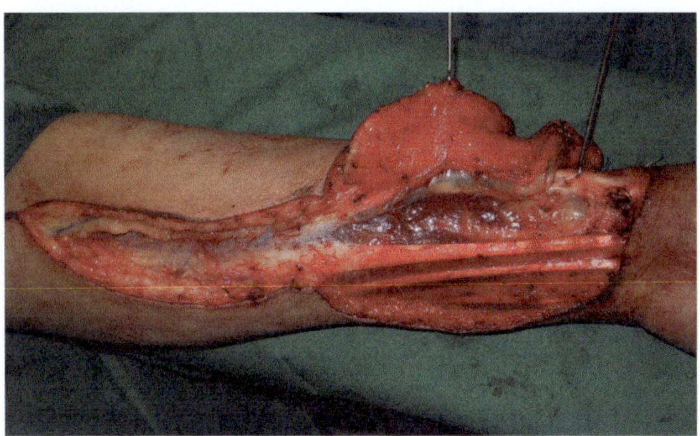

Fig. 16.95 The pedicle is gradually lifted from below ligating all small perforators to deep muscles. All small perforators must be clipped to prevent postoperative hematoma

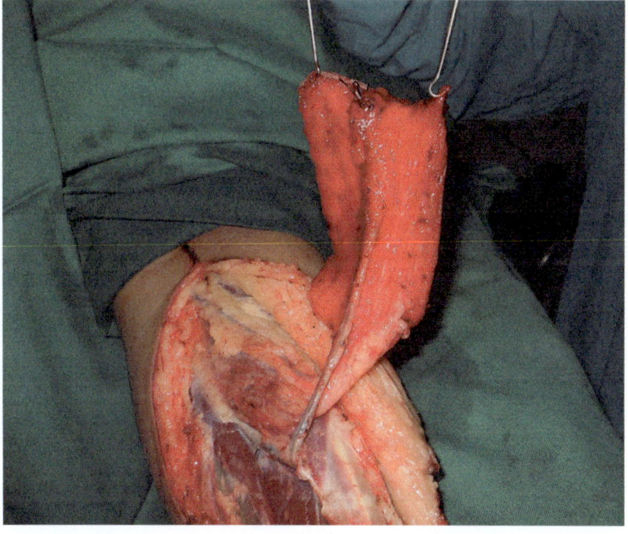

Fig. 16.98 The dissection of pedicle in proximal aspect is continued by detaching brachioradialis and flexor carpi radialis muscles. The pedicle can be traced till origin of the brachial artery but that is usually not needed. The tourniquet is released to check for any small bleeder and hemostasis is secured

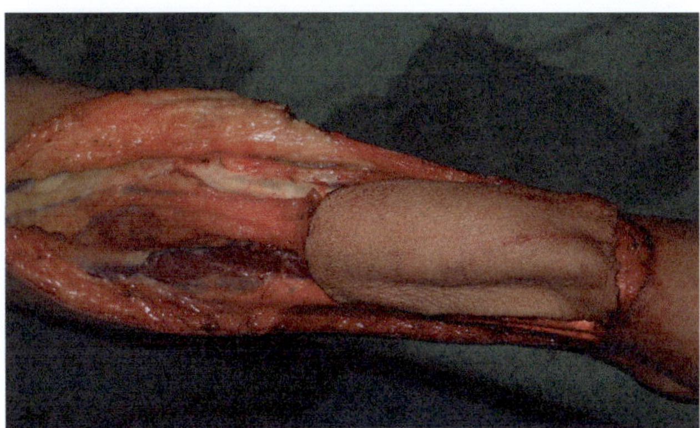

Fig. 16.96 The skin flaps are raised in proximal aspect in subcutaneous planes to preserve cephalic vein which is isolated separately

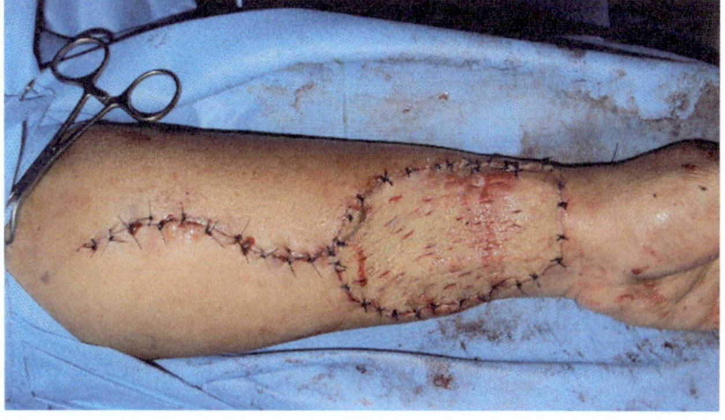

Fig. 16.99 The wound is closed over skin graft. It is better to immobilize the hand for a few days for better graft uptake

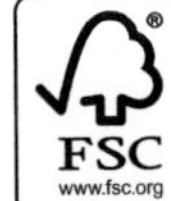

MIX
Papier aus verantwortungsvollen Quellen
Paper from responsible sources
FSC® C105338

If you have any concerns about our products,
you can contact us on
ProductSafety@springernature.com

In case Publisher is established outside the EU,
the EU authorized representative is:
Springer Nature Customer Service Center GmbH
Europaplatz 3, 69115 Heidelberg, Germany

Printed by Libri Plureos GmbH
in Hamburg, Germany